fifth
EDITION

THE MONT REID
SURGICAL
HANDBOOK

fifth
EDITION

THE MONT REID SURGICAL HANDBOOK

The University of Cincinnati Residents
From the Department of Surgery
University of Cincinnati College of Medicine
Cincinnati, Ohio

EDITORS-IN-CHIEF

David R. Fischer, MD
Burnett S. Kelly, Jr., MD

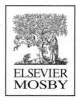

ELSEVIER
MOSBY

ELSEVIER
MOSBY

The Curtis Center
170 S Independence Mall W 300E
Philadelphia, Pennsylvania 19106

The Mont Reid Surgical Handbook   ISBN 0-323-01704-5
Copyright © 2005, 1997, 1994, 1990, 1987 by Mosby, Inc.

NOTICE

First Edition. Fifth Edition.

Library of Congress Cataloging-in-Publication Data

The Mont Reid surgical handbook / the University of Cincinnati residents from the
     Department of Surgery, University of Cincinnati, College of Medicine.—5th ed.
         p. ; cm.
     Includes bibliographical references and index.
     ISBN 0-323-01704-5
     1. Therapeutics, Surgical—Handbooks, manuals, etc. I. Title: Surgical handbook. II.
Reid, Mont. III. University of Cincinnati. Dept. of Surgery.
     [DNLM: 1. Surgical Procedures, Operative–Handbooks. WO 39 M747 2005]
     RD49.M67 2005
     617'.9–dc22   2004040348

Acquisitions Editor: Elyse O'Grady
Developmental Editor: Maria Lorusso
Project Manager: Amy Norwitz

Printed in the United States of America

Last digit is the print number: 9   8   7   6   5   4   3   2   1

EDITORS-IN-CHIEF

David R. Fischer, MD

Assistant Professor of Surgery
Division of GI and Endocrine Surgery
University of Cincinnati College of Medicine
Cincinnati, Ohio

Burnett S. Kelly, Jr., MD

Chief Resident, Department of Surgery
University of Cincinnati College of Medicine
Cincinnati, Ohio

SECTION EDITORS

Richard A. Falcone, Jr., MD

Chief Resident, Department of Surgery
University of Cincinnati College of Medicine
Cincinnati, Ohio

Philip K. Frykman, MD, PhD

Chief Resident, Department of Surgery
University of Cincinnati College of Medicine
Cincinnati, Ohio

Harry T. Papaconstantinou, MD

Chief Resident, Department of Surgery
University of Cincinnati College of Medicine
Cincinnati, Ohio

Sara J. Pereira, MD

Chief Resident, Department of Surgery
University of Cincinnati College of Medicine
Cincinnati, Ohio

Contributors

Steven R. Allen, MD
Assistant Resident, Department of Surgery
University of Cincinnati College of Medicine
Cincinnati, Ohio

Kfir Ben-David, MD
Assistant Resident, Department of Surgery
University of Cincinnati College of Medicine
Cincinnati, Ohio

Parag Bhanot, MD
Assistant Resident, Department of Surgery
University of Cincinnati College of Medicine
Cincinnati, Ohio

Jennifer L. Butterfield, MD
Assistant Resident, Department of Plastic Surgery
University of Cincinnati College of Medicine
Cincinnati, Ohio

Robert M. Cavagnol, MD
Assistant Resident, Department of Surgery
University of Cincinnati College of Medicine
Cincinnati, Ohio

Wilson M. Clements, MD
Assistant Resident, Department of Surgery
University of Cincinnati College of Medicine
Cincinnati, Ohio

James B. Colombo, MD
Assistant Resident, Division of Urology
University of Cincinnati College of Medicine
Cincinnati, Ohio

Jaime R. Este-McDonald, MD
Assistant Resident, Department of Vascular Surgery
University of Cincinnati College of Medicine
Cincinnati, Ohio

Richard A. Falcone, Jr., MD
Chief Resident, Department of Surgery
University of Cincinnati College of Medicine
Cincinnati, Ohio

David R. Fischer, MD
Assistant Professor of Surgery
Division of GI and Endocrine Surgery
University of Cincinnati College of Medicine
Cincinnati, Ohio

Philip K. Frykman, MD, PhD
Chief Resident, Department of Surgery
University of Cincinnati College of Medicine
Cincinnati, Ohio

Gyu Il Gang, MD
Assistant Resident, Department of Surgery
University of Cincinnati College of Medicine
Cincinnati, Ohio

Eric Hungness, MD
Assistant Resident, Department of Surgery
University of Cincinnati College of Medicine
Cincinnati, Ohio

Marcus D. Jarboe, MD
Assistant Resident, Department of Surgery
University of Cincinnati College of Medicine
Cincinnati, Ohio

Scott R. Johnson, MD
Assistant Resident, Department of Surgery
University of Cincinnati College of Medicine
Cincinnati, Ohio

Russell J. Juno, MD
Assistant Resident, Department of Surgery
University of Cincinnati College of Medicine
Cincinnati, Ohio

Burnett S. Kelly, Jr., MD
Chief Resident, Department of Surgery
University of Cincinnati College of Medicine
Cincinnati, Ohio

Joseph Kim, MD
Assistant Resident, Department of Surgery
University of Cincinnati College of Medicine
Cincinnati, Ohio

Nancy Y. Kim, MD
Assistant Resident, Division of Urology
University of Cincinnati College of Medicine
Cincinnati, Ohio

David M. Kitchens, MD
Assistant Resident, Division of Urology
University of Cincinnati College of Medicine
Cincinnati, Ohio

Andrew W. Knott, MD
Assistant Resident, Department of Surgery
University of Cincinnati College of Medicine
Cincinnati, Ohio

Jeffrey Larson, MD, PhD
Resident, Department of Neurosurgery
University of Cincinnati College of Medicine
Cincinnati, Ohio

Jefferson M. Lyons, MD
Assistant Resident, Department of Surgery
University of Cincinnati College of Medicine
Cincinnati, Ohio

Grace Z. Mak, MD
Assistant Resident, Department of Surgery
University of Cincinnati College of Medicine
Cincinnati, Ohio

Joshua M.V. Mammen, MD
Assistant Resident, Department of Surgery
University of Cincinnati College of Medicine
Cincinnati, Ohio

Kelly McLean, MD
Assistant Resident, Department of Surgery
University of Cincinnati College of Medicine
Cincinnati, Ohio

CONTRIBUTORS

Lindsey A. Nelson, MD
Assistant Resident, Department of Anesthesia
University of Cincinnati College of Medicine
Cincinnati, Ohio

Son Thanh Nguyen, MD
Assistant Resident, Department of Surgery
University of Cincinnati College of Medicine
Cincinnati, Ohio

David P. O'Brien, MD
Assistant Resident, Department of Surgery
University of Cincinnati College of Medicine
Cincinnati, Ohio

Thaddeus P. O'Neil, MD
Assistant Resident, Department of Surgery
University of Cincinnati College of Medicine
Cincinnati, Ohio

Harry T. Papaconstantinou, MD
Chief Resident, Department of Surgery
University of Cincinnati College of Medicine
Cincinnati, Ohio

George Papacostas, MD
Assistant Resident, Department of Orthopedic Surgery
University of Cincinnati College of Medicine
Cincinnati, Ohio

Sara J. Pereira, MD
Chief Resident, Department of Surgery
University of Cincinnati College of Medicine
Cincinnati, Ohio

Susan M. Pike, MD
Assistant Resident, Department of Plastic Surgery
University of Cincinnati College of Medicine
Cincinnati, Ohio

Timothy A. Pritts, MD, PhD
Assistant Resident, Department of Surgery
University of Cincinnati College of Medicine
Cincinnati, Ohio

Gina Quaid, MD
Assistant Resident, Division of Trauma
University of Cincinnati College of Medicine
Cincinnati, Ohio

Bruce W. Robb, MD
Assistant Resident, Department of Surgery
University of Cincinnati College of Medicine
Cincinnati, Ohio

Amod A. Sarnaik, MD
Assistant Resident, Department of Surgery
University of Cincinnati College of Medicine
Cincinnati, Ohio

Marc Shapiro, MD
Assistant Resident, Department of Surgery
University of Cincinnati College of Medicine
Cincinnati, Ohio

Donn H. Spight, MD
Assistant Resident, Department of Surgery
University of Cincinnati College of Medicine
Cincinnati, Ohio

Melissa McCarty Statham, MD
Assistant Resident, Department of ENT
University of Cincinnati College of Medicine
Cincinnati, Ohio

Lawrence E. Stern, MD
Assistant Resident, Department of Surgery
University of Cincinnati College of Medicine
Cincinnati, Ohio

Amit D. Tevar, MD
Transplant Fellow, Department of Surgery
University of Cincinnati College of Medicine
Cincinnati, Ohio

KuoJen Tsao, MD
Assistant Resident, Department of Surgery
University of Cincinnati College of Medicine
Cincinnati, Ohio

Konstantin Umanskiy, MD
Assistant Resident, Department of Surgery
University of Cincinnati College of Medicine
Cincinnati, Ohio

Curtis J. Wray, MD
Assistant Resident, Department of Surgery
University of Cincinnati College of Medicine
Cincinnati, Ohio

Foreword

It is a testament to the quality of previous editions of *The Mont Reid Surgical Handbook*, as well as evidence of the progression of surgical practice, that we now see a fifth edition. Since joining the Department of Surgery at the University of Cincinnati College of Medicine in 2001 as the sixth Christian R. Holmes Professor and Chairman, I continue to marvel at the talents of our surgical residents and their commitment to excellence in the care of the surgical patient. Year after year, in our increasingly complex and specialized healthcare system, the surgical residents at the University of Cincinnati keep pace with rapid advances in knowledge of the basic biology of human disease as well as the ever-increasing armamentarium of technological tools available for diagnosis, management, and treatment.

The Mont Reid Surgical Handbook reflects the art and science of surgery at the University of Cincinnati Medical Center as practiced by our senior surgical residents, who adopt what they have learned from the faculty, place this knowledge in the context of available supportive evidence, and translate this into a written compendium that is passed down to succeeding generations of interns, junior residents, and senior medical students, who rely upon this during the formative years of their surgical training. Each edition reflects the improvements in day-to-day practice gained from current experience at the bedside. Included in this fifth edition are guidelines for preoperative and postoperative care for a wide spectrum of surgical diseases whose pathophysiology is exquisitely detailed, as well as surgical management that encompasses state-of-the-art technology and recent innovations in technique and instrumentation. Emphasis is placed on minimally invasive techniques, including important coverage of laparoscopic cholecystectomy, appendectomy, and herniorrhaphy, as well as advanced laparoscopic procedures. Finally, bearing in mind the additional administrative dimensions of modern surgical practice required by malpractice and HIPAA considerations, guidelines are provided for proper medical record-keeping as well as other medicolegal aspects of surgical care.

The residents who served as co-editors for this edition—David R. Fischer, MD, and Burnett S. Kelly Jr., MD—exhibited great dedication to this task, and we extend our appreciation to them and their understanding families. We also thank the junior residents who contributed chapters, and we offer a special thanks to Dr. Fischer, a graduate of our program and now a faculty member, for his willingness to take on the final coordination of this volume. *The Mont Reid Surgical Handbook* reflects a residency training program whose excellence is largely due to the leadership of Robert H. Bower, MD, Director of the General Surgery Training Program and the Division of Surgical Education, and to the hardworking staff of Surgical Education at UC.

It is an honor to be associated with these outstanding surgical residents, and I hope that you will benefit from their accumulated knowledge and experience.

Jeffrey B. Matthews, MD, FACS
Christian R. Holmes Professor of Surgery
and Chairman of the Department of Surgery
University of Cincinnati Medical Center
Cincinnati, Ohio

Foreword
to the first edition

Dr. Mont Reid was the second Christian R. Holmes Professor of Surgery at the University of Cincinnati College of Medicine. Trained at Johns Hopkins, he came to Cincinnati as the associate of Dr. George J. Heuer, the initial Christian R. Holmes Professor, in 1922, and became responsible for the teaching in the residency. He assumed the Chair in 1931 and died in 1943, a great tragedy for both the city and the University of Cincinnati College of Medicine. He was beloved by the residents and townspeople. A very learned, patient man, he was serious about surgery, surgical education, and surgical research. His papers on wound healing are still classics and can, to this day, be read with profit.

It was under Mont Reid that the surgical residency first matured. In his memory, the new surgical suite built in 1948 was named the Mont Reid Pavillion. Part of the surgical suite is still operational in that building, as are the residents' living quarters. *The Mont Reid Handbook* is written by the surgical residents at the University of Cincinnati hospitals for residents and medical students and thus is appropriately named. It represents a compilation of the approach taken in our residency program, of which we are justifiably proud. The residency program as well as the Department reflect a basic science physiological approach to the science of surgery. Metabolism, infection, nutrition, and physiological responses to the above as well as the physiological basis for surgical and pre-surgical interventions form the basis of our residency program and presumably will form the basis of surgical practice into the twenty-first century. We hope that you will read it with profit and that you will use it as a basis for further study in the science of surgery.

Josef E. Fischer, MD
Christian R. Holmes Professor of Surgery
and Chairman of the Department of Surgery
University of Cincinnati Medical Center
Cincinnati, Ohio
1987

Preface
to the fifth edition

We are proud to present the fifth edition of *The Mont Reid Surgical Handbook*. This edition has been made possible by the hard work of the residents in the general surgery program at the University of Cincinnati as well as the residents of neurosurgery, plastic surgery, urology, anesthesia, pharmacy, and orthopedics.

Each chapter represents the generalized practice at the University of Cincinnati. The residents have extensively researched these chapters to make them as comprehensive as possible. While this edition is not meant to be a comprehensive overview, we hope that it serves as a ready guide to most clinical situations encountered by the surgeon. We hope that this book continues to be a valuable companion in the search for excellence by all students of surgery.

David R. Fischer, MD
Burnett S. Kelly, Jr., MD

Preface
to the first edition

We can only instill principles, put the student in the right path, give him methods, teach him how to study, and early to discern between essentials and non-essentials.

Sir William Osler

The surgical residency training program at the University of Cincinnati Medical Center dates back to 1922 when it was organized by Drs. George J. Heuer and Mont R. Reid, both students of Dr. William Halsted and graduates of the Johns Hopkins surgical training program. The training program was thus established in a strong Hopkins mode. When Dr. Heuer left to assume the chair at Cornell University, Mont Reid succeeded him as chairman. During Reid's tenure (1931-1943), the training program at what was then the Cincinnati General Hospital was brought to maturity. Since then, the training program has continued to grow and has maintained the tradition of excellence in academic and clinical surgery which was so strongly advocated by Dr. Reid and his successors.

The principal goal of the surgical residency training program at the University of Cincinnati today remains the development of exemplary academic and clinical surgeons. There also is a strong tradition of teaching by the senior residents of their junior colleagues as well as the medical students at the College of Medicine. Thus, the surgical house staff became very enthused when Year Book Medical Publishers asked us to consider writing a surgical handbook which would be analogous to the very successful pediatrics handbook, *The Harriet Lane Handbook* (now in its 11th edition). We readily accepted the challenge of writing a pocket "pearl book" which would provide pertinent, practical information to the students and residents in surgery. The six chief residents for 1985–1986 served as editors of this handbook and the contributors included the majority of the surgical house staff in consultation with other specialists who are involved in the direct care of surgical patients and the education of residents and medical students.

The information collected in this handbook is by no means exhaustive. We have attempted simply to provide a guide for the more efficient management of prevalent surgical problems, especially by those with limited experience. Therefore, this is not a substitute for a comprehensive textbook of surgery, but is rather a supplement which concentrates on those things that are important to medical students and junior residents on the wards, namely the initial management of common surgical conditions. Much of the information is influenced by the philosophies advocated by the residents and faculty at the University of Cincinnati and thus reflects a certain bias. In areas of controversy, however, we have also provided other views and useful references. The index has been liberally cross-referenced in order to provide a rapid and efficient means of locating information.

This handbook would not have been possible without the enthusiastic support and advice of our chairman, Dr. Josef E. Fischer, whose commitment to excellence in surgical training serves as an inspiration to all of his residents.

We also would like to acknowledge the invaluable advice provided by several of the faculty members of the Department of Surgery: Dr. Robert H. Bower, Dr. James M. Hurst, and Dr. Richard F. Kempczinski. The authors gratefully acknowledge the helpful input of Dr. Donald G. McQuarrie, Professor of Surgery at the University of Minnesota, for his review of each chapter in the handbook. Also we would like to thank Mr. Daniel J. Doody, Vice President, Editorial, Year Book Medical Publishers, for his patience and guidance in the conception and writing of this first edition of *The Mont Reid Handbook*.

None of this would have been possible were it not for the word processing expertise and herculean efforts of Mr. Steven E. Wiesner. His assistance in the typing and editing of the manuscript was invaluable.

Finally, this handbook is the result of the cumulative efforts of the surgical house staff at the University of Cincinnati as well as those residents who preceded us and taught us many of the principles that are advocated in this book. We wish to thank all of those who worked so diligently on this manuscript in order to make the first edition of *The Mont Reid Handbook* a reality.

Michael S. Nussbaum, MD
Editor-in-Chief
Cincinnati, Ohio
1987

Contents

PART II   Specialized Protocols in Surgery

CONTENTS

PART I

Perioperative Care

Medical Record

Kelly McLean, MD, and Son Thanh Nguyen, MD

I. THE SURGICAL HISTORY AND PHYSICAL EXAMINATION

A. MEETING THE PATIENT

1. Initial contact—Gain his or her confidence and convey assurance that help is available.
2. Put the patient at ease—Be gentle and considerate, creating an atmosphere of sympathy, personal interest, and understanding. Be certain that the patient is as comfortable as possible and make yourself comfortable; demonstrate that you are *interested* and concerned about the patient.
3. Listen to your patient—He or she is trying to tell you the diagnosis. Much can be learned by letting the patient "ramble" a little. Discrepancies and omissions in the history are often due as much to overstructuring and leading questions as to an unreliable patient.
4. Ensure the patient's privacy.

B. HISTORY

1. Chief complaint—This should be in the patient's own words.
2. History of present illness (HPI)
a. Main symptom—A careful analysis of the nature of a symptom is an important feature of a surgical history.

> **O** – Onset: When did it start? How did it start? What was the patient doing when it started? Was it a gradual or sudden onset?
> **P** – Position: Where is it? Does it radiate? Has it moved?
> **Q** – Quality: What is it like? Is it sharp, dull, crampy? Does it wax and wane?
> **R** – Related symptoms
> **S** – Severity: How bad is it?
> **T** – Timing/triggers: What makes it better/worse? How long does it last?

A complete review of symptoms helps identify missed symptoms, but the following symptoms require extra focus in general surgery.
b. Fever—The onset of fever and cyclical patterns are important for excluding certain disease states.
c. Vomiting—Inspect vomitus when possible. What did the patient vomit? What did it look like? How much? How often? Was the vomiting projectile? Was it associated with pain? Was it bilious or bloody? Was it associated with eating? The relationship between onset of abdominal pain and onset of vomiting, as well as the quality of the emesis, suggests the level of obstruction.
d. Bowel habits—Any change? Last bowel movement? Flatus? Hard/soft/runny? Chalky/black? For example, intermittent constipation and diarrhea must lead one to suspect colon cancer or diverticular disease.

e. Bleeding
  (1) A past history of bleeding is the best indicator of potential bleeding tendencies.
  (2) Any abnormal bleeding from any orifice must be carefully evaluated and should never be dismissed as due to some immediately obvious cause (e.g., hemorrhoids causing rectal bleeding).
  (3) Hematemesis or hematochezia—Character of blood helps differentiate between pathologic states. Does it clot? Is it bright or dark red blood? Is it changed in any way? Coffee-ground vomitus is indicative of slow gastric bleeding; dark, tarry stool is characteristic of upper GI bleeding.
f. Trauma—When a patient is subjected to trauma, the details surrounding the injury must be established as precisely as possible (see Chap. 14).
g. Medications—Ask the patient what medications have been tried and whether the medications helped. It is very important to impress on the patient that all medications tried must be related to the medical team, especially over-the-counter drugs, herbals, diuretics, corticosteroids, and cardiac drugs. Indicate dose, route, frequency, and duration of usage.
3. **Past medical history (PMH)—Always obtain old records/reports. The PMH is particularly important in assessing patients for potential anesthetic and perioperative complications.**
a. Chronic illnesses—Diabetes mellitus, hypertension, myocardial infarction, chronic obstructive pulmonary disease, etc?
b. Acute illness/hospitalizations—Pneumonia, asthma attacks, diabetic ketoacidosis?
c. Injuries/accidents—Broken bones, trauma?
4. **Past surgical history—Again, obtain old records/operative reports.**
a. Type, date, and place (hospital) of surgery?
b. Reason for the surgery, if known?
c. Any difficulties with anesthesia; any family history of difficulties?
5. **Allergies—Specify drug reaction (e.g., rash, edema, stridor, anaphylaxis).**
6. **Social history—Alcohol, tobacco, or other substance abuse (how much and how long?)**
7. **Family history—A significant number of surgical disorders are familial in nature (e.g., colonic polyposis, multiple endocrine neoplasia syndromes, carcinoma of the breast).**

C. REVIEW OF SYSTEMS (ROS)
To make certain that important details of the history are not overlooked, this system review must be formalized and thorough. Nutritional deficiencies, particularly acute fluid and electrolyte losses, recent weight loss, and anorexia, must be noted. Record all pertinent positive and negative findings.

D. PHYSICAL EXAMINATION
1. Put the patient at ease.
2. Develop a system—The examiner must develop his or her own method of examining a patient in a detailed and orderly fashion in exactly the

same sequence with each patient so that no step is omitted and no details are excluded.

3. Assess the patient—Look at the patient prior to the "laying on of hands"; many clues to the diagnosis may be obtained. For example, a patient who is thrashing about and cannot seem to get comfortable may be suffering from renal or biliary colic. Very severe pain due to peritoneal inflammation or vascular disease usually forces the patient to restrict all movement as much as possible. Observe the patient's general physique, habitus, and affect. Carefully inspect the hands, because many systemic diseases (e.g., cirrhosis, hyperthyroidism, Raynaud's disease, pulmonary insufficiency, heart disease, nutritional disorders) may involve them.

4. Use inspection, auscultation, percussion, and palpation—Essential steps in evaluating both the normal and abnormal ("look, listen, feel")
a. Compare both sides of the body.
b. Auscultation, particularly of the abdomen and peripheral vessels, is essential in evaluating surgical disorders.
c. Palpation and percussion should be performed gently, carefully, and precisely.

5. Cover all systems.
a. Vital signs
b. General
c. Head, eyes, ears, nose, throat (HEENT)
d. Chest
e. Heart
f. Abdomen
g. Genitourinary (GU)
h. Extremities
i. Musculoskeletal
j. Pulses
k. Neurologic
l. Mental status/psychological
m. Skin

6. Examination of the body orifices—Complete inspection of the ears, mouth, eyes, rectum, and pelvis is an essential part of every complete examination.

E. RECAP
After the history and physical exam, recap to the patient *your* understanding of the patient's problems and/or findings. This gives the patient a chance to clarify or correct any misconceptions. Also, after the physical exam, new questions or clarifications of the history might be warranted.

F. ANCILLARY STUDIES
1. Objectives of laboratory examination
a. Confirm the suspected diagnosis.

MEDICAL RECORD

1

b. Screen for asymptomatic disease that may affect the surgical result.
c. Screen for diseases that may contraindicate elective surgery or require treatment before surgery.
d. Diagnose disorders that require surgery.
e. Evaluate the nature and extent of metabolic or septic complications.

2. Routine lab studies—CBC, electrolyte profile, BUN, creatinine, prothrombin time/international normalized ratio (PT/INR), partial thromboplastin time (PTT), urinalysis, and ECG (>40 years of age or history of cardiac disease); hepatic profile if known liver problems or hepatic surgery planned

3. Radiologic evaluation—A chest radiograph is indicated in most patients undergoing major surgery. Special radiographs and studies are required in certain specific clinical situations. It is essential when sending a patient for a particular study that the radiologist be provided with an adequate account of the patient's history and physical examination and your specific reason for ordering the study.

G. ASSESSMENT AND PLAN

Following a thorough history and physical exam, one should be able to make a reasonable assessment of the patient's problem and form a differential diagnosis, construct a problem list, and develop a diagnostic and therapeutic plan.

1. Problem list—List in order of importance the particular problems identified in the history and physical examination.

2. Assessment—A concise and precise summary of the important data relevant to the patient's problem that supports the tentative conclusions and diagnosis. Delineate fully the thought process, including major decision-making points, deviations from the norm, "red herrings," and complicating factors.

3. Plan—List specific plans for further diagnostic evaluation and therapeutic measures.

H. EMERGENT HISTORY AND PHYSICAL EXAMINATION

In cases of emergency, the routine history and physical exam must often be truncated with initial efforts directed toward resuscitating the patient. The history may be limited to a single sentence or obtained from family or friends, rescue or ambulance personnel.

1. History—The mnemonic is AMPLE
   - *A*llergies
   - *M*edications
   - *P*ast medical history
   - *L*ast meal
   - *E*vents preceding injury or illness

2. Physical examination—The mnemonic is ABCDE
   - *A*irway
   - *B*reathing

Circulation
Disability
Exposure

II. PHYSICIAN ORDERS

A. ADMISSION

A helpful mnemonic is ADCA-VAN-DIMLS.

*A*dmit to ward, intensive care, or postanesthesia care unit; surgery service; attending/resident.

*D*iagnosis (illness/disease)

*C*ondition (I = excellent; II = good; III = fair; IV = serious; V = critical)

*A*llergies

*V*ital signs and frequency—Specify neurologic or vascular checks. Include parameters to notify physician (systolic blood pressure [SBP] <90, >180 mm Hg; diastolic blood pressure [DBP] >110 mm Hg; pulse [P] >110, <60 beats/min; temperature [T] >101.5°F; urine output <30 mL/h or <250 mL/8 h; change in neurologic/vascular status; respiratory distress; respiratory rate [RR] <10, >30 breaths/min)

*A*ctivity or position (weight-bearing status; type of bed; elevation of head or foot of bed as needed; footboard; measures for prevention of decubitus and thromboembolism (e.g., turn side to side q 2 h, out of bed to chair t.i.d., ambulate with assistance in the halls b.i.d.)

*N*ursing orders
   Strict intake and output measurements
   Tubes—Nasogastric, bladder catheter, chest tubes, drains
   Dressings
   Monitors/arterial line/central venous pressure
   Respiratory care—Supplemental O_2, ventilator settings, incentive spirometry
   Compression boots or thromboembolic disease stockings (TEDS)

*D*iet—When in doubt, keep the patient NPO until decisions about patient disposition are finalized.

*I*V orders (e.g., D-5 $\frac{1}{2}$ NS + 20 mEq KCl/L at 125 mL/h)

*M*edications (dose, route, frequency; sedatives, hypnotics, analgesics, laxatives, antiemetics, antipyretics, antibiotics, patient's regular medications, thromboembolism prophylaxis)

*L*aboratory tests

*S*pecial (radiographs, special tests)

B. PREOPERATIVE

The preoperative orders are very important, since operations may be canceled if the orders are inappropriately written.

1. NPO after midnight, including tube feeds

2. Adjust insulin.

3. Hydration (D-5 $\frac{1}{2}$ NS + 20 mEq KCl/L at 100 mL/h)
4. Antibiotics/steroids on call to OR if needed
5. Bowel prep
6. Lab studies
7. Blood
8. Special studies

C. POSTOPERATIVE

Include the following orders.
1. Pain meds
2. Deep venous thrombosis (DVT) prophylaxis
3. Perioperative antibiotic prophylaxis
4. GI prophylaxis
5. Incentive spirometer
6. Bowel regimen
7. PRNs—Antinausea, temp, sleep, antipyretic

III. NOTES

Record the *date* and *time* of all medical record entries.

A. PREOPERATIVE NOTES (see also Chap. 6)

1. Preoperative diagnosis
2. Procedure planned
3. Surgeons
4. Anesthesia anticipated
5. Laboratory data
a. Minor operations—CBC and urinalysis required
b. Major operations—CBC, renal profile, urinalysis, PT, PTT, ECG if patient > 40 years old; chest radiograph if patient has not had a normal chest radiograph in past 6 months; type and screen or crossmatch if needed for specific procedure (verify crossmatch with the blood bank); arterial blood gases, hepatic profile, bone profile, and other lab studies or specific radiographs as indicated by the patient's disease processes
6. Identify any specific risk factors related to cardiac, renal, pulmonary, hepatic, coagulation, and nutritional status.
7. Current medications or allergies; major medical illnesses
8. Preoperative order checklist
a. Blood on hold
b. Antiseptic scrub
c. Incentive spirometry training
d. Thromboembolic prophylaxis
e. Prophylactic antibiotics
f. IV fluid overnight
g. Special medications (e.g., steroids, insulin, antihypertensives)
h. NPO after midnight

9. Document that potential risks and benefits of intended operation have been explained to the patient (and family or guardian), questions answered, and patient (or guardian) has consented to the procedure. Check that the signed consent is in the chart.

B. POSTOPERATIVE NOTES
1. Subjective—Patient's concerns
2. Mental status—Neurologic exam, adequacy of pain control, nausea/emesis
3. Vital signs, urine and drain outputs
4. Physical exam—Including inspection of surgical dressings, wounds, drains
5. Laboratory data
6. Assessment of condition
7. Plan

C. PROGRESS NOTES
Use Weed's problem-oriented approach to medical records (see Recommended Reading).
1. Daily notes—Written to document status of current problems and identify new problems. Include data such as the postoperative day number, hospital day number, and antibiotic or hyperalimentation day number.
2. SOAP notes
   Subjective data (patient's complaints, nurses' observations)
   Objective data (vital signs, physical findings, lab data)
   Assessment
   Plans (diagnostic, therapeutic, patient education)
3. Flow sheets—For complex data and time relationships, e.g., hyperalimentation data, diabetes control, hemodynamic parameters

IV. DICTATION
Always dictate immediately after an operation.

A. OPERATIVE REPORT
1. Name
2. Medical record/account numbers
3. Date of procedure
4. Dictator
5. Attending surgeon/surgical service
6. Copies—Attending physician, assistants, billing, referring physician
7. Assistants
8. Anesthesia
9. Preoperative diagnosis
10. Postoperative diagnosis—Accurate record imperative for both patient's medical record and billing

11. Procedure—Dictate in list format, not paragraph format
12. Complications
13. Specimens
14. Indications for surgery—Brief history (reason for surgery). Document explanation of risks and benefits and acquisition of informed consent.
15. Details of operation—Patient position, skin prep and draping, type and location of incision and technique, operative findings, specific details of procedure, audit of abdomen, hemostatic technique, closure technique, dressings, disposition of patient, condition of patient, estimated blood loss, presence of attending physician, and sponge and needle counts. Include any difficulties with the procedure or confounding situations that made the procedure more difficult, e.g., Redo, extensive loss of appetite (LOA).

Note: *The "operative report" just described is a formal, dictated note. A more concise written note including any photos or drawings should be recorded in the chart immediately after all procedures.*

B. DISCHARGE SUMMARY
1. Name
2. Medical record/account numbers
3. Date of admission/date of discharge
4. Dictator
5. Attending physician/service
6. Copies—Attending physician, dictator, billing office, referring physician
7. Discharge diagnoses—Remember that "history of" implies that the condition is no longer active.
8. Operations/procedures performed
9. Consultations
10. Allergies
11. Discharge medications—Include all home medications that the patient should resume.
12. Reason for admission—Pertinent physical exam finding, lab values, and studies
13. Hospital course
14. Condition on discharge—Pertinent physical exam, lab values
15. Discharge instructions—Diet, activity, follow-up

Note*: Many hospitals require a simple written note consisting of these "discharge summary" items to be included in the medical record. This is useful in follow-up visits if the dictated summary is not yet in the chart.*

V. BILLING

In addition to being the primary vehicle for communication about patient care, the medical record is also the documentation on which level of billing is based. As health care costs have increased and reimbursements have decreased, hospitals and insurance companies have found it financially advantageous to audit medical records. Including confounding factors in operative notes (e.g., describing difficulty with adhesions, listing comorbid conditions, and detailing complexities of thought processes) justifies a higher level of patient billing. Medicare publishes cards listing the minimum physical exam/patient interaction required for each organ system. Here is a synopsis of the various levels:

Problem focused	Brief HPI	0 P/F/SH	0 ROS	1-5 exam elements
Expanded	Brief HPI	0 P/F/SH	Pertinent ROS	6 exam elements
Detailed	Full HPI	1 P/F/SH	2+ ROS	12 exam elements
Comprehensive	Full HPI	3 P/F/SH	10+ ROS	2 elements from any 9 organ areas

HPI = history of present illness; P/F/SH = past/familial/social history; ROS = review of systems.

Level	Decision Making
New/Consult	
Level I: Problem focused	Straightforward
Level II: Expanded	Straightforward
Level III: Detailed	Low complexity
Level IV: Comprehensive	Moderate complexity
Level V: Comprehensive	High complexity
Established	
Level II: Focused	Straightforward
Level III: Expanded	Low complexity
Level IV: Detailed	Moderate complexity
Level V: Comprehensive	High complexity

Medicare defaults to the least complex section unless each part is well documented.

VI. HEALTH INFORMATION PORTABILITY AND ACCOUNTABILITY ACT

No chapter on the medical record would be complete without mentioning the Health Information Portability and Accountability Act (HIPAA).

A. PROTECTS PRIVACY OF PATIENT INFORMATION

B. WHAT DOES IT MEAN?
1. Reasonable efforts must be made to limit disclosure of protected health information to the minimum necessary to accomplish an intended purpose.
2. Information may be shared as required to provide services.
3. Research falls outside of "necessary for treatment."
4. Each patient must sign a notice of privacy practices and must give permission to share information outside the given system.

MEDICAL RECORD

1

5. All identifying waste must be shredded and computer systems protected.
6. Don't discuss patient care in elevators or other public places.

C. PROTECTED HEALTH INFORMATION (PHI)
1. Demographic information
2. Information relating to past/present/future physical or mental health
3. Provision of health care
4. Payment for health care

D. SHARING OF INFORMATION ALLOWED
1. To provide treatment
2. To obtain payment
3. For health care operations
4. To research with permission
5. In incidental disclosure
6. In compliance with laws
7. For public health reporting
8. In judicial/law enforcement
9. For coroners and organ donation

E. PENALTIES
1. Civil
a. $100/violation
b. Up to $25,000/yr
2. Criminal
a. Up to $250,000
b. Possible prison time

VII. SUMMARY

A. COMMUNICATION
The goal for all documentation is to provide a continuing commentary of the patient's care. This commentary is used by all the health care team members in providing the best care for the patient. Therefore, your notes must effectively communicate to health care workers your impression of the patient and your plans for the patient.

B. STANDARD DOCUMENTATION
1. Admission history and physical exam
2. Daily SOAP notes
3. Procedure notes
a. Include any bedside procedures
b. Describe complications and findings
4. Operative notes
a. Preoperative note to include consent

b. Operative note written and dictated. Check with your department/ institution for any required format or elements. Dictate notes *immediately* after operation for optimal accuracy.

c. Postoperative note is a documented examination of the patient after surgery.

5. Description of discussions with patients and their families, especially as it pertains to decisions regarding patient care

6. Crucial occurrences—Write a note any time you're called to see a patient for a serious symptom, e.g., chest pain, shortness of breath. Document the condition of the patient and any treatment given or ordered.

7. Consult notes—Indicate your thorough review of the patient's history, physical exam, pertinent lab studies, and findings. Detail your impression and recommendations; include references to patient input and relevant discussion with other clinicians.

8. Discharge summary

C. LITIGATION

Remember, in the event of litigation, nothing can be supported without written and legible documentation in the chart. To be convicted of malpractice, you must be found negligent, wanton, and willful.

Special thanks are offered to Drs. Bower and Shaughnessy for their invaluable knowledge and guidance.

RECOMMENDED READING

Weed L: Medical Records, Medical Education, and Patient Care: The Problem-Oriented Record as a Basic Tool. Chicago, Year Book, 1970.

1

MEDICAL RECORD

Fluids and Electrolytes

Joshua M. V. Mammen, MD

I. BASIC PHYSIOLOGY

A. BODY FLUID COMPARTMENTS
1. Total body water (TBW)
a. 50-70% of total body weight
b. Higher in males (60%) than in females (50%); normal variation, 15%
c. Decreases with age due to declining muscle mass and constituent proportion of intracellular fluid
d. Highest in the newborn (70%)
2. Intracellular fluid (ICF)
a. 30-40% TBW
b. Primarily in muscle
3. Extracellular fluid (ECF)
a. Interstitial water—15% TBW
b. Intravascular water—5% TBW
    (1) Plasma volume—50 mL/kg body weight
    (2) Blood volume—70 mL/kg body weight

B. FLUID HOMEOSTASIS
Management considerations include (1) baseline requirements, (2) replacement of ongoing losses, (3) increased requirements, and (4) correction of abnormalities.
1. Baseline requirements
a. Adult—35 mL/kg/day or 1500 mL/m^2/day
b. Pediatric
    (1) 0-10 kg = 100 mL/kg/day
    (2) 10-20 kg =1000 mL + 50 mL/kg/day
    (3) >20 kg = 1500 mL + 20 mL/kg/day
2. Fluid turnover
a. GI tract (Table 2-1)
    (1) 6000-9000 mL/day
    (2) 250 mL/day lost in stool
b. Renal
    (1) 800-1500 mL/day
c. Insensible losses
    (1) 400 mL/m^2/day or 600 mL/day for adults (≈10 mL/kg/day)
    (2) 75% via water evaporation through the skin; remaining 25% via respiratory exchange
3. Increased requirement in patients with abnormal losses
a. Fever—250 mL/day per degree of fever or 15% increase in insensible losses for each 1°C above 37°C
b. Tachypnea—50% increase for each doubling of respiratory rate
c. Evaporation—Perspiration, ventilator, open abdominal wound

TABLE 2-1

COMPOSITION OF GI SECRETIONS

Secretion	Volume in mL/24 h (Range)	mEq/L Na (Range)	mEq/L K (Range)	mEq/L Cl (Range)	mEq/L HCO₃ (Range)
Salivary gland	1500 (500-2000)	10 (2-10)	26 (20-30)	10 (8-18)	30 —
Stomach	1500 (100-4000)	60 (9-116)	10 (0-32)	130 (8-154)	— —
Duodenum	140 (100-2000)	140 —	5 —	80 —	— —
Ileum	3000 (100-9000)	140 (80-150)	5 (2-8)	104 (43-137)	30 —
Colon	— —	60 —	30 —	40 —	— —
Pancreas	— (100-800)	140 (99-185)	5 (3-7)	75 (54-95)	115 —
Bile	— (50-800)	145 (99-164)	5 (3-12)	100 (89-180)	35 —

d. GI—Diarrhea, fistula, tube drainage (see Table 2-1 for composition of losses)
e. Third-space losses
f. Operative losses—May be 600-1000 mL/h in major abdominal operations

C. ELECTROLYTE COMPOSITION
1. Sodium
a. Major determinant of body tonicity; primary extracellular cation
b. Serum value not indicative of total body sodium or volume status
c. Requirements—Adult: 100-150 mEq/day; child: 3-5 mEq/kg/day
2. Potassium
a. Important in glucose transport, intracellular protein deposition, and myoneural conduction
b. Major intracellular cation along with magnesium; 97% of potassium in the body is located in the intracellular compartment
c. Serum levels do not reflect intracellular values

$$1 \text{ mEq/L ECF} = 200 \text{ mEq/L ICF}$$

d. Affected by acid-base balance, severe injury, surgical stress, nutritional state, sodium metabolism, renal function, and diuretic use
e. Requirements—Adult: 50-100 mEq/day; child—2-3 mEq/kg/day
3. Bicarbonate (see section V)—Major extracellular anion with chloride
4. Chloride
a. Closely related to sodium metabolism
b. Requirements—Adult: 90-120 mEq/day; child: 5-7 mEq/kg/day

5. Calcium
a. Important in neuromuscular and enzyme physiology
b. Body stores—1-1.2 kg, mostly in bone in the phosphate or carbonate form
c. Requirements—1-3 g/day (PO), or 7-10 mmol/day (IV); 35-40% of ingested calcium is absorbed by the small intestine while the remainder is excreted
d. Metabolism controlled by vitamin D and parathyroid hormone (PTH)
e. Physiologically active form in ionized state; acidosis increases ionized form
f. Protein bound in serum. Correction for albumin level is

Corrected Ca = (3.5 − patient's albumin) × 0.8 + patient's Ca

6. Magnesium
a. Involved in myoneuronal conduction, enzyme phosphorylation, and protein anabolism
b. Second most abundant intracellular cation; distribution similar to potassium
c. Requirement—20 mmol/day; most of the intake excreted by the GI tract

7. Phosphorus
a. Involved in enzyme regulation, energy storage, oxygen transport, proton buffering, and maintenance of cell wall integrity
b. Mostly intracellular; 80% is found in bone
c. Requirement—20-30 mmol/day; 80% is absorbed in the duodenum

II. ASSESSMENT

A. HISTORY
1. Medical conditions that predispose to fluid and electrolyte abnormalities (e.g., congestive heart failure, renal failure, cirrhosis, history of GI losses, nasogastric suctioning, fistula losses)
2. Usual and present weight
3. Significant medications—Steroids, diuretics, cardiac medications

B. PHYSICAL EXAM
1. Tissue turgor decreased by contraction of interstitial fluid secondary to loss of sodium-containing fluids; may take 24-48 hours
2. Jugular venous distention—Indicator of volume status if cardiac disease is absent
3. Orthostatic blood pressure—Changes present with 10% loss of ECF
4. Edema and lung crepitation due to increased body water and sodium

C. LABORATORY
1. Serum electrolytes
2. Hematocrit—Slow reflection of changes in volume and tonicity

3. Serum osmolality—"Tonicity" of body fluids
a. Defined as ions per unit volume, primarily determined by sodium
b. Calculated by

$$\text{Osmolality (mOsm/L)} = 2(Na) + glucose/18 + BUN/2.8$$

4. Urine
a. Volume should be 0.5-1 mL/kg/h if adequate intravascular volume, renal function, and cardiac function
b. Specific gravity and osmolality vary inversely with volume status. Exceptions are diabetes insipidus, diuretic use, congestive heart failure.
c. Urine indices can be obtained from "spot" urine and simultaneous serum samples.

$$F_eNa = (\text{Urine Na} \times \text{serum Cr/Serum Na} \times \text{Urine Cr}) \times 100$$

where F_eNa = fractional excretion of Na and Cr = creatinine.
d. Both hypovolemia and cardiogenic shock can cause prerenal azotemia (Table 2-2), and their urine indices are identical.

5. Arterial blood gas—Acid-base status

TABLE 2-2		
AZOTEMIA		
Value	Prerenal	Renal
BUN	Increased	Increased
BUN/creatinine ratio	Normal	Increased
Urine Na	<10 mEq/L	>20 mEq/L
Urine osmolality	>500	<350
F_eNa	<1%	>1%
Response to fluid	Increased output	No response
BUN = blood urea nitrogen; F_eNa = fractional excretion of Na.		

III. VOLUME DISORDERS

A. HYPOVOLEMIA
1. Clinical setting—Trauma, prolonged GI losses (vomiting, tube suction output, diarrhea), third-spacing (ascites, effusions, bowel obstruction, crush injuries, burns), increased insensible losses
a. Mild—4% loss TBW, 15% of blood volume
b. Moderate—6% TBW loss, 15-30% blood volume
c. Severe—8% TBW loss, 30-40% blood volume
d. Shock—>8% TBW loss, >40% blood volume
2. Signs and symptoms
a. Mental status changes—Sleepiness, slow responses, anorexia, anesthesia of the distal extremities, apathy, coma
b. Cardiac—Orthostatic hypotension, collapsing pulse, distant heart sounds, tachycardia, decreased pulse pressure, decreased central venous pressure and pulmonary capillary wedge pressure

c. Tissue—Decreased skin turgor, atonic muscles, sunken eyes, hypothermia, pale extremities, dry tongue, soft globe, depressed fontanelle in infants

d. GI—Ileus, anorexia, distention, nausea, vomiting

e. Metabolic—Hypothermia

3. Laboratory

a. Increased BUN out of proportion to creatinine (>20:1)

b. Increased hematocrit, 3% rise for each liter deficit

c. F_eNa <1%; increased urine specific gravity and osmolality

4. Treatment (Table 2-3)

a. Acute, life-threatening hypovolemia usually secondary to trauma or major vascular catastrophe; requires rapid infusion of isotonic fluid (crystalloid, plasma, and blood)

b. Nonacute hypovolemia requires determination of volume deficit and associated electrolyte imbalances.

    (1) Hypotonic and isotonic deficits secondary to GI and third-space losses are replaced with isotonic fluid (i.e., normal saline or lactated Ringer's solution).

    (2) Hypertonic deficits result from hyperosmolar nonketotic dehydration and jejunal feeding.

        (a) Replace free water with D-5-W or D-5 ¼ NS.

        (b) Give D-5-W for excess free water losses: ventilator, high fever, tracheostomy, and excessive perspiration

c. Administration of fluid

    (1) Bolus therapy—250-1000 mL of fluid (depending on cardiac status and rate of losses), with frequent monitoring of heart

2

FLUIDS AND ELECTROLYTES

TABLE 2-3

REPLACEMENT THERAPY—PARENTERAL FLUIDS

Solution	Na (mEq/L)	K (mEq/L)	Cl (mEq/L)	Base (mEq/L)	mOsm/L	Dextrose (g/L)	Kcal/L
D-5-W	—	—	—	—	278	50	170
D-10-W	—	—	—	—	556	100	340
D-50-W	—	—	—	—	2780	500	1700
0.9% NaCl	154	—	154	—	286	—	—
0.45% NaCl	77	—	77	—	143	—	—
3% NaCl	513	—	513	—	1026	—	—
D-5 0.9% NaCl	154	—	154	—	564	50	170
D-5 0.45% NaCl	77	—	77	—	421	50	170
D-5 0.2% NaCl	39	—	39	—	350	50	170
LR	130	4	109	28	272	—	9
D-5 LR	130	4	109	28	524	50	170

D-5-W = dextrose 5% in water; D-10-W = dextrose 10% in water; D-50-W = dextrose 50% in water; LR = lactated Ringer's solution.

rate, blood pressure, urine output. Use bolus therapy to achieve euvolemia.

(2) Adjust rate and composition of fluids for maintenance, replacement of deficits, and ongoing losses to maintain euvolemia.

B. HYPERVOLEMIA

1. Usually iatrogenic or secondary to renal failure, cirrhosis, or congestive heart failure
2. In the elderly, there may be a quick progression to pulmonary edema secondary to heart failure.
3. Clinical findings
a. Cardiovascular—Distended peripheral veins, increased cardiac output, loud heart sounds, functional murmurs, bounding palpable pulses, gallop, high pulse pressure, pulmonary edema
b. Tissue—Pitting edema, anasarca
c. GI—Vomiting, diarrhea
4. Laboratory findings
a. Decreased hematocrit and albumin
b. Serum sodium level may be low, normal, or elevated, but total body sodium is usually increased.
5. Treatment
a. Water restriction to 1500 mL/day
b. Judicious use of diuretics
c. Sodium restriction to 0.5 g/day
d. Anasarca may respond to colloid (albumin) infusion followed by parenteral loop diuretics.
e. Dialysis may be required to remove excess fluid.

IV. COMPOSITIONAL DISORDERS

A. HYPONATREMIA

Lower than normal sodium levels may be secondary to free water excess or salt deficit.
1. Forms
a. Hypotonic
   (1) Hypovolemic due to loss of isotonic fluids—Vomiting, diarrhea, thermal injury, salt-losing nephritis, or replacement with inadequate volume of excessively hypotonic fluid
   (2) Hypervolemic due to fluid-retaining states—Congestive heart failure, nephrosis, hepatic failure, malnutrition, certain medications (indomethacin, barbiturates, morphine, carbamazepine, vincristine, vinblastine, cyclophosphamide, and nicotine derivatives)
   (3) Isovolumic—Due to iatrogenic free water overloading, syndrome of inappropriate antidiuretic hormone (SIADH), renal insufficiency, hypokalemia (sensitizes kidney to antidiuretic hormone)

b. Isotonic (pseudohyponatremia)—Occurs in presence of hypertriglyceridemia and hyperproteinemia

c. Hypertonic
   (1) Due to nonsodium osmotic substances with intracellular water osmotic redistribution (glucose, mannitol)
   (2) For each 100 mg/dL of serum glucose >100 mg/dL, serum sodium is decreased 3 mEq/L.

2. Signs and symptoms

a. Neurologic—Muscle twitching, hyperactive deep tendon reflexes (DTRs), seizures, and hypertension secondary to increased intracranial pressure

b. Tissue—Salivation, lacrimation, watery diarrhea, "fingerprinting" of the skin

c. Renal—Oliguria that progresses to anuria

d. Usually asymptomatic if develops slowly to <120 mEq/L. Symptoms may appear at 130 mEq/L in children or in rapid onset of hyponatremia.

3. Treatment

a. Correct the underlying disorder.

b. Water restriction to <1500 mL/day

c. Loop diuretics followed by hourly potassium and sodium replacement

d. Hypertonic saline (3%, 5%) is reserved for symptomatic patients. Rate of infusion should increase sodium by 2-3 mEq/h, up to a serum Na of 125-130 mEq/h. Maximum rate of infusion is 100 mL/h of 5% saline. Rapid correction may produce central demyelination.

B. HYPERNATREMIA

Hypernatremia occurs when there is a free water deficit or water loss is > salt loss. It is always associated with a hyperosmolar state.

1. Forms

a. Hypovolemic due to loss of hypotonic fluids with inadequate volume replacement or hypertonic fluids. Each 3-mEq rise in serum Na reflects a 1-L loss of free water.

b. Isovolemic—Actually subclinical hypovolemia; frequent with diabetes insipidus

c. Hypervolemic is usually iatrogenic (large amounts of parenteral sodium bicarbonate, certain antibiotics); also seen in disorders of adrenal axis, Cushing's syndrome, Conn's syndrome, congenital adrenal hyperplasia, steroid use, dialysis error

2. Signs and symptoms

a. Neurologic—Restlessness, seizures, coma, delirium, mania

b. Tissue—Sticky mucous membranes, decreased salivation and lacrimation, increased temperature, and red, swollen tongue

c. Cardiovascular—Tachycardia, hypertension

d. Other—Thirst, weakness

3. Treatment

a. Reversal of underlying disorder

b. Provision of free water. Water deficit is

$$(0.6 \times \text{kg body weight})(\text{Serum Na}/140 - 1)$$

Hypotonic fluids, such as D-5-W, are metabolized in the liver to leave electrolyte-free water.

c. Replacement should be slow, half the calculated deficit over 8 hours, with the remaining half over the next 16-24 hours to avoid cerebral edema.

C. HYPOKALEMIA

1. Etiology

a. Redistribution losses from intracellular uptake of potassium; significant in acute metabolic alkalosis, insulin therapy, anabolism

b. Depletion due to, for example, external losses from GI tract, renal losses (diuretics), steroid use, renal tubular acidosis

c. Prolonged administration of low potassium fluids in the presence of the obligatory 20 mEq/day renal potassium loss

2. Signs and symptoms

a. Musculoskeletal—Weakness, cramps, myalgia, rhabdomyolysis

b. GI—Constipation, ileus

c. Renal—Polyuria, nocturia

d. Neurologic—Thirst, paresthesias, decreased DTRs

e. ECG findings include low voltage, flattened T waves, ST segment depression, and prominent U waves; may lead to arrhythmias

3. Treatment

a. Ensure adequate renal function prior to repletion.

b. Deficit usually greater than serum value indicates, due to depleted body stores

c. Treat alkalosis, decrease sodium intake.

d. Enteral replacement preferred—20-40 mEq doses

e. Parenteral replacement—7.5 mEq KCl in 50 mL D-5-W over 1 hour with peripheral IV; 20 mEq KCl/h with central line; may increase amount of KCl in maintenance IV fluids; rate of administration should not be >40 mEq/h unless telemetry is present

D. HYPERKALEMIA

1. Etiology

a. Pseudohyperkalemia in leukocytosis, hemolysis, thrombocytosis; often occurs when patients clench their fist during a blood draw

b. Redistribution—Acidosis, hypoinsulinism, tissue necrosis (crush injury, burn, electrocution), reperfusion syndrome, digoxin poisoning, β blockers

c. Elevated total body potassium in renal insufficiency, excessive intake, mineralocorticoid deficiency, diabetes mellitus, spironolactone use

2. Signs and symptoms

a. Clinical—Nausea/vomiting, intestinal colic, weakness, diarrhea

b. ECG changes include peaked T waves, decreased ST segments, widened QRS complex progressing to sine wave formation and ventricular fibrillation.

c. Cardiac arrest occurs in diastole.

3. Treatment

a. Remove exogenous source—Medications, IV fluids, diet

b. Emergent measures—If >7.5 mEq/L or ECG changes present
   (1) 1 g of 10% calcium gluconate
   (2) Sodium bicarbonate—1 ampule, repeat in 15 minutes
   (3) D-50-W (1 ampule = 50 g) and regular insulin 10 units IV piggyback
   (4) Emergent hemodialysis or peritoneal dialysis

c. Hydration and forced diuresis to promote renal excretion

d. Kayexalate 20-50 g in 100-200 mL 20% sorbitol PO q 4 h, 50 g in 200 mL water with 50 g sorbitol as retention enema, repeat q h as needed

e. Kayexalate and dialysis deplete total body potassium. Other measures only temporize by producing intracellular shifts of potassium.

E. HYPOCALCEMIA

1. Etiology

a. Frequently seen in hypoalbuminemic patients with normal ionized fraction

b. Usually asymptomatic until serum level < 8 mEq/dL

c. Ionized calcium may be subnormal with normal serum calcium in acute alkalosis.

d. If albumin is normal, check PTH level.
   (1) Low PTH—Hypoparathyroidism, magnesium deficiency
   (2) High PTH—Pancreatitis, hyperphosphatemia, hypovitaminosis D, pseudohypoparathyroidism, massive citrated blood transfusion, certain drugs (gentamicin, furosemide), renal insufficiency, small bowel fistulas, massive soft tissue infection

2. Signs and symptoms

a. Numbness and tingling in extremities, circumoral paresthesias, muscle and abdominal cramps, tetany, increased DTRs, and seizures

b. Chvostek's sign—Twitching of facial muscles after percussion over masseter muscle

c. Trousseau's sign—Carpopedal spasm induced by inflation of blood pressure cuff > systolic blood pressure for 3 minutes

d. ECG findings—Prolonged QT interval

3. Treatment

a. Acute management (IV)
   (1) Calcium chloride 10 mL 10% solution = 6.5 mmol calcium (potential for tissue necrosis if infiltrated)
   (2) Calcium gluconate 10% solution = 2.2 mmol calcium

b. Chronic management (PO)
   (1) Calcium carbonate
      (a) Titralac—1 mL = 1 g $CaCO_3$ = 400 mg Ca
      (b) Os-Cal—1 tab = 1.25 g $CaCO_3$ = 500 mg Ca
      (c) Tums—1 tab = 0.5 g $CaCO_3$ = 200 mg Ca
   (2) Phosphate-binding antacids improve GI absorption of calcium

2

FLUIDS AND ELECTROLYTES

(3) Vitamin D (calciferol)—Begin once serum phosphate is normal. Start at 50,000 units/day and increase up to 200,000 units/day as needed.

F. HYPERCALCEMIA

1. Etiology

a. Usually secondary to malignancy or hyperparathyroidism

b. Other causes include medications (thiazide diuretics, vitamins A and D, lithium), pheochromocytoma, acromegaly, factitious (hemoconcentration, postprandial), milk-alkali syndrome, granulomatous disease, acute adrenal insufficiency, hyperthyroidism, prolonged immobilization in young patient, and Paget's disease of bone.

c. Acute crisis with serum calcium >12 mg/dL; critical levels at 16-20 mg/dL; requires immediate treatment

2. Signs and symptoms include nausea, vomiting, anorexia, abdominal pains, constipation, polyuria, confusion, lethargy, and mental status changes ("bones, stones, abdominal groans, and psychic overtones")

3. Treatment

a. Most patients have an extracellular volume deficit, so begin with hydration with normal saline (dilution).

b. Oral or IV inorganic phosphate inhibits bone resorption and forms calcium-phosphate complexes; IV administration should be slow, over 12 hours, to avoid abrupt hypocalcemia.

c. Diuresis using loop diuretic promotes renal excretion.

d. Steroids—Used in lymphomas, multiple myeloma, non-PTH-secreting tumors metastatic to bone, vitamin D intoxication; may take several days to work; decrease resorption of bone and reduce intestinal vitamin D absorption

e. Mithramycin—Used in malignant-induced hypercalcemia unresponsive to other treatments; use 15-25 µg/kg IV piggyback over 4-6 hours; onset of action at 12 hours, peak action at 36 hours, duration of action 3-7 days; bone marrow suppression is main side effect; effectiveness decreases with repeated administration

f. Calcitonin—Used in malignancy-associated increased PTH. Skin test 1 unit SQ. Usual dosage is 4 units/kg SQ or IM q 12-24 h.

g. Hemodialysis

h. Primary treatment of hypercalcemic crisis due to hyperparathyroidism— Parathyroidectomy

G. HYPOMAGNESEMIA

1. Etiology—Malnutrition of any type (e.g., alcoholism, prolonged fasting, total parenteral nutrition [TPN] without adequate replacement, short gut syndrome, malabsorption, fistulas), burns, pancreatitis, SIADH, vigorous diuresis, amphotericin B therapy, after parathyroidectomy, primary hyperaldosteronism

2. Signs and symptoms—Weakness, fasciculations, mental status changes, seizures, hyperreflexia, cardiac dysrhythmias

3. Treatment

a. Parenteral—1-2 g $MgSO_4$ (8-16 mEq) IV as 10% solution over 15 minutes; continue with 1 g IM or IV piggyback q 4-6 h. Monitor replacement closely in oliguric patients.

b. Oral—Magnesium oxide 35-70 mg/day

c. Follow replacement with decreasing patellar reflexes, serial serum measurements, and resolution of symptoms. ECG monitoring is recommended for large doses.

d. Should be administered very cautiously in the setting of renal insufficiency and severe volume deficit

H. HYPERMAGNESEMIA

1. Etiologies—Renal insufficiency, early thermal injury, early traumatic or surgical stress, severe extracellular volume deficit, severe acidosis, magnesium-containing antacid or laxative overuse, adrenal insufficiency, hypothyroidism, excessive intake (e.g., treatment of eclampsia)

2. Signs and symptoms

a. Clinical—Nausea, vomiting, weakness, mental status changes, loss of DTRs, hyperventilation

b. ECG findings include atrioventricular block and prolonged QT interval.

3. Treatment

a. Discontinue or remove external sources; large amounts found in antacids and cathartics

b. IV calcium gluconate for emergent symptoms

c. Correct acidosis and extracellular volume deficit.

d. Dialysis in renal failure patients

I. HYPOPHOSPHATEMIA

1. Etiologies—Hyperalimentation, recovery from severe thermal injury, hypothyroidism, vitamin D deficiency, alkalosis, pregnancy, nutritional recovery after starvation, diabetic ketoacidosis, malabsorption, phosphate-binding antacids, alcoholism, acute tubular necrosis, prolonged alkalosis, hemodialysis, starvation

2. Signs and symptoms

a. Myocardial depression secondary to low adenosine triphosphate levels

b. Shift in oxyhemoglobin curve secondary to decreased 2,3-diphosphoglycerate levels

c. Clinical—Anorexia, bone pain, weakness, rhabdomyolysis, CNS changes, hemolysis, platelet and granulocyte dysfunction, cardiac arrest

3. Treatment

a. Parenteral $NaPO_4$ or KPO_4 if unable to take PO or if severe hypophosphatemia (1 mg/dL)

   (1) Recent onset—0.08-0.2 mmol/kg over 6 hours

   (2) Prolonged—0.16-0.24 mmol/kg over 6 hours

b. Enteral
   (1) Neutra-Phos—2 caps b.i.d.-t.i.d. (250 mg phosphorus/tab)
   (2) Phospho-Soda—5 mL b.i.d.-t.i.d. (129 mg phosphorus/mL)

J. HYPERPHOSPHATEMIA
1. Etiology—Renal insufficiency, hemodialysis, antacids, acidosis, hypoparathyroidism, catabolism, vitamin D metabolites
2. May produce metastatic calcification
3. Treatment
a. Restrict external sources.
b. Phosphate-binding antacid (Amphojel, ALternaGEL)

K. ZINC
1. Amount is 1-2 g in body, with high concentrations in brain, pancreas, liver, kidney, prostate, testis
2. Functions as enzyme activator and cofactor in enzymatic reactions
3. Absorbed via ligand binding
4. Deficiencies seen in malnutrition, malabsorption, trauma, inflammatory bowel disease, refeeding syndrome, cancer, diarrhea
5. Signs and symptoms
a. 4 Ds—Diarrhea, Dermatitis, Depression, Dementia
b. Others—Alopecia, night blindness, tremor, loss of taste
6. Treatment with zinc sulfate 3-6 mg/day if patient having normal number of stools

V. ACID-BASE DISORDERS

A. PHYSIOLOGY
1. Most enzymatic reactions occur in a narrow pH range.
2. Metabolism accounts for large proton load.
3. Three primary systems to buffer pH
a. Buffer systems
   (1) Bicarbonate-carbonate system in red blood cells is the most important and rapid buffer system:

   $$HCl + NaHCO_3 \rightleftarrows NaCl + H_2CO_3 \rightleftarrows H_2O + CO_2$$

   (2) Others include intracellular proteins and phosphates, hemoglobin (intracellular buffer in red blood cells), and bone minerals.
   (3) Henderson-Hasselbach equation

   $$pH = pK + \log BHCO_3/H_2CO_3$$

b. Respiratory system eliminates carbon dioxide ("volatile acid") generated during reduction of bicarbonate by metabolism; provides rapid and inexhaustible source of acid elimination as long as ventilation is not compromised
c. Renal system responsible for excretion of acid salts as well as reclamation of filtered bicarbonate and generation of de novo bicarbonate

B. DISORDERS
1. Metabolic acidosis
a. Etiology—Due to overproduction or underexcretion of acids or depletion of buffer stores; characterized by anion gap; normal anion gap = 8-12; anion gap = Na − (Cl + HCO$_3$)

    (1) Increased anion gap—Renal failure, ketoacidosis, alcohol intoxication, lactic acidosis, various toxins (methanol, ethylene glycol, ethanol salicylates, paraldehyde)

    (2) Normal anion gap (hyperchloremic)—Renal tubular acidosis, diarrhea, biliary or pancreatic fluid losses, Sulfamylon, small bowel fistula, dilutional acidosis, acetazolamide, ureteral diversions

b. Treatment

    (1) Correct underlying disorder.

    (2) Mild to moderate acidosis requires no treatment unless complications ensue; excessive use of sodium bicarbonate can lead to volume overload, hypernatremia, hyperosmolar state, and central alkalosis.

    (3) For pH <7.25 or HCO$_3$ <15, treatment may be required. Enzymes and catecholamines function poorly below pH 7.2.

    (4) Base deficit 0.4 × wt (kg) × (25 − measured HCO$_3$)

    (5) Correct half deficit, then recheck laboratory tests.

    (6) 1 ampule bicarbonate = 50 mEq NaHCO$_3$

2. Metabolic alkalosis
a. Etiology

    (1) Due to loss of acid or gain in base, aggravated by hypokalemia and volume contraction

    (2) Chloride-responsive—Contraction alkalosis, diuretic induced, protracted vomiting or nasogastric suction, exogenous bicarbonate loading, villous adenoma

    (3) Chloride-unresponsive—Severe potassium depletion, mineralocorticoid excess

b. Diagnosis—Elevated bicarbonate and pH, and compensatory hypercapnia are frequently associated with hypokalemia

c. Treatment

    (1) Correction of underlying disorder

    (2) Correction of hypovolemia with chloride-containing solutions (0.9% NaCl)

    (3) Correction of hypokalemia (ensure adequate renal function first)

    (4) Provision of acid solutions in refractory cases

       (a) Chloride deficit

$$\text{Weight (kg)} \times 0.4 \times (100 - \text{measured Cl})$$

       (b) Calculate amount of 0.1 N HCl acid solution required to replace deficit; replace slowly over 6-24 hours with frequent re-evaluations.

    (5) Acetazolamide (Diamox) (dosage 500 mg q 6 h) inhibits carbonic anhydrase, preventing renal reclamation and synthesis of bicarbonate; loses effect as serum bicarbonate decreases

(6) For prolonged gastric suctioning, H_2 antagonists may decrease gastric acid production and minimize acid loss.

3. Respiratory acidosis

a. Etiology—Results from acute or chronic hypercapnia secondary to inadequate ventilation: depression of the respiratory center (narcotics, CNS injury), pulmonary disease (pleural effusion, atelectasis, abdominal distention, emphysema, pneumonia), or failure to ventilate secondary to pain (upper abdominal incision)

b. Diagnosis
  (1) Characterized by increased P_{CO_2}, decreased pH
  (2) Acutely, HCO_3 may be normal, whereas in chronic states there is a compensatory increase in HCO_3.

c. Treatment
  (1) Any measure designed to improve alveolar ventilation—Aggressive pulmonary toilet, treatment of pneumonia, removal of obstruction (foreign body, secretions, and misplaced endotracheal tube), bronchodilators, avoidance of respiratory depressants
  (2) Mechanical ventilation if conservative methods fail
  (3) Maximize minute ventilation on ventilator—Tidal volume of 12-15 mL/kg, then increase rate

4. Respiratory alkalosis

a. Etiology
  (1) Secondary to acute or chronic hyperventilation
  (2) Caused by anxiety, pain, assisted ventilation, metabolic encephalopathy, CNS infections, cerebrovascular accidents, early sepsis, pulmonary embolism, hypoxia, early asthma, pneumonia, congestive heart failure, cirrhosis, or severe head injury

b. Diagnosis—Characterized by hypocapnia and elevated pH; the danger of respiratory alkalosis is hypokalemia and shifting of oxyhemoglobin curve to the left

c. Treatment
  (1) Treat underlying disorder.
  (2) In ventilated patients, keep the Pa_{CO_2} no less than 30 mm Hg.
  (3) If symptomatic, use rebreather device.
  Note: *5% CO_2 was used in past, but this practice is hazardous and is not recommended.*

C. EVALUATION OF ACID-BASE DISORDERS (Table 2-4)

1. Obtain simultaneous blood gas and electrolyte panel.
2. Calculate anion gap.
3. Calculate expected compensation from chart and locate on acid-base nomogram.
4. If compensation not within predicted values, suspect "mixed" disorder.
5. Correlate suspected diagnosis with clinical picture.

TABLE 2-4

ACID-BASE DISORDERS

Disorder	Primary Change	Secondary Change	Effect
Metabolic acidosis	↓ HCO_3	↓ Pco_2	Last 2 digits pH = Pco_2
			$HCO_3 + 15$ = last 2 digits pH
Metabolic alkalosis	↑ HCO_3	↑ Pco_2	$HCO_3 + 15$ = last 2 digits pH
Respiratory acidosis			
Acute	↑ Pco_2	↑ HCO_3	Δ pH = 0.08 per 10 Δ in Pco_2
Chronic	↑ Pco_2	↑↑ HCO_3	Δ pH = 0.03 per 10 Δ in Pco_2
Respiratory alkalosis			
Acute	↓ Pco_2	↓ HCO_3	Δ HCO_3 = 0.2 × Δ in Pco_2
Chronic	↓ Pco_2	↓↓ HCO_3	Δ HCO_3 = 0.3 × Δ in Pco_2

2

FLUIDS AND ELECTROLYTES

Shock

Timothy A. Pritts, MD, PhD

Shock is *not* hypotension but rather a state of inadequate tissue perfusion, leading to cellular hypoxia and injury.

I. PATHOPHYSIOLOGY

Inadequate oxygen delivery relative to local oxygen demand leads to conversion from aerobic to anaerobic metabolism, with production and accumulation of lactic acid, leading to metabolic acidosis. Eventually, cellular adenosine triphosphate is depleted, leading to leakage of sodium and potassium from the cell with loss of the transmembrane potential. In the presence of continued energy depletion, cellular death occurs.

II. HEMODYNAMIC CONSIDERATIONS

Modifying intravascular volume forms the basis of the treatment of shock. This requires an understanding of basic hemodynamic relationships.

A. IMPORTANT RELATIONSHIPS

1. $MAP = CO \times SVR$
   where MAP = mean arterial pressure, CO = cardiac output, and SVR = systemic vascular resistance.
2. $CO = HR \times SV$
   where CO = cardiac output, HR = heart rate, and SV = stroke volume.
3. Frank-Starling curve relates left ventricular end-diastolic volume (LVEDV; preload) to stroke volume. Up to a certain level (the "flat" portion of the curve), increased preload leads to increased stroke volume, with subsequently increased cardiac output. With the exception of septic shock, all forms of shock have low cardiac outputs.
4. Stroke volume is determined by preload, myocardial contractility, and afterload.
5. For a given end-diastolic volume, stroke volume increases with increased myocardial contractility and decreased afterload.

B. PRELOAD

1. Preload reflects filling of the ventricle and, theoretically, the LVEDV.
2. In the absence of right ventricular dysfunction, central venous pressure (CVP) can be used as an indirect measurement of central blood volume. In many elderly patients with cardiac disease or pulmonary dysfunction, CVP is an inaccurate assessment of left-sided filling volume.
3. Pulmonary artery (Swan-Ganz) catheters measure pulmonary capillary wedge pressure (PCWP), an estimation of left ventricular end-diastolic pressure (LVEDP), which in turn should reflect LVEDV. These assumptions may be inaccurate in patients with mitral valve disease, aortic

insufficiency, pulmonary venous pathology, and altered left ventricular (LV) compliance. Optimal PCWP is often 8-15 mm Hg, but this varies with the individual.

C. AFTERLOAD

1. Defined as the resistance against which the heart muscle must contract
2. Afterload of the ventricle is estimated by systemic vascular resistance (SVR), a calculated value.

$$SVR = [(MAP - CVP) \times 80] \div CO$$

where MAP = mean arterial pressure, CVP = central venous pressure, and CO = cardiac output.
3. Afterload reduction can optimize cardiac output for a given preload and contractility. In cardiogenic shock with reduced myocardial function, a reduction in afterload can greatly improve cardiac output.
4. Hypovolemic patients may also demonstrate elevated afterload. This reflects compensatory peripheral vasoconstriction to maintain adequate blood flow to vital organs. Afterload reduction is inappropriate until volume status has been corrected.
5. In neurogenic shock, there is an inappropriate decrease in afterload due to loss of vasomotor tone. There is also decreased afterload in septic shock, with inappropriate vasodilation and relative hypovolemia. In these instances, vasopressors are often used to improve vascular tone to help maintain adequate perfusion.

D. MYOCARDIAL CONTRACTILITY

1. Defined as the strength of myocardial contraction at a given preload and afterload
2. Determined by velocity of shortening, force of contraction, and length of displacement
3. Affected by changes in myocardial perfusion
4. Compromised myocardial contractility is the chief pathology in primary cardiogenic shock. Treatment is directed toward increasing myocardial function with various inotropic agents.

E. VASOACTIVE AGENTS

1. Inotropic agents and vasopressors
   Note: *These agents should not be used as a substitute for adequate volume resuscitation.*
a. Dopamine—Effects are dose dependent.
   (1) 3-5 µg/kg/min (renal dose)—Renal artery vasodilation may enhance splanchnic perfusion and promote diuresis.

(2) 5-10 µg/kg/min—Stimulation of cardiac β receptors, with increased contractility and cardiac output. Increased heart rate is seen with increasing dosage.

(3) >10 µg/kg/min—Increasing α adrenergic effects, with increased MAP and SVR due to peripheral vasoconstriction

b. Dobutamine—Synthetic dopamine analog with β_1 and β_2 effects; also acts as a mild vasodilator in addition to its inotropic effects; usual dosage is 5-15 µg/kg/min

c. Amrinone—Phosphodiesterase inhibitor with inotropic effects; also reduces afterload

d. Norepinephrine—Exerts both α and β effects. β effects predominate at lower doses, with increased heart rate and contractility; dose-dependent increases in α effect seen, with vasoconstriction at increasing dosages

e. Epinephrine—At lower dosages (0.01 µg/kg/min), there are β_1-mediated increases in heart rate and contractility. Vasoconstriction occurs with increasing dosages. Concerns about increased myocardial oxygen demands may limit its usefulness in adults.

f. Phenylephrine (Neo-Synephrine)—α_1 effect (vasoconstriction)

2. **Vasodilators**

a. Nitroglycerin—Primary effect is venodilation via direct action on vascular smooth muscle; increases venous capacitance

b. Nitroprusside—Acts directly on both arterial and venous smooth muscle

III. SHOCK STATES

Blalock (1934) divided shock states into four basic categories, based on etiology, as (1) hypovolemic shock; (2) septic shock; (3) neurogenic shock; and (4) cardiogenic shock. With some additional subcategories, these divisions are still useful. The basic hemodynamic profiles of each type of shock are outlined in Table 3-1 and described in greater detail in this section.

A. HYPOVOLEMIC SHOCK

1. Further divided into hemorrhagic, traumatic, and nonhemorrhagic (e.g., burn shock)

Signs and symptoms depend on degree of volume depletion, rapidity of volume depletion, duration of shock, and the body's compensatory reactions. Severity of hemorrhagic shock and clinical presentation can be stratified according to the amount of fluid lost. Although the classifications presented in Table 3-2 are generally applied to hemorrhagic shock, they are useful in estimating volume depletion.

Note: *Inebriated or cirrhotic patients maintain skin perfusion despite inadequate cardiac indices, making early shock difficult to assess. In addition, young patients, who have particularly effective compensatory responses, may be able to maintain a normal blood pressure and heart rate up to the point of cardiovascular collapse and arrest. It is important to recognize early signs of shock in these patients.*

3

SHOCK

TABLE 3-1

HEMODYNAMIC PROFILES IN SHOCK

Type of Shock	HR	CVP	PCWP	CO	SVR
Hypovolemic	↑	↓	↓	↓	↑
Septic					
Hyperdynamic	↑	↓	↓	↑	↓
Hypodynamic	↑↓	↑↓	↑↓	↓	↑
Neurogenic	↑	↓	↓	↓	↓
Cardiogenic	↑↓	↑	↑	↓	↑

HR = heart rate; CVP = central venous pressure; PCWP = pulmonary capillary wedge pressure;
CO = cardiac output; SVR = systemic vascular resistance.

2. Hemorrhagic shock
a. Remember ABCs—Establish airway; ensure adequate oxygenation and ventilation.
b. Control of external hemorrhage, if present
c. IV access and administration of crystalloid, preferably lactated Ringer's solution. Lactate buffers hydrogen ions from ischemic tissues that are washed out with reperfusion.
d. Blood products as needed
e. Operative control of hemorrhage if necessary
f. Avoid hypothermia.

3. Traumatic shock
a. Initially caused by both internal and external volume losses, i.e., loss of blood or plasma externally from wound or burn surface, loss of blood or plasma into the damaged tissues; worsened by plasma extravasation into tissues distal to injured areas
b. Débridement of ischemic or nonviable tissue may be necessary.
c. Immobilize fractures to prevent further tissue damage.
d. Pulmonary artery catheterization may be necessary for fluid management, especially in elderly patients.

4. Nonhemorrhagic shock
a. Similar to hemorrhagic shock, except that blood transfusion is usually not necessary
b. Examples include third-space losses in bowel obstruction, GI losses from diarrhea, emesis, biliary drainage, pancreatic fistula, and burns.
c. Replacements should be crystalloid with appropriate electrolyte composition of fluid lost. Usually D-5 ½ NS + 10 mEq KCl/L for GI losses proximal to ligament of Treitz, lactated Ringer's for losses distal

B. SEPTIC SHOCK
1. Implies hemodynamic instability due to host inflammatory response to infection
2. Local response to infection includes rubor, calor, dolor, and tumor. Systemic responses in this setting include vasodilation, altered mental status, fever, capillary leak, and organ dysfunction.

SHOCK

3

TABLE 3-2

CLASSES OF HYPOVOLEMIC SHOCK

Class	Amount of Blood Loss (mL)	Blood Loss (%)	Heart Rate (beats/min)	Blood Pressure	Pulse Pressure	Respiratory Rate (breaths/min)	Urinary Output (mL/h)	Mental Status
I	<750	<15	<100	NL	NL to ↑	14-20	>30	Slightly anxious
II	750-1500	15-30	>100	NL	→	20-30	20-30	Mildly anxious
III	1500-2000	30-40	>120	→	→	30-40	5-15	Anxious, confused
IV	>2000	>40	>140	→	→	>35	Negligible	Confused, lethargic

NL = normal.

3. Host mediators implicated in pathogenesis of septic shock include multiple cytokines (e.g., tumor necrosis factor α and interleukin 1), reactive oxygen radicals, vasoactive peptides, the complement cascade, and platelet-activating factor.
4. May result from infection with gram-positive or gram-negative bacteria, fungi, virus, or protozoa, initiating inflammatory, metabolic, endocrinologic, and immunologic pathways
5. Response (see Table 3-1) may be hyperdynamic (compensated) or hypodynamic (uncompensated)
6. Gram positive—Massive fluid losses secondary to dissemination of potent exotoxin, often without bacteremia
   a. Causative organisms include *Clostridium, Staphylococcus,* and *Streptococcus* spp.
   b. Characterized by hypotension with normal urine output and unaltered mental status. Acidosis is infrequent.
   c. The prognosis is generally good with treatment.
   d. Treatment—Appropriate antibiotics, surgical drainage or débridement if necessary, and IV fluids to correct volume deficit
7. Gram negative—Initiated by endotoxins in cell walls of gram-negative bacteria
   a. Causative organisms—GI flora, including coliforms and anaerobic bacilli, e.g., *Klebsiella*, *Enterobacteriaceae*, *Serratia*, and *Bacteroides*
   b. Common sources in order of decreasing frequency—Urinary tract, pulmonary, alimentary tract, burns, and soft tissue infections. Always consider line sepsis.
   c. Endotoxin, or lipopolysaccharide (LPS), in the outer membrane of gram-negative bacteria can elicit marked host inflammatory response even in the absence of viable bacteria.
   d. Treatment
      (1) Early identification of source of infection and appropriate antibiotic treatment
      (2) Foley catheter to monitor urine output
      (3) Invasive hemodynamic monitoring
      (4) IV fluid resuscitation to achieve normal filling pressures
      (5) Vasopressors, inotropes as needed
      (6) Support of individual organ systems
   e. Newer therapies directed at specific inflammatory mediators of sepsis include antibodies against LPS and modulation of host cytokines and mediators; they have met with mixed results in clinical and animal trials, likely due to the redundancy of the inflammatory cascade.
8. Fungal—Causative organisms are commonly *Candida* spp.
   a. Seen in neutropenic, immunosuppressed, multitrauma, or burn patients
   b. Risk factors include parenteral nutrition, invasive monitors, and broad-spectrum antibiotics.
   c. When *Candida* organisms reach the intravascular compartment, widespread dissemination can occur.

(1) Fungi lodge in the microcirculation, forming microabscesses.
(2) Characterized by high fevers and rigors
(3) Blood cultures negative in 50% of patients
(4) Ophthalmologic evaluation may reveal evidence of ocular involvement in dissemination.

d. Treatment—Antifungal agent, e.g., amphotericin B

C. NEUROGENIC SHOCK

1. Usually results from spinal cord injury, regional anesthetic agent, or autonomic blockade. Diagnosis is based on history and neurologic exam.
2. Mechanism
a. Loss of vasomotor control
b. Expansion of venous capacitance bed with peripheral pooling of blood
c. Inadequate ventricular filling
3. Manifestations
a. Warm, well-perfused skin
b. Low blood pressure
c. Low or normal urine output
d. Bradycardia may be present if adrenergic nerves to heart are blocked.
4. Treatment
a. Correct ventricular filling pressure with IV fluids.
b. Vasoconstrictors to restore venous tone

   Note: *Vasculature to those parts of the body with an intact autonomic nervous system may constrict excessively, resulting in ischemia to vital organs or necrosis of fingers.*

c. Trendelenburg position if necessary
d. Maintain body temperature.

D. CARDIOGENIC SHOCK

Differentiate between myocardial dysfunction from primary (e.g., myocardial infarction) and from secondary (e.g., compressive) etiologies.

1. Primary myocardial dysfunction
a. Includes myocardial infarction, dysrhythmias, valvular dysfunction, and myocardial failure
b. Treatment
   (1) Identification and correction of hemodynamically significant arrhythmias
   (2) Optimization of filling pressures (PCWP should be >15 mm Hg)
   (3) If SVR is elevated, initiate afterload reduction with nitroglycerin or nitroprusside.
   (4) If SVR is low or normal, initiate inotropic support with dopamine, dobutamine, or amrinone.
   (5) In practice, afterload reduction and inotropic support are often performed concurrently.

3

SHOCK

(6) If inotropic support fails, consider intra-aortic balloon pump or ventricular assist device.

(7) In the setting of acute myocardial infarction, consider interventional cardiac catheterization, thrombolytic therapy, or surgical treatment.

2. Secondary myocardial dysfunction

a. Includes tension pneumothorax, cardiac tamponade, vena cava obstruction, and pulmonary embolus

b. Treatment of the underlying problem should alleviate shock.

c. In the setting of trauma, distended neck veins should suggest secondary myocardial dysfunction (cardiac compression) and should be acted on immediately. Absence of distended neck veins does not rule out cardiac compression in the hypovolemic patient. Distention may become evident only after adequate fluid resuscitation.

(1) Common causes

(a) Tension pneumothorax—Shift of trachea to uninvolved side, decreased breath sounds, distended neck veins. This is not a radiographic diagnosis!

(b) Cardiac tamponade—Hypotension, muffled heart sounds, distended neck veins (Beck's triad); low voltage on ECG and enlarged cardiac silhouette on chest radiograph (classic "water bottle" shape)

(2) Associated findings may include pulsus paradoxus (drop in systolic blood pressure > 10 mm Hg with inspiration) and Kussmaul's sign (rise in CVP with inspiration [infrequently present]).

(3) Treatment is by fluid administration and correction of underlying mechanism.

(a) Tension pneumothorax—Decompress with 14-gauge angiocatheter in 2nd intercostal space, midclavicular line; definitive treatment by chest tube placement in 5th intercostal space, anterior axillary line

(b) Acute cardiac tamponade—If hemodynamically stable, perform pericardiocentesis or pericardial window (Trinkle maneuver [incision over xyphoid, exposing pericardium, which is then incised]). If the patient is hemodynamically unstable, consider prompt operative thoracotomy or sternotomy.

IV. MULTIORGAN DYSFUNCTION SYNDROME

A. DEFINITION

Multiorgan dysfunction is a syndrome of progressive but potentially reversible dysfunction involving two or more organs or organ systems that arises after resuscitation from an acute disruption of normal homeostasis.

B. CAUSES

1. Can result from prolonged or inadequately controlled shock
2. Is the most common cause of mortality in the surgical ICU

C. PREVENTIVE MEASURES

1. Hemodynamic support—Maintenance of adequate tissue oxygenation and substrate delivery
2. Nutritional support—Provision of adequate nutrition and reversal of catabolism
3. Prevention of infection—Maintenance of optimal antimicrobial defenses and prompt antimicrobial therapy at first sign of infection

3

SHOCK

Blood Component Therapy

Jefferson M. Lyons, MD

The judicious use of blood products is critical in the care of surgical patients. Because of the risk of metabolic, immunologic, and infectious complications, the clinician must be aware of the indications and contraindications of blood product use. The recommendations herein are derived from guidelines established by the American Association of Blood Banks, the American Red Cross, the U.S. Food and Drug Administration (Center for Biologics Evaluation and Research), the Hoxworth Blood Center (at the University of Cincinnati Medical Center), and the Council of Community Blood Centers.

4

I. ESTIMATION OF VOLUMES

A. TOTAL BLOOD VOLUME (TBV)
1. ≈7.5% of total body weight
2. Slightly higher (8-8.5%) in males and newborns
3. TBV—Adults = 70 mL/kg total body weight; newborns = 80 mL/kg total body weight

B. RED BLOOD CELL

RBC volume = TBV × hematocrit (expressed as a decimal)

where RBC = red blood cell and TBV = total blood volume.

C. PLASMA VOLUME

PV = TBV − RBC volume or PV = (1.0 − hematocrit) × TBV

where PV = plasma volume, TBV = total blood volume, and RBC = red blood cell.

II. BLOOD COMPONENTS

Blood should be thought of in terms of its separate components (Table 4-1). Therapy should be directed at the specific deficit.

A. VOLUME
Adequate intravascular volume maintains cardiac preload, cardiac output, and mean arterial perfusion pressure. Oxygen-carrying capacity is the responsibility of the RBC. Hypovolemia without significant RBC mass deficit is managed with volume expanders.
1. Crystalloid—Volume expander of choice in the acute setting. Isotonic fluids are lactated Ringer's solution or normal saline. Remember that three times the volume lost is required because crystalloid extravasates into the extracellular fluid. Potassium should not be added until adequate urine output is established.

TABLE 4-1

SUMMARY OF BLOOD COMPONENTS

Component	Major Indications	Action	Not Indicated For	Special Precautions	Hazards	Rate of Infusion
Whole blood	Symptomatic anemia with large volume deficit	Restoration of oxygen-carrying capacity, restoration of blood volume	Condition responsive to specific component	Must be ABO identical; labile coagulation factors deteriorate within 24 h after collection	Infectious diseases; septic/toxic, allergic, febrile reactions; circulatory overload	For massive loss, as fast as patient can tolerate
Red blood cells	Symptomatic anemia	Restoration of oxygen-carrying capacity	Pharmacologically treatable anemia; coagulation deficiency	Must be ABO compatible	Infectious disease; septic/toxic, allergic, febrile reactions	As patient can tolerate, but <4 h
Red blood cells, leukocytes removed	Symptomatic anemia, febrile reactions from leukocyte antibodies	Restoration of oxygen-carrying capacity	Pharmacologically treatable anemia; coagulation deficiency	Must be ABO compatible	Infectious diseases; septic/toxic, allergic reactions (unless plasma also removed, e.g., by washing)	As patient can tolerate, but <4 h
Red blood cells, adenine-saline added	Symptomatic anemia with volume deficit	Restoration of oxygen-carrying capacity	Pharmacologically treatable anemia; coagulation deficiency	Must be ABO compatible	Infectious diseases; septic/toxic, allergic, febrile reactions; circulatory overload	As patient can tolerate, but <4 h

Fresh frozen plasma	Deficit of labile and stable plasma coagulation factors and TTP	Source of labile and nonlabile plasma factors	Condition responsive to volume replacement	Should be ABO compatible	Infectious diseases; allergic reactions, circulatory overload	<4h
Liquid plasma and plasma	Deficit of stable coagulation factors	Source of nonlabile factors	Deficit of labile coagulation factors or volume replacement	Should be ABO compatible	Infectious diseases; allergic reactions	<4h
Cryoprecipitated AHF	Hemophilia A, von Willebrand's disease, hypofibrinogenemia, factor XIII deficiency	Provides factor VIII, fibrinogen, vWF, factor XIII	Conditions not deficient in contained factors	Frequent repeat doses may be necessary	Infectious diseases; allergic reactions	<4h
Platelets: pheresis	Bleeding from thrombocytopenia or platelet function abnormality	Improves hemostasis	Plasma coagulation deficits and some conditions with rapid platelet destruction (e.g., ITP)	Should not use some microaggregate filters (check manufacturer's instructions)	Infectious diseases; septic/toxic, allergic, febrile reactions	<4h

Continued

BLOOD COMPONENT THERAPY

4

TABLE 4-1

SUMMARY OF BLOOD COMPONENTS—cont'd

Component	Major Indications	Action	Not Indicated For	Special Precautions	Hazards	Rate of Infusion
Granulocytes	Neutropenia with infection	Provides granulocytes	Infection responsive to antibiotics	Must be ABO compatible; do not use depth-type microaggregate filters	Infectious diseases; allergic, febrile reactions	One pheresis unit over 2-4 h period; closely observe for reactions

AHF = antihemophilic factor; ITP = idiopathic thrombocytopenia purpura; TTP = thrombotic thrombocytopenia purpura; vWF = von Willebrand's factor.
From American Red Cross, Council of Community Blood Centers, and American Association of Blood Banks: Circular of Information for the Use of Human Blood and Blood Components, Washington, DC, American Red Cross, Publication #1751, Feb. 15, 1991, pp. 14-15. Used by permission.

2. Colloid solutions—Same hemodynamic effects as crystalloid in $1/3$ the volume

a. 5% or 25% albumin—For patients with hypovolemia and hypoalbuminemia. Its intravascular half-life is short. The only proven benefit of albumin is the earlier return of bowel motility in postoperative patients with hypoalbuminemia. It may also lead to increased morbidity by increasing pulmonary edema in inflammatory states secondary to capillary leak.

b. Fresh frozen plasma (FFP)

c. Purified protein fraction (Plasmanate)—83% albumin, 17% globulin

d. Hetastarch (Hespan)—Artificial colloid of 6% hetastarch in saline; effectiveness decreases over 24 hours; exacerbates bleeding disorders and congestive heart failure

B. WHOLE BLOOD

Whole blood is generally separated into components for directed therapy. Whole blood is rarely available for use in any setting. It is used by the military in trauma scenarios for acute massive hemorrhage and it is regularly used in burn patients for acute intraoperative blood loss replacement, because it is rich in plasma, platelets, and clotting factors. One unit of whole blood is generally 500 mL and has a minimum hematocrit of 38%. It may be stored for 21-35 days, depending on the preservative in which it was collected.

C. AUTOLOGOUS BLOOD

Hemodilution, intraoperative salvage, and preoperative donation should be considered when feasible to reduce the risk of disease transmission and immune reactions.

1. Cell salvage—Involves reinfusion of blood from body cavities not contaminated by bacteria or malignant cells; once processing is complete, the salvaged product contains RBCs only; must be used within 4 hours and is devoid of clotting factors

2. Intraoperative hemodilution—Candidates for this process must have the capacity to compensate for acute RBC loss by increasing their cardiac output. One to three units of blood are removed at the beginning of a procedure with concurrent volume replacement using a mixture of colloid and crystalloid solutions. The whole blood is then infused during the case or postoperatively. Platelets and coagulation factors are present. The theory behind the use of this practice is the decreased loss of RBC mass from intraoperative hemorrhage.

3. Preoperative donation 2-5 weeks prior to a planned procedure—This blood is screened for infectious agents. If positive testing occurs (e.g., hepatitis, HIV), the units may still be suitable for use in some centers but will likely be discarded to prevent inadvertent transmission.

D. RED BLOOD CELLS

RBCs are given when inadequate oxygen-carrying capacity exists.

4

BLOOD COMPONENT THERAPY

1. If the intravascular volume is adequate (see section II. A), a hemoglobin of 8 g/dL will provide adequate oxygen-carrying capacity for most patients. In the compromised elderly and in patients with an acute cardiovascular event (myocardial infarction), a hemoglobin of 10 g/dL may be more appropriate. Do not use RBCs when anemia can be corrected with specific medications (iron, vitamin B_{12}, folate, erythropoietin).
2. In the trauma setting, immobilize and apply direct pressure to control hemorrhage, provide volume repletion with crystalloid, then restore oxygen-carrying capacity with RBCs, in that order of priority.
a. If hemostasis and volume replacement with 2 L of crystalloid stabilize the patient, transfusion can await specific indications.
b. If 2 L of crystalloid fails to produce hemodynamic stability, this suggests that >30% blood volume loss and transfusion should begin immediately with O-negative RBCs or type-specific (ABO-compatible, Rh-compatible) RBCs.
c. Each unit of packed RBCs has a volume of ≈350 mL and a hematocrit of 60-65% and should raise the patient's hematocrit by 3 percentage points.

E. FRESH FROZEN PLASMA
FFP should be used for the normalization of coagulation factors. FFP is prepared from whole blood that is centrifuged, rapidly aliquoted, and frozen to at least −18°C within 8 hours of collection. To use, the plasma must be thawed at 30-37°C. It may be stored for 24 hours at 1-6°C. Has all possible side effects as a blood transfusion.

F. COAGULATION FACTORS (Fig. 4-1)
Blood vessels, platelets, and soluble protein coagulation factors all are critically important in hemostasis. Failure of any of these three can lead to life-threatening hemorrhage.
1. The most common cause of postoperative bleeding is poor surgical hemostasis, followed by thrombocytopenia, thrombocytopathy, acquired coagulation defects, and congenital coagulation defects.
2. A medical history is the single best screening test available for detecting bleeding problems.
a. Family history of coagulopathy (hemophilia A or B, von Willebrand's factor [vWF])
b. Abnormal bleeding during minor trauma, teeth extractions, or menses
c. Medications—Aspirin, warfarin (Coumadin), clopidogrel (Plavix), bile salt binders, dipyridamole, nonsteroidal anti-inflammatory drugs, cephalosporins
d. Concurrent illnesses—Liver disease, biliary obstruction, renal disorders, blood dyscrasias, colon cancer with obstruction
e. Medical/surgical history—Malabsorption, ileal resection, or prosthetic valves
3. Laboratory tests
a. Platelet count

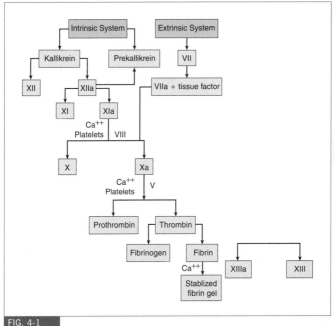

FIG. 4-1

Coagulation cascade.

b. Bleeding time—Evaluates platelet function and blood vessel integrity

c. Prothrombin time (PT)—Evaluates production of the vitamin K–dependent clotting factors and therefore is used to monitor warfarin therapy and the extrinsic pathway

d. Activated partial thromboplastin time (PTT)—Evaluates the intrinsic pathway and heparin therapy

e. Thrombin time measures polymerization of fibrinogen—Prolonged with heparin, disseminated intravascular coagulation (DIC), dysfibrinogenemia, and primary fibrinolysis

f. Fibrinogen level—Decreased in DIC, primary fibrinolysis, and hereditary disorders

g. Fibrin split products—Measure fibrinolysis and are increased in DIC and primary fibrinolysis

4. **Congenital coagulopathy states—Absence of each of the factors has been reported, only some of which have clinical significance (see Fig. 4-1)**

a. Hemophilia A (classic hemophilia)—Prolonged PTT. X-linked recessive deficiency of factor VIII. Surgery and trauma require 75-100% factor VIII activity for 7-10 days.

Calculation for number of factor VIII from a commercial concentrate:

$$1\% \text{ factor VIII activity} = 1 \text{ factor VIII unit/dL}$$

Desired factor VIII % activity:

Current factor VIII % activity × plasma volume (mL)/100 = number of factor VIII units to be infused

Factor VIII should be given every 8 hours to maintain hemostasis.

b. Hemophilia B ("Christmas disease")—Prolonged PTT; X-linked recessive deficiency of factor IX; treated using factor IX concentrates; for factor IX, 1% activity = 1.5 units

c. von Willebrand's disease—Most common congenital bleeding disorder manifested by a prolonged PTT and a prolonged bleeding time; autosomal dominant deficiency of factor VIII:vWF; treat with commercial factor VIII concentrates that contain vWF or with desmopressin (DDAVP)

5. Acquired coagulopathy states

a. Vitamin K deficiency—Due to inadequate intake, reduction of normal flora, malabsorption, biliary obstruction, total parenteral nutrition, antibiotics, warfarin therapy; treat with vitamin K 10 mg SQ/IV q a.m. × 3; takes days to weeks to correct, whereas FFP corrects the coagulopathy rapidly; provide $1/3$ of plasma volume as rapidly as the patient will tolerate the infusion

b. Hypothermia—Especially in the trauma patient; treat with fluid warmers and heating blankets

c. Liver failure—Due to decreased clotting factors except VIII; treat with FFP

d. Heparin acts with antithrombin III to prolong PTT; protamine 1 mg/100 units of heparin rapidly reverses heparin effects; half-life is 4 hours

e. Renal failure—Leads to uremic bleeding secondary to platelet dysfunction; treatment is dialysis and desmopressin; transfusion of cryoprecipitate and platelet concentrates has also been useful in these patients

f. DIC—Secondary to release of thromboplastic substances with simultaneous clotting and lysis, with secondary microangiopathic hemolytic anemia and thrombocytopenia, with associated bleeding. DIC may occur with trauma, sepsis, malignancy, burns, obstetric accidents (e.g., amniotic fluid embolus, abruptio placentae, retained fetus), envenomation, and anaphylaxis. Large amounts of fibrin degradation products (FDP) complicate the coagulopathy by inhibiting fibrin polymerization. DIC is characterized by diffuse bleeding, prolonged PT, PTT, decreased platelets, decreased fibrinogen, elevated FDP level, and D-dimers. Treatment is supportive with transfusions directed by specific deficits: FFP, cryoprecipitate for fibrinogen, vitamin K, and treatment of the underlying disease. Withhold platelets until the platelet count is <50,000 mm^3 because platelets contribute to thrombotic pathophysiology.

g. Primary fibrinolysis—Occurs acutely with heat stroke, hypoxia, and hypotension and chronically with neoplasms or cirrhosis; consists of a hemorrhagic state characterized by a shortened euglobulin lysis time, decreased fibrinogen, and elevated FDP level without thrombocytopenia; may be treated with aminocaproic acid (Amicar)

6. Components
a. FFP—Contains 200 units of factors VIII, V, and all other coagulation factors; no crossmatch is necessary for this product. The plasma must be ABO compatible; the Rh type is unimportant. No RBCs are in the component. FFP is used for disorders of coagulation, e.g., dilution, liver disease, DIC.
b. Cryoprecipitate—Each unit contains ≥80 units of factor VIII, 150 mg of fibrinogen in 15 mL volume. Indicated for hemophilia A, low fibrinogen states, and von Willebrand's disease. Compatibility testing is unnecessary; ABO compatibility is preferred. Rh type need not be considered. May develop a positive direct antiglobin test and, rarely, hemolysis if large amounts of ABO-incompatible cryoprecipitate are used. Cryoprecipitate must be thawed, then kept at room temperature and transfused within 4 hours.

G. PLATELETS

Platelets are active in normal hemostasis. Masses of platelets occlude breaks in small blood vessels and are a source of phospholipid, which is required for coagulation of blood. Preferred use is of ABO-compatible platelets, but out-of-group components can be used. No crossmatch is required for their use.

1. Indicated in patients actively bleeding owing to thrombocytopenia or thrombocytopathy
2. Indicated to raise platelet count to 80,000 in preoperative patients
3. Indicated to keep platelet counts >50,000 in thrombocytopenic postoperative patients
4. Do not use platelets in patients with thrombotic thrombocytopenia purpura or idiopathic thrombocytopenia purpura unless life-threatening hemorrhage is occurring, because the infused platelets will be rapidly degraded and contribute to the underlying pathophysiology.
5. One unit of platelets raises the platelet count by 5000-10,000/mm^3.
a. Usually platelets are pooled in a package that contains 6 units or as a single-donor apheresis product.
b. Each platelet product also contains the equivalent of stable clotting factors (all except factors V, VIII) in 1-2 units of FFP.
c. Platelet infusion needs to be repeated q 1-3 days due to the platelet half-life and consumption.
d. Platelets are rarely contaminated by bacteria but are the most likely of blood components to be contaminated.
e. Platelet alloimmunization can occur to multiple antigens, most often human leukocyte antigen (HLA). In sensitized individuals, apheresis platelets from an HLA-matched individual may replace pooled platelets.

4

BLOOD COMPONENT THERAPY

H. GRANULOCYTES

Granulocyte therapy is controversial. It is used as supportive therapy in neutropenic patients (<500 neutrophils/L of blood) with a documented bacterial or fungal infection.

1. Usually prepared by pheresis of a single donor's blood
2. Rarely increases the patient's granulocyte count
3. If bone marrow recovery is not anticipated, granulocyte infusion is unlikely to alter the patient's course.
4. Granulocyte colony-stimulating factor has supplanted most uses of granulocyte infusions.
a. Recombinant DNA technology, infectious transmissions are nonexistent.
b. Stimulates the patient's own marrow to produce native granulocytes, so sensitization and graft vs. host disease (GVHD) are not seen.

I. SIDE EFFECTS AND HAZARDS

1. Immunologic complications, immediate
a. Acute hemolytic transfusion reaction—Occurs when donor RBCs and recipient plasma are incompatible. Most common cause is ABO incompatibility caused by identification error at the time of sample acquisition or transfusion and subsequent transfusion of an incompatible product. The reaction is characterized by fever, chills, back pain, chest pain, dyspnea, abnormal bleeding, headache, and shock. In anesthetized patients, hypotension and bleeding (DIC) may be the only signs. Hemoglobinemia, hemoglobinuria, hyperbilirubinemia, and renal failure all may ensue. The transfusion should be stopped with institution of volume expansion and diuresis. Patient and donor blood samples should be collected for evaluation. A positive antiglobin test (direct agglutination test [DAT]) may be present if residual incompatible RBCs are still present in the circulation.
b. Immune-mediated platelet destruction may occur when a patient has become alloimmunized and develops antibodies to platelets.
c. Febrile nonhemolytic reactions occur in 1-2% of recipients and are usually caused by antibodies to leukocytes. Generally a 1°C increase in temperature occurs during or shortly after a transfusion and in the absence of other pyretic stimuli. The incidence of this reaction is reduced with the use of leukoreduced blood components. Occurrence is more likely in alloimmunized patients.
d. Allergic reaction may consist of urticaria, wheezing, and angioedema, which may occur about 1% of the time. Pretransfusion premedication with antihistamines and acetaminophen decreases the incidence of this complication.
e. Anaphylactoid reaction consists of bronchospasm, dyspnea, and pulmonary edema. This may occur in those with IgA deficiency and circulating anti-IgA or those with previous history of transfusion with multiple units of plasma-containing components. Treatment is with epinephrine and steroids.

f. Transfusion-related acute lung injury (TRALI)—Reaction presents with rapid increase in pulmonary capillary permeability leading to massive leakage of fluid and plasma proteins into the pulmonary parenchyma that presents as pulmonary edema. Generally occurs within 6 hours of transfusion. Patients are dyspneic, exhibit decreasing Po_2, and may require mechanical ventilatory support for 2-4 days while the insult resolves. TRALI has been associated with the presence of HLA or granulocyte antibodies either in the donor blood or the recipient.

2. Immunologic complications, delayed

a. Delayed hemolytic reaction usually occurs in patients previously alloimmunized with RBCs, 2-14 days after transfusion. Continued anemia despite transfusions, fever, hemoglobinuria, and hyperbilirubinemia all suggest a delayed hemolytic transfusion reaction. A positive DAT is confirmatory. Most delayed hemolytic reactions are self-limiting and require no treatment. DIC and renal failure may be a significant complication of delayed hemolytic transfusion reactions.

b. Alloimunization to RBC, white blood cell, platelet, or protein antigens can occur. It does not cause immediate problems but sensitizes the recipient to future transfusions, which continues to decreased circulating time for that component or an adverse event for the recipient.

c. Post-transfusion purpura (rare) manifests as the sudden development of self-limited, severe thrombocytopenia with purpura. This is seen typically 7-10 days after blood transfusion in a sensitized patient (transfusion or pregnancy). IV immune globulin may restore the platelet count.

d. GVHD may occur in immunocompromised recipients as a result of infused lymphocytes attacking host tissue. Irradiation of the blood product eliminates this risk.

3. Nonimmunologic complications

a. Transmission of infectious disease
   (1) Viral hepatitis 1:1,000,000 units for hepatitis C and 1:137,000 units for hepatitis B
   (2) HIV <1:1,900,000 units
   (3) Human T-cell lymphotropic virus (HTLV)-I, HTLV-II viruses— 1:160,000 units
   (4) Cytomegalovirus (CMV)—Generally only a concern in immunosuppressed patients. Risk is 1:12 in unscreened, unfiltered products. Leukoreduced or CMV-seronegative products reduce risk to 2-4%.
   (5) West Nile virus—First case contracted from transfusion occurred in 2002. There is an increased risk in recipients of organ transplants.
   (6) Others—*Babesia*, *Bartonella*, *Borrelia*, *Brucella*, Colorado tick fever, plasmodia, and some trypanosomes

b. Bacterial contamination—Contamination is seen most frequently in platelet concentrates. The most commonly reported contaminants are gram-positive cocci, gram-positive bacilli, and gram-negative bacilli.

Gram-negative bacilli can lead to production of endotoxin that causes patients' symptoms.

c. Circulatory overload—Can occur in patients with congestive heart failure or if the component is infused too rapidly. Blood should be given over 3-4 hours in this situation, and IV furosemide should be given between units.

d. Hemosiderosis—Occurs with prolonged RBC transfusion requirements. Each unit of packed RBCs contains 250 mg iron. Desferrioxamine may be helpful in chelating iron to promote its excretion.

e. Depletion of coagulation proteins and platelets—May occur if more than 1 or 2 blood volumes of fluids are administered in <24 hours. Therapy is with specific components as directed by clinical and laboratory evaluation, but in general repletion with FFP and cryoprecipitate should be considered.

4. **Metabolic complications—Can occur when large volumes of banked blood products are transfused**

a. Hypothermia—Most common, may lead to cardiac arrhythmias or a coagulopathy. Warming the blood to 37°C decreases this risk.

b. Acidosis—Can occur in patients with liver failure because of citric acid build-up

c. Alkalosis—More common as the citrate is metabolized to pyruvate and HCO_3 in patients with renal failure and normal liver function. Plasma-containing products are the primary contributors to this complication.

d. Potassium abnormalities—During RBC storage, K^+ moves from the intracellular to the extracellular space secondary to dysfunction of the Na^+,K^+ pump. K^+ accumulates in the supernatant. When large volumes of RBCs are administered, this supernatant potassium may cause an initial serum potassium elevation. However, once the RBCs are transfused, the Na^+,K^+ pump becomes functional and patients may experience a secondary hypokalemia as potassium moves back to the intracellular space.

e. Hypocalcemia—A result of citrate toxicity due to complexing of ionized calcium can occur in patients with liver failure who are unable to metabolize citrate to pyruvate and HCO_3. This is seen when large volumes of plasma-containing components such as FFP or platelets are administered to such patients. Treatment is with IV calcium.

f. Nonimmune hemolysis—This complication can occur in three situations: (1) administration of nonosmolar fluids through the same IV line as the blood component; (2) storage or administration of RBCs in an environment that is too cold or too warm; and (3) administration of RBCs in a setting of increased pressure. All of these scenarios contribute to RBC lysis. The only IV fluid that can be administered the same time as any blood component should be normal saline.

Nutrition

Timothy A. Pritts, MD, PhD

Forty to 60% of hospitalized patients are malnourished to some degree. This may be due to inadequate intake, impaired absorption, or increased requirements.

I. NUTRITIONAL ASSESSMENT

A. SUBJECTIVE GLOBAL ASSESSMENT
1. Clinical impression performed on the basis of history (attention to recent reduction in oral intake, recent unintentional weight loss of >7-10 lb, underlying disease, and functional status)
2. Presence of low serum albumin (<3 g/dL)
3. Physical examination—Wasting of muscle mass (temporalis muscle) and fat, presence of edema or ascites, glossitis, skin lesions (vitamin deficiencies)
4. Weight change or unintentional weight loss is important.
a. Weight loss of >10% of ideal body weight suggests mild to moderate malnutrition.
b. Weight loss of >20% suggests severe malnutrition.
c. Weight loss of >30% is premorbid.

B. BIOCHEMICAL INDICATORS OF MALNUTRITION
1. Visceral proteins
a. Albumin—Adequate indicator of malnutrition in absence of other causes of hypoalbuminemia (hepatic insufficiency, protein-losing nephropathy, or enteropathy). Synthesis decreases with malnutrition.
   (1) Long half-life (21 days) and extravascular space distribution make it unreliable as a short-term index of nutrition.
   (2) Albumin >3.5 g/dL suggests adequate nutritional status; <3 g/dL suggests malnutrition.
2. Rapid-turnover proteins—Shorter half-life; early indicator of nutritional depletion; falling levels suggest ongoing malnutrition.
a. Transferrin—Half-life of 8 days; a sensitive indicator of malnutrition, although anemia may stimulate transferrin synthesis. Level <220 mg/dL suggests malnutrition.
b. Thyroxin-binding prealbumin—Half-life of 2 days
c. Retinol-binding protein—Half-life of 12 hours
3. Nitrogen balance
a. Calculate from intake and excretion of nitrogen.

Total nitrogen loss (g/day) = 24-hour UUN (g/day) + 4 g/day fecal and nonurinary nitrogen loss

where UUN = urinary urea nitrogen.

b. Requires accurate 24-hour urine collection and assessment of grams of nitrogen given daily, in conjunction with the appropriate amount of carbohydrate for proper nitrogen utilization (calorie:nitrogen ratio)

C. IMMUNOLOGIC FUNCTION

Malnutrition is associated with decreased cellular and humoral immunity.

1. Delayed cutaneous hypersensitivity—Reflects cellular immunity. Anergy to antigens suggests malnutrition. Anergy may also occur with cancer, severe infection, or renal or hepatic failure and after chemotherapy or radiation therapy.
2. Total lymphocyte count—Calculated as white blood cell count × % lymphocytes. Count <1500 cells/mm^3 suggests severe malnutrition (must rule out other causes such as hematologic disorder or AIDS).
3. Complement levels, measurements of neutrophil function, and opsonic index may be useful measurements of response to infection but are not widely available for clinical use.

D. PATIENT AT RISK

When all factors are considered, the two most important factors are likely recent weight loss and serum albumin <3 g/dL. Other parameters are used for corroborative purposes.

II. NUTRITIONAL REQUIREMENTS IN STRESS

A. BASIC CONCEPTS

1. Three sources of energy for bodily processes (normally carbohydrates and fat provide 85% of daily energy expenditure, with protein supplying 15%)
2. Glucose yields 4 kcal/g, dextrose 3.4 kcal/g, protein 4 kcal/g, and fat 9 kcal/g.
3. Brain, red blood cells, white blood cells, and renal medulla are dependent on glucose in early fasting. Other tissues can use fat as an energy source.
4. One gram of nitrogen equals 6.25 g of protein.
5. Protein needs are 0.8-1 g protein/kg/day.
6. Stressed, burned, or multiple-trauma patients may need increases up to 50 kcal/kg/day and 2 g protein/kg/day.
7. Adequate calories in relation to nitrogen are needed to allow protein synthesis and minimize protein catabolism. Calorie:nitrogen ratios are as follows.

a. Most disease states, 100-150:1
b. Uremic patients, 300-400:1
c. Septic patients, 100:1

B. DETERMINATION OF INDIVIDUAL CALORIC NEEDS

1. Rough estimate, 35 kcal/kg/day

2. Calculate basal energy expenditure (BEE) using the Harris-Benedict equation:

$$BEE\ (men) = 66.47 + 13.75W + 5H - 6.76A$$

$$BEE\ (women) = 655.1 + 9.56W + 1.85H - 4.68A$$

where W = weight in kg; H = height in cm; and A = age.

3. Calculate increase in energy needs imposed by illness or injury (i.e., BEE × activity factor × injury factor) using Calvin-Long injury factor.
a. Minor operation—1.2 (20% increase)
b. Skeletal trauma—1.35 (35% increase)
c. Major sepsis—1.60 (60% increase)
d. Severe thermal injury—2.10 (110% increase)

4. Calculate increase in energy needs imposed
a. Confined to bed—1.2
b. Out of bed—1.3

5. Indirect calorimetry—Measurements of the patient's oxygen consumption and carbon dioxide production
a. Determines resting energy expenditure by measuring respiratory gas exchange (i.e., O_2 consumption, CO_2 production)
b. Gives index of fuel utilization

$$RQ = V_{CO_2}/V_{O_2}$$

where RQ = respiratory quotient, V_{CO_2} = carbon dioxide consumption, and V_{O_2} = oxygen consumption. RQ of 0.8-1.0 is desirable, <0.7 suggests underfeeding, and >1.0 is overfeeding. Some RQs are listed as follows.
  (1) Carbohydrate = 1.0
  (2) For mixed substrate = 0.8
  (3) Lipid = 0.70; lipogenesis >1.0 (also induced spuriously by hyperventilation)
  (4) Ketogenesis < 0.7

III. INDICATIONS FOR NUTRITIONAL SUPPORT

A. FACTORS
1. Age—In a previously healthy adult, adequately hydrated and mildly catabolic
a. ≤ Age 60 years tolerate ≤10 days of starvation
b. 60-70 years tolerate ≤7 days of starvation
c. >70 years tolerate 5 days of starvation
2. Previous state of health—Including prior nutritional status. Patients with chronic medical problems (e.g., diabetes mellitus; chronic obstructive pulmonary disease; renal, cardiac, or hepatic insufficiency) are probably at more nutritional risk than those patients described in section III. A. 1.
3. Current condition—Metabolic demands per section II

5

NUTRITION

B. PREOPERATIVE NUTRITIONAL SUPPLEMENTATION

Preoperative nutritional supplementation requires consideration of the factors in section III. A and anticipated duration of dietary deprivation. If evidence of moderate to severe malnutrition exists, 7-10 days of preoperative nutritional support may be beneficial.

C. POSTOPERATIVE NUTRITIONAL SUPPLEMENTATION

In the malnourished patient, postoperative nutrition is necessary until adequate oral intake is resumed. For the healthy patient, follow guidelines in section II. A.
1. If the GI tract is functional, enteral nutrition is preferable. Placement of a nasoenteric feeding tube for short-term feeding is recommended.
2. If prolonged support is anticipated, a feeding gastrostomy or jejunostomy should be considered (see section IV. C).

IV. ENTERAL NUTRITION

A. INDICATIONS
1. Prolonged period without caloric intake
2. Functional GI tract
3. Inadequate oral intake
4. Avoid gut mucosal atrophy.
5. In major burns and trauma, may decrease hypermetabolism

B. SHORT-TERM SUPPLEMENTATION

For nasogastric or nasointestinal feedings, use small-bore (7-9 Fr) soft tubes to improve patient comfort.
1. Nasogastric
a. Adequate gastric emptying is required.
b. Alert patient with intact gag reflex is necessary.
c. Maintain gastric residuals < 50% of total infusion over last 4 hours.
2. Nasointestinal—Patients with higher risk of aspiration (i.e., neurologic impairment, poor gastric motility)

C. LONG-TERM SUPPLEMENTATION (>6 weeks)
1. Gastrostomy—Placed operatively or percutaneously
a. Adequate gastric emptying required
b. Evidence of reflux or impaired gag reflex is contraindication
c. Intermittent bolus feeds or continuous infusion
2. Jejunostomy—Placed operatively
a. Anticipate long-term enteral supplementation in patient for whom gastrostomy is contraindicated
b. Requires continuous infusion

D. PRODUCTS
1. Oral supplements

a. Indications—Supplementation for inadequate caloric intake
b. Must be palatable (flavoring increases osmolarity and cost)
c. Examples—Ensure, Ensure Plus, Sustacal, Carnation Instant Breakfast

2. Tube feedings
a. Blenderized food
b. Blenderized (pureed) diet—Complete B
   (1) Primarily used with gastrostomy
c. Polymeric—Isocal, Osmolite, Jevity, Ultracal
   (1) Complete diet, with intact protein; generally lactose free
   (2) Iso-osmolar, fairly well tolerated
   (3) 1 kcal/mL
d. High-caloric density (2 kcal/mL)—Magnacal, TwoCal HN
   (1) Complete diet, with intact protein; generally lactose free
   (2) Hyperosmolar—May provoke diarrhea
   (3) Patients with increased caloric needs and decreased volume tolerance
e. Monomeric—Vivonex T.E.N., Criticare HN
   (1) Amino acids with or without peptides as protein source
   (2) Requires no digestion
   (3) Essentially complete small bowel absorption (low residue)
   (4) Hyperosmolar
f. Disease-specific formulas—Most of unproven benefit
   (1) Renal failure—Amin-Aid, Nepro, Suplena
      (a) Elemental diet, essential L-amino acids, reduced nitrogen
      (b) Hyperosmolar, 2 kcal/mL
      (c) Best when administered by tube (not very palatable)
   (2) Acute or chronic hepatic failure—Hepatic-Aid II
      (a) Enriched with branched-chain amino acids (valine, leucine, isoleucine)
      (b) Low in aromatic and sulfur-containing amino acids
      (c) May be used as tube feeding or to supplement a protein-restricted oral diet
   (3) Immunomodulatory—Impact, Alitraq
      (a) Enriched with immunostimulatory amino acids, lipids, and nucleic acids
      (b) May benefit critically ill patients by reducing infectious complications

E. ADMINISTRATION
1. Generally, all types of tube feedings should be iso-osmolar (i.e., 300 mOsm) for initial administration. Hypertonic feeds require dilution.
2. Gastric feeding—Due to the greater diluting capacity of the stomach and the protective mechanism of the pylorus, concentration is advanced first, then rate is advanced. Bolus feeds may be used.
3. Intestinal feeding by continuous infusion—Increase first rate, then concentration

5

NUTRITION

4. Elevate the head of the bed 30 degrees and check gastric residuals every 4 hours (>50% of total administered over the past 4 hours is a high residual).
5. Metoclopramide (Reglan) 10 mg IV or PO q 6 h may aid gastric emptying.
6. Most feeds can be started at 40 mL/h and advanced by 20 mL/h increments at 12-h intervals as tolerated.
7. If the infusion is stopped for any prolonged period, the tube must be flushed with water to prevent clogging.
8. The position of the tube should be confirmed radiographically prior to use.

F. MAJOR COMPLICATIONS OF ENTERAL FEEDING
1. Aspiration pneumonia—May be minimized by jejunal feeding and by precautions indicated in section III. E
2. Feeding intolerance—Evidenced by vomiting, abdominal distention, cramping, diarrhea. Treat by decreasing infusion rate or diluting feedings.
3. Diarrhea—Defined as >5 stools per day
   a. Minimized by a continuous, appropriate administration schedule, assuming intact GI function and no pancreatic insufficiency. Rule out antibiotic-associated colitis.
   b. May be a symptom of too rapid advancement of hyperosmolar tube feedings
   c. Minimized by clean technique in formula preparation and administration (avoid bacterial overgrowth in formulation). Time limits on formula life and duration of administration should be observed.
   d. Treatment—Depending on severity, one may either decrease administration rate or add an antidiarrheal agent when infectious cause is ruled out.
      (1) Kaolin pectin (Kapectolin) safe to use even in infectious diarrhea
      (2) Diphenoxylate (Lomotil) elixir 2.5-5 mg per gastrostomy tube q 6 h p.r.n.
      (3) Loperamide (Imodium) elixir 2-4 mg q 6 h p.r.n.
      (4) Psyllium seed (Metamucil) 1 package in 6 oz of water b.i.d. (bulking agent)
4. Metabolic—In general, the metabolic complications are the same as for parenteral nutrition. Hyperglycemia should be treated with frequent short-acting insulin or a peripheral drip. Sepsis should be ruled out for new-onset hyperglycemia.
5. Hyperosmotic nonketotic coma—Caused by too many calories without enough free water to excrete the obligatory renal osmotic load

V. PARENTERAL NUTRITION

A. INDICATIONS
1. Prolonged period without caloric intake
2. Enteral feeding contraindicated or not tolerated
3. Presence of malnutrition

B. ROLE IN PRIMARY THERAPY

1. **Efficacy demonstrated in the following situations.**
a. GI fistula—Allows for total bowel "rest" while providing adequate nutrition; rate of spontaneous closure is increased, but overall mortality is not affected
b. Short bowel syndrome—Maintain nutritional status until remaining bowel can undergo hypertrophy. This is the nonoperative strategy for long-term survival.
c. Acute tubular necrosis—Mortality rate is decreased, with earlier recovery from renal failure. Hypercatabolism of renal failure is met by total parenteral nutrition (TPN).
d. Acute-on-chronic hepatic insufficiency—Normalization of amino acid profiles results in improved recovery from hepatic encephalopathy and possibly decreased mortality.

2. **Efficacy not completely established for the following**
a. Inflammatory bowel disease—Crohn's disease limited to small bowel responds best; course of ulcerative colitis not affected but allows for bowel rest and improved postoperative course when given prior to ileoanal pull-through operations
b. Anorexia nervosa

C. SUPPORTIVE THERAPY

1. **Efficacy established for**
a. Radiation enteritis
b. Acute GI toxicity due to chemotherapeutic agents
c. Hyperemesis gravidarum

2. **Efficacy not yet established for**
a. Preoperative nutritional support for malnourished patients. Studies have shown improvement in metabolic endpoints but no statistically significant improvement in mortality or complication rate.
b. Cardiac cachexia
c. Pancreatitis
d. Respiratory insufficiency with need for prolonged ventilatory support
e. Prolonged ileus (>5 days)
f. Nitrogen-losing wounds

D. INDICATIONS CURRENTLY UNDER INVESTIGATION

1. Cancer—Generally, nutritional support indicated in patients undergoing antineoplastic therapy (e.g., surgery, radiation, chemotherapy) during times of ileus, GI mucosal damage, etc. The goal of nutritional support is for weight maintenance, not gain.
2. Sepsis—Some evidence exists concerning the use of enriched branched-chain amino acid solution to improve hepatic protein synthesis and improve septic encephalopathy.

E. BASIC COMPOSITION OF FORMULATIONS (Tables 5-1 and 5-2)

1. Carbohydrate—Dextrose used exclusively in the United States. Concentrations range from 15-47%.

5

NUTRITION

TABLE 5-1

TPN SOLUTIONS: COMPOSITION

Type of Solution	Amino Acid	Glucose	Nonprotein Calories
Standard	4.25% (42.5 g/L)	D-15 (150 g/L)	510 kcal/L
	5% (50 g/L)	D-25 (250 g/L)	850 kcal/L
Renal	1.7% (17 g/L)	D-47 (470 g/L)	1598 kcal/L
Hepatic	3.5% (35 g/L)	D-35 (350 g/L)	1190 kcal/L
Peripheral	3% (30 g/L)	D-10 (100 g/L)	340 kcal/L

For patients receiving solutions with dextrose concentrations of 25% and higher, lipids can be given twice weekly—all others should get daily lipids.
TPN = total parenteral nutrition; D-15 = 15% dextrose, etc.

2. Amino acids—Either balanced or disease specific (renal, hepatic, stress formulations)
3. Lipid emulsions
a. Available as 10% or 20% solutions (1 kcal/mL or 2 kcal/mL, respectively)
b. Infusion of 100 mL of 10% solution per week is adequate to prevent essential fatty acid deficiency.

TABLE 5-2

ADDITIONAL COMPONENTS TO TPN SOLUTION

	Dose	Type
Trace elements (add to 1st bottle q. day)		
Zn	3.0 mg	
Cu	1.2 mg	Stress formula
Cr and	12 µg, and	Hepatic formula
Se	60 mg	
Mn	0.3 mg	
Vitamins (add to 1st bottle q. day)		
M.V.I.	1 ampule (10 mL)	
K (add to 2nd bottle q. Monday)	5 mg (for patients not requiring anticoagulants)	

	Usual	Range
Electrolytes and insulin		
Na$^+$ (mEq/L)	20-80	0-150
K$^+$ (mEq/L)	13-40	0-80
Cl$^-$ (mEq/L)	10-80	0-150
Ca^{2+} (mEq/L)	4.7	0-10
Mg^{2+} (mEq/L)	8	0-15
P (mmol)	14	0-21
Acetate (mEq/L)	45-81	45-220
Human regular insulin (units/L)	0-25	0-60

Electrolytes may be adjusted as appropriately. Some patients with ongoing electrolyte losses may require up to 140 mEq/L NaCl and 80 mEq/L K+.
TPN = total parenteral nutrition.

c. Important to check baseline measurements of serum triglycerides to avoid exacerbation of preexisting hypertriglyceridemia

d. Lipid emulsion substituted for carbohydrate calories in certain situations (decrease overall volume given, carbohydrate overfeeding, TPN hepatotoxicity)

e. Safe to provide 20-60% of total calories as lipid

4. Minor components

a. Vitamins—Including 5 mg vitamin K weekly

b. Trace elements—Zinc, copper, chromium, manganese, selenium

c. Insulin and electrolytes as ordered

F. CENTRAL FORMULAS

Administer into the vena cava.

1. Standard central formula—Most patients requiring parenteral nutrition can use formula containing 15-25% dextrose.

2. Renal formulation

a. Nephramine (essential L-amino acids only)

b. Indicated in patients with acute renal failure who are not being dialyzed

c. Electrolyte composition offsets abnormalities in acute renal failure; useful in preventing rise in potassium and BUN, and may delay dialysis

d. Higher glucose base (D-47) serves to reduce volume.

e. Once the patient has converted to chronic dialysis, parenteral nutrition should be changed to standard.

3. Hepatic formulation

a. Indicated for patients with grade 2 (impending stupor) or greater (grade 3 = stupor, 4 grade = coma, unresponsive to pain) hepatic encephalopathy

b. Hepatic formulation is enriched with 35% branched-chain amino acids, alanine, arginine, and reduced amounts of aromatic and sulfur-containing amino acids

G. PERIPHERAL PARENTERAL NUTRITION

1. Contains 3% amino acids in 10% dextrose

2. To provide adequate calorie:nitrogen ratio, the equivalent of 500 mL of 10% lipid emulsion should be administered with each liter of peripheral formulation to a maximum of 100 g fat/day. Monitoring lipid profile avoids hyperlipidemia.

3. Indicated in patients in whom central venous catheterization is contraindicated (*Candida* sepsis, blood dyscrasias, thrombosis)

4. Difficulties include increased cost and difficulties with long-term venous access due to phlebitis from administration of hypertonic solution.

5. Peripheral parenteral nutrition may be indicated for 3-5 days of nutritional support in patients who may not be able to take an adequate oral intake and are thought to be at increased risk for complications of malnutrition.

6. Only major advantage is elimination of risks associated with central venous catheterization

H. ADMINISTRATION

1. The institution of central formulation should always be via a new central line.
2. The tip of the catheter should reside within the innominate vein, or preferably the superior vena cava (SVC), due to increased blood flow and mixing (*not* right atrium or subclavian vein to avoid perforation or thrombosis, respectively); location of catheter tip should be documented in the patient's chart.
3. Long-term catheters (Hickman, port-A-Cath) may be placed in the SVC to avoid catheter clotting.
4. Insertion of a central venous catheter for parenteral nutrition is *never* an emergency; the patient should be stable, well hydrated, and without serious coagulopathy.

I. INFUSION

1. Rate
   a. All formulations begin at 40-50 mL/h with exception of renal formulation, which generally begin at 30 mL/h due to higher glucose content, and peripheral formulation, which begins at target rate.
   b. Rate increased in increments of 20-25 mL/h per 8-24 hours (if blood sugar is well controlled) until caloric needs are matched
   c. With renal formula, advance in increments of 10 mL/h each day
2. With exception of lipid emulsion, single-lumen catheters should not be used for any other infusion of maintenance fluid, medication, blood products, or central venous pressure readings.

J. MONITORING

1. Vital signs q 6 h for initial 24-48 hours
2. Fingerstick glucose determinations q 6 h to monitor for hyperglycemia
3. Intake and outputs recorded q 8 h
4. Weigh patient every other day
5. Twice-weekly blood work—Electrolytes, glucose, liver enzymes, calcium, phosphorus, prothrombin, partial thromboplastin time, CBC, short-turnover proteins, if available

K. COMPLICATIONS

1. Technical (placement)
   a. Pneumothorax—<3% of all insertions in elective, well-prepared patients
2. Late technical—Thrombosis of subclavian vein or SVC
   a. Clinically silent in ≤ 35% of patients
   b. If clinically apparent, treat with
      (1) Local heat
      (2) Catheter removal
      (3) Heparinization until symptoms resolve

(4) Long-term anticoagulation is usually unnecessary but should be considered for continued symptoms.

c. Prophylactic heparin is of little benefit in preventing thrombosis.

3. Septic complications (Fig. 5-1)

a. Catheter sepsis—Clinical sepsis in a patient receiving parenteral nutrition for which no anatomic septic focus is identified, and which resolves following removal of the catheter

b. The major source of catheter sepsis is bacteria from the skin around the insertion site of the catheter; catheter sepsis is best prevented by *meticulous* adherence to dressing change and catheter access protocols.

4. Metabolic complications

a. Disorders of glucose metabolism

(1) Hyperglycemia (blood sugar >200 mg/dL)

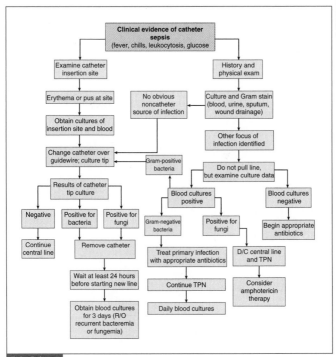

FIG. 5-1

Algorithm for management of suspected total parenteral nutrition (TPN) catheter sepsis. D/C, discontinue; R/O, rule out.

       (a) May be associated with either parenteral or enteral nutrition and may lead to hyperosmolar, hyperglycemic, nonketotic dehydration with shock/death resulting if untreated

       (b) If blood sugar is >200 mg/dL, the rate of infusion of the formulation should not be increased; SQ regular insulin should be administered acutely and the amount of insulin in each liter of solution should be increased appropriately. Causes of sepsis should be ruled out.

    (2) Hypoglycemia—Rare complication

       (a) If TPN is suddenly discontinued for any reason, IV administration of any 5% dextrose solution is sufficient to prevent hypoglycemia.

       (b) Rarely occurs with endogenous insulin response to very high rates of infusion. Treat by slowing the infusion.

  b. Liver dysfunction

    (1) Excess carbohydrate stored in liver as fat

    (2) Reversible, self-limited in adults

  c. Deficiency states

    (1) Requirements for electrolytes, vitamins, and trace elements vary according to age, previous nutritional state, disease, and external losses.

    (2) As patients become anabolic, there is an increased requirement for intracellular ions (potassium, magnesium, phosphate).

    (3) Deficiencies of trace elements and vitamins are generally avoided by the administration (daily) of recommended amounts.

Preoperative Preparation

Konstantin Umanskiy, MD

Preparation of a patient for surgery begins with establishing a diagnosis and determining the course of surgical management. This requires thoughtful consideration of both the risks and benefits of a contemplated operation. Much of preoperative care involves optimizing the patient's physiologic status and taking steps to prevent perioperative complications.

I. NEED FOR OPERATION

6

A. RELATIVE RISKS AND BENEFITS OF SURGERY

Determination of the relative risks and benefits of surgery requires consideration of the following factors.

1. Natural history of disease if left untreated
2. Benefit of surgical therapy vs. medical therapy
3. Urgency of operation—May limit the time available for preoperative preparation
4. Patient's physiologic reserve and overall ability to undergo anesthesia and operation
5. Potential complications of the procedure

II. ASSESSMENT OF OPERATIVE RISK

The patient's age, preoperative physiologic status, and the urgency and magnitude of the planned operation are major determinants of operative morbidity and mortality.

A. AGE

1. Elderly patients often have either limited reserve or impaired function of the major organ systems—immune, cardiovascular, pulmonary, renal, and hepatic
2. True even for "healthy" septuagenarian—"There is nothing like an operation or an injury to bring a patient up to chronological age" (W. R. Howe).

B. URGENCY OF OPERATION

In one study, emergent nature of the surgery doubled the risk of operative mortality in low- and moderate-risk patients.

C. RELATION OF PHYSICAL STATUS TO ANESTHETIC MORTALITY

Impairment of more than one organ system, disease severity, and adequacy of control profoundly influences the risk of operative mortality. See the American Society of Anesthesiologists (ASA) classification of physical status in Chapter 7.

D. CARDIOVASCULAR RISK

1. Coronary artery disease, congestive heart failure (CHF), presence of arrhythmias, peripheral vascular disease, or severe hypertension
2. Goldman cardiac risk in noncardiac surgery
a. Computation of the cardiac risk index (Table 6-1)
b. General concepts (Table 6-2)
   (1) Class III and IV patients warrant routine preoperative cardiology consultation.
   (2) Class IV—life-saving procedures only
   (3) 28 of the 53 points are potentially correctable preoperatively.
   (4) Index correctly classified 81% of the cardiac outcomes.
   (5) Criticisms—Cardiac risks only and based on mixed patient population (e.g., vascular patients have higher morbidity and mortality)

E. PULMONARY RISK (see section III. C)

1. Smoking history—>20 pack-years, morbid obesity, preexisting pulmonary disease, thoracic or upper abdominal surgery, pulmonary hypertension
2. Tests to identify pulmonary risk factors
a. Inability to blow out a match with unpursed lips from a distance of 20-25 cm
b. Shortness of breath on 1-2 flights of steps
c. Pco_2 >45 mm Hg and Po_2 <60 while inspiring room air

TABLE 6-1

COMPUTATION OF CARDIAC RISK INDEX

Category	Description	Score (Points)
History	Age >70 yr	5
	Myocardial infarction within 6 mo	10
Physical examination	S_3 gallop or JVD	11
	Important valvular aortic stenosis	3
ECG	Rhythm other than sinus or PACs *or*	7
	>5 PVCs/min at any time prior to surgery	7
Poor general medical status	Po_2 <60 or Pco_2 >50 mm Hg	3
	K^+ <3.0 or HCO_3^- <20 mEq/L	
	BUN >50 or creatinine >3 mg/dL	
	Abnormal SGOT	
	Chronic liver disease	
	Bedridden due to noncardiac cause	
Operation	Intraperitoneal, intrathoracic, aortic surgery	3
	Emergency surgery	4

JVD=jugular vein distention; PAC=premature atrial contraction; PVC=premature ventricular contraction; SGOT=serum glutamic-oxaloacetic transaminase.

TABLE 6-2

GOLDMAN CLASSIFICATION

Class	Point Total	Major Complication (%)	Cardiac Death (%)
I	0-5	0.6	0.2
II	6-12	3	1
III	13-25	11	3
IV	≥26	12	39

Adapted from Goldman L, Caldera DL, Nussbaum SR, et al: Multifactorial index of cardiac risk in noncardiac surgical procedures. N Engl J Med 297:845, 1977.

d. Ratio of forced expiratory volume in 1 second to forced vital capacity (FEV_1/FVC) < 65% predicted

F. RENAL RISK
1. Renal insufficiency (BUN >50 mg/dL; creatinine >3 mg/day)
2. Highest risk in acute renal failure

G. HEPATIC RISK
1. Cirrhosis, hepatitis
2. Surgical mortality significantly increased in patients with bilirubin >2 mg/dL, albumin <3 g/dL, prothrombin time >16 seconds, presence of encephalopathy, presence or history of varices (advanced Child-Pugh classification)

H. ENDOCRINE RISK
1. Diabetes mellitus, steroid therapy (adrenal insufficiency)
2. Hyperthyroidism or hypothyroidism

I. HEMATOLOGIC RISK
1. Anemia, leukopenia, thrombocytopenia, coagulopathy

III. INTERVENTION TO REDUCE OPERATIVE RISK

A. EMERGENT OPERATIONS
1. Procedure should not be delayed for most situations.
2. Exception is volume-depleted patients (e.g., those with intestinal obstruction, peritonitis, perforated viscus) should undergo fluid and electrolyte repletion prior to operation.

B. CARDIOVASCULAR
1. Coronary artery disease
a. Evaluated by ECG, exercise or dipyridamole thallium scan, multigated acquisition (MUGA), or echocardiogram. Coronary angiography may be indicated.
b. Coronary artery bypass grafting has been shown to decrease risk of postoperative myocardial infarction.

c. Patients with severe disease should undergo major operations with perioperative pulmonary artery monitoring to assess cardiac output and filling pressures (see Chap. 8).

2. CHF—Risk factors for postoperative CHF are coronary artery disease, old age, and major operations.

a. Preexisting CHF should be optimally controlled (e.g., diuretics, digoxin).

b. Preoperative pulmonary artery pressure monitoring and intraoperative transesophageal echocardiogram guides perioperative fluid management and monitoring of hemodynamic performance (i.e., need for fluids, inotropes, or vasodilators).

3. Arrhythmias—Optimal medical control required prior to operation (see Chap. 8). High-grade block and bradyarrhythmias may require preoperative temporary or permanent pacing.

4. Hypertension—No increased risk for nonlabile mild hypertension and diastolic blood pressure <110 mm Hg.

a. Antihypertensive agents should be continued to time of surgery, except monoamine oxidase inhibitors (discontinue 2 weeks before surgery).

b. New-onset hypertension, severe hypertension with diastolic blood pressure >110 mm Hg, systolic blood pressure >250 mm Hg, or suspicion of unusual causes of hypertension should lead to further work-up and treatment.

c. Should check for evidence of end-organ deterioration (e.g., renal insufficiency, CHF)

5. Carotid endarterectomy often performed to prevent intraoperative or postoperative stroke in patients with symptomatic or critical carotid stenosis

C. RESPIRATORY

1. Patient should discontinue smoking as long before surgery as possible; may take up to 8 weeks to decrease risk of pulmonary complications

2. Initiate or continue use of bronchodilators (e.g., inhalants, theophylline) for patients with bronchospastic disease (chronic obstructive pulmonary disease or asthma).

3. Use chest physical therapy, incentive spirometry, and deep-breathing exercises preoperatively.

4. Pneumonia, bronchitis—Delay elective surgery; treat with pulmonary toilet and antibiotics.

D. RENAL

1. Reduce azotemia—Peritoneal or hemodialysis

2. Correct electrolyte abnormalities.

3. Optimize volume status—Ultrafiltration, diuretics. Consider use of pulmonary artery monitoring.

E. HEPATIC (see Chap. 41)

F. ENDOCRINE (see section VII and Chap. 11)

G. HEMATOLOGIC (see Chap. 4)

H. NUTRITION (see Chap. 5)

IV. GENERAL PREOPERATIVE PREPARATION

A. OVERALL ASSESSMENT
For discussion of the patient, history, physical examination, and operative risk, see section II.

B. DOCUMENTATION
For discussion of documentation of indications for the procedure and informed consent, see Chapter 1.

C. ROUTINE PREOPERATIVE LABORATORY AND IMAGING EVALUATION
Although several studies have documented that certain preoperative lab studies are not cost effective, these are the standard preoperative studies performed at our institution.
1. Lab studies—CBC, urinalysis, electrolytes, BUN, creatinine, prothrombin time, partial thromboplastin time
2. Room-air arterial blood gas if at risk for respiratory insufficiency (see section II), or if prolonged postoperative ventilator support is anticipated
3. Radiographs—Posteroanterior and lateral chest radiograph unless previously normal within the past 6 months or patient <35 years of age; radiographs of specific areas of interest in relation to the upcoming procedure
4. ECG if patient >35 years of age or if otherwise indicated by past cardiac history

D. BLOOD ORDERS
Type and screen or type and crossmatch for the number of units appropriate to the procedure.

E. SKIN PREPARATION
1. Hair removal is best performed the day of surgery with an electric clipper. Shaving the night prior to surgery is associated with an increased risk of infection.
2. Provide preoperative (night-before) scrub or shower of the operative site with a germicidal soap (e.g., Hibiclens, pHisoHex).

6

PREOPERATIVE PREPARATION

F. PREOPERATIVE ANTIBIOTICS

1. When used, should have an established blood level at the time of initial skin incision. Administer prophylactic antibiotics 30 minutes prior to incision.
2. Indications for prophylactic antibiotics
a. Clean procedures—Most cardiac, noncardiac thoracic, vascular, neurosurgery, orthopedic, and ophthalmic; use cefazolin 1-2 g IV or vancomycin 1 g IV
b. Clean/contaminated procedures—GI/GU tract, gynecologic, respiratory tract, head and neck, use cefazolin 1-2 g IV; for colorectal procedures, use oral neomycin and erythromycin, and cefoxitin or cefotetan 1-2 g IV
c. Dirty/ruptured viscus—Cefoxitin or cefotetan 1-2 g IV ± gentamicin 1.5 mg/kg q 8 h IV, or clindamycin 600 mg IV q 6 h and gentamicin 1.5 mg/kg q 8 h IV
d. Traumatic wound—Cefazolin 1-2 g IV
e. Special consideration must be given to patients with prosthetic heart valves or history of valvular heart disease (see section VI).

G. RESPIRATORY CARE

1. Preoperative incentive spirometry on the evening prior to surgery when indicated (upper abdominal operations, thoracic operations, predisposed to respiratory insufficiency)
2. Bronchodilators for moderate to severe chronic obstructive pulmonary disorders

H. DECOMPRESSION OF GI TRACT

The patient should be ordered NPO after midnight.

I. INTRAVENOUS FLUIDS

Administer a maintenance rate overnight for IV fluids.

J. ACCESS AND MONITORING LINES

1. At least one 18-gauge IV line needed for initiation of anesthesia
2. Arterial catheters and central or pulmonary artery catheters, when indicated (see Chap. 8)

K. THROMBOEMBOLIC PROPHYLAXIS, WHEN INDICATED
(see Chap. 12)

L. VOID ON CALL TO THE OPERATING ROOM

M. PREOPERATIVE SEDATION AS ORDERED BY ANESTHESIOLOGIST
(see Chap. 7)

N. SPECIAL CONSIDERATIONS

1. Maintenance medications (e.g., antihypertensives, cardiac medications, anticonvulsants) may be given the morning of surgery with a sip of water before routine operations.

2. Preoperative diabetic management (see Chap. 11)
3. Subacute bacterial endocarditis prophylaxis (see section VI)
4. Perioperative steroid coverage (see section VII)

O. STOMAS
The site for the stoma may be marked by the stomal therapist in elective situations.

P. PREOPERATIVE NOTE (see Chap. 1)

V. BOWEL PREPARATION
The purpose of a bowel preparation is (1) to remove all solid and most liquid from the bowel and (2) to reduce the bacterial population in anticipation of procedures or complications of procedures that may contaminate the wound and the peritoneal cavity.

A. NONBOWEL SURGERY
1. Stomach decompression prior to induction of anesthesia by patient remaining NPO after midnight before surgery or by nasogastric suction
2. Bowel prep required if any of the upper or lower GI tract is to be opened or if there is a risk of enterotomy (e.g., complicated ventral hernia repair)
a. Surgery may involve the colon (e.g., extensive surgery for gynecologic malignancy or abdominal masses that impinge on the colon or where there is a potential for mechanical or ischemic bowel damage [aneurysmectomy])
b. Achlorhydria, gastric carcinoma, prolonged H_2 blocker usage, and obstructive peptic ulcer disease allow bacterial growth in the stomach. Consider using an oral antibiotic prep (e.g., neomycin) for gastric surgery in these patients.

B. BOWEL SURGERY
Many variations exist. For large and small bowel resection, we now use the following standard bowel prep.
1. Clear liquid diet 48 hours prior to the procedure
2. Day before surgery

10:00 a.m.	45 mL Fleet Phospho-soda, PO followed by 8 oz of water
11:00 a.m.	8 oz of water PO
12:00 p.m.	8 oz of water PO
1:00 p.m.	8 oz of water PO and neomycin 500 mg and metronidazole 750 mg PO
2:00 p.m.	8 oz of water PO
3:00 p.m.	neomycin 500 mg and metronidazole 750 mg PO
5:00 p.m.	4 bisacodyl 5-mg tablets PO
7:00 p.m.	1 bisacodyl 10-mg suppository by rectum
10:00 p.m.	neomycin 500 mg and metronidazole 750 mg PO

3. If stool contains solid material, the patient can be given 1 bottle of magnesium citrate PO.
4. Perioperative IV antibiotics used in conjunction with oral antibiotic prep (see section V. B. 1)

VI. BACTERIAL ENDOCARDITIS PROPHYLAXIS

A. INDICATIONS
Patients with the following conditions are particularly vulnerable to bacteriologic seeding during transient bacteremia.
1. Prosthetic valve
2. Congenital valve disease
3. Rheumatic valve disease
4. History of endocarditis
5. Idiopathic hypertrophic subaortic stenosis
6. Mitral valve prolapse with murmur (Barlow's syndrome)

B. ANTIBIOTIC RECOMMENDATIONS
Table 6-3 presents information about the use of antibiotics for endocarditis prophylaxis in dental, upper respiratory, GU, and GI procedures.

TABLE 6-3
PREVENTION OF BACTERIAL ENDOCARDITIS*

Drug	Adult Doses	Pediatric Doses
Oral amoxicillin	3 g 1 h before and 1.5 g 6 h after procedure	50 mg/kg 1 h before and 25 mg/kg 6 h after procedure
Oral erythromycin (if allergic to penicillin)	1 g 2 h before and 500 mg 6 h after procedure	20 mg/kg 2 h before and 10 mg/kg 6 h after procedure
IV/IM ampicillin and	2 g 30 min before procedure	50 mg/kg 30 min before procedure
IV/IM gentamicin	1.5 mg/kg 30 min before procedure	2 mg/kg 30 min before procedure
IV vancomycin (if allergic to penicillin)[†]	1 g 1 h before procedure	20 mg/kg 1 h before procedure

*In dental, upper respiratory, GU, and GI procedures.
[†]Add gentamicin to IV vancomycin for GI and GU procedures.
From Medical Letter 31(807):112, 1989.

Notes: *1. Antibiotic prophylaxis as described in Table 6-3 is used for patients with valvular heart disease, prosthetic heart valves, most forms of congenital heart disease (but not uncomplicated secundum atrial septal defect), idiopathic hypertrophic subaortic stenosis, and mitral valve prolapse with regurgitation.*

2. Data are limited on the risk of endocarditis with a particular procedure. For a review of the risk of bacteremia with various procedures, see Everett ED,

Hirschmann JV: Transient bacteremia and endocarditis prophylaxis: A review. Medicine 56:61, 1977; and Shorvon PJ, Eykyn SJ, Cotton PB: Gastrointestinal instrumentation, bacteraemia, and endocarditis. Gut 24:1078, 1983. For useful guidelines on which procedures justify prophylaxis, see Shulman ST, Amren DP, Bisno AL, et al: Prevention of bacterial endocarditis. A statement for health professionals by the Committee on Rheumatic Fever and Infective Endocarditis of the Council on Cardiovascular Disease in the Young. Circulation 70:1123A, 1984.

3. Oral regimens are more convenient and safer. Parenteral regimens are more likely to be effective; they are recommended especially for patients with prosthetic valves, those who have had endocarditis previously, or those taking continuous oral penicillin for rheumatic fever prophylaxis.

4. A single dose of the parenteral drugs is adequate for most dental and diagnostic procedures of short duration. However, one or two follow-up doses may be given at 8-12 h intervals in selected high-risk patients.

VII. STEROIDS

A. INDICATIONS
1. Any patient currently on steroids, or those who have taken them within 1 year
2. Preoperative for adrenalectomy
3. Known history of adrenal insufficiency
3. History of adrenal or pituitary surgery or surgery for renal cell carcinoma
4. Inflammatory bowel disease, steroid dependent

B. ENDOGENOUS CORTISOL OUTPUT
1. Normal unstressed adult—8-25 mg/day
2. Adult undergoing major surgery—75-100 mg/day

C. GUIDE TO STEROID COVERAGE
1. Correct electrolytes, blood pressure, and hydration if necessary.
2. Hydrocortisone phosphate or hemisuccinate—100 mg IV piggyback on call to OR
3. Hydrocortisone phosphate or hemisuccinate—100 mg IV piggyback in postanesthesia care unit and q 6 h for the first 24 hours
4. If progress is satisfactory, reduce dosage to 50 mg q 6 h for 24 hours, then taper to maintenance dosage over 3 to 5 days. Resume previous fluorocortisol or oral steroid dose when patient is taking oral medications.
5. Maintain or increase hydrocortisone dosage to 200-400 mg/24 h if fever, hypotension, or other complications occur.

6. If patient has potassium wasting, may switch to methylprednisolone (Solu-Medrol).

   Note: *High-dose (300-600 mg/day) methylprednisolone regimens are potentially deleterious secondary to impaired wound healing, increased catabolism, electrolyte abnormalities, and increased infectious complications.*

Anesthesia

Lindsey A. Nelson, MD

Although an anesthetist or anesthesiologist plays an integral role in the perioperative management of most patients, the surgeon should be familiar with the various anesthesia techniques and their potential impact on the surgical patient. Communication between the surgeon and the anesthesiologist is paramount to improved perioperative outcomes.

I. PREOPERATIVE ASSESSMENT AND PREPARATION

A. CHART REVIEW

7

B. HISTORY
1. Anesthesia history
2. Current medications
3. Drug allergies (including latex)
4. Complete review of symptoms

C. PHYSICAL EXAMINATION
1. American Society of Anesthesiologists classification (Table 7-1)
2. Central nervous system
3. Cardiovascular system
4. Respiratory system
5. Upper airway
a. Size of tongue vs. pharynx (Mallampati classes I-IV)
b. Cervical spine mobility
c. Anterior mandibular space—Distance from the notch of the thyroid cartilage to the tip of the mentum (thyromental distance) while the head is maximally extended; <6 cm (receding mandible, short muscular neck) increases the difficulty during intubation

D. LABORATORY DATA

TABLE 7-1			
RELATION OF PHYSICAL STATUS TO ANESTHETIC MORTALITY			
Physical Status	No. Patients	No. Deaths	Ratio
I	16,192	0	0/16,000
II	12,154	7	1/1740
III	4,070	11	1/370
IV	720	17	1/40
V	87	4	1/20

Data from Dripps RD, Lamont A, and Eckenhoff JE: The role of anesthesia in surgical mortality. JAMA 178(3):216, 1961, American Medical Association, with permission.

E. DETERMINE APPROPRIATE ANESTHETIC TECHNIQUE
(see section II)
1. Explain associated risks and benefits to patient/guardian and document conversation in the chart.

F. INDICATIONS FOR DELAYING OR POSTPONING ELECTIVE SURGERY
1. Uncontrolled medical disease (cardiac, respiratory, hepatic, renal, endocrine)
2. Upper respiratory infection
3. Patient noncompliance with fasting guidelines
4. No informed consent

G. FASTING GUIDELINES FOR ELECTIVE SURGERY
1. Oral medications with sips of water—1 hour
2. Clear liquids (water, pulp-free juices, carbonated beverages, clear tea, black coffee)—2 hours
3. Breast milk—4 hours
4. Infant formula, nonhuman milk, solid food (low-fat content)—6 hours
5. Solid foods—8 hours

H. PREOPERATIVE MEDICATION GOALS
1. Anxiety relief, sedation, analgesia, amnesia
2. Control oral and bronchial secretions
3. Increase gastric pH and decrease gastric secretions, antiemetic effects

II. TECHNIQUES OF ANESTHESIA

A. GENERAL ANESTHESIA
1. Inhalational
a. Nasotracheal—blind vs. fiberoptic guidance
b. Orotracheal—direct visualization vs. fiberoptic guidance
2. IV
3. Inhalational/IV combination
4. Laryngeal mask airway

B. REGIONAL ANESTHESIA
1. Spinal
2. Epidural
3. Combined spinal/epidural
4. Caudal
5. Peripheral nerve blocks; local/field blocks with or without sedation

C. MONITORED ANESTHESIA CARE
1. Sedation
2. Analgesia
3. Monitoring

III. IV ANESTHESIA

IV anesthesia may be used as the induction agent, the supplemental anesthesia agent, or the sole anesthetic agent.

A. ULTRASHORT-ACTING BARBITURATES

1. **Thiopental (Pentothal) dosage—3-5 mg/kg over 30 seconds**
   a. Onset—Immediate; duration, prompt awakening may occur due to redistribution
   b. Side effects—Respiratory depression, peripheral vasodilation; use with caution in patients with coronary artery disease and hypovolemia; may induce histamine release; decreases cerebral blood flow and intracranial pressure
2. **Methohexital (Brevital) dosage—1-2 mg/kg**
   a. Onset—Immediate; used for induction and intubation; respiratory depression may be prolonged
   b. Side effects—Myocardial depression, significant hypotension
   c. *Contraindicated* in patients with porphyrias

B. ETOMIDATE (AMIDATE)

1. Dosage—0.1-0.4 mg/kg
2. Onset—30-60 seconds; induction and intubation
3. Side effects—Adrenocortical suppression lasting 4-8 hours, myoclonus
4. Organ effects—Cardiovascular stability maintained; potent cerebral vasoconstrictor

C. KETAMINE (KETALAR)

1. Dosage—2.5-5 mg/kg IM, 0.5-2 mg/kg IV
2. Dissociative anesthesia with good analgesia; acts as a bronchodilator and maintains airway reflexes; does not relieve visceral sensation; useful for brief anesthetic procedures (e.g., burn dressing changes)
3. Side effects—Apnea with rapid administration, tachycardia, hypertension, increased cardiac output and myocardial oxygen demand; cerebral vasodilator and may increase cerebral blood flow and intracranial pressure; emergence hallucinations prevented by pretreatment with a benzodiazepine

D. PROPOFOL (DIPRIVAN)

1. Dosage—2-2.5 mg/kg, 0.1-0.2 mg/kg/min constant infusion IV
2. IV hypnotic with immediate onset and rapid return with minimal CNS effects; lacks analgesic and amnestic properties
3. Metabolism
   a. Conjugation in the liver to inactive metabolites that are excreted by the kidney; extrahepatic metabolism expected as well
   b. Pharmacokinetics not changed by chronic hepatic or renal failure
4. Uses—Induction of anesthesia, sedation, antipruritic effect, anticonvulsant effects

7

ANESTHESIA

5. Side effects—Pain on injection (inject 20-30 mg lidocaine prior to infusion); decreases mean arterial pressure ≈20%

E. NARCOTICS

Narcotics are useful for both analgesia and anesthesia.

1. **Fentanyl (Sublimaze) dosage—1-10 µg/kg IV**
a. Short-acting agent, 75 times more potent than morphine; minimal myocardial effects make fentanyl useful in cardiac surgery
b. Side effects—Respiratory depression, possible bradycardia
c. Reversible with naloxone (Narcan) 1-4 µg IV push
   Note: *Be cautioned that the short half-life of naloxone can result in a return of the opioid effect; analgesic effects are reversed as well. Titrate to response; may repeat at 2-3 minute intervals, to a maximum of 10 mg.*

2. **Morphine sulfate dosage—0.1-0.2 mg/kg IV**
a. Side effects—Hypotension, bradycardia, respiratory depression, biliary tract spasm

3. **Meperidine (Demerol) dosage—0.5-2 mg/kg IV/IM/PO**

F. BENZODIAZEPINES

Benzodiazepines provide good anterograde amnesia, anxiolysis, and sedation and act as an anticonvulsant.

1. **Diazepam (Valium) dosage—0.1-0.2 mg/kg per dose; do not exceed 2.5 mg/min for sedation**
a. Use as preoperative medication and sedation for endoscopic or minor surgical procedures. Use cautiously in elderly or cachectic patients.
b. Side effects—Respiratory depression, disorientation, unpredictable IM absorption

2. **Midazolam (Versed) dosage—0.5-2 mg/dose deep IM 1-2 hours preoperatively; or 0.07-0.1 mg/kg IV for sedation**
a. Short duration of action; useful as preoperative medication or for minor surgical procedures; water soluble, predictable IM absorption
b. Use cautiously in the elderly (reduce dosage 50%).

3. **Lorazepam (Ativan) dosage—0.05 mg/kg deep IM up to 4 mg 2 hours preoperatively**
a. Contraindicated in patients with egg allergy
b. Adverse reactions
   (1) Pain at injection site
   (2) Hypotension
   (3) Apnea

IV. NEUROMUSCULAR-BLOCKING DRUGS

Patients must be adequately anesthetized because neuromuscular-blocking drugs are *without* analgesic or anesthetic effects. The choice of neuromuscular-blocking agent depends on the desired speed of onset, duration of effect, route of elimination, and potential side effects. Clinically, the degree of neuromuscular blockade is monitored by visually monitoring a twitch response following electrical stimulation of a peripheral motor nerve (ulnar or facial nerve branch).

A. DEPOLARIZING AGENTS
1. Mimic the action of acetylcholine, producing depolarization of the postjunctional membrane
2. Succinylcholine (Anectine) dosage—1 mg/kg
a. Onset of action—30-60 seconds; duration, 3-5 minutes; metabolized by pseudocholinesterase
b. Most commonly used agent
c. Side effects—May cause hyperkalemia and subsequent dysrhythmias in patients with severe muscle denervation (i.e., burns, crush injury, spinal cord injury); can cause bradycardia and hypotension as well as postoperative muscle pain (secondary to fasciculations); potent trigger of malignant hyperthermia
d. *Contraindicated* in eye injury due to increased intraocular pressure

B. NONDEPOLARIZING AGENTS
Nondepolarizing agents are classified clinically as long-acting, intermediate-acting, and short-acting. They compete with acetylcholine for postjunctional receptors and prevent changes in membrane ion permeability.
1. Pancuronium (Pavulon) dosage—0.1 mg/kg
a. Onset of action—1-3 minutes; duration, 40-65 minutes
b. Renal and hepatic elimination
c. Side effects—Interacts with halothane to increase ventricular irritability; may cause tachycardia and hypertension due to vagolytic effect
2. Atracurium (Tracrium) dosage—0.5-0.6 mg/kg
a. Onset of action—2-3 minutes; duration, 20-40 minutes
b. Hoffmann elimination; can use in hepatic or renal failure
c. Side effects—Metabolite; laudanosine may build up and cause seizures
3. Vecuronium (Norcuron) dosage—0.1 mg/kg
a. Onset of action—2-3 minutes; duration, 20-40 minutes
b. Hepatic elimination
c. Very little histamine release, fewer cardiovascular effects than other neuromuscular-blocking agents
4. Rocuronium (Zemuron) dosage—0.6-1.2 mg/kg IV
a. Onset of action—1 minute (only rapid-onset nondepolarizing agent); duration, 20-35 minutes

C. REVERSAL OF NEUROMUSCULAR BLOCKADE
Nondepolarizing agents can be antagonized by anticholinesterase drugs. Atropine (0.6-1.2 mg) or glycopyrrolate (Robinul) should be added to block muscarinic side effects (e.g., salivation, bronchospasm, and bradycardia).

7

ANESTHESIA

1. Edrophonium (Tensilon) dosage—0.75-1 mg/kg IV
a. Always use with atropine because onset and duration are similar.
2. Neostigmine (Prostigmine) dosage—0.4-1 mg/kg IV
a. Onset of action—7-10 minutes
b. Always use with glycopyrrolate 0.01 mg/kg.
3. Pyridostigmine (Mestinon) dosage—0.1 mg/kg IV
a. Onset of action—12-15 minutes
b. Must add either atropine or glycopyrrolate

V. INHALATIONAL ANESTHESIA

A. **GENERAL COMMENTS**
1. Minimum alveolar concentration (MAC) is the minimum concentration of anesthesia that prevents movement in 50% of patients in response to a noxious stimulus (skin incision).
2. Speed of onset depends on alveolar partial pressure (P_A) of the anesthetic, blood solubility, cardiac output, and alveolar-to-venous partial pressure difference.

B. **NITROUS OXIDE (MAC = 104% with O_2)**
1. Commonly used; nonflammable and odorless (good patient acceptability); rapid recovery with low potency; decreases MAC of volatile agents; potent analgesia but decreased myocardial contractility
2. Complications
a. Diffusion anoxia—O_2 administration postoperatively to prevent hypoxia
b. Expansion of air-filled cavities, e.g., bowel (dangerous in bowel obstruction), pneumocephalus, pneumothorax

C. **HALOTHANE (FLUOTHANE) (MAC = 0.77%)**
1. Potent, rapid onset of action; bronchial smooth muscle relaxant (excellent for asthmatics)
2. Complications
a. May cause vagal stimulation, leading to bradycardia
b. Sensitizes myocardium to catecholamines with increased risk of ventricular arrhythmias
c. Potent vasodilator, increases cerebral perfusion and intracranial pressure (harmful with CNS space-occupying lesions)
d. Halothane hepatitis (cumulative with repeat exposures)—Marked elevation of liver function tests 2 to 5 days postoperatively and preceded by fever and eosinophilia; more common in females
e. History of unexplained jaundice and pyrexia following previous administration is an *absolute contraindication.*

D. **SEVOFLURANE (ULTANE) (MAC = 2.05%)**
1. Rapid induction and emergence, inhalational induction
2. Complications

a. Similar cardiovascular effects as isoflurane
b. Interacts with CO_2 absorbers (soda lime, barium lime) to produce compound A that is toxic to the brain, liver, and kidneys

E. ISOFLURANE (FORANE) (MAC = 1.2%)
1. Potent muscle relaxant, with minimal hepatic, CNS, or renal impairment; less cardiovascular depression than with enflurane or halothane
2. Complications—Coronary steal; pungent; not suitable for inhalational induction

F. DESFLURANE (SUPRANE) (MAC = 6-7%)
1. New inhalation agent with very rapid induction and rapid recovery (similar to that of N_2O)
2. Low toxic potential
3. Hemodynamic effects similar to isoflurane
4. Potent muscle relaxant

VI. MALIGNANT HYPERTHERMIA

Malignant hyperthermia, characterized by a hypermetabolic state, has a genetic predisposition and associated incidence of 1:40,000 in adults and 1:12,000 in children. It is presumed that a defect in the calcium release channel sustains higher concentrations of calcium in the myoplasm, causing persistent skeletal muscle contraction following administration of succinylcholine and/or volatile anesthetics. Definitive diagnosis is by muscle biopsy.

A. PROPHYLAXIS
1. Avoid malignant hyperthermia–triggering drugs in patients with suspected family history.
2. Dantrolene sodium (2-10 mg/kg)—May be used in addition to drug avoidance

B. CLINICAL SIGNS
1. Masseter rigidity following succinylcholine administration
2. Unexplained tachycardia and tachypnea
3. Arrhythmias
4. Cyanosis
5. Metabolic and/or respiratory acidosis (increased end-tidal CO_2)
6. Fever is a *late* sign (may reach 107°F).

C. TREATMENT
1. Terminate anesthetic agent and administer nonmalignant hyperthermia–inducing agent.
2. Hyperventilate with 100% O_2.
3. $NaHCO_3$—Guided by arterial pH
4. Hyperkalemia—Treat with $NaHCO_3$, insulin (0.15 mg/kg), 20% dextrose.
5. Initiate active cooling—Cooled saline, cold gastric lavage, surface cooling

D. LATE COMPLICATIONS
1. Consumptive coagulopathy
2. Acute renal failure
3. Hypothermia
4. Pulmonary edema
5. Skeletal muscle swelling
6. Neurologic sequelae

VII. LOCAL ANESTHETICS

A. USES
1. Analgesia/anesthesia without risks of general anesthesia
2. Used in spinal, regional, and local anesthesia

B. DOSAGE CONSIDERATIONS
1. Limit total anesthetic dosage to prevent seizures.
2. Add vasoconstrictor to slow vascular absorption.
3. Avoid inadvertent vascular injection by preinjection aspiration.
4. Impending toxicity—Muscle twitching, restlessness, sleepiness

C. TREATMENT OF TOXICITY AND PRECAUTIONS
1. Trendelenburg position, O_2, IV diazepam (5-10 mg),
   thiopental (50-100 mg)
2. Never inject solutions containing epinephrine into digits, ear, tip of
   nose, or penis—May cause local ischemic necrosis

D. COMMONLY USED LOCAL ANESTHETICS
1. Procaine (Novocaine, Planocaine) dosage—14 mg/kg;
   duration, 0.5 hours
2. Lidocaine (Xylocaine, Xylotox) dosage—7 mg/kg; duration, 1-2 hours
3. Mepivacaine (Carbocaine, Polocaine) dosage—7 mg/kg;
   duration, 1-2 hours
4. Tetracaine (Pontocaine, Pantocaine) dosage—1.5 mg/kg;
   duration, 2-3 hours
5. Bupivacaine (Marcaine) dosage—3 mg/kg; duration, 5-7 hours

E. SYSTEMIC TOXICITY EFFECTS
Systemic toxicity effects include numbness of the tongue, visual
disturbances, unconsciousness, seizures, CNS depression, coma, and
respiratory arrest.

VIII. SPINAL ANESTHESIA

A. INJECTION OF LOCAL ANESTHETIC INTO SUBARACHNOID SPACE
1. Order of blockade—Preganglionic sympathetic fibers, somatic sensory
   fibers, somatic motor fibers

2. Denervation can extend about two spinal segments above the anesthetic areas.

B. LEVEL OF ANESTHESIA
1. Controlled by specific gravity of injected mixture (hyperbaric solution, e.g., D-10-W), contour of the spinal canal, and patient position

C. BEST FOR PROCEDURES BELOW THE UMBILICUS
1. T4 dermatome—Nipple
2. T6 dermatome—Xiphoid
3. T10 dermatome—Umbilicus
4. L1 dermatome—Pubic crest

D. COMPLICATIONS
1. Diminished sympathetic tone, vasodilation, hypotension, and decreased cardiac output
2. Spinal headache produced by leakage of cerebrospinal fluid from puncture site occurring about 36-48 hours after spinal puncture
a. Most frequent after use of large-bore spinal needles in young adults; uncommon when rounded, finer-point needles used (Sprotte and Whitacre)
b. Treatment includes bedrest, hydration, prone position, IV hydration, "epidural blood patch" (patient's blood injected into epidural space)
3. Hypoventilation—Intercostal paralysis if agent extends into thoracic area
4. Spinal block of cardiac nerves (T2-T4) can produce hypotension and bradycardia.
5. Total spinal (above C3) block of all intercostal and phrenic nerves requires ventilatory and hemodynamic support.
6. Urinary retention

E. ADVANTAGES OF SPINAL AND EPIDURAL ANESTHESIA
1. Blunts "stress response" to surgery
2. Reduces intraoperative blood loss and thromboembolic complications
3. Provides means of postoperative pain control
4. Maintains upper airway reflexes, protecting against aspiration

F. CONTRAINDICATIONS
Contraindications to spinal anesthesia include coagulopathy, infection at site, current neurologic dysfunction, and uncorrected hypovolemia.

IX. EPIDURAL ANESTHESIA

A. EPIDURAL SPACE
1. Bordered by the dura mater internally and the spinal canal periosteum
2. Contains fat and blood vessels

7

ANESTHESIA

B. ANESTHETIC INJECTION

Anesthetic injection blocks sympathetic/parasympathetic ganglia and motor/sensory impulses. These opioid receptors in the spinal cord allow opioid epidural administration for acute and chronic pain states.

C. OTHER CHARACTERISTICS

1. Less dependent on position of patient than spinal anesthesia
2. Larger amounts of local anesthetic required (vs. spinal)
3. More technically difficult

F. SURGICAL ADVANTAGES (see section VII. E)

1. Blockade of all nerve functions without requirements for endotracheal intubation
2. In combination with light general anesthesia, lessens postoperative complications

G. COMPLICATIONS

1. Profound hypotension if block above T5
2. Infection of indwelling catheter (especially immunocompromised patients)
3. Respiratory depression (especially epidural opioid administration); may last much longer than equivalent IV dosage
4. Urinary retention
5. CNS toxicity

X. COMBINED SPINAL/EPIDURAL ANESTHESIA

Combined spinal/epidural anesthesia takes advantage of the beneficial aspects of both, i.e., a rapid, reliable block with spinal anesthesia and the ability to supplement the block and provide postoperative pain relief with an epidural.

XI. CAUDAL ANESTHESIA

A. DEFINITION

1. Injection at S5 through sacrococcygeal ligament (ligamentum flavum equivalent)

B. USES AND ADVANTAGES

1. No spinal headache
2. Continuous anesthesia for long procedures; useful for rectal surgery, circumcision
3. Similar degree of hypotension as with spinal anesthetic; lessened amount of motor paralysis

XII. REGIONAL NERVE BLOCKS

A. CERVICAL BLOCK (ANTERIOR DIVISIONS OF C1-C4)

1. Indications—Carotid endarterectomy, lymph node biopsies

2. Provides anesthesia in anteroposterior cervical triangles between jaw and clavicles with relaxation of strap musculature
3. Lateral-approach injection at midpoint of posterior border of sternocleidomastoid (SCM) muscle to anesthetize superficial cervical plexus; fan out with 10-20 mL 1% lidocaine
4. 2nd, 3rd, and 4th nerves are individually blocked at anterior tubercles of transverse processes using 5 mL 1% lidocaine at 4th process just above midpoint of posterior border of SCM where external jugular crosses the muscle

Note: *Cervical block also blocks the phrenic nerve. Bilateral block produces phrenic paralysis and hypoventilation.*

B. **INTERCOSTAL BLOCK (12 THORACIC NERVES)** (Figs. 7-1 and 7-2)
1. Intercostal nerve courses from intervertebral foramen to rib angle along subcostal groove—Nerve = inferior; artery = middle; vein = superior
2. May also provide anesthesia of abdominal wall (T5-T11 must be blocked)
3. Technique
a. Prone position for bilateral block; lateral position for unilateral block
b. Insert needle over selected rib at 5 cm from posterior midline until needle point touches rib; walk down rib (2-3 cm); aspirate (no air or blood); and inject 3-4 mL 1% lidocaine
c. For successful intercostal space block, three intercostal nerves (one on each side) must be anesthetized.
4. Complications—Pneumothorax, intravascular injection

C. **WRIST AND HAND BLOCKS** (Figs. 7-3 to 7-6)
1. Hand procedures may be performed through blockage of the median, ulnar, and radial nerves, or with wrist bracelet infiltration. Minor procedures in digits can be accomplished using a digital block.
2. General considerations
a. Always complete the sensory exam prior to injection.
b. Do *not* use epinephrine or inject into an infected area.
c. Always aspirate first to avoid intra-arterial injection.
3. Median nerve—Located between tendons of palmaris longus (PL) and flexor carpi radialis (FCR) with wrist flexed; enter 2 cm proximal to the distal crease and just radial to the PL tendon or 1 cm medial to the FCR tendon; penetrate to a length of 1 cm and inject 5 mL 1% lidocaine (see Figs. 7-3 and 7-4)
4. Ulnar nerve—Medial to ulnar artery and lateral to flexor carpi ulnaris (FCU); enter to the ulnar side of the FCU and just proximal to the pisiform bone, aiming about 1.5 cm below tendon; aspirate, then inject 5 mL 1% lidocaine (see Figs. 7-3 and 7-4)

7

ANESTHESIA

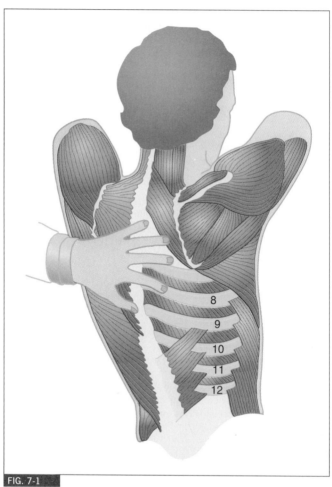

FIG. 7-1
Intercostal nerve block position.

5. Radial nerve—Superficial branch of radial nerve located in anatomic "snuff box"; inject 5 mL 1% lidocaine in snuff box (see Figs. 7-3 to 7-5)
6. Wrist bracelet—Achieved by individual block of median, ulnar, and radial nerves and SQ infiltration of wrist circumferentially
7. Digital block—Inject 1-2 mL 1% lidocaine into the web space just dorsal to the palmar (plantar) and dorsal skin junction. Then redirect

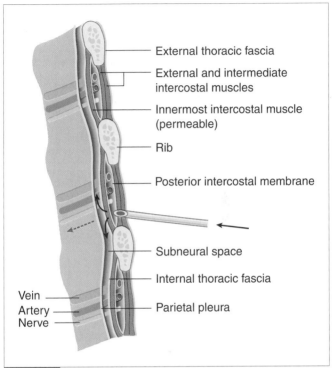

External thoracic fascia

External and intermediate intercostal muscles

Innermost intercostal muscle (permeable)

Rib

Posterior intercostal membrane

Subneural space

Internal thoracic fascia

Vein

Artery

Nerve

Parietal pleura

FIG. 7-2

Diagrammatic representation of intercostal nerve block position (*arrow*).

the needle dorsally and inject an additional 1 mL to include dorsal branch. Avoid circumferential injections in the digits (see Figs. 7-3 and 7-6).

D. FEMORAL NERVE BLOCK
1. Level below inguinal ligament
2. Nerve-artery-vein—Lateral to medial
3. Lateral to artery with 10-20 mL 1% lidocaine
4. Most combine lateral femoral cutaneous nerve block (L2, L3)—Inject 5-10 mL 1% lidocaine beneath inguinal ligament, 2 cm medial and 2 cm inferior to the anterior superior iliac spine

E. ANKLE NERVE BLOCK
1. Must block anteroposterior tibial nerves
2. Knee flexed with sole of foot on table

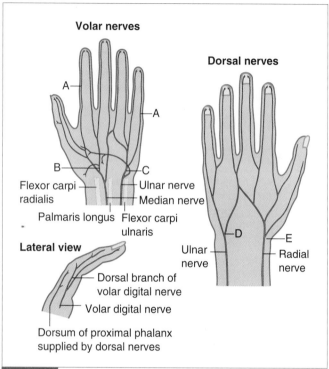

Volar nerves

A

A

B

C

Flexor carpi radialis

Ulnar nerve

Median nerve

Palmaris longus Flexor carpi ulnaris

Dorsal nerves

D

E

Ulnar nerve

Radial nerve

Lateral view

Dorsal branch of volar digital nerve

Volar digital nerve

Dorsum of proximal phalanx supplied by dorsal nerves

FIG. 7-3

Anatomy of sensory nerve blocks and sites for injection. A, Volar digital nerve; B, median nerve; C, ulnar nerve; D, dorsal branch of ulnar nerve; E, dorsal branch of radial nerve.

3. Deep peroneal nerve located between tendons of tibialis anticus and extensor hallucis longus, with liberal infiltration of 1% lidocaine
4. Posterior tibial nerve located medial to calcaneal tendon, lidocaine as in section XII. E. 3
5. Add superficial "bracelet" cutaneous block and posterolateral compartment block (deep infiltration) for sural nerve block

F. BIER BLOCK (IV REGIONAL ANESTHESIA)
1. Excellent for forearm, hand, or foot procedures
2. Usually limited to 1 hour
3. Double pneumatic tourniquet applied above elbow (or calf)
4. Initially inflate above venous pressure to distend vein, then venipuncture with 22-gauge IV

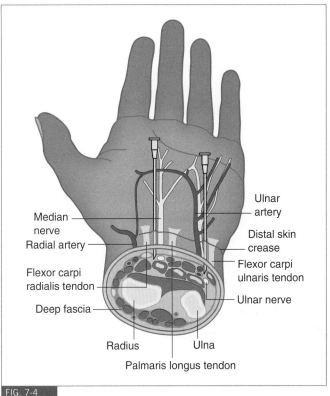

FIG. 7-4

Diagram of anatomy for wrist blocks, volar view.

5. Release tourniquet, exsanguinate extremity with elevation and wrap with elastic bandage, and inflate distal tourniquet then proximal tourniquet (>100 mm Hg above arterial).
6. Inject catheter with 0.5% lidocaine injection IV 3 mg/kg.
7. With onset of tourniquet pain (at 45 minutes), inflate distal tourniquet and release proximal tourniquet for slow release of lidocaine into systemic circulation.

XIII. LOCAL ANESTHESIA FOR INGUINAL/FEMORAL HERNIA REPAIR

A. 7 STEPS

1. Intraepidermal wheal 2-3 cm above and slightly lateral to anterior superior iliac spine (Fig. 7-7)

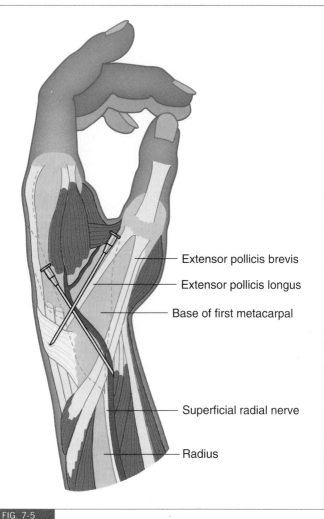

Extensor pollicis brevis

Extensor pollicis longus

Base of first metacarpal

Superficial radial nerve

Radius

FIG. 7-5

Diagram of anatomy for wrist blocks, radial view.

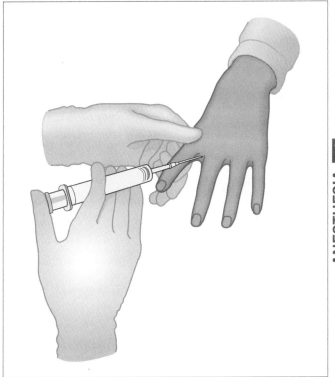

FIG. 7-6

Drawing of hand block injection.

2. At least 5 mL of anesthetic is injected superiorly, horizontally, and inferiorly (fanwise) deep to the external oblique muscle to anesthetize the ilioinguinal and iliohypogastric nerves that lie deep to the external and internal oblique muscles (see Fig. 7-7).

3. Anesthetic is injected SQ and intradermally in a medial direction toward the umbilicus (anesthetize the 11th thoracic nerve), inferiorly toward the anterior superior iliac spine, and obliquely in the direction of the proposed line of incision (Fig. 7-8).

4. Multiple injections of small amounts placed just under the external oblique fascia (Fig. 7-9)

5. Injections about the base of the spermatic cord (Fig. 7-10)

6. 3-5 mL of anesthetic injected into the pubic tubercle and in the area in proximity to Cooper's ligament (Fig. 7-11)

7. Injections of the peritoneal sac under direct vision (Fig. 7-12)

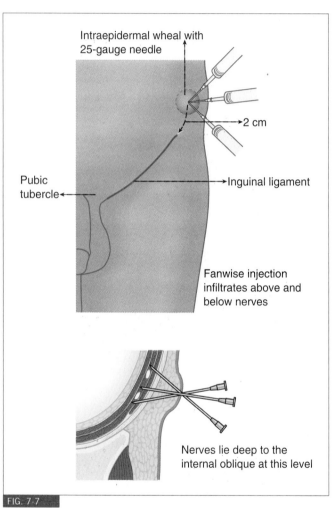

FIG. 7-7

Drawing of the first step in local anesthesia for inguinal/femoral hernia repair.

Labels within figure:
- Intraepidermal wheal with 25-gauge needle
- 2 cm
- Pubic tubercle
- Inguinal ligament
- Fanwise injection infiltrates above and below nerves
- Nerves lie deep to the internal oblique at this level

XIV. ACUTE POSTOPERATIVE PAIN MANAGEMENT

A. PATIENT-CONTROLLED ANALGESIA (PCA)

1. Allows patient to self-administer narcotics with a programmable infusion pump

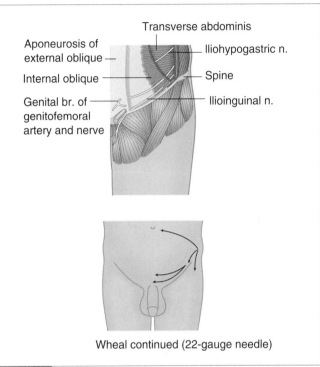

Transverse abdominis
Aponeurosis of external oblique
Iliohypogastric n.
Internal oblique
Spine
Genital br. of genitofemoral artery and nerve
Ilioinguinal n.

Wheal continued (22-gauge needle)

FIG. 7-8

Another step in local anesthesia for inguinal/femoral hernia repair.

2. Attempts to provide optimal pain relief and safety by avoiding peak and trough levels out of the therapeutic range caused by delays in administration, improper dosage, and pharmacokinetic and pharmacodynamic variability
3. Pumps are programmable to be able to deliver intermittent boluses on demand, a continuous infusion, or a continuous background infusion with intermittent bolus doses.
4. The dose, dose interval, and infusion rate are determined by the physician.
5. Morphine and meperidine are used often for intermittent dosing because of an intermediate duration of action. Typical morphine bolus dosages are 0.5-2 mg with a 5-20 minute lockout interval.
6. A loading dose is administered postoperative in the postanesthesia care unit prior to starting PCA therapy. When fully awake, the patient

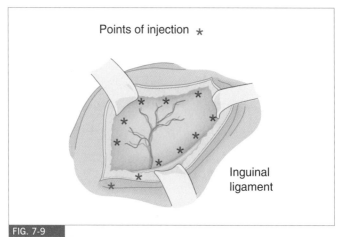

Points of injection ★

Inguinal ligament

FIG. 7-9
Drawing of local anesthesia injections being placed under the external oblique fascia.

is given the control button. Dose and interval can be adjusted as needed to achieve adequate analgesia.

7. Bolus doses and/or infusion rates can be increased at night to provide more sedation and rest.

8. Potential complications are respiratory depression, tolerance, physical dependence, nausea, vomiting, and pruritus.

B. INTRATHECAL ANALGESIA
1. Provides short-term analgesia (24 hours)
2. Morphine is the drug of choice; dosage is 0.5 mg or less.
3. Local anesthetics are not used because of a shorter duration of action and dose-dependent side effects of hypotension and motor block.
4. Limited to single-dose administration by risk of spinal headache and nerve damage from multiple punctures
5. Side effects are respiratory depression, nausea, and vomiting.

C. EPIDURAL ANALGESIA
Epidural analgesia attempts to provide pain relief without high systemic levels and side effects of analgesics. Narcotics and/or local anesthetics can be used.
1. Advantages
a. Prevents muscle spasm and splinting, avoiding pulmonary complications
b. Allows earlier ambulation
c. Possible earlier return of GI function postoperatively
d. Excellent for patients with chest trauma, including rib fractures, pulmonary contusion, and flail chest

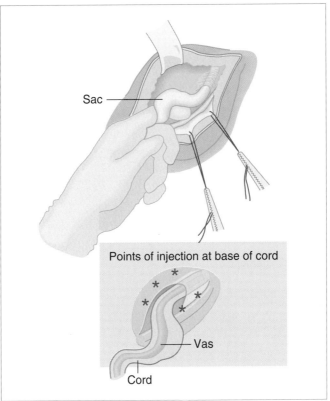

FIG. 7-10

Drawing of local anesthesia injections around the base of the spermatic cord.

2. Catheter tip placed at vertebral level corresponding to targeted dermatome
3. Narcotic analgesics
a. Effect is most likely by direct action on spinal cord.
b. Number of nerve roots involved affected by lipid solubility, infusion rate (continuous infusion), and volume of dose (intermittent dosing)
c. Narcotics with poor lipid solubility (morphine) have greater nerve root spread, slower onset of action, and longer duration of action.
d. Side effects—Respiratory depression, pruritus, nausea, vomiting, urinary retention
e. Chronic obstructive pulmonary disease is a relative contraindication.

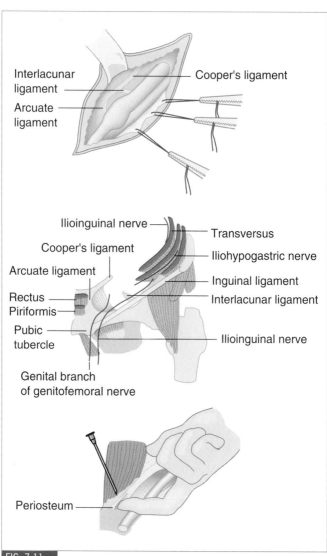

FIG. 7-11

Drawing of local anesthesia injection into the pubic tubercle and near Cooper's ligament.

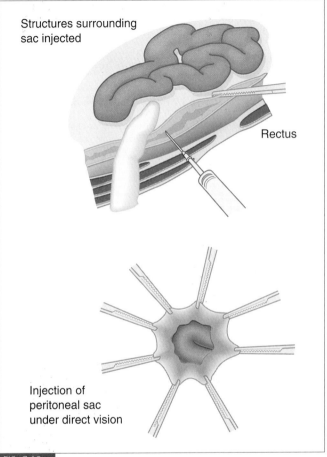

Structures surrounding
sac injected

Rectus

Injection of
peritoneal sac
under direct vision

FIG. 7-12

Drawing of local anesthesia injections of the peritoneal sac.

4. Local anesthetics
a. Blocks conduction and operation of nerve impulses of spinal nerves and spinal cord
b. Number of nerve roots involved affected by infusion rate, volume of intermittent dose
c. Bupivacaine is used most frequently because of rapid onset of action, good analgesia, long duration, and absence of motor block.

    d. Side effects—Hypotension, motor block, systemic toxicity, urinary retention; epidural blocks above T5 may cause bradycardia and cardiac failure

    e. Contraindications are severe heart disease, shock, and hypovolemia.

5. Dosing

    a. Intermittent dosing causes peak systemic levels above those required for analgesia, causing more side effects.

    b. Continuous infusion prevents peaks and troughs of intermittent dosing.

    c. Combining infusions of local anesthetics and narcotics lowers the total dose of each, reducing the chance of side effects.

    d. Continuous infusion of local anesthetics should be weaned off slowly over 2-4 hours because increased fluid mobilization secondary to vasoconstriction can precipitate pulmonary edema.

Cardiopulmonary Monitoring

David P. O'Brien, MD

I. MONITORING

The effective use of monitoring is a basic principle of periodic objective assessment of a patient's clinical condition. Ideal monitors are noninvasive and reliable, and they accurately convey physiologic information in "real-time." Often, in critically ill patients, noninvasive monitors are either unreliable or inaccurate, and invasive techniques are required.

A. VITAL SIGNS

1. Evaluation of pulse, blood pressure, temperature, respiratory rate—In their simplest form, these parameters are measured using a watch, thermometer, and sphygmomanometer.
2. Although such assessments made at 4- or 8-hour intervals are adequate for the "stable" patient, the seriously ill patient requires closer evaluation on a more frequent schedule.
3. Continuous assessment is the ideal situation.

B. MONITORING TECHNIQUES: INVASIVE VS. NONINVASIVE

1. Noninvasive

a. Continuous ECG monitoring—Heart rate, rhythm
b. Apnea monitoring—Respiratory drive
c. Pulse oximetry—Arterial O_2 saturation
d. Capnography—End-tidal CO_2
e. Ultrasonic blood pressure monitor (Dynamap)—Blood pressure
f. Doppler ultrasonography—Presence or absence of nonpalpable pulse

2. Invasive

a. Arterial catheterization—Blood pressure, arterial waveform, continuous arterial blood gas analysis
b. Central venous catheterization—Central venous pressure (CVP)
c. Pulmonary artery catheterization—CVP, pulmonary artery systolic and pulmonary artery diastolic pressures, pulmonary capillary wedge pressure (PCWP), cardiac output

3. In practice, a combination of noninvasive and invasive techniques is applied. Invasive monitoring (placement of intravascular catheters) provides more direct measurement and data from which other measurements can be calculated.

C. CATIONS FOR INVASIVE MONITORING

1. Complex surgical procedures associated with large-volume shifts
2. Circulatory instability
3. Fluid management problems
4. Deteriorating cardiac function
5. Deteriorating pulmonary function

6. Inappropriate response to volume challenge
7. Unexplained hypoxemia
8. Severe head injury
9. Surgical procedures in patients with baseline poor cardiac, respiratory, or renal function

II. PULMONARY MONITORING

A. APNEA MONITORING
Apnea monitors display respiratory rate by sensing chest wall motion. Alarms are usually set for bradypnea or apnea.

B. PULSE OXIMETRY
Pulse oximetry is noninvasive; it is the transcutaneous measurement of arterial oxygen saturation by light absorption technique. The probe is attached to body areas where capillary beds are accessible (i.e., fingernail bed, ear lobes, toes). It does not function under conditions of hypoperfusion (such as in hypothermia) or inadequate pulsatile flow or in situations in which light pulse cannot reach capillaries such as with stained fingernails.

C. CAPNOGRAPHY
Capnography provides direct measurement of end-tidal CO_2.

D. ARTERIAL BLOOD GAS
Arterial blood gas determination is the direct measure of a patient's ability to exchange O_2 and CO_2 and support oxidative metabolism. It reflects oxygenation, ventilation, and acid-base disturbances.

III. HEMODYNAMIC MONITORING TECHNIQUES

A. INDIRECT MONITORING OF BLOOD PRESSURE
Indirect monitoring of blood pressure is done by sphygmomanometer (which is notoriously inaccurate in hypotensive conditions and has wide interobserver variation) or ultrasonic blood pressure monitor. These methods work best in euvolemic patients. Doppler devices give no measure of diastolic pressure.

B. ARTERIAL CATHETERIZATION
Arterial catheterization provides direct measure of arterial pressure as well as arterial access for blood sampling. In conjunction with continuous ECG monitor, it affords indirect evaluation of electromechanical function of the heart.
1. Arterial pressure—The displayed pressure tracing is a synthesis of harmonics of the ejection pressure of the ventricular stroke volume into the elastic arterial tree. Diastolic run-off pressures represent the relationship among systemic vascular resistance, arterial pressure, and

intravascular blood volume. An undampened arterial pressure tracing shows a distinct dichrotic notch separating the systolic and diastolic pressures.

a. In hypovolemia with decreased stroke volume, a smaller pressure wave is generated.

b. If myocardial contraction is diminished, there will be prolongation of the upslope of the arterial pressure tracing.

2. Access for arterial blood samples

a. Sequential analysis of blood gas tensions and acid-base status in the arterial blood is necessary in any acute illness involving cardiovascular or respiratory dysfunction. Continuous arterial blood gas analysis via an arterial line is available; however, it is not widely used.

b. Access to other blood samples is necessary to chart the progression of multisystemic illness.

c. Arterial blood cultures

   (1) Fungal organisms may be more reliably cultured from arterial blood.

   (2) Risk of catheter-induced sepsis is a danger with any invasive monitoring—Sequential arterial cultures are necessary whenever these catheters are maintained for a long period. Arterial catheter colonization occurs much less frequently than with venous catheters.

3. Pitfalls

a. Kinked catheters or inappropriately zeroed transducers may give misleading information.

b. Arterial blood pressure is not the sine qua non of shock and should not be used as the sole criterion of effectiveness of therapy.

c. Blood pressure measurement alone is inadequate to assess the relationship between systemic resistance and cardiac output. If there is a question about low cardiac output or the level of peripheral resistance, then cardiac output should be determined.

C. CENTRAL VENOUS PRESSURE MONITORING

CVP monitoring permits assessment of the ability of the right ventricle (RV) to accommodate the volume being returned to it.

1. Accurate method of estimating RV filling pressure (relevant in interpreting RV function)

2. CVP is a function of four independent forces.

a. Volume and flow of blood in the central veins

b. Compliance and contractility of the right side of the heart during filling of the heart

c. Venomotor tone of central veins

d. Intrathoracic pressure

3. Clinical uses of CVP catheter

a. Infusion of total parenteral nutrition, vasoactive substances, hypertonic solutions, or chemically irritating medications for prolonged period

b. Monitoring of right atrial pressures

c. Aspiration of venous samples for chemical analysis (cannot be used as a substitute for true mixed venous blood)

d. Head injury—Increasing right atrial pressure results in increased intracranial blood volume and may increase intracranial pressure

e. Sensitive in reflecting increased transmyocardial pressure in pericardial tamponade

4. Pitfalls of using CVP in critically ill patient

a. Water manometer system cannot reliably represent RV filling pressure—Transducer-monitor system is necessary; transducer systems also need to be accurately zeroed; i.e., the position of the transducer is critical.

b. Misinterpretation of CVP data when extrapolating information relative to left ventricular (LV) performance in critically ill patients

   (1) In normal situations RV filling pressure may correlate with LV filling pressures.

   (2) In specific pathophysiologic states (e.g., acute respiratory distress syndrome, cor pulmonale, pulmonary fibrosis, pulmonary hypertension, myocardial contusion, septic shock), when invasive monitoring is used, right and left atrial pressures may differ significantly. CVP cannot be substituted for assessment of LV filling pressures in these situations. Thus, in a critically ill patient, placement of a pulmonary artery catheter is more appropriate.

D. BALLOON-TIPPED PULMONARY ARTERY (SWAN-GANZ) CATHETER

1. Advantages over CVP measurements

a. Allows independent assessment of RV and LV function, which may be dissimilar during critical illness

b. Permits measurement of pulmonary arterial diastolic and wedge pressures that approximates left atrial filling pressure (preload)

c. Continuous monitoring of pulmonary artery systolic and mean pressures reflects changes in pulmonary vascular resistance secondary to hypoxemia, pulmonary edema, pulmonary emboli, and pulmonary insufficiency. It helps distinguish cardiogenic from noncardiogenic pulmonary edema.

d. Allows sampling of global mixed venous blood

   (1) Global mixed venous blood saturations ($S\bar{v}O_2$) provide an index of tissue perfusion and oxygenation. Increasing $S\bar{v}O_2$ correlates with increasing cardiac output and tissue perfusion or decreased oxygen extraction (in sepsis or liver failure). Decreasing $S\bar{v}O_2$ signifies decreasing cardiac output or tissue perfusion with increased oxygen extraction. $S\bar{v}O_2$ cannot, however, reflect the changes in regional perfusion, which are often present in critically ill patients.

   (2) Allows calculation of arteriovenous oxygen content difference ($AVDo_2$) and physiologic shunt (Qsp/Qt), which is helpful in the management of respiratory failure (see appendix, later)

e. Permits accurate, reproducible measurement of cardiac output by thermodilution technique

f. Permits monitoring of RV filling pressure through the CVP access port

g. Evaluation of myocardial function—Preload, contractility, and afterload (Table 8-1)

   (1) Myocardial perfusion pressure can be estimated from the difference between systemic diastolic pressure and PWCP.

   (2) Heart rate and systolic pressure can be combined to provide a "time tension index."

   (3) Systemic vascular resistance as an estimation of aortic impedance (afterload) can be calculated.

   (4) Effect of therapeutic interventions can be quantitated in terms of physiologic cost.

h. Specialized pulmonary artery catheter permits atrial, ventricular, or sequential atrioventricular (A-V) pacing simultaneously.

2. **Clinical indications for pulmonary artery catheter—Myocardial infarction, acute respiratory failure, sepsis, peritonitis, multiple trauma, noncardiogenic pulmonary edema, near-drowning, overdoses, pulmonary edema in pregnancy, fat emboli, and elderly or critically ill patients undergoing noncardiac surgical procedures (see Chap. 6)**

3. Pitfalls

a. PCWP is at best an estimation of LV filling pressures. The gold standard for measuring preload is LV end-diastolic volume, which is not practical clinically. PWCP is an extrapolation of left atrial pressure, which in turn is an estimate of LV end-diastolic pressure. Thus, in cardiac disease states with changes in myocardial compliance or valvular function, PCWP may be an inaccurate estimation of preload.

b. Catheter artifact (whip) and high positive end-expiratory pressures may produce inaccurate measurements.

c. Catheters may be difficult to "float" in patients with cardiomegaly or low cardiac output. Placing the patient upright and with the left side down may alleviate this problem. Fluoroscopy may also be helpful.

d. Arrhythmias during insertion include ventricular irritability (premature ventricular complexes [PVCs] and ventricular tachycardia [VT]) and right bundle branch block (RBBB). Catheter placement in a patient with previous left bundle branch block (LBBB) may produce complete heart block. If pulmonary artery monitoring is essential, preparation for emergency pacing should be made.

IV. CARDIAC MONITORING

Surgeons should be versed in basic ECG interpretation and dysrhythmia recognition.

A. RATE

At a standard paper speed of 25 mm/sec, each 5-mm block is 0.2 seconds in duration. Bradycardia is <60 beats/min, whereas tachycardia is >100 beats/min.

8.

CARDIOPULMONARY MONITORING

TABLE 8-1

DETERMINANTS OF CARDIAC OUTPUT

Determinant	Definition	Effect on Cardiac Output	Measurement	Treatment
Preload	Length of myocardial fibers at end-diastole, which is the result of ventricular filling pressure	Direct, up to physiologic limit	End-diastolic volume and pressure of the ventricles Pulmonary diastolic pressure Pulmonary capillary wedge pressure Direct left atrial pressure measurements CVP (right atrial)	Volume expansion Pericardiocentesis Reduction of PEEP
Contractility	The inotropic state of the myocardium; length/tension/velocity relationship of the myocardium independent of initial length and after-load	Direct	Ventricular function curves Ejection fraction V_{max} Vcf PEP/LVET dP/dt	Dopamine Norepinephrine Epinephrine Isoproterenol Dobutamine Digitalis Glucagon GKI
Afterload	Systolic ventricular wall stress, which is produced by the force against which the myocardial fibers must contract	Inverse, as long as coronary flow is maintained Pulmonary artery pressure for right ventricle	Aortic pressure for left ventricle	Diuretics Phentolamine Sodium nitroprusside Nitroglycerine Intra-aortic balloon pumping External counter-pulsation

| Pulse rate | The number of cardiac systoles per minute | Direct, >60 and <180 per minute | ECG Count pulse | Bradycardia Atropine Pacemaker Epinephrine Tachycardia Digitalis Lidocaine Electroversion |

CVP = central venous pressure; PEEP = positive end-expiratory pressure; V_{max} = peak velocity; Vcf = velocity of circumferential fiber shortening; PEP = pre-ejection period; LVET = left ventricular ejection time; dP/dt = rate of change of left ventricular pressure; GKI = glucose-potassium-insulin.

From Hardy JD: Textbook of Surgery. Philadelphia, JB Lippincott, 1983, p 54.

CARDIOPULMONARY MONITORING 8

B. RHYTHM
Cardiac rhythm is described as *regular* or *irregular*.

C. AXIS (Fig. 8-1)
An estimate of the cardiac axis can be obtained from line leads I and aVF.
1. Normal axis is between +120 and −30 degrees. The QRS complex is positive (above the isoelectric line) in leads I and aF (+I, +aF).
2. Left axis deviation is −30 to −90 degrees; QRS is positive in lead I and negative (below isoelectric line) in aVF (+I, −aF).
3. Right axis deviation is +120 to −90 degrees; QRS is negative in I, and above or below isoelectric line in aVF (−I, +/−aVF).
4. Alternatively, the mean cardiac axis is perpendicular to a frontal QRS complex with a net amplitude of 0.

D. WAVES, INTERVALS, AND SEGMENTS
By analyzing the P-QRS-T complex in systematic fashion, ECG interpretation is simplified, and pathology can be readily identified.
1. P Waves
a. P waves reflect electrical activity of the atria. Abnormalities include "P pulmonale" or tall P waves (>2.5 mm) in leads II, III, and aVF. This reflects right atrial pathology in some conditions, e.g., pulmonary hypertension, chronic obstructive pulmonary disease, pulmonary embolus, and tricuspid stenosis or insufficiency.

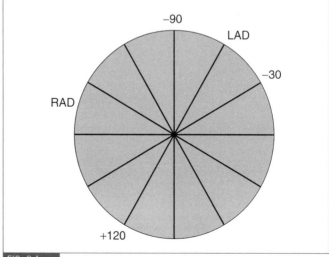

FIG. 8-1

Diagram useful for estimating cardiac axis. LAD = left axis deviation; RAD = right axis deviation.

b. "P mitrale" is wide P waves (>0.10 second) in lead II, or a notched P wave in lead V_1. Left atrial pathology, secondary to mitral stenosis or regurgitation, may cause P mitrale.

2. **PR interval—Normally 0.12 to 0.20 seconds, but may be as long as 0.14 seconds in young patients; A-V block reflected in the PR interval**

a. First degree—Delayed A-V conduction, with prolonged PR

b. Second degree

    (1) Type I (Wenckebach)—PR interval is progressively prolonged until a QRS complex is dropped.

    (2) Type II—PR intervals are constant, but QRS complexes are unexpectedly dropped.

c. Third degree—Atrial and ventricular activity are independent; conduction is interrupted; also termed *complete heart block*

3. **QRS complex—Reflects ventricular activity; normal QRS width, up to 0.09 seconds.**

a. LV hypertrophy—Increased leftward forces result in large R waves in leads I, aVL, V_5, and V_6 ("large" ≥20 mm high in limb leads and >30 mm in precordial leads). Inverted T waves and depressed ST segments accompany this finding; this is called a *strain pattern*.

b. RV hypertrophy—Increased rightward forces lead to large S waves in I, aVL, V_5, and V_6, as well as tall R waves in V_1 and/or V_2. Again, an RV strain pattern is manifested by inverted T waves and depressed ST segments in leads with dominant R waves.

c. LBBB—A mid-conduction delay causes prolonged ventricular depolarization in LBBB; the QRS interval is >0.12 seconds. Note that ventricular hypertrophy criteria are invalid if LBBB is present (see section IV. D. 3. a and b). The following is seen in LBBB.

    (1) Broad R waves in I, aVL, V_5, and V_6

    (2) Broad S waves in V_1 and/or V_2

    (3) Absent septal Q waves in I, aVL, V_5, and V_6

d. RBBB—A terminal delay in ventricular conduction results in characteristic changes. Again, the QRS is >0.12 seconds in duration and has the following.

    (1) Broad R waves in V_1

    (2) Broad S waves in I, aVL, V_5, and V_6

e. Incomplete block defined as QRS between 0.10 and 0.12 seconds in duration

4. **ST segment changes—May be the only changes seen in infarction or ischemia**

a. ST depression seen in subendocardial infarction and myocardial ischemia and in patients on digitalis

b. ST elevation seen in transmural infarction, LV aneurysm, and pericarditis

5. **T waves—This indicator of depolarization changes the morphology in several clinical settings.**

a. Ventricular hypertrophy (see section IV. D. 3. a and b)

8

CARDIOPULMONARY MONITORING

b. Transient ischemia
c. Late transmural infarction
d. High/low serum potassium

V. DYSRHYTHMIAS: RECOGNITION AND MANAGEMENT

A. BRADYCARDIA (RATE <60 beats/min)

1. Sinus bradycardia
a. Decreased rate from within the sinus node, e.g., disease, increased parasympathetic tone, drugs (digitalis or β blockers)
b. Rhythm—Regular
c. Therapy—Immediate treatment is required only when accompanied by hypotension, angina, dyspnea, altered mental status, myocardial ischemia, or ventricular ectopy.
2. Second-degree A-V block, Mobitz type I (Wenckebach) occurs at level of A-V node and is often due to increased parasympathetic tone or drug effect (digitalis, propranolol). Usually transient. Characterized by progressive prolongation of the PR interval, which is indicative of decreasing conduction velocity through the A-V node before an impulse is completely blocked. Usually only a single impulse is blocked, then the cycle is repeated. The atrial rhythm is usually regular. There is no risk of progression to complete heart block.
3. Second-degree A-V block, Mobitz type II occurs below level of A-V node either at the bundle of His (uncommon) or at the bundle branch level. Associated with an organic lesion in the conduction pathway. Poor prognosis; the development of complete heart block should be anticipated. The PR interval does not lengthen prior to a dropped beat. Atrial rhythm is usually regular. Placement of a transvenous pacemaker is usually required.

B. SINUS TACHYCARDIA

1. Increased rate within sinus node from demands for higher cardiac output (e.g., exercise, fever, anxiety)
2. Rate >100 beats/min
3. P wave—Upright in I, II, aVF
4. Therapy—Usually none, other than to treat underlying cause. In older patients with cardiac disease, β blockers or calcium channel blockers may be needed acutely to prevent the increase in myocardial oxygen demand that occurs at high heart rates.

C. PAROXYSMAL SUPRAVENTRICULAR TACHYCARDIA/PAROXYSMAL ATRIAL TACHYCARDIA

1. Sudden onset of tachycardia originating in atria, lasting minutes to hours
2. Rate—Atrial rate, 160-200 beats/min
3. Rhythm—Regular

4. P waves—May not be present, i.e., buried in previous T wave
5. PR—Normal or prolonged
6. QRS—Normal with rapid rate
7. RBBB, or less often LBBB, with paroxysmal supraventricular tachycardia/ paroxysmal atrial tachycardia may appear like VT but can be discerned by presence of P waves and BBB.
8. Therapy
  a. For symptomatic (unstable) patients, use low-voltage DC cardioversion.
  b. For stable patients with preserved cardiac function, calcium channel blockers, β blockers, or amiodarone is indicated.
  c. For stable patients with compromised cardiac function (ejection fraction <0.40 or congestive heart failure), amiodarone is first-line therapy. DC cardioversion is contraindicated.

D. PREMATURE ATRIAL CONTRACTION
1. Originates in atria, not in sinus node; may be caused by stimulants (caffeine, tobacco, ethyl alcohol), drugs, hypoxia, digitalis intoxication
2. Rate—Variable
3. Rhythm—Irregular
4. P wave—Abnormal, premature; may be buried in preceding T
5. PR—Normal or prolonged (premature atrial contraction with first-degree A-V block)
6. QRS—Normal or wide if aberrancy (usually RBBB); QRS absent with complete block
7. Therapy—Discontinue the stimulating factor (drug) and correct hypoxia.

E. ATRIAL FLUTTER (Fig. 8-2)
Atrial rate is 250 beats/min and the rhythm is regular. Every other F (flutter) wave is conducted to ventricles (2:1 block), resulting in regular ventricular rhythm at rate of 125 beats/min.
1. "F-wave," "sawtooth," or "picket-fence" waves between QRS complexes with varying conduction ratios, best seen in leads II, III, and aVF; seen in organic heart disease (mitral or tricuspid valve) or coronary disease
2. Rate—Atrial rate about 300 beats/min (220-350 beats/min); ventricular rate about 150 beats/min but varies with ratio (2:1, 3:1, etc.)
3. Rhythm—Atrial, regular
4. P waves—Absent
5. Flutter waves between QRS complexes
   Note: *A hint is to turn the ECG upside down to see waves.*
6. QRS—Normal, may be aberrant
7. Therapy
  a. If hemodynamically unstable, low-voltage DC cardioversion
  b. For stable patients with preserved cardiac function, use calcium channel blockers and β blockers to control rate.

8

CARDIOPULMONARY MONITORING

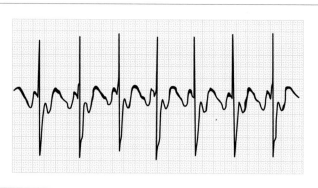

FIG. 8-2

Atrial flutter. *(From Cummins RO [ed]: Textbook of Advanced Cardiac Life Support. Dallas, American Heart Association, 1994, pp 3-12.)*

c. For stable patients with compromised cardiac function, use amiodarone, digoxin, or diltiazem to control rate.
d. For rhythm conversion in patients with duration <48 hours with normal cardiac function, consider DC cardioversion or one of following agents: amiodarone, flecainide, ibutilide, or procainamide.
e. For rhythm conversion in patients with duration <48 hours with compromised cardiac function, consider DC cardioversion or amiodarone.
f. For rhythm conversion in patients with duration >48 hours, anticoagulation must be performed prior to cardioversion to prevent embolization of arterial thrombi.

F. ATRIAL FIBRILLATION (Fig. 8-3)
1. Originates from multiple areas within atria, with only a small area of depolarization; multiple etiologies, e.g., valvular heart disease, pulmonary embolus, digitalis intoxication, pulmonary disease, electrolyte abnormalities, idiopathic

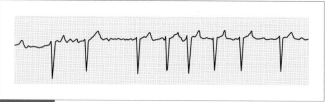

FIG. 8-3

Atrial fibrillation. *(From Cummins RO [ed]: Textbook of Advanced Cardiac Life Support. Dallas, American Heart Association, 1994, pp 3-11.)*

2. Rate—Atrial rate 400-700 beats/min (may not be clearly seen); ventricular rate 60-180 beats/min (variable)
3. Rhythm—Irregularly irregular
4. P waves—Absent
5. QRS—Normal
6. Therapy (see section IV. E. 7)

G. **PREMATURE VENTRICULAR COMPLEX** (Fig. 8-4)
1. Early depolarization arising within a ventricle from one or more sites; ventricles depolarize sequentially, followed by a compensatory pause (usually twice the regular sinus interval)
2. Rate—Variable
3. Rhythm—Variable, irregular
4. P wave—Usually obscured in previous S or T wave, or may be present
5. QRS—Prolonged, bizarre ≥0.12 seconds. Complexes may have different appearances with different ectopic sites.
6. ST segments—Slope away from QRS (inverted)
7. T waves—Inverted
8. Variations
a. Bigeminy—Alternating normal beats and PVCs
b. Trigeminy—Every third beat is a PVC
c. R-on-T—PVC falls on previous T wave; is especially dangerous because it may precipitate VT or ventricular fibrillation
9. Therapy
a. Acute treatment for frequent or multifocal PVCs is usually a lidocaine drip, titrated to maintain suppression.
b. Procainamide is recommended if lidocaine is unsuccessful. Bretylium is then used if ectopy continues or progresses to VT.

H. **VENTRICULAR TACHYCARDIA** (Fig. 8-5)
1. Three or more PVCs together; may or may not cause clinical symptoms
2. Rate—>100 beats/min; usually <220 beats/min
3. Rhythm—Variable, usually regular
4. P waves—May or may not be present
5. QRS—Wide; usually no Q in V_5, V_6

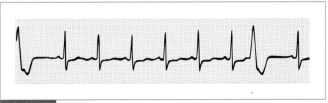

FIG. 8-4

Premature ventricular complex. *(From Cummins RO [ed]: Textbook of Advanced Cardiac Life Support. Dallas, American Heart Association, 1994, pp 3-8.)*

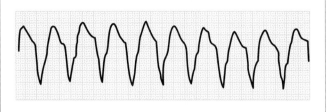

FIG. 8-5

Ventricular tachycardia. *(From Cummins RO [ed]: Textbook of Advanced Cardiac Life Support. Dallas, American Heart Association, 1994, pp 3-6.)*

6. Fusion beats—Early sinus-like, later like PVC. These occur prior to and at the end of a run of VT and thus are characteristic.
7. Therapy
a. Stable patient—Determine if tachycardia is monomorphic or polymorphic. If polymorphic, consider torsades de pointes if the baseline QT interval is prolonged. Additionally, if cardiac function is impaired, use amiodarone or lidocaine followed by synchronized cardioversion.
b. Unstable patient—Immediate cardioversion
8. Unstable—Symptoms (e.g., chest pain, dyspnea), hypotension (systolic blood pressure <90 mm Hg), congestive heart failure, ischemia, or infarction
9. Sedation should be considered for all patients, including those defined as unstable, except those who are hemodynamically unstable (e.g., hypotensive, in pulmonary edema, or unconscious).
10. If the patient is hemodynamically stable, a precordial thurnp may be employed prior to cardioversion.
11. Once VT has resolved, begin IV infusion of the antiarrhythmic agent that has aided in resolution of the VT. If the patient is hemodynamically unstable, use lidocaine if cardioversion alone is successful.

I. TORSADES DE POINTES
1. A form of VT characterized by gradual alteration in the amplitude and direction of the electrical activity
2. Treated differently than other types of VT
a. Correct electrolytes.
b. Magnesium sulfate
c. Consider overdrive pacing with or without β blocker.
d. Isoproterenol (as temporizing measure to pacing)
e. Phenytoin or lidocaine
f. Quinidine-like drugs are *contraindicated.*

3. Polymorphic VT (PVT) can masquerade as torsades de pointes—Pay close attention to the length of the QT interval of complexes preceding the tachycardia.

a. When QT interval is long, consider torsades de pointes.

b. If QT interval is normal, the arrhythmia is more likely to be PVT and may therefore respond to antiarrhythmics, including β blockers, lidocaine, amiodarone, procainamide, and sotalol.

J. VENTRICULAR FIBRILLATION (Figs. 8-6 and 8-7)

1. There are multiple areas of ectopic ventricular activity but no effective contraction of the heart, hence no cardiac output. It is a common cause of cardiac arrest due to ischemia or infarction. Amplitude of activity determines "coarse" vs. "fine" ventricular fibrillation.

2. Rate—Rapid, disorganized

3. Rhythm—None

4. P, QRS, ST, T waves all indefinable

5. Therapy—Cardioversion, then epinephrine or vasopressin. If unsuccessful, consider amiodarone, magnesium, and/or procainamide.

6. Pulseless VT should be treated identically to ventricular fibrillation.

7. Check pulse and rhythm after each shock. If ventricular fibrillation recurs after transiently converting (rather than persists without ever converting), use whatever energy level has previously been successful for defibrillation.

8. The value of sodium bicarbonate is questionable during cardiac arrest, and it is *not* recommended for the routine cardiac arrest sequence. Consideration of its use in a dose of 1 mEq/kg is appropriate at the point noted in the algorithm. One half of the original dose may be repeated q 10 min if it is used.

K. VENTRICULAR ASYSTOLE (AGONAL RHYTHM)

1. No effective electrical activity, resulting in no cardiac contraction

2. P waves, QRS, ST, T waves may appear in ever-increasing intervals until no impulses or only isolated impulses are seen.

3. Asystole should be confirmed in two leads.

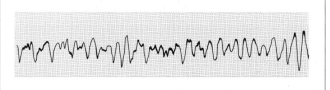

FIG. 8-6

Ventricular fibrillation (coarse). *(From Cummins RO [ed]: Textbook of Advanced Cardiac Life Support. Dallas, American Heart Association, 1994, pp 3-5.)*

8

CARDIOPULMONARY MONITORING

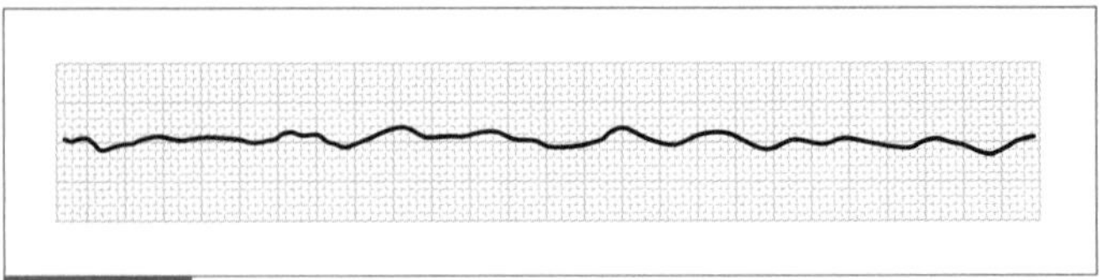

FIG. 8-7
Ventricular fibrillation (fine). *(From Cummins RO [ed]: Textbook of Advanced Cardiac Life Support. Dallas, American Heart Association, 1994, pp 3-5.)*

L. PULSELESS ELECTRICAL ACTIVITY

Pulseless electrical activity, formerly known as *electrical-mechanical dissociation*, is electrical activity (usually QRS type) depicted on the ECG, but there is no pulse. Consider the following possible causes.

1. Hypovolemia—Volume infusion
2. Hypoxia—Ventilation
3. Cardiac tamponade—Pericardiocentesis
4. Tension pneumothorax—Needle decompression followed by thoracostomy tube
5. Hypothermia—Warming
6. Massive pulmonary embolism—Surgery, thrombolytics
7. Drug overdoses such as tricyclics, digitalis
8. Hyperkalemia
9. Acidosis—Sodium bicarbonate
10. Massive myocardial infarction

RECOMMENDED READINGS

Durham R, Neunaber K, Vogler G, et al: Right ventricular end-diastolic volume as a measure of preload. J Trauma 39:218-223, 1995.

Ermakov S, Hoyt JW: Pulmonary artery catheterization. Crit Care Clin 8:773-806, 1992.

Guidelines 2000 for Cardiopulmonary Resuscitation and Emergency Cardiovascular Care. Part 6: Advanced Cardiovascular Life Support. The American Heart Association in collaboration with the International Liaison Committee on Resuscitation. Circulation 102(8 Suppl): I-136–I-165, 2000.

APPENDIX: FORMULAS USED IN CARDIOPULMONARY CRITICAL CARE

1. **Mean arterial pressure** (MAP):

$$MAP = DP + \tfrac{1}{3}(SP - DP)$$

where DP = diastolic pressure and SP = systolic pressure
[normal = 80-90 mm Hg]

2. **Stroke volume** (SV):

$$SV = CO/HR$$

where CO = cardiac output and HR = heart rate [normal = 50-60 mL]

3. **Cardiac index** (CI):

$$CI = CO/BSA$$

where CO = cardiac output and BSA = body surface area
[normal = 3.5-4 in ICU population]

4. **Stroke index** (SI):

$$SI = SV/BSA$$

where SV = stroke volume and BSA = body surface area
[normal = 35-40 in ICU population]

5. **Right ventricular stroke work** (RVSW):

$$RVSW = SV \times (MAP - CVP) \times 0.0136$$

where SV = stroke volume, MAP = mean arterial pressure, and
CVP = central venous pressure [normal = 10-15 g/m]

6. **Left ventricular stroke work** (LVSW):

$$LVSW = SV \times (MAP - PAO) \times 0.0136$$

where SV = stroke volume, MAP = mean arterial pressure, and
PAO = pulmonary artery occlusion [normal = 60-80 g/m]

$$Ratio = LVSW/PAO$$

7. **Systemic vascular resistance** (SVR) (also referred to in the literature as total peripheral resistance):

$$SVR = [(MAP - CVP) \times 80] \div CO$$

where MAP = mean arterial pressure, CVP = central venous pressure,
and CO = cardiac output [normal = 800-1200 dynes/sec/cm^{-5}]

8. **Pulmonary vascular resistance** (PVR):

$$PVR = [(MAP - PAO) \times 80] \div CO$$

where MAP = mean arterial pressure, PAO = pulmonary artery occlusion,
and CO = cardiac output [normal = 100-200 dynes/sec/cm^{-5}]

9. **Myocardial oxygen consumption—correlate** (MVo_2C):

$$MVo_2C = (SP \times HR)/100$$

where SP = systolic pressure and HR = heart rate; this term is a fair
calculated measure of how much O_2 the heart is requiring) [higher
values = greater consumption]

8

CARDIOPULMONARY MONITORING

10. **Alveolar P_{O_2} (P_{AO_2}):**

$$P_{AO_2} = (P_B - P_{H_2O}) \times F_{IO_2} - P_{ECO_2}/R$$

where P_B = barometric pressure (760 mm Hg at sea level), P_{H_2O} (at body temperature) = water pressure (47 mm Hg), P_{ECO_2} = P_{ACO_2}, and R = 0.8 (assumed).
Thus,

$$P_{AO_2} = (760 - 47)F_{IO_2} - P_{ACO_2}/0.8$$

where F_{IO_2} = fraction of inspired oxygen and P_{ACO_2} = partial pressure of carbon dioxide, arterial.

11. **Capillary O_2 content (Cc'_{O_2}):**

$$Cc'_{O_2} = (P_{AO_2} \times 0.0031) + Hb \times 1.39 \times 1$$

where P_{AO_2} = alveolar partial pressure and Hb = hemoglobin (assumes 100% Hb saturation) [normal = 18.3 mL/100 mL]

12. **Mixed venous O_2 content ($C\bar{v}_{O_2}$):**

$$C\bar{v}_{O_2} = P\bar{v}_{O_2} \times 0.0031 + (Hb \times 1.39 \times Ven\ Sat)$$

where $P\bar{v}_{O_2}$ = partial pressure of mixed venous oxygen, Hb = hemoglobin, and Ven Sat = venous saturation [normal = 13 mL/100 mL]

13. **Arterial O_2 content (Ca_{O_2}):**

$$Ca_{O_2} = Pa_{O_2} \times 0.0031 + (Hb \times 1.39 \times Art\ Sat)$$

where Pa_{O_2} = partial pressure of oxygen, arterial; Hb = hemoglobin; and Art Sat = arterial saturation [normal = 18 mL/100 mL]

14. **O_2 delivery (O_2 Del):**

$$O_2\ Del = C_A \times CO \times 10$$

where C_A = arterial oxygen content and CO = cardiac output [normal = 1000 mL/min]

15. **Arteriovenous O_2 difference (AVD_{O_2}):**

$$AVD_{O_2} = Ca - Cv$$

where Ca = arterial content and Cv = venous content [normal = 3.5-4.5 mL/100 mL]

16. **O_2 consumption (O_2 Cons):**

$$O_2\ Cons = (Ca - Cv) \times CO \times 10$$

where Ca = arterial content, Cv = venous content, and CO = cardiac output [normal = 250 mL/min]

17. **O_2 utilization (% Util):**

$$\%\ Util = Ca - Cv/Ca$$

where Ca = arterial content and Cv = venous content [normal = 0.2-0.25]

18. **Intrapulmonary shunt (Qsp/Qt):**

$$Qsp/Qt = (Cc'_{O_2} - Ca_{O_2})/(Cc'_{O_2} - Cv_{O_2})$$

where $Cc'o_2$ = capillary O_2 content, Cao_2 = arterial O_2 content, and Cvo_2 = mixed venous O_2 content [normal < 0.10]

19. **Body surface area** (BSA)—use the DuBois formula:

$$BSA = (W^{0.425} \times H^{0.725}) \times 0.007184$$

where W = weight and H = height

Wound Healing, Care, and Complications

Susan M. Pike, MD

Healing and tissue repair are central to the science of surgery. The surgeon's goal is to create an environment where healing can proceed in an optimal fashion. Accomplishing this goal requires an understanding of the physiologic mechanisms involved in the wound healing process. Although healing generally proceeds without complication, impaired wound healing and infection are leading causes of morbidity in surgical patients.

9

I. THE PHYSIOLOGY OF WOUND HEALING

Wound healing can be divided into four phases, each with specific biologic processes. However, healing results from a continuum of events that overlap in time.

A. EARLY PHASE (0-4 DAYS)

1. Hemostasis—In response to tissue injury, the body acts to control hemorrhage by vasoconstriction and clot formation, which consists of aggregated platelets and fibrin. Platelet aggregation results in degranulation of α granules and release of biologically active factors, including matrix glycoproteins (fibrinogen, fibronectin, and thrombospondin) and cytokines (platelet-derived growth factor [PDGF] and transforming growth factor [TGF]-β). These platelet products play a pivotal role in wound healing by mediation of cell migration, recruitment, and differentiation in the phases that follow.

2. Inflammation—Tissue damage initiates the inflammatory response. The transient vasoconstriction to aid hemostasis is followed by vasodilation, which is mediated by histamine, kinins, prostaglandins, and complement components. Inflammatory cells reach the site of injury by migration and chemotaxis. *Polymorphonuclear leukocytes* begin migration a few hours after injury and predominate in the first 48-72 hours. Although they are not essential for wound healing, their role is to cleanse the area of bacteria, foreign particles, and necrotic tissue via phagocytosis. *Macrophages*, the next wave of inflammatory cells, are derived from circulating monocytes and enter the wound approximately 72 hours following injury. Macrophages are essential in controlling and regulating wound healing. In addition to their phagocytic role, macrophages are the primary source of cytokines such as PDGF and TGF-β. These cytokines stimulate fibroblast proliferation and collagen production and therefore play a pivotal role in the transition from inflammation to repair.

B. INTERMEDIATE PHASE (4-30 DAYS)

1. Fibroblast migration and proliferation are cytokine-directed processes that begin 4-5 days following injury. Fibroblasts migration is

facilitated by extracellular matrix proteins and occurs along a fibrin framework.

2. Angiogenesis is the growth of new capillary blood vessels in areas of damage or new tissue formation. Increased lactate levels, acidic pH, and decreased oxygen tension serve as stimulators. Angiogenesis provides a pathway for delivery of nutritional factors and oxygen, which are essential for wound healing.

3. Epithelialization is essential to re-establish the barrier function of the skin. In partial-thickness wounds (abrasions or partial-thickness burns), the epidermis and a portion of the dermis are damaged. Epithelial migration begins almost immediately and proceeds from both wound margins and from the epidermal appendages. In contrast, an incisional or full-thickness wound involves the migration of epithelial cells from only the wound margins. Incisional wounds are usually re-epithelialized in 24-48 hours.

C. LATE PHASE

The main feature of the late phase is collagen deposition. Clinically, this is the most important phase of healing because the rate, quality, and quantity of collagen deposition determine the strength and character of the scar.

1. Matrix deposition—Fibroblasts produce an amorphous medium composed of glycosaminoglycans, proteoglycans, and hyaluronic acid that serves as the matrix for collagen deposition.

2. Collagen synthesis—Collagen is the principal building block of connective tissue. *Type I* is most common and accounts for 80-90% of the collagen found in normal skin. Collagen synthesis begins 3-5 days following injury, and the rate of synthesis increases rapidly for up to 4-5 weeks. At this time the number of fibroblasts and, hence, the rate of collagen synthesis declines. The collagen fibers gradually thicken and organize along the stress lines of the scar; these changes are accompanied by an increased scar tensile strength. The collagen fibers in a healed wound never become as organized as that of intact dermis, and maximum breaking strength is only 90% that of normal tissue.

3. Wound contraction—The process begins with collagen synthesis and continues for 12-15 days. Wound contraction is the approximation of the wound edges, by the action of migrating fibroblasts and myofibroblasts, and occurs from the wound edges toward the center. This process plays a trivial role in the repair of incisions; however, it plays a significant role in the closure of full-thickness open wounds in areas such as the back and abdomen.

D. FINAL PHASE (30 DAYS-2 YEARS)

1. Scar remodeling or maturation—Defines the final phase of wound healing. This is characterized by a peak and plateau in collagen

content at 4 weeks with continued changes in the density and organization of the collagen fibers. As the scar becomes relatively avascular and acellular, visible changes are appreciated in terms of texture, thickness, and color of the healing wound.

2. Wound strength—As the wound enters the intermediate proliferative phase, the strength of the wound parallels the rapid rise in collagen content for about 4 weeks. Following the plateau of collagen content, there is an increase in the number of intramolecular and intermolecular cross links that contribute to the increasing strength of the wound. By 6 weeks the scar has reached 85% of its eventual strength, and at 6 months it achieves a bursting strength of 90% in comparison to normal skin. Through remodeling, the scar increases in strength for 2 years, but the ultimate strength never reaches that of unwounded tissue.

II. CYTOKINES AND GROWTH FACTORS IN WOUND HEALING

Cytokines are polypeptides with multiple regulatory roles in cell growth and differentiation. Cytokines have emerged as the primary mediators of most wound healing events. The carefully regulated release of specific cytokines at appropriate intervals following injury appears to orchestrate the wound healing process. The terms *cytokine* and *growth factor* are used interchangeably; both are proteins that mediate cellular function by binding receptors located on cell membranes. However, technically, growth factors only stimulate cell proliferation, whereas cytokines can mediate all types of cellular processes.

Careful orchestration of growth factors is responsible for normal healing at a near-maximal rate. Alterations in the production and responsiveness to these potent compounds likely contribute to a large number of proliferative disorders such as excessive scarring and neoplasms, as well as impaired wound healing.

A. EPIDERMAL GROWTH FACTOR
Epidermal growth factor (EGF) was the first growth factor identified. The primary function of EGF is to stimulate proliferation of epithelial cells, endothelial cells, and fibroblasts. It also serves as a chemotactic factor for epithelial cells and fibroblasts. EGF has been shown to stimulate fibroplasia, increase collagenase activity, and promote angiogenesis and fibronectin synthesis.

B. TRANSFORMING GROWTH FACTOR β
TGF can be isolated from macrophages, platelets, and lymphocytes. It is found in high concentrations in the α granules of platelets and is released at the site of injury during platelet degranulation. TGF acts on monocytes to synthesize other growth factors including fibroblast growth factor (FGF),

PDGF, tumor necrosis factor (TNF), and interleukin 1. TNF-β stimulates chemotaxis and proliferation of fibroblasts and may be the most potent stimulator of collagen synthesis.

C. PLATELET-DERIVED GROWTH FACTOR
PDGF is localized to the α granules of platelets and is secreted by platelets, macrophages, and endothelial cells. PDGF is most active in fibroplasia and collagen synthesis and contributes to chemotaxis and proliferation of fibroblasts.

D. FIBROBLAST GROWTH FACTOR
FGF has been found to be the primary stimulant of angiogenesis. Endothelial cells can both produce and respond to FGF. Applied topically to wounds, FGF has been found to stimulate wound contraction and play a role in collagen, proteoglycan, and fibronectin synthesis.

III. WOUND CLOSURE

A. PRIMARY HEALING (BY FIRST INTENTION)
Primary healing is wound closure by direct approximation.

B. SPONTANEOUS HEALING (BY SECOND INTENTION)
In spontaneous healing, wound closure is dependent on contraction and epithelialization.

C. TERTIARY HEALING (BY THIRD INTENTION)
Tertiary healing is delayed wound closure after several days, an intentional disruption of healing that began as secondary intention. Closure can occur any time after granulation tissue is formed in the wound. Delayed closure should be performed only when the wound is not infected.

IV. FACTORS INFLUENCING WOUND HEALING

A. LOCAL FACTORS (CONTROLLED BY THE SURGEON)
1. Tissue trauma—Must be kept to a minimum by gentle handling of tissues
2. Hematoma/seroma—Associated with an increased rate of infection and wound dehiscence
3. Blood supply
4. Temperature
5. Infection
6. Technique and suture materials

B. GENERAL FACTORS (ANEMIA, HYPOXIA)
1. Systemic effects of steroids—Decreases the inflammatory response and therefore impairs every phase of wound healing

2. Malnutrition—Deficiencies in basic cellular building blocks
3. Chemotherapy—Detrimental to early stages of healing and should be delayed for at least 1 week after surgery
4. Radiation—Wounds from this source are dose related; both acute and chronic effects are seen. Waiting 1 week significantly decreases the incidence of wound complication.
5. Chronic illness
6. Obesity—Poorly vascularized fatty tissue is prone to infection and breakdown.
7. Diabetes—Peripheral vascular disease, neuropathy, and poor leukocyte function all contribute to poor wound healing in diabetic patients.

V. MANAGEMENT OF SOFT TISSUE WOUNDS

A. TRAUMATIC WOUND CARE
1. ABCs—Address more urgent problems first. Bleeding is initially controlled with direct pressure.
2. Obtain radiographs for suspected fracture or foreign bodies.
3. Before closure, a careful neurovascular exam and local wound exploration should be undertaken to identify injury to nerves, vessels, tendons, joints, or other structures in anatomic proximity.
4. Cleanse the skin surrounding the wound. Use antibacterial soap or povidone-iodine (Betadine). These agents are damaging to exposed tissues and should be kept out of the wound and eyes. Cut the hair as needed, but never shave the eyebrows because they occasionally fail to grow back.
5. Anesthetize with local agents if there is no history of allergy (see Chap. 7, section VII). Epinephrine is useful to control skin bleeding, particularly on the face, but avoid areas where distal ischemia may occur, e.g., fingers, toes, nose, ear, and penis.
6. Débridement—Remove clot, debris, and necrotic tissue. Copious saline irrigation will remove gross contaminates; no amount of irrigation sterilizes the wound. Perform careful, sharp débridement of all devitalized tissue. Bleeding vessels should be clamped and tied under direct vision.

B. WOUND CLOSURE
1. Most traumatic wounds can be closed primarily following adequate débridement, hemostasis, and copious irrigation. Use atraumatic technique. Minimize wound tension.
a. Buried sutures should be used to minimize wound edge tension. Use the least number of sutures possible to accomplish this goal, as each suture is a foreign body that increases the risk of infection.
b. Skin sutures of monofilament material should be used to approximate the skin edges in an interrupted fashion.
c. Let anatomic landmarks serve as guides for closure, e.g., aligning the vermilion border, the eyebrow, or the helical rim of the ear.

9

WOUND HEALING, CARE, AND COMPLICATIONS

d. Observe periodically, q 24 h, for drainage or infection.

e. Remove sutures on the face in 4-5 days; all other sutures should be removed within 7 days.

f. Wounds that are left open should be cleaned, débrided, and packed with normal saline-moistened gauze. The dressing should then be changed q 8-12 h.

g. Antibiotics are indicated for cellulitic or infected wounds, immunocompromised or diabetic patients, and all bites.

h. Delayed primary closure may be performed after several days of dressing changes, when the wound is free of devitalized tissue and infection.

C. EXCEPTIONS (CONSIDER LEAVING WOUND OPEN)

1. Human bites—Heavy bacterial inoculums
2. >8 hours elapsed since wounding (the face is an exception)
3. Obviously inflamed or infected wounds
4. Crushed or ischemic tissue—Contusion avulsion injury
5. Sustained high-level steroid use

D. WOUND DRESSINGS

1. Protect the wound from trauma.
2. Provide an environment for healing.
3. Antibacterial ointments (bacitracin, Neosporin, Polysporin, etc.)—Provide a moist environment conducive to epithelialization.
4. Clean surgical wounds—Dressings should be left in place for 48 hours to allow epithelialization to occur. The ideal dressing is sterilely applied and provides absorption, protection, immobilization, and compression if needed. Dressings should be removed earlier if saturated by blood or serosanguineous fluid, or for suspicion of infection.
5. Contaminated wounds—Following thorough cleansing and sharp débridement, the wound should be packed open to promote hemostasis and drainage. Wet-to-dry dressings should be changed every 8-12 hours for further mechanical débridement of the wound.

a. Normal saline is isotonic and nontoxic.

b. Dakin's solution, 0.25% acetic acid, and povidone-iodine may inhibit formation of granulation tissue. However, in heavily contaminated, colonized, or infected wounds, their antiseptic benefits often justify their use.

E. TETANUS AND RABIES PROPHYLAXIS

1. Tetanus is caused by the toxin of *Clostridium tetani.*

a. Tetanus-prone wounds are old (>6 hours), deep (>1 cm), devitalized, and contaminated, especially those involving rusty metal, feces, or soil.

b. In children <7 years of age, immunization requires four injections of diphtheria-pertussis-tetanus vaccine. A fifth dose may be given at 4-6 years of age. Thereafter, adult type (Td) is recommended for routine or wound boosters.

2. Specific measures for patients with wounds

a. Previously immunized individuals

    (1) If the patient is fully immunized and the last dose of toxoid was given within 10 years, for nontetanus-prone wounds no booster of toxoid is indicated. For tetanus-prone wounds and if >5 years have elapsed since the last dose, 0.5 mL of adsorbed toxoid should be given IM.

    (2) When the patient has had 2 or more prior injections of toxoid and received the last dose more than 10 years previously, 0.5 mL of adsorbed toxoid should be given for both tetanus-prone and nontetanus-prone wounds. Passive immunization is not required.

b. Individuals *not* adequately immunized (or unknown)

    (1) For nontetanus-prone wounds, 0.5 mL of adsorbed toxoid should be given.

    (2) For tetanus-prone wounds, 0.5 mL of adsorbed toxoid and ≥250 units of human tetanus immune globulin should be given using different needles, syringes, and sites of injection. Administration of antibiotics should be considered, although their effectiveness in prophylaxis is unproven.

3. Rabies is a potentially fatal disease caused by the rabies virus, a single-stranded RNA virus of the rhabdovirus group. Generally <5 cases are reported in the United States each year.

a. Prophylaxis is indicated for bites by carnivorous wild animals (especially skunks, raccoons, foxes, coyotes, and bats). Prophylaxis is not indicated for bites by domestic animals (unless they are thought to be rabid or are unable to be supervised for the emergence of rabid characteristics) or rodents, e.g., mice, rats, or squirrels.

b. Previously nonimmunized persons should receive one 1-mL dose of human diploid cell vaccine (HDCV) by IM injection on days 0, 3, 7, 14, and 28 (a total of five doses). Rabies immune globulin (RIG) 20 IU/kg (preferable) or equine antirabies serum (ARS) 40 IU/kg should be given prior to day 8, with half the dose infiltrated in the area of the wound and the remainder given IM. RIG or ARS is not indicated after day 8.

VI. MANAGEMENT OF WOUND COMPLICATIONS

1. Wound infection—50% of all postoperative complications are wound related. Most of these are infections.

a. Incidence is increased in prolonged preoperative stay, breaks in surgical technique, long operation, abdominal procedures, and any factor that adversely affects wound healing.

b. Most commonly occur 3-7 days after surgery with advent of fever. Wound is red, warm, tender, and fluctuant and often has drainage.

c. Wound infections within 24-48 hours are frequently caused by clostridia or group A streptococci.

d. Common pathogens are staphylococci and streptococci. If a hollow viscus has been entered, consider gram-negative bacteria.

9

WOUND HEALING, CARE, AND COMPLICATIONS

e. Necrotizing fasciitis—Aggressive surgical débridement is essential in the treatment of this polymicrobial infection that spreads in the plane of the SQ tissue and fascia.

f. Treatment of wound infections includes opening the wound and drainage and débridement as necessary. The fascia should be visually and manually inspected for integrity. Cultures should be obtained and dressing changes should be initiated. Broad-spectrum antibiotics are indicated until results of cultures have been obtained.

2. Seromas and hematomas—Fluid collections

a. Use closed-suction drains (Jackson-Pratt) when flaps are elevated. Seromas can be aspirated with sterile technique. Drains minimally increase the incidence of infection but are effective in preventing seromas.

b. Expanding hematomas must be evacuated and bleeding controlled, usually in the operative arena. Small, nonexpanding hematomas may be left alone but should be watched for signs of infection. Evacuated hematomas may be closed if otherwise clean.

3. Ischemic necrosis—Caused by compromised arterial inflow or venous outflow, or by tension at the site of closure that may strangulate tissues. Necrotic tissue should be débrided.

4. Wound dehiscence

a. Superficial—Separation of skin edges; may be reclosed if not infected; otherwise treat as an open contaminated wound

b. Fascial—Separation of fascia with potential for evisceration; associated with 15% mortality

   (1) The most common causes are local ischemia, increased intra-abdominal pressure, underlying or concomitant illness, and technical problems. Typical occurrence at postoperative days 5-8 is heralded by sudden drainage of pink, serosanguineous, "salmon-colored" peritoneal fluid.

   (2) If evisceration occurs, cover the wound with sterile saline-soaked towels and arrange immediate operative intervention and repair. Minor fascial separation without evisceration may be treated expectantly with later repair of the resultant hernia.

c. Retention sutures are used to prevent evisceration in the event of fascial dehiscence and have no influence on whether dehiscence will or will not occur. They are usually placed in high-risk patients and should be removed around postoperative day 21.

VII. PRINCIPLES OF DRAIN MANAGEMENT

A. INDICATIONS

Drains are rarely indicated in uninfected wounds unless flaps have been or fluid collections are anticipated. Closed-suction drains have the lowest incidence of infection and are removed as drainage decreases.

B. INTRA-ABDOMINAL DRAINS

Use closed-suction drains. Penrose drains work best with the help of gravity, but they provide a two-way route for bacteria.

1. Infection—Drains are placed in abscess cavity or dependent areas for drainage and to produce a tract. They are usually left in place for at least 7-10 days and then are slowly advanced out over 2 days.

2. Peritonitis—Drains are not effective in draining the whole peritoneal cavity and should not be used for generalized infection.

9

WOUND HEALING, CARE, AND COMPLICATIONS

Surgical Infections

Gina Quaid, MD

I. DEFINITIONS

A. SURGICAL INFECTION
A surgical infection is an infection that requires operative treatment or results from operative treatment.
1. Nonoperative infections
a. Necrotizing soft tissue infections
b. Body cavity infections
   (1) Peritonitis
   (2) Suppurative pericarditis
   (3) Empyema
c. Confined tissue, organ, or joint infections
   (1) Abscess
   (2) Septic arthritis
d. Prosthetic infections
2. Operative infections
a. Wound infection
b. Postoperative abscess
c. Tertiary peritonitis
d. Other postoperative body cavity infections
e. Prosthetic device–related infection
f. Other hospital-acquired infections
   (1) Pneumonia
   (2) Urinary tract infection
   (3) Vascular catheter–related infections

II. DETERMINANTS OF INFECTION

A. MICROBIAL PATHOGENICITY AND NUMBER
1. Virulence of organism
2. Number of organisms present

B. HOST DEFENSES
1. Local
a. Epithelial layer protects underlying tissues
b. Lack of moisture in skin
c. Flushing action of tears and urine
d. Cilia
e. Mucus
f. pH
g. Local immunity
2. Systemic
a. Phagocytic cells

b. Immune system
c. Molecular cascades
   (1) Complement system
   (2) Coagulation system
   (3) Kinin system

C. LOCAL ENVIRONMENTAL FACTORS
1. Devitalization of tissue
2. Foreign bodies
3. Fluid collections
4. Edema
5. Comorbid conditions (peripheral vascular disease)
6. Shock

D. SURGICAL TECHNIQUE
1. Prevention of infection
a. Handle tissues gently.
b. Remove devitalized tissues, blood, and other substances that promote microbe growth.
c. Use drains appropriately.
d. Avoid excessive cautery.
e. Do not do anastomoses under tension or with inadequate blood supply.

III. POSTOPERATIVE FEVER

A. FEVER AT 0-48 HOURS
1. Atelectasis—Treat with incentive spirometry, cough and deep breathing, ambulation, and/or pulmonary toilet.
2. Wound infection—Soft tissue infection with clostridia or group A streptococcus
a. Rapidly spreading wound erythema and lymphangitis
b. Treatment is immediate opening of wound and administering antibiotics. All wounds should be examined in patients with early postoperative fever, because these infections spread rapidly and have high mortality rates if treatment is delayed.
3. Leakage of bowel anastomosis
a. Diffuse abdominal tenderness
b. Immediate demonstration with diagnostic radiographs
c. Treat with celiotomy
4. Aspiration pneumonia
a. Cough, decreased breath sounds, and rhonchi
b. Chest radiograph with infiltrates
c. Pulmonary toilet and antibiotics

B. AFTER POSTOPERATIVE DAY 3
1. Urinary tract infection

a. Especially common in instrumented patients
b. Diagnose by both urinalysis and culture.
c. Antibiotic treatment

2. Wound infection—Usually not seen until postoperative day 3-5 (see section III. A. 2 for treatment)

3. Catheter infections

a. Local catheter-related infection
   (1) Manifestations may include redness, streaking, tenderness, purulence, and lymphangitis.
   (2) Removal of catheter is usually adequate. Culture the tip.

b. Catheter-related sepsis
   (1) Manifestations—Signs of local catheter infection and isolation of same organism from blood and catheter, signs of systemic toxicity, and no other source of septicemia
   (2) Treat by removal of catheter. If temperature and white blood cell (WBC) count return to normal within 24 hours, no antibiotics are needed.

c. Septic thrombophlebitis
   (1) Should be suspected when signs of sepsis, positive blood cultures, and local inflammation persist after removal of offending catheter
   (2) Surgical removal of the affected vein is required.

4. Intra-abdominal abscess

a. Manifests between 3-5 days with abdominal pain and associated clinical signs of infection
b. Diagnosis and possible percutaneous drainage via CT scan

5. Deep venous thrombosis

a. Usually postoperative days 7-10, but can occur anytime
b. Diagnose with duplex Doppler ultrasound and impedance plethysmography.
c. Treatment with heparin and concomitant warfarin initially, followed by 3-6 months of warfarin therapy, depending on site of thrombus

6. Cholecystitis

a. Acalculus—Seen in critically ill patients, associated with NPO status and parenteral nutrition
b. Calculus—Occurs postoperatively in patients with known cholelithiasis
c. Diagnosis by ultrasound with or without hepatobiliary iminodiacetic acid (HIDA) scan

7. Other causes—Pulmonary embolus, sinusitis (especially in patients with endotracheal or nasogastric tubes), salivary/parotid glands (check amylase), prostate, perirectal abscess, drug fevers, inflammation in ears or throat, factitious fever

8. New and unrelated diseases should be considered, e.g., appendicitis, neoplasm.

10

SURGICAL INFECTIONS

IV. DIAGNOSIS

A. HISTORY AND PHYSICAL EXAM

B. SIGNS AND SYMPTOMS
1. Five cardinal signs
a. Dolor—Pain
b. Rubor—Redness
c. Calor—Heat
d. Tumor—Swelling
e. Functio laesa—Loss of function
2. Other tissue response
a. Fluctuance
b. Crepitance
c. Drainage
3. Systemic response
a. Fever
b. Rigors
c. Tachycardia
d. Tachypnea

C. LABORATORY
1. WBC count with differential
a. Increased in presence of infection
b. Differential—Left shift: presence of bands and immature WBCs in the blood
c. Neutropenia may be seen in overwhelming sepsis.
2. Renal panel or arterial blood gas determination—Evaluation of HCO_3 or pH for signs of sepsis

D. SPECIMEN COLLECTION
1. Aspiration of fluid collection
2. Aspiration of *edge* of cellulitic area (instillation of 1-2 mL of sterile nonbacteriostatic saline may increase yield)
3. Wound or fluid swab
4. Tissue biopsy
5. Blood cultures
a. 2 sets each time from a peripheral vein and/or indwelling catheters
b. Must obtain at time of fever or at timed intervals
c. 30% are positive
6. Urine and sputum cultures

E. CULTURE TECHNIQUES
1. Obtain Gram stain on all specimens.
2. Aerobic and anaerobic cultures—Remember to obtain pertinent sampling vehicles for specimens prior to collection.

3. Identification of specific organisms
a. Viral infections
    (1) Immunofluorescent methods of scraped cells
    (2) Immunologic studies of serum
    (3) Molecular techniques (polymerase chain reaction?)
b. Fungal infections
    (1) Gram stains
    (2) Tissue biopsy
    (3) Retinal exams for systemic disease (e.g., fluffy white retinal infiltrates that extend into the vitreous)

F. IMAGING TECHNIQUES
1. Radiograph
a. Air-fluid levels
b. Gas in tissues or portal system
c. New opacities
2. CT scan
a. Evaluation for intra-abdominal or intrathoracic pathology
b. Therapeutic interventions are possible.
3. Ultrasound
a. Localizes intra-abdominal abscess
b. Characterizes fluid collections
c. Therapeutic interventions are possible.
4. Tagged (radiolabeled) or gallium WBC scan
a. Patient's WBCs labeled with indium or gallium and reinfused
b. Cells pool at site(s) of inflammation.
c. Very nonspecific and poor localization
d. Require 12-72 hours for completion

10

SURGICAL INFECTIONS

V. PRINCIPLES OF THERAPY

A. OPERATIVE INTERVENTION
1. Incision and drainage of fluid collections
2. Débridement of necrotic tissue and foreign bodies
3. Removal of contaminated foreign bodies

B. WOUND MANAGEMENT
1. Left open when contaminated
2. Dressing
a. Moist to dry—Some cases use antimicrobial saturated dressings.
b. Changed at least b.i.d., but could be as often as q 4 h with necrotizing wounds

C. ANTIBIOTICS THERAPY
1. Types of antibiotics

a. Bacteriostatic—Prevents growth and multiplication of bacteria but does not kill them; rely on defense mechanisms of the host to clear infection

b. Bactericidal—Kills bacteria; must be employed in immunocompromised patients

2. Selection of antibiotics

a. Empiric choices—Based on likely infecting organism, often related to endogenous flora of involved organ

b. Specific choices—Based on culture results and sensitivities

c. Other factors
   (1) Ensure adequate contact between the drug and the infecting agent.
      (a) Adequate dosage
      (b) Adequate tissue perfusion
      (c) Drugs reach the site or organism via routes such as biliary excretion and CNS penetration.
   (2) Minimize potential side effects.
   (3) Maximize host defenses.

d. Treatment failure is considered after 24-72 hours of treatment without improvement.

3. Antibiotic prophylaxis

a. Prevention of surgical infection

b. Indications
   (1) Traumatic wounds with contamination, delay of treatment, injury to a hollow viscus
   (2) Clean-contaminated, and contaminated operations
   (3) Resection/anastomosis of colon or intestine
   (4) Prosthetic devices are or will be present.
   (5) Valvular heart disease
   (6) Immunocompromised patient
   (7) Shock
   (8) Ischemic tissue present
   (9) Open fractures, penetrating joint injuries

c. Duration of 24-48 hours with no complications

d. Intestinal preparation prior to surgery
   (1) Mechanical cleansing with systemic antibiotics
   (2) Oral antibiotics slowly falling out of favor secondary to systemic antimicrobial therapy

4. Complications of antibiotic therapy

a. Drug toxicity
   (1) Presents with drug fever, rashes, or anaphylaxis on starting agent
   (2) Neurologic complications (seizures, neuropathy), GI symptoms, renal dysfunction, blood/bone marrow dyscrasias, visual and auditory losses

b. Emergence of resistant strains

c. Superinfection with microorganisms resistant to current regimen (gram-negative bacteria or *Candida* spp)

VI. SOFT TISSUE INFECTION

A. FOCAL INFECTIONS

1. Cutaneous abscesses

a. Furuncle ("boil")—Abscess in a sweat gland or hair follicle

b. Carbuncle—Multilocular suppurative extension of a furuncle into adjacent SQ tissue; usually caused by staphylococci

c. Impetigo—Intraepithelial abscesses, usually caused by contagious staphylococci or streptococci

2. Pyoderma gangrenosum—Rare

a. Painful, raised pustule with necrotic center, which progresses to spreading ulceration

b. 60-80% are associated with underlying condition—Inflammatory bowel disease, polyarthritis, or leukemia

c. Treat by local wound care and antimicrobials. Treatment of underlying condition is essential.

3. Meleney's progressive synergistic gangrene

a. Appears after injury or operation on purulent pleural or peritoneal infection, usually after ≥2 weeks

b. Characterized by necrotic center, bluish undermined edges, and surrounding erythema

c. Synergistic infection with *Staphylococcus aureus* and microaerophilic *Streptococcus* spp

d. Treat by wide excision, open wound care, and high-dose penicillin or vancomycin

B. DIFFUSE NON-NECROTIZING INFECTIONS

1. Cellulitis

a. Nonsuppurative inflammation of SQ tissues

b. Presents with redness, swelling, pain, often fever and chills

c. Streptococci and staphylococci are the most common organisms. Gram-negative bacilli may be present, especially in diabetic patients.

d. Failure to improve after 72 hours of antibiotics suggests abscess formation or necrotizing process (see section VI. C), requiring incision and drainage

2. Lymphangitis

a. Inflammation of lymphatic channels manifested by erythematous streaks

b. Often accompanies cellulitis, usually associated with streptococcal infections

c. Regional lymphadenopathy usually seen

d. Appropriate antibiotic therapy is usually sufficient treatment.

3. Erysipelas

a. Acute spreading streptococcal cellulitis and lymphangitis. Lesions are raised with defined margins.

b. Usually responds well to antibiotic therapy

10

SURGICAL INFECTIONS

C. DIFFUSE NECROTIZING INFECTIONS

1. Nonclostridial

a. A spectrum of life-threatening necrotizing infections, including necrotizing fasciitis, Fournier's gangrene (necrotizing fasciitis of the perineum), gram-negative synergistic necrotizing cellulitis that manifests as extensive necrosis of SQ tissue, and superficial fascia with widespread undermining of surrounding tissues and severe systemic toxicity; more common in diabetic patients

b. Causal organisms are anaerobic *Streptococcus* spp, *Staphylococcus* spp, and *Bacteroides* spp.

c. Characterized by erythematous skin, edema beyond erythema, crepitance, hemodynamic derangements due to systemic sepsis

d. Diagnosis—Confirmed by serosanguineous exudate, necrotic fascia with extensive undermining; Gram stain demonstrates gram-positive organisms, WBCs

e. Treatment—Emergent aggressive wide débridement and broad-spectrum antibiotics; hyperbaric oxygen may be helpful, but used as secondary treatment; may require daily operative débridement to prevent ongoing infection

2. Clostridial myonecrosis (gas gangrene)

a. Rapidly progressive invasion of muscle by anaerobic *Clostridium* spp

b. Treatment—Emergent wide débridement or amputation, and antibiotics (IV high-dose penicillin). Delay of treatment may be fatal. Hyperbaric oxygen may be helpful but, again, as secondary treatment.

VII. OTHER INFECTIONS

A. INTRA-ABDOMINAL ABSCESS

1. Localized collection of pus walled off from the rest of the peritoneal cavity by inflammatory adhesions and viscera
2. Usually polymicrobial, with aerobic and anaerobic organisms
3. Clinical manifestations
a. Fever, tachycardia, and anorexia
b. Paralytic ileus and/or abdominal pain
c. Elevated WBC with shift
4. Diagnosis—Ultrasound or CT scan
5. Treatment
a. Drainage—Percutaneous, transrectal, transvaginal, or open surgical
b. Antibiotic therapy should cover aerobic and anaerobic organisms.

B. ANTIBIOTIC-ASSOCIATED (PSEUDOMEMBRANOUS) COLITIS

1. Overgrowth of *Clostridium difficile*—Can be caused by any antibiotic, and can be induced after one dose
2. Clinical manifestation
a. Watery, nonbloody diarrhea
b. Fever, leukocytosis, abdominal pain, and distention may be present.

3. Diagnosis
a. Organism, toxin, and fecal leukocytes detected in stool
b. Sigmoidoscopy reveals yellow-white, exudative pseudomembranes.
4. Treatment
a. Discontinue offending antibiotic.
b. IV or PO metronidazole—Oral vancomycin has also been used, but it is falling out of favor as first-line therapy due to the emergence of vancomycin-resistant *Enterococcus* spp.

C. WOUND INFECTIONS
1. **Conditions associated with increased wound infection rates**—Extremes of age, malnutrition, decreased blood flow to wound, cirrhosis, steroids, immunosuppression, leukopenia, foreign body, devitalized tissue, fluid collections, cancer, irradiated tissue, diabetes mellitus
2. **Classification of surgical wounds and expected wound infection rates**
a. Clean (skin, vascular)—1.5-5%
b. Clean-contaminated (GI, GU, gynecologic, respiratory tract surgery)—≈7% if prophylactic antibiotics used
c. Contaminated (penetrating trauma, bowel spillage)—10-15%
d. Dirty/infected (gross pus, gangrene, bowel perforation)—15-40%
3. **Superficial wound infections**—75% of wound infections
a. Involve skin and SQ tissues, superficial to fascia and muscle
b. Clinical manifestation—Wound erythematous with seroma, drainage with or without bacteria, fluctuance, tenderness, and nonhealing
c. Management—Open wound
   (1) Wound may be opened and cultured (aerobic and anaerobic) at the bedside.
   (2) Fascia should be palpated to prove it is intact.
   (3) Complicated wounds (extreme obesity, uncooperative patient, wound failure, fistula) should be explored in the OR.
   (4) Begin wet-to-dry saline dressing changes t.i.d. Showers may be helpful to clean the wound.
   (5) Systemic antibiotics if patient has systemic manifestation of infection and/or associated cellulites, is immunocompromised, or has prosthetic devices
   (6) Wound may be closed secondarily when infection has cleared and healthy granulation tissue is present.
4. **Deep wound infections**
a. Involves muscles, fascia, and/or structures deep to them
b. Clinical manifestation—As in section VII. C. 3. b, plus fascial dehiscence, drainage between fascial sutures, evisceration, and ileus
c. Management
   (1) Explore in the OR.
   (2) For fascial dehiscence—Explore abdominal wound to rule out fistula or abscess, débride necrotic fascia, and primarily close. Consider retention sutures to prevent evisceration if there is subsequent

dehiscence. Retention sutures may not prevent dehiscence, however. Leave skin and SQ tissue open.

   (3) Antibiotics

5. Prevention

a. Preoperative antimicrobial shower

b. Remove hair immediately before operation by clipping.

c. Administer prophylactic antibiotics 30 minutes before incision, and maintain therapeutic levels throughout the case.

d. Vigilance for breaks in aseptic technique

e. Appropriate skin preparation and sterile draping

f. Meticulous surgical technique

   (1) Monofilament sutures

   (2) Minimize sutures and ligatures (foreign bodies).

   (3) Do not strangulate tissues.

   (4) Meticulous skin closure

g. Avoidance of postoperative hypoxia

h. Surveillance of wounds for early signs of infection

VIII. ANTIMICROBIAL AGENTS

Antibiotics should be targeted toward an organism, not a disease.

A. PENICILLINS

Penicillins are bactericidal, with a β-lactam ring that blocks bacterial cell wall synthesis.

1. Streptococcal penicillins

a. Penicillins G, V

b. Drug of choice for *Streptococcus pyogenes* and clostridia

2. Staphylococcal penicillins—β-lactamase resistant

a. Methicillin, nafcillin, oxacillin, and dicloxacillin

b. *S. aureus* and *Staphylococcus epidermidis* only

3. Enterococcal penicillins—Ampicillin and amoxicillin

4. Antipseudomonal and gram-negative penicillins

a. Piperacillin, carbenicillin, mezlocillin, and ticarcillin

b. Used in conjunction with an antipseudomonal triple-drug regimen

5. Penicillin/β-lactamase inhibitor combinations

a. Ampicillin-sulbactam, amoxicillin-clavulanate, and ticarcillin-clavulanate

b. Covers gram-positive organisms, most *Bacteroides* spp, and gram-negative aerobes

c. Does not cover methicillin-resistant *S. aureus*

B. CEPHALOSPORINS

Cephalosporins are bactericidal, and their mechanism of action is similar to penicillins.

1. 5-10% allergic cross-reactivity with penicillin-sensitive patients

2. Staphylococcal cephalosporins

a. All cephalosporins, but first-generation best coverage is cefazolin

b. *Staphylococcus* spp, *Streptococcus* spp, and some aerobic coliforms

3. Anaerobe cephalosporins

a. Cefoxitin, cefotetan, cefmetazole, and moxalactam

b. Enhanced activity against aerobic gram-negative organisms and anaerobes, including most *Bacteroides fragilis*

4. Antipseudomonal cephalosporins

a. Cefoperazone, ceftazidime, and cefepime

b. Must be used in conjunction with antipseudomonal regimen

5. Coliform cephalosporins

a. Cefotaxime, ceftizoxime, ceftriaxone, cefoperazone, and cefepime

b. Effective against most coliforms, as well as *S. aureus* and streptococci

c. Enterococci, *Pseudomonas* spp, and *B. fragilis* have shown resistance.

C. MONOBACTAMS

Monobactams are monocyclic β-lactams, and they are bactericidal. Aztreonam is active only against gram-negative aerobes, including *Pseudomonas* spp.

D. CARBAPENEMS

Carbapenems are bactericidal, and the cilistatin prevents breakdown of the antibiotic.

1. Imipenem and meropenem

2. Very broad-spectrum agents; diphtheroids, *P. maltophilia,* and *Proteus mirabilis* are resistant

3. Best use in pancreatic infections

E. AMINOGLYCOSIDES

Aminoglycosides inhibit protein synthesis and are broad-spectrum bactericidal antibiotics.

1. Gentamicin, tobramycin, amikacin, and kanamycin

2. Enterococci and anaerobes are resistant.

3. Significant adverse effects include ototoxicity and nephrotoxicity. Ototoxicity is not reversible. There are significant drug interactions.

4. Avoid complications with 24-hour dosage at 5-7 mg/kg; classic dosage at 1.7 mg/kg q 8 h; must ensure good kidney perfusion prior to use

F. TRIMETHOPRIM AND SULFONAMIDES

Trimethoprim and sulfonamides provide inhibition of folates and pyrimidines, and the combination of drugs is bactericidal. These are the drug of choice for *Pneumocystis carinii* and *Nocardia* spp and first-line treatment of uncomplicated urinary tract infections.

G. FLUOROQUINOLONES

Fluoroquinolones provide inhibition of DNA synthesis, have a broad spectrum of activity, and are bactericidal.

10

SURGICAL INFECTIONS

1. Ciprofloxacin, levofloxacin, and moxifloxacin
2. First-line therapy in intra-abdominal infections
3. Useful as PO broad-spectrum agent and for refractory urinary tract infection

H. TETRACYCLINES

Tetracyclines inhibit protein synthesis, have variable broad-spectrum coverage, and are bacteriostatic.

1. Tetracycline and doxycycline
2. Frequently used with ceftriaxone in the empiric treatment of gonococcal/chlamydial sexually transmitted diseases
3. Should not be used in children or lactating mothers due to dental discoloration

I. OTHER AGENTS

1. Vancomycin and teicoplanin—Treat gram-positive organisms by bactericidal activity
   a. Drug of choice for methicillin-resistant *S. aureus* and useful orally for *C. difficile* pseudomembranous colitis refractory to metronidazole
   b. May cause ototoxicity and phlebitis at IV site; need to monitor serum levels
2. Macrolides—Inhibits protein synthesis, has a narrow spectrum, and is bacteriostatic (bactericidal for some gram-positive organisms)
   a. Erythromycin, azithromycin, and clarithromycin
   b. Drug of choice for *Legionella* spp and *Mycoplasma* spp. Erythromycin base is used for preoperative oral bowel prep (Nichols-Condon prep).
   c. Resistance common with long-term treatment; cause GI upset when given orally
   d. Also used as a motilin agonist
3. Metronidazole—Covers anaerobic, few gram-negative bacteria, amoebae, and trichomonads; bactericidal
   a. Key for abdominal infections, *C. difficile* colitis, and preoperative preparation for abdominal surgery
   b. Disulfuram (Antabuse)-like activity with alcohol intake; stocking-glove peripheral neuropathy and convulsions with long-term use
4. Clindamycin—Covers anaerobic and gram-positive cocci; is bacteriostatic
   a. Primarily used for anaerobic coverage in intra-abdominal infections and aspiration pneumonia
   b. Overgrowth of enteric *C. difficile* leading to pseudomembranous enterocolitis is major adverse effect.

J. ANTIFUNGAL AGENTS

1. Amphotericin B
   a. The only fungicidal drug available; effective against all species of fungus
   b. Begin therapy with 1-mg test dose, and if well tolerated, increase dose by 5-10 mg/day up to maximum of 15-30 mg/kg total dose.

Pretreatment with acetaminophen and diphenhydramine and perhaps hydrocortisone is recommended.

c. Major toxicity is renal. Dosing interval may have to be extended to every other day or every third day to avoid renal insufficiency.

2. Imidazoles and triazoles—Inhibit synthesis of ergosterol
a. Clotrimazole, miconazole, ketoconazole, fluconazole, and itraconazole
b. Active against most pathogenic fungi of surgical importance
c. Administered PO or IV
d. Less toxicity than associated with amphotericin

3. Flucytosine
a. For serious *Candida* spp and *Cryptococcus* spp infections
b. May act synergistically with amphotericin

4. Nystatin—Nonabsorbed oral agent used prophylactically in the immunosuppressed patient or those on broad-spectrum antibiotics to prevent GI overgrowth of *Candida* spp

IX. ACQUIRED IMMUNODEFICIENCY SYNDROME (AIDS)

A. GENERAL
1. Retro RNA virus attacks the CD4 receptor of T4 lymphocytes.
a. Internalized and incorporated into cellular DNA
b. Replication of the virus leads to cell destruction and infection of other cells.
2. Seropositivity 6-8 weeks after infection with the virus
3. T4 helper cell diminishes to a generalized state of immunocompromise
4. Serotesting
a. Enzyme-linked immunosorbent assay—Good screening test
b. Western blot—Definitive confirmatory test

B. EPIDEMIOLOGY
1. Homosexual males—10-70% HIV positive
2. IV drug abusers—5-60% HIV positive
3. Hemophiliacs—A, 70% HIV positive; B, 35% HIV positive
4. Sexual partners of 1-3 above—5% HIV positive
5. Study in Baltimore revealed 3% of critically ill patients and 16% of young trauma patients were HIV positive.

C. CLINICAL STAGES
The Centers for Disease Control and Prevention AIDS classification system is the following.
1. Category A—Asymptomatic carrier (largest group), generalized lymphadenopathy, acute retroviral infection (mononucleosis-like illness)
2. Category B—AIDS-related complex: endocarditis, oral candidiasis, herpes zoster, idiopathic thrombocytopenia purpura, tuberculosis; diseases must be attributed to HIV infection

10

SURGICAL INFECTIONS

3. Category C—AIDS: disseminated candidiasis, coccidioidomycosis, cytomegalovirus, Kaposi's sarcoma, lymphoma, *P. carinii* pneumonia, atypical mycobacterium

D. RISK TO HEALTH CARE WORKERS

1. Studies of needle sticks with contaminated needles demonstrate a seroconversion rate of 0.3-0.5% per stick
2. Risk to surgeons may be underestimated. Factors that determine the surgeon's risk are the following.
a. Number of contaminated needle sticks
b. Percentage of HIV-positive patients in a surgeon's patient population
c. Number of years at risk
3. Precautions
a. Wear gloves when at risk for body fluid exposure.
b. Protective clothing, mask, and goggles during procedures are required where material may be aerosolized or body fluid exposure is likely.
c. Wash hands after body fluid contact.
d. Treat all sharps as infected. Do not recap needles.
e. Clean up sharps after procedures to prevent injury to others.
f. Clean spills with ammonia, bleach, or other sterilizing agents.
g. Double-bag and label infective fluids.
4. Postexposure prophylaxis—Immediate administration of zidovudine after injury with a contaminated sharp may prevent infection. Confirmatory studies are pending.

E. RISK TO PATIENTS

1. Transfusion
a. Whole blood, packed red blood cells, platelets, plasma, cryoprecipitate, and leukocytes can carry HIV.
b. With antibody testing, the risk of transfusion-related transmission is now 1 in 36,000-100,000 per unit transfused.
2. Transplantation—Potential donor tissues must be tested.
3. Surgeon to patient—A theoretical risk; no documented cases

F. SURGICAL CONSIDERATIONS

1. Role of surgeons involves performing diagnostic biopsy procedures, providing supportive care, and managing complications of infectious and malignant processes.
2. Some surgical problems in HIV patients
a. Central venous access for chemotherapy
b. Acute cholecystitis, cholangitis secondary to cryptosporidiosis and cytomegalovirus infection
c. Splenectomy for marked splenomegaly or thrombocytopenia
d. GI perforations and obstructions from infectious agents and malignancies
e. Spontaneous pneumothorax due to *Pneumocystis* pneumonia

3. **Patients' risk of postoperative complications is related to their underlying condition.**
a. Patients with CD4 counts ≥500 are not at increased risk of opportunistic infections.
b. Asymptomatic HIV patients are not at increased risk of wound-healing complications.
c. Emergent procedures in AIDS patients are associated with high rates of morbidity and mortality.

10

SURGICAL INFECTIONS

The Diabetic Patient

Robert M. Cavagnol, MD

Diabetes mellitus is the most common metabolic disease that surgeons encounter. Not only do these patients suffer from acute problems such as increased susceptibility to infections, poor wound healing, diabetic ketoacidosis, and nonketotic hyperosmolar coma, but they present with the chronic problems of retinopathy, neuropathy, nephropathy, and advanced atherosclerosis, all of which may complicate their perioperative management.

I. GENERAL PRINCIPLES

11

A. DIAGNOSIS
Patients can be diagnosed with diabetes mellitus based on a fasting plasma glucose >140 mg/dL on two separate occasions or an abnormal glucose tolerance test. Patients can develop glucose intolerance in response to stress (trauma, surgery, infection, pregnancy). Glycosylated hemoglobin indicates mean blood glucose values over the long term and is useful for follow-up.

B. CLASSIFICATION
1. Type 1—20% of all diabetics; due to lack of insulin production; childhood or adolescent onset; prone to hyperglycemia and ketoacidosis
2. Type 2—Onset usually after 30 years of age; usually obese; due to insulin resistance and relative insulin deficiency; prone to nonketotic hyperosmolar coma (ketoacidosis is rare); patients usually require exogenous insulin during stress or perioperative period
3. Secondary diabetes
a. Pancreatic insufficiency—Chronic pancreatitis, hemochromatosis, postpancreatic resection
b. Hormonal excess—Cushing's disease, adrenocortical tumors
c. Medications—Steroids, thiazide diuretics

C. PREOPERATIVE EVALUATION
Preoperative evaluation for the presence and severity of diabetic complications include the following.
1. Cardiovascular
a. Atherosclerosis; history of angina, myocardial infarction, congestive heart failure, hypertension, claudication, and stroke or transient ischemic attacks
b. Examine to find evidence of congestive heart failure and bruits and to document distal pulses.
c. Labs—Baseline ECG; multiple gated acquisition (MUGA) scan or echocardiogram, and dipyridamole-thallium scan for major procedures in patients with symptoms of angina, congestive heart failure, or previous myocardial infarction. Remember that diabetic patients may also have "silent" or asymptomatic myocardial ischemia.

2. Nephropathy
a. Evidence of proteinuria or elevated creatinine level
b. Sensitive to nephrotoxic effects of IV contrast agent; hydrate before study and follow renal function afterward. *N*-acetylcysteine has been shown to be protective against the nephrotoxic effect of IV contrast agent.

3. Neuropathy—Autonomic and somatic nerves
a. Peripheral—Examine for lower extremity neuropathy (e.g., Charcot's joint).
b. Gastrointestinal—Gastroparesis with resulting gastric dilation may require metoclopramide, erythromycin, and/or nasogastric decompression during stress/surgery.
c. Hemodynamic—Postural hypotension

4. Infections
a. Leukocyte dysfunction (decreased chemotaxis and phagocytic activity) occurs when blood glucose >250 mg/dL.
b. Evidence of urinary tract infection (most common), pneumonia, bronchitis, skin infections, diabetic foot ulcers
c. At risk for development of candidiasis—Should be treated with nystatin for signs and symptoms of thrush and single PO dose of fluconazole for vaginal yeast infection while on antibiotics

5. Metabolic
a. Duration of diabetes, need for oral hypoglycemics, insulin dosage and schedule
b. History of episodes of hypoglycemia, diabetic ketoacidosis, and hyperglycemic coma

II. PERIOPERATIVE MANAGEMENT

In general, hospitalized diabetic patients are maintained at a slightly higher blood glucose level than at home because the consequences of prolonged hypoglycemia are much more severe than those of mild hyperglycemia.

A. PREOPERATIVE
1. Patients on oral hypoglycemic agent—Discontinue 1 day preoperatively.
2. Schedule early morning operation, if possible.
3. Start IV containing dextrose (i.e., D-5 ½ normal saline [NS]) the day of surgery at 50-75 mL/h (the minimum carbohydrate requirement is 100 g/day).
4. Give ⅓ of usual dose and type (i.e., NPH, Lente, Regular) of insulin SQ the morning of surgery.
5. Continuous IV infusion of regular insulin may be preferred for perioperative control of the brittle diabetic.

B. POSTOPERATIVE
1. Continue IV dextrose.
2. Follow glucose q 4-6 h with finger-stick blood sugar (FSBS) (must be correlated initially with serum glucose). Use insulin sliding scale

(see section IV) to maintain serum glucose between 100-180 mg/dL. A recent *New England Journal of Medicine* study[1] showed that tighter blood glucose control (90-140 mg/dL) using an insulin drip in critically ill patients improved survival. Absorption may be erratic with SQ administration in patients with poor peripheral perfusion (i.e., hypotensive, hypothermic).

3. Adjust insulin dose with resumption of oral diet or enteral feeding. Convert to intermediate (NPH) regimen by giving 80% of the previous 24-hour insulin requirements as $2/3$ NPH and $1/3$ Regular. Continue to monitor FSBS.

4. Resume oral hypoglycemic agent when the patient is tolerating solid food.

III. MANAGEMENT OF COMPLICATIONS

A. HYPOGLYCEMIA (<60 mg/dL)

Hypoglycemia occurs most commonly in brittle diabetics. It must be suspected in obtunded patients receiving insulin.

1. Treat with oral carbohydrates (milk or orange juice). If the patient is obtunded, give 1 ampule of D-50 IV push and repeat as needed; failure to respond at this point should lead one to question the diagnosis. Start D-5-W via a peripheral IV and continue to monitor FSBS.

2. Adjust insulin sliding scale or infusion.

B. NONKETOTIC HYPEROSMOLAR HYPERGLYCEMIA

Nonketotic hyperosmolar hyperglycemia is a condition of extreme hyperglycemia (>600 mg/dL) and hyperosmolality with mental status changes. It is usually precipitated by stress, trauma, surgery, sepsis, or total parenteral nutrition.

1. Findings—Include CNS changes from lethargy to coma and/or seizures, hypotension, tachycardia (extreme dehydration secondary to osmotic diuresis), and nausea/vomiting (ileus)

2. Therapy

a. The patient may require an ICU setting for invasive monitoring. Place a nasogastric tube and Foley catheter to facilitate output measurements.

b. Begin hydration with NS solution to correct extreme dehydration. Urine output cannot be used as an indicator of fluid resuscitation due to osmotic diuresis.

c. Serial electrolyte, glucose, and arterial blood gas determinations

d. Give 10 units insulin IV and begin insulin drip at 5-10 units/h; should not decrease serum glucose >100 mg/dL per hour to avoid cerebral edema

e. Once serum glucose is <300 mg/dL, add D-5 to IV fluids.

f. Replace potassium, magnesium, and phosphate levels as needed.

g. Investigate precipitating cause (e.g., infection).

11

THE DIABETIC PATIENT

C. DIABETIC KETOACIDOSIS

Diabetic ketoacidosis is similar to nonketotic hyperglycemia except that the patient is severely acidotic secondary to ketone production.

1. Findings—Include CNS changes, tachycardia, hypotension secondary to dehydration, dysrhythmias secondary to hypokalemia, Kussmaul respirations (rapid deep breathing), and abdominal pain; serum potassium level may be high initially secondary to acidosis but falls with hydration and correction of acidosis.

2. Therapy—See treatment of nonketotic hyperosmolar hyperglycemia (section III. B. 2). May need to correct acidosis with $NaHCO_3$ IV if pH < 7.20. Continue insulin therapy until ketonemia is resolved.

IV. INSULIN SLIDING SCALE

The insulin sliding scale varies among patients, but this is good starting point.

A. RECOMMENDATIONS FOR SQ

Serum Glucose (mg/dL)	When to Give SQ
<50	1 ampule D-50 IV push and call house officer
50-150	0 units
151-200	3 units Regular SQ
201-250	6 units Regular SQ
251-300	9 units Regular SQ
301-350	12 units Regular SQ
351-400	15 units Regular SQ
>400	18 units Regular SQ and call house officer (blood glucose should be rechecked 2 hours after dose is given)

B. RECOMMENDATIONS FOR IV

1. Monitored setting only
2. q 2 h Accu-Cheks
3. Start IV insulin infusions at 5 units/h and increase by 2-3 units/h for blood glucose levels >150 mg/dL; for blood glucose levels >250 mg/dL, give bolus 10 units IV, then increase by 2-3 units/h as needed.

V. TYPES OF INSULIN

A. HUMAN INSULIN (HUMULIN)

Human insulin should be used as the standard class of insulin (as opposed to bovine or porcine). With its recombinant DNA source, it is useful in diabetic patients with antibodies to animal-derived insulin.

B. INSULIN CHARACTERISTICS

Action	Type	Onset (hours)	Peak (hours)	Duration (hours)
Short	Regular	$1/_2$-1	2-4	6
	Semilente	$1/_2$-1	4-8	12-16
Intermediate	NPH	1-2	8-12	18-24
	Lente	1-2	8-12	18-24
Long	Protamine zinc	4-8	12-24	36
	Ultralente	4-8	12-24	36

REFERENCE

1. van den Berghe G, Wouters P, Weekers F, et al: Intensive insulin therapy in the critically ill patients. N Engl J Med 345: 1359-1367, 2001.

11

THE DIABETIC PATIENT

Thromboembolic Prophylaxis and Management of Deep Venous Thrombosis

Steven R. Allen, MD

I. GENERAL REMARKS

A. EPIDEMIOLOGY

Deep venous thrombosis (DVT) is a common problem in surgical patients of all types. Estimates of the occurrence of DVT after various surgical procedures without DVT prophylaxis include the following.

1. Orthopedic procedure—46-66%
2. Prostatectomy—50%
3. General surgery (intra-abdominal)—22-33%
4. Trauma—20%
5. Postpartum—3%

B. ETIOLOGY

The three factors that contribute to the development of venous thrombosis are referred to as *Virchow's triad*.

1. Venous stasis
2. Endothelial injury
3. Hypercoagulable

C. RISK FACTORS FOR THE DEVELOPMENT OF DVT

1. Age >60 years
2. Malignancy (especially prostate cancer, pancreatic cancer, and carcinomatosis)
3. Prior history of DVT, pulmonary embolism (PE), or varicose veins
4. Prolonged immobilization or bedrest
5. Cardiac disease, especially congestive heart failure
6. Obesity
7. Major surgery, especially pelvic surgery
8. Trauma
9. Hypercoagulable, congenital or acquired
10. Pregnancy
11. Oral contraceptives

D. CLINICAL PRESENTATION

The clinical presentation in DVT is nonspecific and may include signs or symptoms of extremity swelling and/or tenderness, calf pain on ankle dorsiflexion (Homans' sign), or fever. Clinical diagnosis is inaccurate.

1. <50% of patients with these signs or symptoms have a DVT.

12

2. Only ≈50% of patients with documented DVT by venography have any signs and symptoms.
3. Diagnosis—Best made with venography (gold standard), Doppler ultrasonography, or impedance plethysmography; radioisotope fibrinogen studies are poor in diagnosing proximal vein thrombosis
4. If the diagnosis of DVT is established in a patient without any risk factors, an occult malignancy should be suspected and worked up.

E. SEQUELAE
1. PE is potentially the most lethal result of DVT. One in 200 patients undergoing a major operation dies from massive pulmonary embolus, accounting for 50,000 deaths/yr. Ten percent of the deaths occur within 60 minutes of the first symptom. This underscores the importance of prophylaxis versus treatment.
   a. Calf vein thrombosis rarely gives rise to PE unless there is propagation into the femoral vein.
   b. Pulmonary emboli can originate from the iliofemoral, pelvic, ovarian, axillary, subclavian and internal jugular veins, as well as the inferior vena cava (IVC) and the cavernous sinuses of the skull.
   c. Clinical manifestations of PE are inconsistent and nonspecific but may include dyspnea, chest pain, hemoptysis, tachycardia, recent fever, rales, and accentuated P_2 heart sound. Also there may be ECG changes such as arrhythmias, enlarged P waves, ST depression, and T-wave inversions (particularly in III, aVF, V_1, V_3, and V_4).
   d. Diagnosis is established by *pulmonary arteriography*. A high probability ventilation/perfusion ($\dot{V}/\dot{Q}$) scan coupled with a high clinical suspicion to PE may obviate the need for arteriography; low probability scans effectively exclude PE. CT of the pulmonary arteries with thin cuts through the pulmonary vasculature is also commonly used for high clinical suspicion, with or without a moderate to high probability $\dot{V}/\dot{Q}$ scan (less invasive than arteriography).
2. Post-thrombotic syndrome—Occurs in 50% of patients with acute DVT and reflects chronic venous insufficiency; brawny, nonpitting edema and ulcer formation eventually occur
3. Severe cases of DVT may cause phlegmasia cerulea dolens (a loss of sensory and motor function secondary to compromised arterial supply to the limb from severe swelling).

F. UPPER EXTREMITY DVT
Upper extremity DVT typically presents with upper extremity swelling and/or pain. Patients may also present with superior venacaval syndrome and loss of upper extremity vascular access. There is a significant incidence of PE. Morbidity and mortality rates from upper extremity DVTs are higher than from lower extremity DVTs.
1. Primary thrombosis—A rare disorder of the upper extremity that occurs in the dominant arm of an otherwise healthy individual

a. Either idiopathic or part of Paget-Schroetter syndrome
b. Occurs spontaneously after strenuous physical exertion
c. Heavy exertion or effort thrombosis is thought to cause microtrauma to the venous intima, leading to initiation and propagation of the coagulation cascade.
2. Secondary thrombosis—Axillary or subclavian vein thrombosis is occurring more frequently in surgical patients due to the increasing use of indwelling catheters for total parenteral nutrition, bone marrow transplant, chemotherapy, and central cardiovascular monitoring.
3. Superior vena cava obstruction is usually related to tumor invasion; however, it may also be due to primary thrombosis, chronic fibrosing mediastinitis, or granulomatous disease.
4. IVC thrombosis in adults is usually a consequence of extension of thrombi from pelvic or thigh veins. Tumor thrombus is a consequence of tumor invasion (e.g., renal, hepatic, adrenal, soft tissue) into the vena cava. There is an increased incidence of tumor thrombus embolization.

II. METHODS OF PROPHYLAXIS

A. MECHANICAL
1. Leg elevation—Has been advised historically but without substantive support
2. Graduated compression stockings—Must be well fitted; however, they have a modest if appreciable effect
3. Early ambulation—Simple and effective
4. Pneumatic compression boots—Intermittently inflate and deflate; cause compression of the limb, usually the calves
a. Mechanism of action is by both propulsion of blood flow proximally and activation of fibrinolytic system. Boots are effective even when placed on the arms.
b. Reduce risk of DVT by 50-75% in general surgery patients and 66% in neurosurgery patients
c. Confer an increased risk of bleeding and are therefore especially important in neurosurgical and ophthalmologic patients

B. PHARMACOLOGIC AGENTS
1. Aspirin acts by irreversibly inactivating platelet cyclooxygenase and has been shown to be effective in patients undergoing hip surgery. It is not currently recommended as adequate DVT prophylaxis.
2. Dextran solution (40 and 70) is a branched polysaccharide solution that causes decreased platelet adhesiveness, aggregation, and release reaction in addition to red blood cell and factor VIII and plasma volume effects.
a. Disadvantages
   (1) Increased rate of bleeding

(2) Pulmonary edema due to volume overload in patients with cardiac compromise

(3) Allergic reactions in 1% of patients

b. Recommended perioperative dosage is 15-20 mL/h continuous IV infusion

3. Warfarin (Coumadin)

a. Shown to decrease incidence of DVT by 66% and PE by 80% in patients undergoing hip surgery

b. Disadvantages

(1) Severe hemorrhage in 2-7% of patients

(2) Must be started 2-3 days preoperatively

(3) Must monitor prothrombin time (PT) closely

4. Heparin (unfractionated) accentuates antithrombin III inhibition of factor X and thrombin and may also potentiate the disintegration of thrombi that form while it is being administered.

a. "Low-dose" regimen of 5000 units SQ 2 hours preoperatively, then q 12 h postoperatively until the patient is fully ambulatory, has been shown to decrease the incidence of DVT by $2/3$ and PE by $1/2$ in general, urologic, and orthopedic surgical patients.

b. For morbidly obese patients, a "microheparin" drip at 1 unit/kg per hour is believed to be more effective. Alternative effective regimens include 5000 units SQ q 8 h, or 8000 units SQ q 12 h.

c. Disadvantages

(1) Risk of bleeding—4-6%

(2) Rarely, associated with thrombocytopenia at this dose

(3) Contraindicated in patients with active peptic ulcer disease, uncontrolled hypertension, evidence of bleeding disorders, current aspirin use

5. Heparin and dihydroergotamine (DHE) combinations

a. DHE at low dosages causes preferential vasoconstriction of capacitance vessels and increased venous return.

b. Shown to be as effective as heparin alone; particularly effective in orthopedic procedures

c. Contraindicated in patients with hypotension, ischemic heart disease, and peripheral arterial occlusive disease

6. Low-molecular-weight heparins (LMWHs) (Enoxaparin, Fragmin)—Heparin fragments are made by depolymerizing a heparin ester. Standard (unfractionated) heparin is a mixture of compounds of varying molecular weight and anticoagulant activity. Characteristics of LMWH are the following.

a. Equivalent inhibition of factor X but less inhibition of thrombin and platelet aggregation

b. A smaller increase in partial thromboplastin time (PTT)—In orthopedic studies, LMWH is more effective than standard heparin in DVT prophylaxis but is not associated with a higher risk of hemorrhagic complications.

c. Studies in general surgery patients have been inconclusive in demonstrating a reduction in DVT and/or a decrease in bleeding complications.

d. Longer half-life and daily dosing

e. More expensive than standard heparin

7. Alternative anticoagulation—Lepirudin, danaparoid sodium, and argatroban (synthetic thrombin inhibitor) are alternatives for anticoagulation in patients who develop heparin-induced thrombocytopenia.

a. Lepirudin—Half-life depends on renal function; must dose on an individual basis

b. Argatroban—Preferred in patients with renal failure because of its hepatic elimination

c. Disadvantages—Risk for bleeding if not dosed appropriately; must closely monitor clotting time

8. Prophylactic IVC (Greenfield) filter placement may be performed in patients at extremely high risk (e.g., quadriplegics, severe closed head injury) who have contraindications to other forms of prophylaxis and/or cannot be anticoagulated. It prevents only PE, not DVT.

III. AN APPROACH TO PROPHYLAXIS

A. DETERMINE THE PATIENT'S RISK
1. Low risk—Age <40 years; ambulatory or minor surgery
2. Moderate risk—Age >40 years; abdominal, pelvic, or thoracic surgery
3. High risk—Age >40 years; prior DVT or PE, malignancy, hip and other orthopedic surgery, immobility, hypercoagulable states

B. PROPHYLAXIS OF CHOICE
1. Encourage early ambulation in all patients.
2. Low-risk patients probably do not need prophylaxis.
3. Moderate-risk patients should have pneumatic compression boots, low-dose heparin prophylaxis, or LMWH.
4. High-risk patients should have a combination of treatment consisting of pneumatic compression boots plus low-dose heparin or dextran. Full anticoagulation with warfarin or IVC filter placement can be considered in this population.
5. Prophylaxis should be started prior to the institution of anesthesia.
6. Ophthalmologic and neurosurgical patients with intracranial or spinal lesions are not candidates for prophylaxis with anticoagulants because minor bleeding may have disastrous consequences.
7. High-risk patients should be watched closely for clinical signs and symptoms of DVT in addition to frequent (q 3-4 day) objective testing. Duplex scanning is the least invasive of these methods. Its sensitivity is 88% in the lower extremity.

THROMBOEMBOLIC PROPHYLAXIS

12

IV. TREATMENT OF DVT AND PULMONARY EMBOLUS

A. PREVENT DEATH FROM PULMONARY EMBOLUS
1. Intubate and give mechanical ventilatory support if necessary.
2. Aggressive respiratory care and monitoring often are obtainable only in an ICU setting.
3. Consider anticoagulation vs. thrombolytic therapy.

B. ANTICOAGULATION
Anticoagulation is done for treatment of both PE and DVT. It prevents propagation of the thrombus and minimizes the late complication of post-thrombotic syndrome in the leg.
1. Heparin bolus with 100-150 units/kg IV followed by constant infusion (starting at 1000 units/h). Titrate the drip to maintain the PTT at 50-70 seconds. The PTT should be checked every 4-6 hours after a bolus or rate change. Once the PTT is therapeutic and stable, it should be checked daily. Continue the heparin until the patient's warfarin dose is manipulated into the therapeutic range (usually 7-10 days).
2. Warfarin is started when the heparin is therapeutic (generally 3-5 days) and continued 3-6 months. The PT should be maintained at 1.5 times normal (17-20 seconds) or an INR 2.0-2.5.
3. Absolute contraindications
   a. Recent neurosurgical or ophthalmologic surgery or hemorrhage
   b. Serious active bleeding
   c. Malignant hypertension
4. Relative contraindications
   a. Severe hypertension
   b. Recent major surgery or trauma
   c. Recent stroke
   d. Active GI bleeding
   e. Bacterial endocarditis
   f. Severe hepatic or renal failure

C. THROMBOLYTIC THERAPY (STREPTOKINASE, UROKINASE, TISSUE PLASMINOGEN ACTIVATOR)
1. Promotes rapid clot lysis and may preserve venous valve function
2. Useful in cases of massive PE or in patients who are hypertensive or severely hypoxic due to the mechanical effect of clot producing occlusion of a significant portion of the pulmonary circulation
3. Indicated in patients who have occlusive iliofemoral DVT or in patients who have free-floating caval thrombus after IVC filter placement
4. May require subsequent percutaneous or open thrombectomy to remove residual thrombus

D. **VENA CAVAL INTERRUPTION (GREENFIELD FILTER)**
1. Prevents further embolism of thrombi >3 mm; vena cava must be <24 mm (measured by venography) to deter migration of the filter postoperatively; filter can be placed from either internal jugular or nonthrombosed femoral approach
2. Indications
a. Recurrent thromboembolism despite adequate anticoagulation
b. PE in a patient with contraindications to anticoagulation
   (1) Hemorrhage
   (2) Thrombocytopenia
c. Chronic recurrent PE with ensuing pulmonary hypertension
d. Possible complications from anticoagulation
   (1) Pending orthopedic procedure
   (2) Pending bariatric surgery
   (3) Condition after trauma
   (4) Multiple long bone fractures
   (5) Pregnancy
   (6) Complex pelvic/facial fractures
3. Complications include malpositioning, peristrut vena caval leak, filter thrombosis, and filter migration.

E. **VENOUS THROMBECTOMY**
Venous thrombectomy is not indicated for routine iliofemoral DVT; however, it may be necessary in cases of venous gangrene or in the event of septic thrombosis.

F. **PULMONARY EMBOLECTOMY**
1. Open embolectomy, usually through median sternotomy with cardiopulmonary bypass; associated with >50% mortality and high morbidity
2. Transvenous embolectomy with a suction cap–tipped catheter passed via jugular or femoral vein; especially useful in massive PE in which there is a contraindication to fibrinolytic therapy

12

THROMBOEMBOLIC PROPHYLAXIS

Universal Precautions

Konstantin Umanskiy, MD

"It only needs to happen once."

Universal precautions, as defined by the Centers for Disease Control and Prevention (CDC), are a "set of precautions designed to prevent transmission of human immunodeficiency virus (HIV), hepatitis B virus (HBV), and other blood-borne pathogens when providing first aid or health care. Under universal precautions, blood and certain body fluids of *all* patients are considered potentially infectious for HIV, HBV, and other blood-borne pathogens."

13

I. APPLICATIONS

A. PRECAUTIONS APPLY
Universal precautions apply to blood and other body fluids such as the following.
1. Semen
2. Vaginal secretions
3. Cerebrospinal fluid
4. Synovial fluid
5. Pleural fluid
6. Peritoneal fluid
7. Pericardial fluid
8. Amniotic fluid

B. PRECAUTIONS DO NOT APPLY
Universal precautions *do not* apply to the following substances (unless they contain visible blood).
1. Feces
2. Nasal secretions
3. Sputum
4. Sweat
5. Tears
6. Urine
7. Vomitus
8. Saliva, except when visibly contaminated with blood or in the dental setting where blood contamination of saliva is predictable

II. GUIDELINES

A. BEDSIDE
1. Use gloves when touching blood and body fluids requiring universal precautions, mucous membranes, or nonintact skin of *all* patients.
a. Change gloves after contact with each patient.
b. Wash hands immediately after gloves are removed.

c. Gloves cannot prevent penetrating injuries caused by needles or other sharp instruments.

d. Use gloves in situations where contamination with blood may potentially occur.

2. Masks and protective eyewear or face shields must be used during procedures that are likely to generate droplets of blood or body fluids requiring universal precautions.

3. Gowns or aprons should be worn during procedures that are likely to generate splashes of blood or body fluids requiring universal precautions.

B. OPERATING ROOM

1. Wear gloves preoperatively and postoperatively for all patient contact.

2. At the end of the operation, remove first the gown, then the gloves.

3. Remove gown and gloves as soon as the operation is over; wash hands, then put on clean gloves.

4. Wear protective eyewear with side shields at *all times* while in the OR.

5. Double-gloving is recommended when operating on a patient whose body fluids are known to be infectious.

C. TRAUMA RESUSCITATION

1. Gloves, eyewear with side protectors, mask, and gown or apron are required.

D. NEEDLE STICK/SHARP INSTRUMENT INJURY

According to the CDC, most needle stick injuries do not result in exposure to an infectious disease, and of those that do, most do not result in the transmission of infection. Nevertheless, needle stick injuries may expose the physician to blood-borne pathogens such as HIV, HBV, and/or HCV.

1. HIV—The risk of transmission from a single percutaneous exposure, such as a needle stick or a cut with a sharp object, to HIV-infected blood is ≈0.3%.

2. Hepatitis B—Most physicians are now immune to HBV due to pre-exposure vaccination. However, studies done before the availability of hepatitis B vaccine showed rates of HBV transmission ranging from 6-30% after a single needle stick exposure to an HBV-infected patient.

3. Hepatitis C—Epidemiologic studies of health care workers exposed to HCV through a needle stick or other percutaneous injury have found that the incidence of infection averages 1.8% per injury.

E. CIRCUMSTANCES LEADING TO NEEDLE STICK INJURY

1. ≈38% of percutaneous injuries occur during use, when a needle or other sharp being manipulated in a patient becomes accidentally dislodged.

2. During clean-up, disposal of a sharp device

3. Recapping contaminated needles

4. Transferring a body fluid between containers
5. Failure to properly dispose of used needles in puncture-resistant "sharps" containers

F. ACTUAL NEEDLE STICK INJURY

In the event of a needle stick or other sharps injury or exposure to the blood or other body fluid of a patient, follow these steps.
1. Wash needle sticks and cuts with soap and water.
2. Flush splashes to the nose, mouth, or skin with water.
3. Irrigate eyes with clean water, saline, or sterile irrigation.
4. Report the incident to your supervisor.
5. Immediately seek medical treatment.

13

G. COMPLIANCE

1. Educate about and frequently revisit main principles of universal precautions.
2. Provide adequate and convenient supply of protective equipment.
3. Lead by example—Junior physicians are more likely to exercise universal precautions if compliance is demonstrated by their seniors.
4. One study[1] reports that experienced trauma care team members are cavalier regarding blood-borne disease exposure risks.
5. Enforce adherence to universal precautions.

REFERENCE

1. Evanoff B, Kim L, Mutha S, et al: Compliance with universal precautions among emergency department personnel caring for trauma patients. Ann Emerg Med 33:160-165, 1999.

UNIVERSAL PRECAUTIONS

PART II

Specialized Protocols in Surgery

Trauma

Marc Shapiro, MD

I. GENERAL OVERVIEW OF TRAUMA CARE

A. **BRIEF HISTORY**
1. Egypt (6000-3500 BC)—Surgeons performed various procedures including cataracts, amputations, and general wound care.
2. Edwin Smith Papyrus (3000-1600 BC)—Surgical treatise of 48 cases of trauma to the entire body
3. Plastic surgery seems to have originated in ancient India around 2500-1500 BC.
4. The Greeks named physicians *iatros,* which meant "extractor of arrows."
5. Arabs eventually handed down the knowledge of the Greeks via the Persians, among whom surgery was performed by barbers and even hangmen.
6. The Renaissance brought forth such famous surgeons as Ambroise Paré—Introduction of boiling oil in wounds and cautery
7. 17th century saw the introduction of the idea of IV medication—Attributed to Christopher Wren, more popularly known for his architecture
8. Crawford W. Long (1815-1878) or William Morton (1819-1868) (who was first is controversial)—Introduced general anesthesia
9. Joseph Lister (1827-1912)—British surgeon who developed antiseptic techniques, including carbolic acid spray over surgical field
10. William Beaumont (1785-1853)—In area of gastric physiology, studied bullet wound on his patient Alexis St. Martin with a gastrocutaneous fistula.
11. William Halsted (1852-1922)—Among many things, along with William Osler, the designer of the modern-day surgical residency program
12. Mont Reid—Along with George Heuer (pr. Hoy-er), attended the inaugural class at the Johns Hopkins University under Halsted and Osler
    a. Mont Reid was the second Chief of Surgery at the University of Cincinnati.
    b. George Heuer was the first.

B. **TRAUMA FACTS AND FIGURES, 1994-2002 (FROM NATIONAL TRAUMA DATA BANK REPORT)**
1. 396,445 people received a portion of their care in the emergency department (ED).
   a. 56% of these were admitted directly to the floor.
   b. 12% were <16 years of age.
   c. 24% were >55 years of age.

d. 20% were admitted to the ICU.

e. 22% were admitted to the OR.

2. Motor vehicle crashes (MVCs) and falls made up 70% of all injuries. MVCs were the most common injury (38%) and falls were second most common (30%).

3. Gunshots, stabs, fights made up 11% of injuries.

4. Mortality is highest from gunshot wounds, which are the third most common injury (6.6%).

5. Mortality percentages are relatively constant for injuries of varying severity (Table 14-1) until age 50 years, whereupon there is a demonstrable increase with age.

C. MORTALITY OF THE TRAUMA PATIENT—TRIMODAL DISTRIBUTION

1. First few seconds to minutes after trauma event

a. Deaths result from brain injury; high spinal cord injury; and heart, aorta, great vessels, and airway injuries.

2. The "golden hour" after trauma event

a. Deaths result from intracranial hemorrhage, hemothorax, tension pneumothorax, ruptured spleen, severe liver lacerations, open and/or femur fractures, and other multiorgan injuries.

3. Several days to weeks after trauma event

a. These patients die from sepsis and multiorgan failure.

D. TRAUMA SCORING SYSTEMS

1. Trauma score—Based on the Glasgow Coma Scale (GCS) score and hemodynamic parameters

2. Acute Physiological and Chronic Health Evaluation (APACHE) II

a. 12 physiologic parameters/scores

b. Not accurate with trauma patients

3. Abbreviated Injury Scale (AIS)

a. Hundreds of injuries listed by score—1 = minor to 6 = fatal

b. Complex system not used commonly

TABLE 14-1

MORTALITY RATE FOR INJURIES BASED ON SEVERITY

ISS Group	Severity of Injury Description	Group Mortality Rate (%)	Percentage of All Deaths
1-9	Minor or single system	1.02	14.03
10-15	Moderate	1.9	4.28
16-24	Severe	7.23	15.77
>24	Very severe	35.47	65.92

ISS = Injury Severity Score.

4. Injury Severity Score (ISS)
a. Most often used
b. Based on the AIS
c. Accurate
d. Scored as 1 = minor to 75 = fatal

E. ADULT VS. PEDIATRIC TRAUMA

Some differences, including anatomic types, are noted in the trauma patients themselves. Table 14-2 shows normal ranges of vital signs in the pediatric group.
1. Fontanelle
a. Palpable pulses
b. Increased intracranial domain
2. Endotracheal tube size
a. Size of the 5th digit
b. (16 + age in years)/4
3. Resuscitation—Table 14-3 shows the four classes of hemorrhagic shock and the type of fluid replacement required in each.
a. Pediatric—10-20 mL/kg of crystalloid, 2 boluses before packed red blood cells (RBCs) or whole blood is transfused
b. Adult—2 L lactated Ringer's (LR) solution or normal saline (NS); generally, LR is most suitable for resuscitative fluid. Some may argue for NS in patients with head injury; however, both are isotonic, which is the most important requirement.
c. Albumin has been proven in several studies to lead to a higher mortality, specifically in the trauma patient. Furthermore, in the acutely ill, it does not stay in the vascular space as it has been predicted in animal studies alone. It also has been shown to worsen coagulopathy as well as acute lung injury.
d. Other colloids (hetastarch, pentastarch) have shown mixed results at best, with LR being the gold standard in resuscitative fluid.

F. BLUNT VS. PENETRATING WOUNDS
1. Blunt trauma
a. MVCs

TABLE 14-2

NORMAL RANGE FOR PEDIATRIC VITAL SIGNS

Age Group	Heart Rate (beats/min)	Systolic Blood Pressure (mm Hg)	Respiratory Rate (breaths/min)
Infant	160	80	40
Preschool	120	90	30
Adolescent	100	100	20

TABLE 14-3

CLASSES OF HEMORRHAGIC SHOCK

Variables		Class		
	I	II	III	IV
Blood loss				
Amount (mL)	≤750	750-1500	1500-2000	>2000
Percentage	≤15	15-30	30-40	>40
Heart rate (beats/min)	<100	>100	>120	>140
Blood pressure (mm Hg)	Normal	Normal	Decreased	Decreased
Capillary refill	Normal	Prolonged	Prolonged	Prolonged
Respiratory rate (breaths/min)	14-20	20-30	30-40	>35
Urine output (mL/h)	>30	20-30	5-15	Oliguric-anuric
Mental status	Slightly anxious	Mild anxiety	Anxious-confused	Confused-lethargic
Fluid replacement	Crystalloid	Crystalloid	Crystalloid + blood	Blood

b. Motorcycle crashes
c. Falls
d. Kick by a horse
e. Assaults (e.g., bats, fists)
f. Diving "accidents"

2. Penetrating trauma
a. Stab wounds
b. Gunshot wounds
    (1) Place paper bags over hands *if possible* for evidence purposes.
    (2) High velocity (≥2200 ft/sec)—Includes rifles
    (3) Low velocity—Most handguns
        (a) 45 automatic Colt pistol (ACP), slow heavy round
        (b) 9 mm very fast smaller round
    (4) Shotgun wounds—Damage depends on
        (a) Ammunition (birdshot vs. deer slugs)
        (b) Distance from the victim—Wadding included in the wound
            implies very close range.
        (c) Amount of spread of the shot
c. Plate glass windows
d. Other foreign bodies

II. THE PRIMARY SURVEY

A. HISTORY AND PHYSICAL EXAM
1. These include a brief yet specific history from not only the patient (if possible) but also the paramedics and others who were at the scene or directly involved with the patient, i.e., fellow passengers and witnesses.
2. One must execute the primary survey in lightning speed but be extraordinarily thorough. Just by conversing in the first few seconds, you have already made several keen observations (airway, breathing, mental status, and arguably circulation, to name a few).

B. ABCDEs + F
1. Airway—Patent or not; intubated, compromised with SQ air, foreign body, etc. Maintain cervical spine protection.
2. Breathing—Spontaneous or mechanical; labored or without difficulty
3. Circulation
a. Distal pulses (radial artery, dorsalis pedis artery, posterior tibial artery)—Present or absent
b. IV access
    (1) Large bore (14-16 gauge), in at least two locations
    (2) Central access, usually femoral
        (a) High risk of deep venous thrombosis (DVT) (12-15%)
        (b) It is difficult to maintain a strict sterile environment while placing resuscitation lines.

14

TRAUMA

      (c) Discontinue these lines within 24 hours because of risk of DVT or infection.

c. Control hemorrhage at this time.
    (1) Direct digital control of hemorrhage when possible
    (2) Consider splinting or traction for fracture.

4. Disability

a. Neurologic status
    (1) Person, place, time, situational awareness
    (2) Best exam at patient's initial presentation
    (3) GCS score
        (a) Motor

Obeys	6
Purposeful (crosses midline)	5
Withdraws	4
Flexion	3
Extends	2
No response	1

        (b) Verbal

Oriented speech	5
Confused speech	4
Inappropriate words	3
Incomprehensible words	2
No verbal response	1

        (c) Eye

Spontaneous opening	4
Opens to voice	3
Opens to pain	2
No response	1

5. Exposure

a. Remove all clothing, but prevent hypothermia.
b. Check everywhere!
    (1) Axillae
    (2) Gluteal folds
    (3) Ears
    (4) Nares
    (5) Scalp (injuries may be behind or within the hair)
    (6) Back
    (7) Perineal body

6. Fingers in every orifice and Foley catheter

a. Not every patient needs a Foley catheter
    (1) Bedside decision
    (2) Risk of urinary tract infection, the most common nosocomial infection; urinary infection due to Foley catheter unlikely if used short term
    (3) Urinary output is *not* a determinant of adequate resuscitation— Ethanol and hyperglycemia, e.g., are common reasons that trauma patients may have a brisk diuresis early.

(4) Perform digital rectal exam prior to Foley catheter placement.
    (a) Presence of blood may indicate rectal injury
    (b) Presence of "high-riding prostate" may indicate significant pelvic fracture with urethral injury
(5) Observe for blood at urethral meatus
(6) If clinical suspicion of urethral injury exists, perform urethrogram prior to attempting urinary catheter placement

C. VITAL SIGNS
1. Blood pressure
2. Heart rate
a. More predictable of blood loss than blood pressure
b. Not reliable for the following
    (1) Patients on β blockers and some calcium channel blockers
    (2) Neurogenic shock (e.g., sympathectomy)
    (3) Athletes or those with significant physiologic reserve
3. Respiratory rate
4. Pulse oximetry
a. Needs a good waveform—Difficult to obtain in shock
b. Multiple factors can obscure the value, e.g., some nail polish, fluorescent lighting, and carbon monoxide/methemoglobinemia.
5. Temperature
a. Hypothermia may be underestimated as a source of morbidity.
b. Hypothermia should be corrected to minimize coagulopathy.

III. THE SECONDARY SURVEY

The secondary survey is the opportunity to assess what has been done so far and what else needs to be done to complete the patient's work-up and disposition. The diagnostic work-up and treatment should be guided by findings from a complete physical examination and awareness of the mechanism of injury.

A. LAB AND OTHER STUDIES
1. CBC—Will not see anemia in acute blood loss
2. Arterial blood gas
a. Indicated in those with severe multi-trauma, or if acid-base status is in question
b. Highly recommended for the following
    (1) Mechanical ventilation
    (2) Moderate to severe pelvic fractures
    (3) The elderly
    (4) Extremity injuries (e.g., open fractures)
    (5) Chest injuries
3. Type and screen/type and crossmatch (T&S/T&C)
4. β Human chorionic gonadotropin in females
5. Coagulation profile

14

TRAUMA

a. Elderly on warfarin (Coumadin)
b. Synthetic liver function
c. Few patients come in with a history consistent with a blood dyscrasia
6. Ethyl alcohol/toxicology—Check before one administers a therapeutic dose of a narcotic or anxiolytic.
7. No need for routine liver function test (LFT)
a. LFTs are not cost-effective in this setting.
b. No data have proven that there was a change in management secondary to increased LFTs.
8. ECG
a. Useful for premorbid purposes only, e.g., did the patient have a myocardial infarction that led to the MVC?
b. No serial cardiac isoenzymes are available for blunt cardiac injury.
9. Initial radiographic studies in blunt trauma—Chest, lateral cervical spine, pelvic radiographs
a. Recent data have shown that the hemodynamically stable patient who is awake, alert, and without pelvic tenderness does *not* need a pelvic radiograph.
10. The focused assessment with sonography in trauma (FAST) exam
a. Useful for those patients with blunt trauma who are hemodynamically labile/unstable
b. Quick and noninvasive
c. Four views
   (1) Pericardium
   (2) Right upper quadrant—Morison's pouch/hepatorenal space
   (3) Left upper quadrant—Splenorenal space
   (4) Pelvis
d. Evaluate for the presence of intra-peritoneal free fluid.
e. Inadequate for examining the retroperitoneum
11. CT scan
a. Indications
   (1) Head CT if suspicion of traumatic brain injury, depressed GCS score, or loss of consciousness
   (2) Abdominal CT if suspicion of intra-abdominal or retroperitoneal injury
      (a) Contrast purpose is to fill duodenum only
      (b) Oral contrast vs. no oral contrast is a topic of some debate; recent studies have *not* demonstrated an increased incidence of missed small-bowel injuries secondary to a lack of oral contrast agent; diagnosis was made secondary to free air, mesenteric stranding
      (c) Oral contrast agent has been shown to delay CT scan and increase aspiration complications.
   (3) Chest CT if suspicion of significant thoracic injury, especially the possibility of blunt aortic disruption

B. PROCEDURES

1. Cystogram
a. With or without pelvic fractures
b. Definitely if gross hematuria is present
c. CT cystogram is the most accurate; this is *not* simply a CT scan of the pelvis.

2. Diagnostic peritoneal lavage (DPL)
a. For the unstable patient
b. Can be done in the OR if patient is there for emergent neurosurgical procedure
c. Poor evaluation of the retroperitoneum
d. Risks include bowel and bladder injury.
e. Must place nasogastric (NG) tube and Foley catheter before procedure
f. Pregnant women and patients with pelvic fractures must have DPL performed above the umbilicus/arcuate line.
g. Considered grossly positive if >10 mL of blood is present on initial aspiration
h. After instillation of warmed lactated Ringer's solution, look for >100,000 RBCs in blunt injuries; >10,000 RBCs in penetrating injuries.
i. Look for bile, stool, or food in any injury.
j. Advantages include accuracy ≈95%, low in cost, and speed.

3. Tube thoracostomy—Indicated for evacuation of pneumothorax or hemothorax
a. Decreased risk of empyema
b. Sterile procedure
c. Can lose $\frac{1}{2}$ blood volume in the chest
d. Check for air leak; rolling, vigorous leak could mean bronchial injury.
e. 28-32 Fr chest tubes
   (1) For blood—Place posteriorly
   (2) For air—Place anteriorly
f. If multiple rib fractures, administer nonsteroidal anti-inflammatory drugs, if possible. Also, order an epidural block if no significant spine fractures exist.

4. Pericardiocentesis
a. Beck's triad—Distended neck veins, muffled heart sounds, hypotension.
b. Take off the cervical collar to examine the neck; muffled heart sounds may be difficult to appreciate in the trauma bay
c. If pericardial effusion or tamponade, the patient likely requires a pericardial window (Trinkle procedure) or pericardial exploration

5. Resuscitative thoracotomy
a. Should only be performed in the presence of a surgeon
b. Signs of life (SOL)—Number 1 prognostic factor (Fig. 14-1)
c. Must have SOL within 5 minutes of arrival in the ED, or in the ED in penetrating trauma.
   (1) Heart rate (>40 beats/min), systolic blood pressure (>60 mm Hg), and ECG tracing as compatible with life

14

TRAUMA

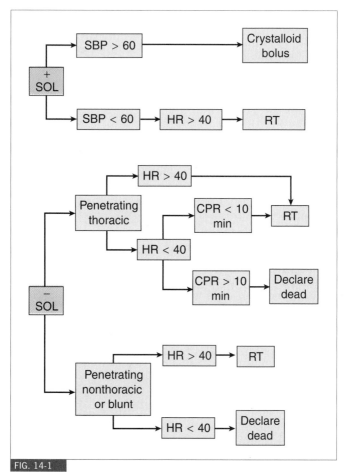

FIG. 14-1

Algorithm for resuscitative thoracotomy (RT) in the presence or absence of signs of life (SOL). SBP = systolic blood pressure; HR = heart rate; CPR = cardiopulmonary resuscitation.

d. Must have SOL *in* the ED for blunt trauma; even then, it is highly controversial to perform at all with blunt trauma
e. Extraordinarily costly
f. Stab wounds have a much better prognosis than gunshot wounds.
g. Pericardial tamponade is a protective mechanism, especially with stab wounds.
h. Outcomes

(1) Survival in adults
  (a) 13% overall in penetrating trauma in a series of 2400 patients, which is an optimistic figure that excludes those with neurologic catastrophes; gunshot wounds, 7% survival; stab wounds, 18% survival
  (b) Blunt trauma in adults—Expect <1-3% survivability, depending on indications and setting.
(2) Survival in the pediatric population—Stab wounds, 9%; gunshot wounds, 4%; blunt trauma, 2%

C. COMPLETE PHYSICAL EXAM

Can you reconstruct the trauma by the history and physical exam? Given the story, do the wounds/injuries match up?

1. Head, eyes, ear, nose, and throat
a. Hemotympanum
b. Otorrhea/rhinorrhea
c. Midface
  (1) Stable or not?
  (2) Malocclusion
d. Trachea
  (1) Deviation or midline
  (2) Crepitance or intact
e. Jugular venous distention
  (1) Do not forget to take off the cervical collar.
  (2) Injuries may be missed here if not checked.

2. Chest
a. Point tenderness
  (1) Clinical evidence of rib fractures
  (2) May not see rib fractures on plain chest radiograph
b. Flail chest
  (1) Paradoxical breathing
  (2) Two or more segments of the same rib or more ribs that are fractured
  (3) Judicious fluid management
  (4) Patients may have an underlying pulmonary contusion.
  (5) Excellent candidates for an epidural block
c. SQ air—Check for tracheal or esophageal injury and pneumothorax.
d. Dull vs. resonant percussion, i.e., hemothorax vs. pneumothorax
e. Seatbelt signs—Seen across the chest, but pathology could be elsewhere
  (1) Carotid stretch injury—Diagnosed by angiography
  (2) Low thoracic/high lumbar spine fracture (Chance fracture)
  (3) Retroperitoneal injury—Duodenum, pancreas

3. Abdomen
a. Nipples to pelvis
b. Acute vs. nonacute—Recognize that an acute abdomen is a surgical abdomen.
c. Is a seatbelt sign present?

14

TRAUMA

4. Pelvis

a. Stable vs. unstable

    (1) Pubic rami fractures are stable fractures generally.

    (2) Open-book fracture and the shear fractures with acetabular fractures can be very unstable.

    (3) One can decrease the pelvic volume by wrapping the pelvis in a bed sheet and clamping it in place with penetrating towel clips or tying it in a knot.

        (a) If this works, an external fixator placed by the orthopedic surgeons is indicated.

        (b) Medical antishock trousers (MAST) can also be used as a temporary measure, but they make it much more difficult to perform angiography and they predispose patients to intra-abdominal hypertension.

    (4) A hemodynamically unstable patient with an unstable pelvic fracture warrants evaluation with a DPL or FAST.

        (a) If the study is positive, immediately transfer the patient to the OR.

        (b) If the study is negative, proceed to order an angiography, with likely angioembolization.

b. Rectal

    (1) Prostate—High-riding prostate?

    (2) Foreign bodies

    (3) Bone chips—Perform an anoscopy or rigid sigmoidoscopy to evaluate for rectal injury.

    (4) Gross hematuria

5. Extremities

a. Open vs. closed fractures

b. Open fractures warrant an irrigation and drainage procedure within 6 hours.

c. Be alert for the development of compartment syndrome.

    (1) >30 mm Hg in any compartment where muscle and fascia exist

        (a) Four compartments in the leg—Anterior, lateral, posterior (deep or superficial)

        (b) Three compartments in the arm—Flexor (deep, superficial), extensor

    (2) Fasciotomies to be performed early and before arterial exploration/reconstruction

    (3) Suspect when ischemia present for >4-6 hours

    (4) Elevate the extremity.

d. Pulses present or not?

    (1) If pulses are not present, obtain Doppler signals and document the exam.

    (2) Effects of shock—Acid washout, myocardial instability

    (3) Evaluate the need for angiography.

        (a) Most of the literature recommends angiography for posterior knee dislocations.

(4) Few physicians obtain a duplex without hard signs.
   (a) Hard signs include active or pulsatile hemorrhage; pulsatile or expanding hematoma; signs of limb ischemia; diminished or absent pulses; presence of a bruit or thrill.
(5) Ankle/brachial Index (ABI)—Difference between sides should be <0.1—ABI is performed by taking the systolic pressure from each ankle and dividing it by the same-sided brachial pressures.
e. Range of motion—Pain? Fracture?
f. If it hurts, obtain a radiograph! If it doesn't hurt, it may still need a radiograph later, so vigilance is required. Check the radiograph for foreign bodies.

6. Cervical/thoracic/lumber/sacral spine exams

a. Emergent vs. nonemergent
(1) Rarely, if ever, is ruling out spine fractures a life-threatening task.
(2) Steroids are to be instituted for *blunt* spine injuries that are symptomatic.
   (a) Standard of care—No strong data proving steroids are of benefit, however
   (b) If within 3 hours of the injury, give methylprednisolone 30 mg/kg bolus, followed by 5.4 mg/kg drip for 48 hours.
   (c) If within 8 hours of the injury, give methylprednisolone 30 mg/kg bolus, followed by 5.4 mg/kg drip for 23 hours.
   (d) Data merely suggest sparing of one or two levels.
   (e) Not indicated for penetrating trauma
b. Radiographic vs. clinical clearance
(1) If patient is awake and not intoxicated and there are no distracting injuries, it is safe to *clinically* clear the spines.
c. Backboard
(1) Patients should be removed from a backboard within 2 hours from being placed on the board.
(2) Lying flat on a hospital bed or gurney is sufficient as long as axial alignment is not compromised.
d. Radiographic evaluation
(1) Cervical spine
   (a) Plain films—Lateral, anteroposterior, Swimmer's, odontoid
   (b) CT scan of questionable areas—If negative, the patient will need temporary cervical stability in the form of a Miami J collar.
   (c) Active flexion (on the patient's part) and extension in 2 weeks
   (d) MRI for longitudinal ligament injury
   (e) Clinical clearance when at all possible
(2) Thoracic/lumbar/sacral spine
   (a) Plain films
   (b) CT scan for suspicious areas
   (c) Clinical clearance when at all possible
(3) Angiography for fractures through the vertebral and carotid foramina

7. Neurologic
a. Components of the GCS score—Document the exam.
(1) Moves all four extremities
(2) Symmetrical vs. asymmetrical motor and sensory exams
(3) Paralysis/paresthesia
(4) Dermatomes
(5) Myotomes
(6) Priapism/bulbocavernosus reflex
(7) Rectal tone
8. Results of other data
a. Radiographic studies
b. Brain stem responses

IV. INJURY SPECIFICS

A. THE FACE AND HEAD
1. Battle's sign or raccoon's eyes—May indicate basilar skull injury
2. Mid-face
a. Generally does not cause airway obstruction
b. LeFort fractures (Fig. 14-2)
    LeFort I—Transverse fracture
    LeFort II—Pyramidal fracture
    LeFort III—Craniofacial disjunction
c. Repair generally performed days to weeks after injury when edema is minimal
3. Fractures/missing teeth—Can obstruct airway if aspirated
4. Ear lacerations—Two-layer closure. Do not use epinephrine with the lidocaine.
5. Head lacerations
a. Very bloody
b. Temporary closure to minimize bleeding during the acute evaluation, followed by definitive closure soon after
6. Skull fracture
a. Open
(1) Depressed skull fracture through inner table
(2) Surgical emergency
(3) Risk of meningitis with this injury
b. Closed—Observe fracture.

B. THE NECK
1. Blunt vs. penetrating mechanism
a. Intervention generally requires hard signs, e.g., crepitance, dysphonia, stridor, bruit, active bleeding, expanding hematoma, neurologic deficit, radiographic evidence of injury (displaced anatomic structures, tracking air or fluid).
b. Zones of the neck (Figs. 14-3 and 14-4)

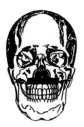 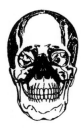

LeFort I
(Transverse fracture)

LeFort II
(Pyramidal fracture)

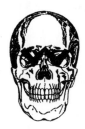

LeFort III
(Craniofacial disjunction)

FIG. 14-2

LeFort fracture classification.

14

TRAUMA

Zone I—Horizontal area between the clavicles and the cricoid
Zone II—Area between the cricoid and the angle of the mandible
Zone III—Area between the angle of the mandible and the base of the
skull
(1) Injuries to areas I and III require angiography for adults; for
pediatric population, should strongly weigh risks secondary to
smaller vessels
(2) Injuries to area II require either *selective management*
(esophagoscopy, esophagram, laryngoscopy, arteriography, bronchoscopy) or *exploration*.

2. Tenderness in blunt cervical spine injuries
a. Cervical spine films
b. CT scan for suspicious areas
c. Consider spine surgery consult
d. Possible MRI

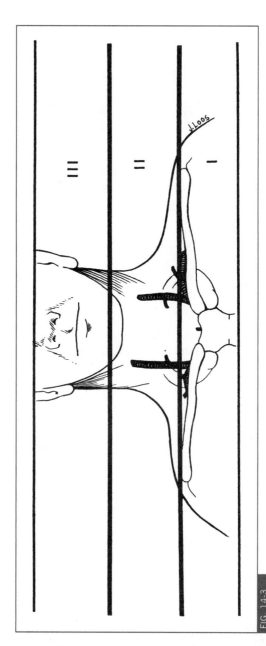

FIG. 14-3

Diagram depicting zones of the neck.

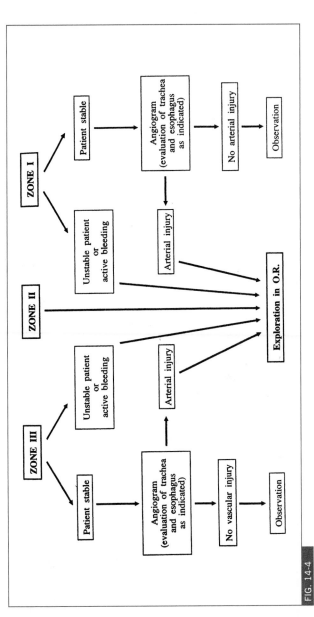

FIG. 14-4
Penetrating neck trauma algorithm.

3. Special issues—In high spinal cord injuries (C3-C5), the patient exhibits "belly breathing"; C3 and higher may not be breathing at all!

C. THE CHEST
1. Auscultate—Be wary of pneumothorax.
2. Flail chest—Paradoxical motion when breathing
3. Needle decompression is an *emergent* procedure for tension pneumothorax.
a. To be followed by tube thoracostomy
b. Anatomically, there are two choices—Area between 2nd and 3rd ribs in the mid-clavicular line *and* anterior axillary line just inferior to axillary fossa
4. **Proximal airway injuries**
a. Needle cricothyroidotomy
   (1) 14-gauge angiocatheter in the cricothyroid membrane followed by jet ventilation—Works for ≈15 minutes
   (2) Next, go to the OR for formal tracheostomy.
b. Emergent cricothyrotomy
   (1) Similar to needle cricothyroidotomy, but place a guide wire into the trachea via the catheter, followed by a tracheostomy tube or 6-Fr endotracheal tube
   (2) Next step usually an urgent trip to the OR within the next 24-48 hours
c. Emergent tracheostomy
   (1) Rare, but requires the presence of a skilled surgeon
   (2) No. 11 blade into the trachea in a vertical fashion, followed by the scalpel handle with a 90-degree twist.
5. **Main stem bronchial injury**
a. Often diagnosed by presence of a pneumothorax and rolling air leak after tube thoracostomy
b. Fiberoptic bronchoscopy—Diagnostic instrument of choice
c. Usually found 2.5 cm (1 inch) from the carina
6. **Blood loss that prompts operative intervention**
a. 1500 mL immediately out of chest tube
b. 200 mL/h for ≥2 consecutive hours
c. Video-assisted thoracic surgery
   (1) Procedure of choice for retained hemothorax not evacuated by tube thoracostomy (e.g., entrapped lung) or persistent air leak (other options include a Heimlich valve or other commercial device)
7. **The wide mediastinum**
a. May suggest aortic injury; 8 cm is the textbook definition
b. Chest radiographs are largely unreliable if they are negative.
c. Should have a relatively low threshold to obtain CT scan of the chest with IV contrast in the appropriate patient
   (1) Appropriate to repeat the chest radiograph as an upright film if possible
   (2) The initial chest radiograph can be inadequate secondary to being an anteroposterior film while the patient is lying supine.

8. Blunt cardiac injuries

a. Obtain ECG—Cardiac isoenzymes may not be diagnostic.

b. Observe 24 hours in monitored setting if arrhythmias—Most common are the tachyarrhythmias

c. Echocardiogram—Diagnostic study of choice

9. Diaphragm injuries

a. Presentation

    (1) Occurs in ≈2-4% of all abdominal injuries

    (2) Likely occurs with equal frequency between blunt and penetrating injuries, although historical reports would favor blunt injuries over penetrating trauma

    (3) Requires high index of suspicion to diagnose

    (4) Dyspnea, orthopnea, chest pain—Can have referred pain to scapula

    (5) Gastric distention with ipsilateral lung collapse in extreme situations

    (6) Diagnosis can be difficult; however, several studies may be employed.

        (a) Look for NG tube in left hemithorax on chest radiograph

        (b) CT scan

        (c) Fluoroscopy—Mobility of left hemidiaphragm (most commonly injured)

        (d) Bowel sounds in the chest on auscultation

        (e) Cardiac displacement

b. Approach

    (1) Early diagnosis

        (a) Repaired via celiotomy with horizontal mattress sutures—Recommend nonabsorbable monofilament, but almost any permanent suture would suffice

    (2) Late diagnosis

        (a) Repair via thoracotomy—Laparoscopic or open; less scar tissue to contend with

10. Other

a. Internal mammary artery

    (1) Capable of high flow (300 mL/min)

    (2) Can lead to hemothorax and/or cardiac tamponade

    (3) Often-missed injury

b. Subclavian artery injury

    (1) Right side control—Approach via median sternotomy and extend up the neck

    (2) Left side control

        (a) Approach through anterolateral thoracotomy for proximal control

        (b) May need to use an "open book" approach combining anterolateral thoracotomy with median sternotomy

        (c) Also possible to approach these through supraclavicular incisions and at times resection of the clavicle

        (d) Be wary of the phrenic nerve.

        (e) Mortality ≈5%

14

TRAUMA

D. THE ABDOMEN—EXPLORATORY LAPAROTOMY: CONDUCT AND RULES OF ENGAGEMENT

Rule 1—Control the bleeding.

Rule 2—Control contamination.

Rule 3—Assume nothing, prove it, i.e., mobilize and inspect it closely.

1. Stomach

2. Hollow viscus injury

a. Free air on chest radiograph

b. Immediate exploration

c. Does not always show signs of peritonitis for hours

3. The duodenum

a. Hematoma—May cause obstruction

(1) Observation is the rule with NG tube decompression.

(2) Explore after 2 weeks if contrast agent unable to pass through.

b. Perforation

(1) Options include primary repair, Roux-en-Y duodenojejunostomy, or partial resection, depending on anatomy

(2) Pyloric exclusion

(a) May be performed with antecolic gastrojejunostomy in order to begin PO intake before the pyloric exclusion opens

(b) Not necessary; often practiced to protect duodenal anastomosis

(c) Can use any suture or even staples because over time, stomach recannulates

(3) Decompress

(a) Stomach with NG tube or gastrostomy

(b) Duodenum with retrograde or lateral duodenostomy tube

(c) Feeding jejunostomy tube

(4) Drain with closed-suction drain

4. Small bowel injuries—Repair vs. resect

a. If the bowel wall is ≥50%, then a resection is warranted, as repair would restrict the lumen diameter.

b. Bowel wall injury <50%, it is prudent to repair the wall

c. No difference in single- or double-layer closure complications

d. Although controversial, stapled and hand-sewn anastomosis have equal number of complications.

(1) May be more difficult to staple a thick, edematous bowel, however

5. Need for damage-control laparotomy

a. Large intraoperative resuscitation

b. Risk of abdominal compartment syndrome—Clinical diagnosis based on

(1) Intra-abdominal hypertension (>25 mm Hg) (as transduced by bladder pressure at the level of the symphysis pubis with 100 mL of sterile crystalloid)

(2) + at least one of the following

(a) Increased peak airway pressures

(b) Decreased urinary output

(c) Intracranial hypertension

6. Colon injuries

a. Primary repair vs. diverting colostomy
b. Civilian injuries are treated differently from those injuries obtained in combat.
   (1) Guidelines for diversion
      (a) Systolic blood pressure <90 mm Hg
      (b) >1 L of blood loss
      (c) Gross contamination
      (d) Operative delay >8 hours
      (e) Significant abdominal wall loss
      (f) More than two organs injured
   (2) Antibiotics—Without gross contamination, antibiotics should not be continued >24 hours.

7. Liver injuries

a. Need for laparotomy
   (1) Most liver parenchymal injuries can be managed nonoperatively.
   (2) Less likely than spleen to have a delayed rupture
b. Angiogram
   (1) For "blush" (active hemorrhage) on CT scan
   (2) Pseudoaneurysms
      (a) Some institutions believe that patients are at a high risk of rebleeding and automatically perform a CT scan 24-48 hours after the injury to look for pseudoaneurysms.
c. Intrahepatic balloon tamponade
d. Fabian tampon—Gelfoam wrapped by Surgicel
e. Omental packing—Excellent technique; often confused for abscess, however, when CT scan is performed on a patient days later for fevers
f. Resection
   (1) Bile leaks—Risk of biloma/bile peritonitis
   (2) Drain or not to drain
      (a) Drains can create up to 100 cm H_2O of negative pressure, thereby creating a fistula; can drain via CT scan or ultrasonography any time if needed
      (b) Controlled leak with a drain

8. Spleen

a. Laparotomy vs. angioembolization vs. observation
   (1) Risks vs. benefits of both laparotomy and angioembolization
   (2) If blush of contrast is present on CT but patient is hemodynamically stable, would advocate angioembolization of spleen
      (a) Angioembolization with Gelfoam so that splenic artery may recannulate over time
      (b) Risk of arterial dissection
      (c) Pseudoaneurysms
   (3) Goal is to decrease the pressure head so the spleen will stop bleeding
   (4) Increased risk for overwhelming postsplenectomy sepsis

14

TRAUMA

(a) Encapsulated bacteria—*Streptococcus* spp, *Haemophilus influenzae* spp, *Meningococcus* spp
(b) Occurs in <0.5% of adults
  b. Nonoperative management
   (1) Increasingly popular among the trauma centers and those institutions equipped for moderate- to high-risk patients
      (a) Must have the staff and the training to support these patients
      (b) Serial exams must mean frequent checks by qualified personnel.
      (c) OR must be prepared.
   (2) Some centers advocate routine follow-up CT scan for pseudoaneurysms 3-5 days after their injury.
   (3) Memphis/Grady/Oregon Health Sciences experience
      (a) Among several centers who have championed and published data on their nonoperative experience with splenic injury
      (b) Data—Success, 30-100%; failure, generally between 48 and 72 hours
      (c) Vaccine issues
         (i) Most efficacious time to receive is 2 weeks before or 2 weeks after splenectomy
         (ii) Impractical for most trauma patients—Cannot predict trauma, and many trauma patients are at risk for poor follow-up habits
         (iii) Most patients receive Pneumovax in the postanesthesia care unit.
         (iv) Poor data concerning the need for *Haemophilus influenzae* type B and *Meningococcus* vaccines
         (v) The University of Cincinnati uses only Pneumovax vaccine currently.
   (4) Patient may return to competitive sports after 6 weeks
   (5) No data to support follow-up CT scan at this time

9. **Renal trauma**
  a. Angiography vs. laparotomy for diagnosis and treatment
  b. IV pyelogram—Mostly for historical purposes
  c. Partial vs. complete nephrectomy
   (1) Generally speaking, nephrectomy reserved for cold coagulopathic patients
   (2) Partial nephrectomies may be difficult if kidney is edematous (pledgeted repair).
   (3) Possible to place a stent for collecting system injuries
  d. Drain—Control fistula if uroma develops.
  e. Hypertension—Delayed complication can occur weeks to years after trauma.

10. **Urinary bladder trauma**
  a. Do not use silk suture for repair—Nidus for calculi formation
  b. Posterior bladder = danger; order a genitourinary consult

c. Suprapubic (SP) and Foley catheters—Trauma data do not support the use of both.
    (1) Increased rate of infected SP sites and urinary tract infections
    (2) Supports use of Foley catheters as sufficient drainage

E. EXTREMITY TRAUMA
1. ABI or arterial pressure index—If <0.9, arteriography indicated
2. Duplex vs. angiography
a. Duplex—Mixed results at mixed institutions; angiography is the gold standard
b. Late thrombosis
3. Compartment syndrome
a. Ischemic reperfusion injury
b. Consider when the patient requests more narcotics to quell the increasing pain.
c. Stryker needle and pressure transducers used to evaluate compartment pressure
d. Diagnostic when compartment pressure >30 mm Hg
4. Myoglobinuria
a. No data exist that demonstrate benefit to a furosemide (Lasix) drip nor adding bicarbonate to the IV fluids.
b. Goal is to hydrate such that urinary output is ≥100 mL/h.
5. Electrical burns
a. Check for cardiac arrhythmias—Somewhat controversial, more probable with high-voltage injuries (>1000 V)
b. Check for entrance and exit wounds.
c. Check for myoglobinuria.
d. Bone has the greatest resistance, and therefore the surrounding tissues are at greatest risk for tissue destruction, i.e., myonecrosis.
6. OR time—Early excision and grafting
a. After initial resuscitation, by day 3 or 4

F. NEUROLOGIC TRAUMA
1. Closed head injuries
a. Greatest cerebral edema days 2-4, with day 3 generally thought of as the time of maximal edema
b. Epidural
    (1) Convex hematoma
    (2) Surgical emergency
    (3) Presentation commonly includes a brief lucid interval followed by unconsciousness
    (4) Middle meningeal artery injury is the etiology
c. Subdural hematoma
    (1) 30-40% occurrence of closed head injuries
    (2) Convex hematoma

14

TRAUMA

(3) Bridging veins are torn

(4) Can be a surgical emergency depending on size, rate of expansion

d. Subarachnoid hemorrhage

(1) No mass effect as the blood is spread in a diffuse pattern

(2) Risk of vasospasm and hydrocephalus

e. Diffuse axonal injury

(1) Also known as "shear" injury

(2) Difficult to interpret on CT scan

(3) Can be a devastating injury if enough neural pathways are disrupted or destroyed

f. Cerebral perfusion pressure (CPP)

$$CPP = MAP - ICP$$

where MAP = mean arterial pressure and ICP = intracranial pressure. Most agree to keep CPP >70 mm Hg (absolutely >60 mm Hg).

g. Most patients receive an intracranial monitor should they have a GCS score ≤8.

h. These patients may have an intense coagulopathy because the intracranial concentration of tissue plasminogen is released in traumatic injury.

i. Hyperventilation for intracranial pressure control is contraindicated, *except for brief instances of intracranial hypertensive spikes*.

(1) Hyperventilation promotes vasoconstriction, which ultimately promotes cerebral embarrassment.

j. Mannitol is acceptable *after* the patient is adequately volume resuscitated.

(1) Keep serum osmolarity <310 mOsm/L.

(2) Serum sodium level rises—Be wary of excessive hypernatremia.

k. With the exception of burn patients, these are the most metabolically active patients in the ICU; therefore, they warrant early nutritional intervention to meet their caloric needs.

2. Spine injuries

a. Neurogenic shock

(1) Disruption of the descending sympathetic pathways in the spinal cord—C5-T1

(2) Loss of vasomotor tone

(3) Includes bradycardia due to unopposed vagal nerve action

(4) Risk of pulmonary edema secondary to overzealous fluid resuscitation

b. Spinal shock

(1) Flaccidity and loss of reflexes following insult to spinal cord

(2) Duration may be variable

(3) No hemodynamic changes

c. Steroid protocol as described in section III. C. 6

d. Syndromes

(1) Anterior cord syndrome

(a) Devastating injury

(b) Paraplegia

(c) Dissociative loss of pain and temperature sensation

(d) Usually due to an infarct of the anterior spinal artery

(2) Central cord syndrome

(a) Cervical extension injury

(b) Disproportionate loss of strength of the extremities, upper being worse than lower

(c) Some may have a congenital stenosis of the cervical region, predisposing them to this type of injury.

(d) The syndrome seems to be due to the ischemic compromise to the distribution of the anterior spinal artery as well.

(3) Brown-Séquard syndrome

(a) Most often seen in children and in penetrating injuries

(b) Rarely seen as a pure form of the disease, i.e., a "textbook case"

(c) Ipsilateral motor loss (corticospinal tract)

(d) Contralateral sensory loss two levels below the injury site (spinothalamic tract)

G. TRAUMA IN WOMEN AND PREGNANCY

1. Anatomic differences

a. In the gravid female, the uterus is a pelvic organ. As the fetus matures, the uterus ascends.

b. In the latter part of pregnancy, the gravid uterus is a protective organ for the mother when she is subjected to abdominal trauma.

2. Physiologic differences

a. Plasma volume increases, resulting in decreased hematocrit.

b. Increased propensity to clot

c. Leukocytosis

d. Increased cardiac output

(1) If the vena cava is compressed by the gravid uterus (supine position); cardiac output can decrease to $\frac{1}{3}$ of the original output

e. Increased minute ventilation—Increased respiratory rate

f. Increased glomerular filtration rate

g. Prolonged gastric emptying time

3. Early involvement of the obstetric/gynecologic team

4. All initial efforts should be guided toward the mother.

a. In 80% of mothers who arrive in shock, the fetus dies.

b. The mother can lose nearly 35% of her blood volume before she shows signs of shock—Much too late for the health of the fetus

c. Even minor injuries are associated with placental abruption and subsequent fetal demise.

d. Fluid loss (blood) should be treated with fluid replacement, *not* vasopressors—The uterus is exquisitely sensitive to vasopressors.

e. Part of the initial assessment of the pregnant female is rolling her 15 degrees to her left in a modified left-lateral decubitus position, keeping her spine in a stable axial alignment. This maintains caval patency.

   f. When indicated, a DPL is performed supraumbilically after an NG tube is placed as well as a Foley catheter—Still difficult to do late in pregnancy, and the patient might best be evaluated in the OR if in extremis

5. Domestic violence

a. A growing problem

b. Physicians are obligated to notify protective services if suspicious.

c. Look for these signs.

   (1) Trauma not consistent with stated history

   (2) Signs of self-abuse

   (3) Self-blame and/or low opinion of self

   (4) Poor eye contact at questioning

   (5) Afraid to have spouse leave room during questioning

   (6) History of substance abuse

6. Oral contraceptives and hormone replacements can increase the propensity to clot. This along with trauma significantly predisposes patients to DVT and potentially pulmonary embolism. The patients when indicated should be placed on a therapeutic regimen of either unfractionated heparin or low-molecular-weight heparin.

V. FUTURE DIRECTIONS IN TRAUMA AND CRITICAL CARE

A. EARLY GOAL-DIRECTED RESUSCITATION
1. Has been shown to decrease mortality in septic patients
2. Invasive
3. Must have the resources available to do so
4. Use Swan-Ganz monitoring on all patients in <6 hours and have their hemodynamics optimized before admission to the ICU.

B. TIGHT GLUCOSE CONTROL
1. Serum glucose level should be maintained between 80 and 110 mg/dL.
2. Usually means an insulin drip
3. Need nursing staff to be able to monitor
4. Usually in an ICU setting

C. DROTRECOGIN ALFA (Xigris)
1. Activated protein C
2. An early study (PROWESS[1]) demonstrated a decrease (6%) in sepsis mortality.
3. Prevents microthrombosis of end organs

D. TELEMEDICINE AS PERTAINING TO TRAUMA AND CRITICAL CARE
1. Several institutions are on the rise for pioneering telemedicine in the field.
2. Rural hospitals have been assisted in obtaining surgical airways from level I trauma centers.

3. Already able to perform physiologic function in extreme, rigorous environments in "real time" to provide up to the second medical/surgical support
a. Has been performed in climbs up Mount Everest and on the battlefield

E. **LOW TIDAL VOLUMES IN ACUTE RESPIRATORY DISTRESS SYNDROME (ARDSNet[2])**
1. Decreases the shearing forces on the alveoli
2. Decreases volutrauma to healthy alveoli
3. Uses higher positive end-expiratory pressure (PEEP) for maintaining oxygenation
4. Permissive hypercapnia as long as adequate pH is maintained
5. Decrease in mortality

F. **PRESSURE/VOLUME CURVES**
1. Measures lower inflection point
a. Determines amount of positive opening pressure of the alveoli
b. Determines amount of PEEP to set the ventilator on
c. More to come with subsequent studies

14

TRAUMA

REFERENCES

1. Bernard GR, Vincent JL, Laterre PF, et al: Efficacy and safety of recombinant human activated protein C for severe sepsis. New Engl J Med 344:699-709, 2001.
2. Ventilation with lower tidal volumes as compared with traditional tidal volumes for acute lung injury and the acute respiratory distress syndrome. The Acute Respiratory Distress Syndrome Network. New Engl J Med 342:1301-1308, 2000.

RECOMMENDED READING

Rivers E, Nguyen B, Havstad S, et al: Early goal-directed therapy in the treatment of severe sepsis and septic shock. New Engl J Med 345:1368-1377, 2001.

Orthopedic Emergencies

George Papacostas, MD

I. FRACTURE ASSESSMENT

As part of the basic trauma evaluation, the patient should be thoroughly examined for fractures, dislocations, ligamentous injuries, neurovascular injuries, and intra-articular lacerations. Systematic inspection and palpation of every bone and joint should be carefully carried out. The following characteristics should be evaluated in every fracture.

A. OPEN VS. CLOSED FRACTURE

B. DEGREE OF SOFT TISSUE INJURY

C. NEUROVASCULAR STATUS

D. LOCATION
1. Intra-articular vs. extra-articular
2. Metaphyseal vs. diaphyseal

E. FRACTURE CONFIGURATION

Pattern	Mechanism
Transverse	Tension
Oblique	Compression
Spiral	Torsion
Butterfly	Bending
Comminuted	High energy

F. DISPLACEMENT

G. DISLOCATION

H. ANGULATION

I. ROTATION

J. LENGTH

II. ORTHOPEDIC EMERGENCIES IN THE TRAUMA PATIENT

A. OPEN FRACTURES
The type of open fracture influences the plan of treatment, the subsequent clinical course, and the overall prognosis for the injury.
1. Classification (Table 15-1)
2. Treatment
a. Wound cultures

TABLE 15-1

GRADES OF FRACTURES AND THEIR DEFINING FACTORS

Grade	Wound	Energy	Contamination	Soft Tissue Injury
I	<1 cm	Low	Clean	Minimal stripping
II	1-10 cm	Moderate	Moderate	Moderate stripping
III*	>10 cm	High	Severe	Extensive stripping
III A	Adequate soft tissue coverage—Able to close			
III B	Soft tissue defect requiring reconstructive procedure—Bone is exposed			
III C	Soft tissue defect and associated vascular injury—Circulation is hosed			

*Special grade III injuries include (1) farm injuries; (2) traumatic amputations; (3) segmental open fractures; (4) high-velocity gunshot wounds; (5) associated neurovascular injury; and (6) open fractures >8 hours old.

(1) Preoperative culture to evaluate initial wound contamination is *not* reliable.
(2) Postirrigation culture to assess residual bacterial flora
b. Antibiotics—Reduce the rate of infection in open fractures
  (1) Cefazolin—1 g q 8 h for all grades I and II open fractures
  (2) Gentamicin—2.5 mg/kg q 12 h or 5-7 mg/kg q 24 h added for contaminated wounds as well as all grade III open fractures
  (3) Penicillin—6 million units q 6 h; required in farm injuries for clostridial coverage
c. Tetanus prophylaxis—See Chapter 9
d. Fracture stabilization
  (1) Povidone-iodine (Betadine)–soaked gauze to minimize further wound contamination; some debate about local tissue necrosis; saline-soaked gauze may be preferable
  (2) Preliminary splinting or traction
    (a) Prevents further soft tissue injury
    (b) Immobilization decreases pain
    (c) Facilitates patient transport
    (d) Helps maintain perfusion to extremity
    (e) Maintains length and facilitates fracture reduction
  (3) Secondary stabilization—Definitive fracture stabilization includes open reduction internal fixation (ORIF), external fixation, intramedullary nailing, or skeletal traction
e. Irrigation and débridement
  (1) Meticulous removal and excision of foreign and nonviable tissue within 6 hours of injury
  (2) Reduces bacterial contamination of wound
  (3) Serial débridement indicated every 24-72 hours to re-evaluate and prepare for wound closure
f. Wound management
  (1) Preliminary evaluation of all wounds is performed in the emergency department (ED); ideally, a photograph is taken to document soft tissue injury.

(2) Secondary evaluation of wound is performed in the OR, and serial photographs are taken to document the extent of soft tissue and bony injury.

(3) Definitive care must provide for coverage of bone, tendons, hardware, and neurovascular bundle.

(4) Primary wound management—Wound left open (standard treatment)

(5) Secondary wound management—No grade II or III open fractures should be closed on initial débridement; all are taken back to the OR in 48 hours for repeat incision and drainage and delayed primary closure vs. coverage procedure.

    (a) Delayed primary closure (common in grades I and II injuries)

    (b) Delayed skin graft (split or full-thickness) or muscle flap (frequent in grade III, characteristic of grade IIIB)

    (c) Healing by second intention (occasional grade I or II)

g. Relative indications for immediate amputation

    (1) Complete anatomic disruption of posterior tibial nerve in adults

    (2) Crush injuries with warm ischemia time >6 hours

    (3) Serious associated polytrauma

    (4) Severe ipsilateral foot trauma

    (5) Anticipated protracted course in soft tissue coverage and bony reconstruction

    (6) Crush injury to both muscles and skin with complete neurovascular injury (Mangled Extremity Severity Score [MESS] >7 and grade IIIB or C injuries)

    (7) Intact neurovascular system with severe muscular deficit and bone loss such that reasonable function is unlikely

    (8) Insensate limb with intact vascular system and limited motor function; heavily debated

B. COMPARTMENT SYNDROME

1. Definition—Compartment syndrome is characterized by increased pressure within a closed space that causes irreversible ischemic damage to the contents of that space.

2. Pathophysiology

a. Any condition that increases the content of a compartment or reduces the space of a compartment can lead to the development of an acute compartment syndrome.

Decreased Space	Increased Pressure
External compression	Hemorrhage
Cast or dressing	Fractures
Medical antishock trousers	Reperfusion secondary to change in capillary permeability

b. Pressure within the compartment continues to rise until capillary perfusion pressure is exceeded. This results in arterial shunting leading to muscle and nerve ischemia that, if untreated, causes irreversible damage.

c. Palpable pulses are invariably present in an acute compartment syndrome unless there is an associated vascular injury. Pressure within a compartment is rarely elevated enough to obstruct the major artery traversing that compartment.

d. One must clinically distinguish among compartment syndrome, vascular injury, and neuropraxia. Each of these diagnoses requires different therapeutic intervention. Keep in mind that any of these injuries may be coexistent with each other.

3. Diagnosis

a. Subjective findings—Pain disproportionate to injury/mechanism

b. Objective findings

  (1) Early

    (a) Pain on palpation of swollen compartment

    (b) Increased pain with passive stretch of compartment musculature

  (2) Late

    (a) Hypoesthesia in the distribution of the nerve traversing the compartment

    (b) Muscle weakness

4. Compartment pressure monitoring

a. Devices

  (1) STIC catheters (Stryker, Ace)—Hand-held device that allows the physician to measure compartment pressures; quick and simple to use

  (2) Arterial line setup—Readily accessible in most EDs and all surgical ICUs

b. Measurements

  (1) Measurement of all compartments of the affected limb is mandatory.

  (2) Low threshold to measure compartment pressures in obtunded, neurologically impaired, or multitrauma patients

5. Indications for fasciotomies (Fig. 15-1)—There is not a universally accepted threshold for fasciotomy, but compartment pressures >30 mm Hg above diastolic pressure appear to be the most commonly recognized standard. These numbers must be evaluated with regard to the patient's mean arterial pressure because in hypotensive patients compartment syndrome may be present with compartment pressures <30 mm Hg. However, clinical findings are most important.

6. Treatment—Release elevated compartment pressure with compartment fasciotomies.

a. Hand

  (1) Commonly occurs secondary to crush injuries with associated metacarpal or carpal fractures

  (2) Symptoms and clinical findings are secondary to the effect on intrinsic muscles.

  (3) Treatment requires release of intrinsic compartments.

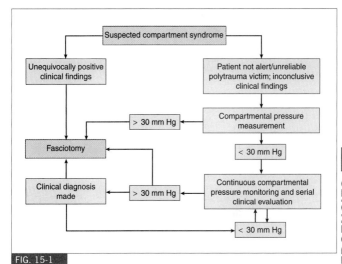

FIG. 15-1

Algorithm of indications for fasciotomy when a compartment syndrome is suspected.

b. Wrist
   (1) Occasionally occurs with fracture of the distal radius or perilunate dislocations
   (2) Clinical findings are consistent with median and ulnar nerve compression.
   (3) Compartment decompression requires fracture reduction, release of transverse carpal ligament, and exploration of carpal tunnel and Guyon's canal.
c. Forearm
   (1) Occasionally occurs with fractures of the radius and ulna
   (2) Forearm contains three compartments—Superficial flexor, deep flexor, and extensor
   (3) Fasciotomies require volar and dorsal incision to release all compartments.
d. Thigh
   (1) Trauma to thigh with or without femoral fracture
   (2) Three-compartment release—Anterior, posterior, and obturator
e. Leg
   (1) Compartment syndrome commonly occurs as a complication of tibial shaft and tibial plateau fractures.
   (2) Four compartments
      (a) Anterior
      (b) Lateral
      (c) Superficial posterior

        (d) Deep posterior
   (3) Fasciotomy techniques
      (a) Subcutaneous fasciotomies—Never indicated
      (b) Fibulectomy—Historical interest only
      (c) Single incision—Rarely indicated
      (d) Double incision—Standard of care (Fig. 15-2); employs two
          vertical incisions separated by a skin bridge of 7 cm; first
          incision is centered between the anterior and lateral compartments
          while second incision is 1-2 cm behind the posterior medial
          border of tibia; underlying fascia over each compartment is then

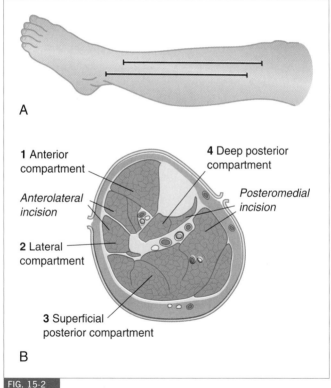

FIG. 15-2

A, Double-incision technique for performing fasciotomies of all four compartments of the lower extremity. *B*, Cross section of lower extremity showing a position of anterolateral and posteromedial incisions that allows access to the anterior and lateral compartments (1 and 2) and the superficial and deep posterior compartments (3 and 4).

released; skin is left open and the patient is brought back to the OR in 48-72 hours for delayed primary wound closure vs. split-thickness skin graft.

C. DISLOCATIONS

Pure dislocations and fracture dislocations represent an orthopedic emergency owing to the associated risk of neurovascular compromise, acute compartment syndrome, chondrolysis, and development of avascular necrosis. It is critical to carefully document the neurovascular status of the limb prior to and following successful reduction maneuvers. After reduction, check the stability of the joint and range of motion, and document where a redislocation occurs. Reduction of all dislocations requires adequate IV sedation. Dislocations frequently found in trauma patients are outlined in the following.

1. Hip dislocations
a. Hip dislocations and fracture dislocations frequently result from loading the hip joint through three mechanisms.
    (1) Flexed knee striking stationary object (dashboard)
    (2) Axial loading of foot with extended ipsilateral knee (floorboard)
    (3) Lateral compression through greater trochanter
b. Diagnosis
    (1) Posterior dislocations (90%)—Classically present with an adducted, flexed, and internally rotated position of the hip and a notably shortened leg
    (2) Anterior dislocations (10%)—Classically present with an extended and externally rotated position of the hip
    (3) Hip dislocations are frequently associated with fractures of the acetabulum, femoral head or neck, and patella.
c. Reduction—Allis maneuver uses traction applied in line with deformity and countertraction to stabilize the pelvis. Reduction is evident with an audible and palpable "clunk." Rochester maneuver uses pressure against the unaffected flexed knee with the forearm under the knee of the affected side. It is important to test the stability of reduction by performing range of motion of the hip. Radiographs are required to confirm concentric reduction and to rule out intra-articular loose fragments.
d. Complications
    (1) Avascular necrosis of femoral head (2-11%)—Incidence is increased with prolonged delay between dislocation and reduction.
    (2) Post-traumatic osteoarthritis
    (3) Sciatic nerve injury (8-19%)
    (4) Heterotopic ossification

2. Ankle
a. Ankle dislocations almost exclusively occur with fracture dislocations. These fractures are clinically unstable and require preliminary stabilization with splinting followed by ORIF.

b. Complications
   (1) Post-traumatic arthritis
   (2) Neurovascular compromise
   (3) Open fracture
c. Reduction—Longitudinal traction and manipulation reversing the injury force followed by a well-molded splint

3. Shoulder
a. Most commonly dislocated joint in body
b. To rule out dislocation requires shoulder anteroposterior (AP), axillary lateral, and scapular outlet (Y) radiographs.
c. Mechanisms
   (1) Anterior dislocation (90%)—Combination of abduction, external rotation, and extension
   (2) Posterior dislocation (10%)—Axial loading of adducted and internally rotated arm and direct force to anterior shoulder; historically associated with electroconvulsive therapy and seizures
d. Complications
   (1) Recurrent instability is the rule (younger > older).
   (2) Neurovascular injury (axillary nerve common, especially in the elderly)
   (3) Osteoarthritis
   (4) Rotator cuff tear
   (5) Avascular necrosis (secondary to chronic dislocation)
e. Reduction
   (1) Modified Stimson technique—Patient is prone with arm hanging over the edge of a table, and gentle downward traction is applied. Gentle scapular rotation may facilitate reduction.
   (2) Traction/countertraction—Gentle longitudinal traction is applied along the axis of the arm while countertraction is applied to the axilla. Avoid internal and external rotation owing to the associated risk for fracture.

4. Knee
a. Associated with complex ligamentous knee injuries
b. Immediate reduction critical to vascular status and peroneal nerve function
c. Arteriogram indicated for all posterior knee dislocations (regardless even with good distal pulses) to rule out popliteal artery injury (40-50% incidence)

5. Elbow
a. Mechanism—The elbow is a highly constrained joint, but dislocations are not uncommon. The exact mechanism is not completely understood.
b. Incidence
   (1) Greatest among 10- to 20-year-old population
   (2) Posterior (most common)
   (3) Anterior (rare)
   (4) Lateral
   (5) Medial
   (6) Divergent

c. Complications
    (1) Heterotopic ossification
    (2) Flexion contraction
    (3) Vascular injury (brachial, radial)
    (4) Nerve injury (median, ulnar, radial, anterior interosseous)
d. Reduction—Performed with elbow in semiflexed position with longitudinal traction applied to the forearm and countertraction applied to the humerus. Postreduction radiographs should be obtained out of plaster to check concentric reduction and rule out intra-articular fracture–coranoid and epicondyle fractures.

D. SPINAL TRAUMA (see Chap. 22)

E. INTRA-ARTICULAR LACERATION—OPEN JOINT
1. Associated with open fractures and joint penetration by foreign objects
2. Surgical emergency because of the associated risk for septic arthritis due to contamination introduced at the time of injury
3. Common locations
a. Knee
b. Elbow
c. Wrist
d. Ankle
4. Diagnosis—Accurate diagnosis requires clinical exam and intra-articular injection of sterile saline. Enough saline to distend the joint capsule must be injected. An open joint laceration is indicated by the extrusion of saline through the laceration.
5. Treatment
a. Intraoperative irrigation and débridement within 6 hours
b. Antibiotics

F. PULSELESS EXTREMITY
1. Encountered frequently in the trauma patient with vascular injuries and occasionally in dislocations and complex fractures
2. Treatment
a. Fracture or dislocation reduced immediately to relieve external vascular pressure
b. Vascular repair
    (1) Acute repair within 6 hours of the time of vascular injury is critical to limb survival.
    (2) Compartment syndrome is common after repair-reperfusion phenomenon. Fasciotomy should be considered at the time of vascular repair.
    (3) In general, fracture reduction and fixation are performed prior to vascular repair. If ischemia time precludes this, intra-arterial shunts may be used to restore blood flow temporarily during fixation.

15

ORTHOPEDIC EMERGENCIES

III. COMMON FRACTURES

A. PELVIC FRACTURES

1. Evaluation—Secondary assessment performed to examine the following.
   a. Fracture stability
   b. Fracture pattern
   c. Soft tissue injury
   d. Neurologic deficits

2. Physical examination
   a. Inspection—Rule out
      (1) Open fracture (rectal and vaginal exam)
      (2) Hemorrhage, hematoma, contusions
      (3) Limb-length discrepancies
      (4) Rotational abnormalities
   b. Palpation
      (1) Rotational stability—Axial loading of anterior iliac spines to assess if pelvis opens or closes
      (2) Vertical stability—Push-and-pull evaluation to determine vertical migration

3. Radiographic assessment
   a. Primary assessment—AP: overview of pelvic injuries used to assess pubic rami, iliac wing, pubic symphysis, sacroiliac (SI) joints, and acetabulum. Sacral fractures are commonly missed with AP views.
   b. Secondary assessment (order based on initial screening AP)
      (1) Inlet view—Used to assess posterior displacement of SI joints, sacrum, iliac wing, and rotational deformities of sacrum and ileum
      (2) Outlet view—Used to assess vertical displacement and to evaluate sacral foramina
      (3) Judet view—Used to assess acetabular fractures
         (a) Obturator oblique—Visualizes anterior column and posterior wall
         (b) Iliac oblique—Visualizes posterior column and anterior wall
      (4) CT scan—Used to evaluate acetabulum and posterior structures of pelvis

4. Associated injuries
   a. Hemorrhage—Frequently results in the loss of several units of blood secondary to bleeding from fracture sites, arterial and venous vessels
   b. Urologic—Associated injuries to bladder, urethra, and genitals (see Chap. 53)
   c. GI—Open fractures and parenchymal injuries are common due to the close anatomic relationship of these structures. Open fractures with GI contamination require immediate diverting colostomy.Wounds are managed with serial wet-to-dry dressing changes. There is a very high associated morbidity and mortality rate (50%) associated with these injuries.
   d. Neurologic—Commonly involves sciatic and sacral nerves

5. **Indications for external fixation**
a. Resuscitation—If pelvic ring is disrupted anteriorly, then may aid with control of hemorrhage
b. Rotationally unstable fracture
c. Adjunct to traction in unstable fractures (type C)

6. **Indications for ORIF**
a. Anterior ring fixation (rotationally unstable type B)
b. Posterior fixation (vertically unstable type C)
   (1) Displaced SI joint or fracture dislocation (C1-C3)
   (2) Failure to obtain reduction in extra-articular SI joint; vertically unstable fracture (C1-C3)
   (3) Multitrauma with unstable pelvis (type C)
   (4) Open posterior fracture with no rectal or perineal injury
c. Anterior and posterior fixation
   (1) Displaced unstable posterior injury with disruption of pubic symphysis
   (2) Displaced unstable posterior injury with displaced or unstable pubic rami fractures
d. Anterior fixation with external fixation
   (1) Pubic symphysis disruption with unstable posterior injury or severe posterior soft tissue injury
   (2) Unstable pubic rami fracture with unstable posterior injury or severe posterior soft tissue injury

B. ACETABULAR FRACTURES

1. **Anatomy**
a. Anterior column—Iliac crest to pubic symphysis and includes anterior wall
b. Posterior column—Descends from superior gluteal notch through acetabulum, including inferior pubic rami, obturator foramen, posterior wall of acetabulum, and ischial tuberosity
c. Acetabular fossa—Medial wall and teardrop

2. **Indications for nonoperative management**
a. Displacement <2-5 mm in dome, depending on fracture location and patient factors
b. Low anterior column fracture
c. Low transverse fracture
d. Minimal posterior column displacement

3. **Indications for operative management**
a. Most displaced acetabular fractures, especially those involving the acetabular dome
b. Retained bone fragments large enough to cause incongruity
c. Unstable posterior wall fracture
d. Displaced fractures of both columns (floating acetabulum)
e. High transverse or T fractures
f. Femoral head fracture with associated acetabular fracture

C. FEMORAL SHAFT FRACTURES

Femoral shaft fractures are usually the result of major trauma. Most fractures are sustained by young adults during high-energy injuries such as vehicular accidents, falls, or gunshot wounds. Patients must therefore have a complete physical exam to evaluate for associated injuries. Radiographic assessment must include an AP view of the pelvis.

1. Treatment

a. A large number of complex associated factors are evaluated in determining the appropriate treatment of different femoral shaft fractures. Some of these factors include the following.

    (1) Open vs. closed

    (2) Fracture location

    (3) Comminution

    (4) Associated injuries and fractures

    (5) Bone quality (degree of osteoporosis)

b. Treatment modalities

    (1) Intramedullary nailing

        (a) Treatment of choice for appropriate femoral shaft fractures

        (b) Advantages include earlier postoperative mobilization and lower pulmonary complications.

    (2) Traction—Treatment of choice in most other countries

    (3) Plating

    (4) External fixator

    (5) Casting

2. Complications

a. Neurovascular injury (peroneal most commonly)

b. Shortening and malrotation

c. Nonunion

d. Stiffness

e. Infection

f. Compartment syndrome

3. Associated injuries

a. Patella and femoral neck fractures

D. ANKLE FRACTURES

1. Evaluation

a. Neurovascular exam—May need intervention for vascular injury or compromise

b. Rule out open fracture.

c. Assess soft tissue swelling and skin compromise.

d. Radiographic evaluation—AP, lateral, and mortise views

e. Preliminary fracture stabilization

2. Treatment

a. Nonoperative treatment

    (1) Closed reduction is obtained by reversing the mechanism of injury and holding this reduction with a well-molded splint.

   (2) Splints are used for acute fracture stabilization to allow for soft tissue swelling.
   (3) Stable fractures typically require treatment in a cast for ≥6 weeks, whereas unstable fractures require longer immobilization.
 b. Operative treatment
   (1) Anatomic reduction of the fracture is the goal.
   (2) Operative treatment is recommended for the following indications.
     (a) Failure to obtain satisfactory closed reduction
     (b) Displaced, unstable, or open fractures
     (c) Multitrauma
     (d) Patient factors—Compliance, age, associated medical problems, etc.

E. DISTAL RADIUS FRACTURES
1. Fracture characteristics
a. Common fracture of the upper extremity
b. Involve both intra-articular and extra-articular injury patterns
c. Most fractures can be managed by closed reduction and casting.
2. Evaluation
a. Neurovascular status—Trauma to adjacent nerves and arteries can lead to ischemia and possible carpal tunnel syndrome.
b. Associated injuries—Energy of impact dissipates at fracture site, but associated injuries are not uncommon and include the following
   (1) Ligamentous injuries of wrist
   (2) Carpal fractures
   (3) Distal radioulnar joint disruption
   (4) Proximal ulna fracture—Radiographs of the entire forearm are mandatory.

F. CLAVICLE FRACTURE
1. Superficial location makes the clavicle the most commonly fractured bone in the body. Most clavicle fractures heal uneventfully with conservative treatment.
2. Treatment
a. Nondisplaced—Sling and swath
b. Displaced—Figure-8 bandage
c. ORIF—Limited indications
   (1) Open
   (2) Skin tenting
   (3) Neurovascular injury
   (4) Some distal fracture types

G. HUMERAL SHAFT FRACTURES
1. Most humeral shaft fractures can be managed nonoperatively with an expected union rate of 90-100%. These fractures are initially stabilized in a coaptation splint and are later changed to Sarmiento fracture

15

ORTHOPEDIC EMERGENCIES

brace at approximately 14 days after injury. Most closed treatments of humeral shaft fractures require patient cooperation and gravity/dependency for alignment.

2. Indications for ORIF
   a. Open fracture
   b. Multitrauma
   c. Pathologic fracture
   d. Vascular injury—Supracondylar fracture
   e. Malreduction or failure of conservative treatment
   f. Floating elbow (humerus and ipsilateral radius or ulna fractures)
   g. Postreduction radial nerve palsy
3. Complications
   a. Nonunion
   b. Malunion
   c. Radial nerve palsy
   d. Volkmann's ischemic contracture—Supracondylar fractures

Burn Care

Bruce W. Robb, MD

I. INDICATIONS FOR HOSPITAL ADMISSION

A. OUTPATIENT SETTING
Some burn injuries may be managed on an outpatient basis.

B. BURN UNIT SETTING
Admission to the burn unit is indicated in the following situations, based on the guidelines of the American Burn Association Injury Severity Grading System.
1. Full-thickness burns of >10% total body surface area (TBSA)
2. Partial-thickness burns >25% in an adult or >20% in a child
3. Involvement of the face, hands, feet, or perineum
4. Presence of electrical, chemical, or inhalation injury
5. High-risk patient—Age >65, <3 years; preexisting medical problems, multitrauma
6. Suspicion of abuse or neglect

II. INITIAL MANAGEMENT
Initial management is directed toward resuscitation, stabilization, and thorough evaluation of injuries.

A. HISTORY
1. Associated with burn—Circumstances such as unconsciousness, arrest, jumped from house
2. Burn agent—Flame, scald, chemical, electrical
3. Open vs. closed space
4. Time of burn
5. Prehospital treatment administered and vital signs during transport
6. Past medical history—Allergies, immunizations, current medications, or medical problems

B. AIRWAY/BREATHING
1. Ensure adequate airway—Prophylactic endotracheal/nasotracheal intubation for significant inhalation injury, extensive (>60%) burns, deep facial burns, supraglottic obstruction, facial fracture, closed head injury with unconsciousness
2. Inhalation injury—Major contributor to mortality
   a. Carbon monoxide (CO) poisoning—CO displaces oxygen (affinity is 200 times higher for hemoglobin and cytochromes) and binds hemoglobin, forming carboxyhemoglobin. Poor oxygen delivery results, and carboxyhemoglobin levels >50% are potentially lethal.
      (1) Diagnosis—Signs and symptoms of hypoxia and/or serum carboxyhemoglobin level >10% (nonsmokers) or >20% (smokers)

16

are diagnostic. Levels of 40-50% are not uncommon in survivors with aggressive care. Oxygen saturation levels are normal despite high levels of carboxyhemoglobin.

(2) Treatment—100% O_2 reduces half-life of CO from 250 to 50 minutes. Follow with carboxyhemoglobin levels, and continue to treat until levels are 10-15%. Persistent metabolic acidosis despite adequate volume resuscitation implies CO poisoning of cellular respiration.

(3) Treatment with hyperbaric oxygen may be of theoretical advantage but is often logistically difficult.

b. Results from exposure to carbon monoxide, chemical irritants, and toxic gases; rarely due to thermal injury (exception is superheated steam). Suspect inhalation injury if the following are present

(1) Closed-space injury (e.g., house fire)

(2) Presence of facial burns, singed nasal hairs, bronchorrhea, carbonaceous sputum, wheezing and rales, tachypnea, progressive hoarseness, and difficulty clearing secretions

c. Upper airway—Obstruction may occur within the ensuing 48 hours (maximal edema $\approx$ 24 hours).

d. Lower airway—Pulmonary edema and chemical tracheobronchitis due to noxious gases

e. Diagnosis

(1) Upper—Direct laryngoscopy; look for carbon deposits, airway edema, oropharyngeal burns

(2) Lower—Fiberoptic bronchoscopy: findings of airway edema, carbon deposits in tracheobronchial tree, and mucosal erythema and necrosis

(3) ^{133}Xenon scan—Evaluates the lower respiratory tract by washout of radioisotope. Incomplete washout by 90 seconds indicates lower airway involvement.

f. Treatment—O_2 supplementation, ventilatory assistance, aggressive pulmonary toilet, O_2 saturation monitor, arterial line for serial arterial blood gases, bronchodilators, and bronchioalveolar lavage to remove debris. Systemic corticosteroids and prophylactic antibiotics are *contraindicated*.

C. BURN EVALUATION
Totally expose the patient and remove any burned clothing and constricting jewelry; examine with suspicion of associated injuries.

1. Depth
a. First degree—Epidermal layer involved, basal layer intact, painful, pink, no blisters

b. Second degree (partial thickness)—Partial dermal layer involved, painful, white to pink, blebs and blisters may be present. If partial-thickness burn is deep, then most epidermal appendages are destroyed and spontaneous re-epithelialization is markedly delayed (similar to third-degree injury).

c. Third degree (full thickness)—Entire dermal layer involved (all dermal appendages destroyed); insensate, white, black, or red; dry and leathery (inelastic) texture

d. Fourth degree—Underlying fascia, muscle, and/or bone involved

e. The estimate of TBSA burn injury is the sum of second- and third-degree burns.

f. Epithelialization occurs in partial-thickness burns from epithelial cells surrounding hair follicles or sweat glands (skin appendages) and from the wound edges.

2. Size estimation—Rule of 9s: 9% head and neck, 9% each upper extremity, 18% each lower extremity, 18% anterior trunk, 18% posterior trunk, 1% perineum

a. Children have a larger head and trunk proportionally and smaller lower body.

b. For final size calculation, use Lund-Browder chart, which is more accurate for patients of any age.

c. Calculate

$$\text{TBSA} = 71.84 \times \text{weight (kg)} \times \text{height (cm)}$$

or use standard nomogram (see Rapid References section).

D. FLUID RESUSCITATION

1. Access

a. Two large-bore (>18-gauge) peripheral catheters—Burned area can be used if necessary

b. Central venous access—More suitable than peripheral catheters

c. Central venous pressure or pulmonary catheters are used in patients with cardiac or pulmonary disease, questionable fluid status, or hemodynamic instability. Catheters are changed every 48-72 hours.

d. In children, recommend femoral or jugular insertion sites.

2. Formulas for fluid resuscitation

a. Parkland formula is the most widely used. The basic formula is lactated Ringer's (LR) solution at 4 mL/kg/% burn, with half the total volume given over the first 8 hours (calculated from the time of burn), and the other half over the following 16 hours (Table 16-1).

b. Remember to include allowance for basal fluid requirements—Especially important in children

c. Initial K^+ supplementation not required, although large amounts are needed in anabolic phase of healing

d. Colloid may be given as early as 12 hours after injury in large burns and usually consists of albumin infused at a constant rate. Fresh frozen plasma may be given if coagulation defects are present.

e. Hypertonic saline appears to replenish intravascular fluid (from intracellular source) more quickly and improves cardiac contractility while decreasing total IV fluid volume and edema—Its use remains controversial. We add

16

BURN CARE

TABLE 16-1	
RESUSCITATION CALCULATIONS	
RESUSCITATION	
Calculated resuscitation and basal requirements	(4 mL × ___ kg × ___ % burn) + (1500 mL × BSA [cm^2]) = ___ mL/24 h (___) + (___) = ___ mL/24 h
Resuscitation fluid per 8 h	1st 8 h = ___ mL; ___ mL/h 2nd 8 h = ___ mL; ___ mL/h 3rd 8 h = ___ mL; ___ mL/h
MAINTENANCE	
Basal fluid requirement: 1500 mL/m^2	Total BSA = ___ m^2 × 24 h = ___ mL h = ___ mL/h
Evaporative water loss	Adults: (25 + % burn)m^2 = ___ mL/h Children: (35 + % burn)m^2 = ___ mL/h Calculated evaporative loss: (___ + ___ % burn) ___ m^2 = mL/hr; ___ mL/24 h
Total maintenance fluids: basal requirement and evaporative water loss	24 h = ___ mL h = ___ ML

BSA = body surface area.

1 ampule of bicarbonate to each liter of LR solution during the first 8 hours of resuscitation for large burns.
f. Blood should not be used for initial resuscitation (unless anemic).
g. Avoid fluid boluses but adjust IV rate as needed. Remember, resuscitation formulas serve only as a *guideline* for *initial* IV fluid administration. Adjust based on physiologic response.
3. **Goals of resuscitation—Maintain adequate tissue perfusion.**
a. Adequate urine output—Best indicator of resuscitation fluid status; goal is to maintain urine output (adults, 0.5 mL/kg/h; children, 1-2 mL/kg/h)
b. Normal mentation
c. Well-perfused extremities (warm, good capillary refill)
d. Normal arterial pH and lactate levels
e. Mixed venous O_2 saturations >70%
4. **Inadequate volume restoration is manifested by oliguria, tachycardia, and persistent or worsening base deficit**

E. INITIAL PROCEDURES
1. Foley catheter—Required for accurate urine output measurements during resuscitation in patients with >20% TBSA burn
2. Nasogastric (NG) tube—Gastric ileus occurs frequently after burns; also a useful route for PO medications
3. Nasojejunal feeding tube—Placed under fluoroscopy beyond the ligament of Treitz, with immediate initiation of enteral feedings
4. Escharotomy—May be required for burns to extremities and chest to prevent compartment syndrome and respiratory compromise

a. Compartment syndrome—Loss of motor and sensory nerve function, diminished pulses, decreased capillary refill, pressure >30 mm Hg by direct measurement
   (1) Incise the lateral and medial aspects of the extremity. The incision must be carried out across the joint and *into normal skin.*
   (2) If symptoms are unrelieved, then fasciotomy may be required.
b. Circumferential chest burns—Reduce compliance of chest wall, but escharotomies are rarely needed. Escharotomies should be performed in the presence of increased peak pressures, increased Pco_2, and decreased compliance.

F. INITIAL TESTS
1. Baseline weight
2. Labs—CBC, electrolytes, arterial blood gas with carboxyhemoglobin (for large burns or suspected inhalation injury), coagulation studies
3. Chest radiograph and ECG (for history of cardiac problems or electric burns)
4. Urinalysis

G. MEDICATIONS
1. Tetanus prophylaxis—Unless received booster within last 5 years
2. Ulcer prophylaxis—May use sucralfate (Carafate) 1 g PO q.i.d. or H_2 blocker (ranitidine 50 mg IV q 8 h), with antacids 30 mL q 2-4 h per NG tube to titrate gastric pH >5.0
3. Fungal prophylaxis—Nystatin 15 mL swish and swallow and 15 mL per NG tube t.i.d.
4. Multivitamins (particularly vitamin C and the other antioxidants) in tube feedings
5. Hemoglobinuria/myoglobinuria—Treat myoglobin based on urine color. If tea colored or reddish, increase urine output to >1 mL/kg/h by increasing IV rates; if there is no improvement, may give mannitol 12.5 g IV, and alkalinize urine with 1 ampule $NaHCO_3$ in IV fluids to keep urine pH >7.0. If not adequately treated, renal failure can occur.
6. Prophylactic antibiotics are contraindicated.

III. PATHOPHYSIOLOGIC CHANGES ASSOCIATED WITH BURNS

A. EDEMA
Edema is maximal at 18-24 hours after the burn owing to the following reasons.
1. Generalized increase in microvascular permeability—Involves nonburned tissue if burn >20% TBSA
2. Generalized impairment in cell membrane function > increased intracellular volume drawn in by increased intracellular Na^+ concomitant with loss of K^+

16

BURN CARE

B. HEMODYNAMICS

1. Initial hypodynamic state with decreased cardiac output/contractility and increased vascular resistance. This usually resolves with adequate resuscitation.
2. By day 2-3 a hyperdynamic state exists with increased cardiac function and decreased vascular resistance.

C. METABOLISM

There is a state of wound-, central nervous system-, and stress hormone-induced hypermetabolism.

1. Begins at 48 hours postburn
2. Caloric needs increased 1.3-2 times normal
3. Characterized by increased oxygen consumption, heat production, elevated body temperature, hypoproteinemia due to catabolism and wound exudate, gluconeogenesis, and hyperglycemia
4. Gradually returns to normal after wound is closed and the inflammation is resolved

D. IMMUNOCOMPROMISE

1. All aspects of the immune function are depressed, including cellular-mediated immunity (T cells), humoral-mediated immunity (B cells), opsonization due to decreased complement and antibodies, decreased phagocytosis and bactericidal activity by macrophages and neutrophils, and loss of natural barrier function of the skin
2. Predisposes the patient to infections and multiorgan failure

IV. BURN WOUND CARE

A. GOALS OF BURN WOUND CARE

1. *Cover wound*
2. Decrease infection
3. Allow for optimal re-epithelialization of partial-thickness burns.
4. Burns (second or third degree) that do not heal by 2-3 weeks produce significantly more scarring; thus, these wounds require excision and grafting for best cosmetic and functional results.
5. The mortality of large burns has been reduced by the expeditious excision of the burn wound followed by coverage with autograft or allograft.

B. TOPICAL AGENTS

Topical agents decrease wound sepsis but do not prevent colonization of eschar.

1. Bacitracin ointment—Useful for partial-thickness burns and facial burns
2. Silver sulfadiazine (Silvadene)—Broad spectrum, includes *Candida*. Intermediate eschar penetration but less than mafenide acetate.

Nonpainful on application. Apply b.i.d. *Contraindicated* in patients with glucose-6-phosphate dehydrogenase deficiency.
3. Mafenide acetate (Sulfamylon) (not used frequently)—Broad spectrum, but little fungicidal activity; penetrates eschar well, but causes pain on application; because this agent is a carbonic anhydrase inhibitor, absorption can cause hyperchloremic metabolic acidosis. Apply b.i.d.
4. Silver nitrate 0.5%—Applied as wet dressing, poor eschar penetration. May result in Na^+, K^+, Ca^{2+}, Mg^{2+} depletion; may cause methemoglobinemia

C. LOCAL CARE
1. First-degree burns—Minor care, symptomatic pain control
2. Partial-thickness burns—Initially wash with antiseptic soap (e.g., chlorhexidine gluconate), remove debris, unroof vesicles. Apply topical agents (bacitracin).
3. Deep partial-thickness, full-thickness burns—Initially treat as for partial-thickness burns. If there is no healing after 2 weeks, grafting is required.

D. EARLY EXCISION AND GRAFTING
Excise eschar in layered fashion to the point of capillary bleeding; perform within 2-7 days of admission for obvious deep second- and third-degree burns. Graft immediately or cover temporarily with homograft or biologic dressing. The physician may excise and then graft the next day (decreases operative blood loss). Advantages include early removal of eschar and coverage, improved joint function, shortened hospitalization, earlier mobilization and rehabilitation, improved immune status, and decreased wound sepsis.

E. GRAFTING
Grafting decreases evaporation pain and protects neurovascular tissue and tendons.
1. Partial-thickness wounds should heal spontaneously by day 14.
2. Without immediate physiologic coverage, fascial desiccation and subsequent infection may occur.
3. Sheet vs. mesh graft—Sheet grafts are optimal for cosmetic appearance but do not expand to cover a large surface area. Mesh grafts are also better for nonoptimal recipient beds. Sheet grafts are preferred for hands, feet, and face.
4. Grafts usually 0.010-0.014 inches thick—Thicker grafts have less scarring but slightly increased risk of graft failure and increased scarring of donor sites.
5. Types of grafting material
a. Autograft (from self)—Optimal; split thickness vs. full thickness, sheet vs. mesh
b. Allograft (same species, i.e., cadaver). Indications for use of allograft are the following.
  (1) Insufficient autologous skin available

16

BURN CARE

(2) Temporary wound coverage prior to autologous grafting

(3) Speeds epithelialization

(4) Prevents infection

c. Xenograft (different species, i.e., porcine)—Used infrequently due to the establishment of skin banks

d. Skin substitutes

    (1) Cultured keratinocytes—Trend is toward decreased use (needs a dermis)

        (a) For use in large burns with little donor skin available

        (b) Poor resistance to infection

        (c) Fragile, easily scars

        (d) Variable take

        (e) Place on dermal allografts

    (2) Dermal substitutes—Cover wound until autograft is available.

        (a) Dermal allograft

        (b) Collagen glycosaminoglycan (GAG)

        (c) Polyglactic acid (Vicryl) mesh

    (3) Skin substitutes (bilayer material)

        (a) Both dermal and epidermal components

        (b) Improved take in recent reports

        (c) Still not as good as split-thickness acute graft (STAG)

6. Priorities—Graft hands, feet joints, extremities, and face first, then trunk

7. Graft care

a. Donor site—Covered with topical antimicrobial (bacitracin, silver sulfadiazine) and biologic dressing such as calcium alginate (Kaldostat) or occlusive dressing

b. Graft site

    (1) Wet—Dressings irrigated with antibiotic solution to be kept constantly damp

    (2) Dry—Nonstick gauze (Adaptic), then pressure dressing over graft

c. Nonadherence of graft is due to avascular or infected graft bed, hematoma, seroma, or graft movement.

V. SUPPORTIVE CARE

A. NUTRITION

When making nutrition decisions, start early. The metabolic rate is proportional to burn size up to 40-50% TBSA burn and may be 1.3-2 times usual. Total body O_2 consumption and water loss are proportional to burn size.

1. Nutrient needs

a. Caloric needs based on Harris-benedict equation using a multiplier (see Chap. 5)

b. Indirect calorimetry is often used.

2. Route

a. Enteral (nasoduodenal) preferred, start during first 12 hours postinjury— Decreased infection and complication rates, decreased cost

b. If IV, *must* change IV site every 48-72 hours. Catheter is used for all infusions, including total parenteral nutrition. Parenteral nutrition is associated with an increased rate of sepsis in burn patients.

B. PHYSICAL AND OCCUPATIONAL THERAPY

Aggressive physical therapy (PT) and occupational therapy (OT) are necessary to prevent contracture and maintain function.

1. Positioning of limbs and joints begins day 1.
2. Splinting is required to prevent contractures.
3. Active exercise program with stretching is greatly superior to passive range of motion.
4. Involve OT early for long-term rehabilitation planning.

C. ANALGESIA

Use methadone for pain management, with IV morphine for acute pain.

VI. MANAGEMENT OF INFECTION IN BURN INJURY

A. MOST COMMON

The most common infection in burn patients is pneumonia.

1. Early pneumonia—Most commonly result of gram-positive organisms
2. Later pneumonia (>7 days after hospitalization)—Most commonly result of gram-negative organisms
3. More common in intubated patients, although can occur in nonintubated patients

B. PATHOGENESIS

In an untreated burn wound, surface bacteria proliferate, migrate through nonviable tissue, pause at the subeschar space, and when microbial invasiveness "outweighs" host defense capability, invade viable tissue with microvascular involvement and systemic dissemination (burn wound sepsis). Avascularity and ischemia of full-thickness burn wound allow microbial proliferation and prevent delivery of systemic antibiotics and cellular components of host defense.

C. CLINICAL SIGNS

1. Conversion of a partial- to full-thickness injury
2. Rapidly spreading ischemic necrosis

D. DIAGNOSIS OF INVASIVE BURN WOUND SEPSIS

1. Cultures of burn wound surface do *not* accurately predict progressive bacterial colonization or incipient burn wound sepsis. Qualitative and

16

BURN CARE

quantitative correlations between flora on the surface of the burn wound and bacterial colonization of the deep layers of the eschar are poor.

2. Bacterial growth is best monitored by semiquantitative burn wound biopsy—Calculate the precise number of organisms per gram of tissue. If biopsy cultures reveal $>10^5$ organisms per gram of tissue or if there is a 100-fold increase in the concentration of organisms per gram of tissue within a 48-hour period, then the organisms have escaped effective control by the topical chemotherapeutic agent, and burn wound sepsis is incipient.

    Note: *False-positive results often occur.*

3. Wound colonization of dead tissue must be differentiated from invasion of viable tissue.

a. Best evaluated by clinical diagnosis

b. Biopsy will find organisms in viable subeschar tissue on histologic examination.

c. Microvascular invasion connotes possible hematogenous dissemination and mandates systemic antibiotic therapy.

4. Wound—Often dry, crusted, black, or violaceous color; may be unchanged

5. Clinical picture of sepsis—Fever, hypoxia, mental status changes, leukocytosis, new-onset ileus, tachypnea, thrombocytopenia, hypotension, oliguria, acidosis, tachycardia, hyperglycemia; bacteremia occurs late in burn sepsis

E. BACTERIOLOGY OF NOSOCOMIAL BURN INFECTION

1. Know your hospital's flora and antibiotic sensitivities of species.

2. Most common pathogens—*Staphylococcus aureus*, group A streptococci (less common), *Pseudomonas aeruginosa*, other gram-negative rods, *Enterococcus* spp, *Candida albicans*

F. PREVENTION OF BURN INFECTION

1. Dressing change b.i.d. and apply topical agents.

2. Use strict handwashing.

G. TREATMENT OF BURN INFECTION

1. Remove *all* devitalized tissue.

2. Surgically drain closed-space abscesses.

3. Apply diffusible topical agent.

4. Empiric antibiotic therapy—Broad-spectrum. Always cover initially for *Pseudomonas* sp. Rarely needs anaerobic coverage. Specific antibiotic therapy on bacteriologic identification requires larger doses than usual (especially aminoglycosides) to provide adequate tissue levels. Our routine triple-antibiotic therapy is nafcillin, piperacillin, and amikacin.

5. Clysis of antibiotic solution under infected burn eschar

H. NONBACTERIAL INFECTION
1. Viral infection—Usually heals with time; virucidal agent recommended for systemic involvement
2. Fungal infection—Topical application of nystatin effectively clears fungi and yeast and may be used prophylactically prior to eschar excision. Amphotericin B is used for systemic involvement. Severe fungal infection may require aggressive débridement.

VII. ELECTRICAL INJURIES

A. TISSUE DESTRUCTION
Tissue destruction is most severe at the points of entry and exit (the points at which the electrical current is most concentrated). Deep tissue damage often greatly exceeds skin injury; it is usually not obvious at the time of initial injury. Electrical resistance of tissues—from least to most—is nerve, blood, and blood vessel, muscle, skin, tendon, fat, and bone.

B. TREATMENT
1. CPR—High-voltage currents usually cause cardiac standstill, whereas low-voltage (<440 V) currents usually produce ventricular fibrillation.
2. Protection against neurologic damage caused by fractures of the spine—Place in cervical spine collar and on a long backboard to immobilize the entire spine. Tetanic contraction of muscle may cause fractures of the cervical and lumbosacral spine and long bones; therefore, perform screening radiographs. Perform frequent examinations.
3. Fluid resuscitation—Cannot be calculated from percentage of skin burns. Give sufficient volume to establish urine output of 1.5 mL/kg/h.
a. High incidence of muscular and blood injury causes hemoglobinuria/myoglobinuria. Hence, larger fluid requirements are needed. If increased fluid resuscitation is not successful, then mannitol (25 g/h) and $NaHCO_3$ are necessary to prevent precipitation of myoglobin/hemoglobin in the renal tubules. Mannitol is continued until the urine color clears.
b. Progressively severe metabolic acidosis occurs with electrical injuries and massive tissue destruction. Use IV sodium bicarbonate to correct base deficit.
4. Early débridement of grossly necrotic tissue; amputation may be needed if unable to control acidosis
5. Immediate extremity fasciotomy is frequently required; check compartment pressures.

VIII. CHEMICAL INJURIES

A. PROBLEMS
A major problem in patients with chemical injuries is the failure to recognize ongoing destruction of tissue.

16

BURN CARE

B. MANAGEMENT
Initial management is dilution with copious amounts of water, not neutralization of the chemical burn, because the heat of neutralization can extend the injury (may need to irrigate >1 hour for alkali burns).
1. Avoid hypothermia.
2. Special precautions
a. Lithium—Remove particles prior to irrigation.
b. Hydrofluoric acid—Apply 10% calcium gluconate cream in most cases; can inject calcium gluconate SQ for severe burns
c. Phenol—Irrigation must be vigorous (shower) since absorption increases when spread over a large area.
d. Tar/asphalt—Use Medisol, bacitracin, or other petroleum-based product.

IX. OUTPATIENT AND CLINIC TREATMENT

A. SELECTION
If the patient does not meet admission criteria, he or she can be treated as an outpatient.

B. TREATMENT
1. Tetanus prophylaxis
2. Wounds washed with mild soap
3. Debris and blisters should be débrided.
4. Apply antibiotic ointment (bacitracin, Neosporin, Polysporin) and nonstick porous gauze (Adaptic), and wrap with gauze.

C. FOLLOW-UP CARE
1. Dressing care b.i.d.—Wash with mild soap (to remove debris and fibrinous exudate) and reapply dressing.
2. Vigorous range-of-motion exercises
3. Return to clinic and/or physical therapy as needed.

D. WOUNDS
If the wounds are deep partial- or full-thickness burns, the patient may be treated as an outpatient until excision and grafting are required.
1. If the wound is not re-epithelialized by 2 weeks, it should undergo excision and grafting.
2. Longer healing time increases scarring.
3. If scarring is a problem, the patient should be fitted for pressure garments and wear them 23 hours a day until wounds no longer blanch.
4. Use moisturizing cream on healing skin.
5. As long as the healed wound is hyperemic and blanches, the patient should vigorously put pressure on (massage-pressure) the wound daily to help prevent scarring.
6. Avoid sun exposure to graft or burn, since it may cause hyperpigmentation.

7. Pruritus is treated with moisturizing cream and PO diphenhydramine (Benadryl) or hydroxyzine (Vistaril) p.r.n.

X. COMPLICATIONS OF BURN INJURY

A. GI
1. Adynamic ileus—Especially large burns; gastric and colonic involvement; generally resolves within 24 hours with IV hydration and NG suction; may be early signs of sepsis
2. Ulcers—"Curling's ulcer" occurs anywhere in the GI tract, though mostly stomach, duodenum, and jejunum. Etiology unknown, but thought to be due to hypovolemia, hypoperfusion, not necessarily related to burn size. Incidence is rare now with early antacids and H_2 blockers and with early enteral feeding. Initial nonoperative management and indications for surgical intervention are essentially the same as those for hemorrhage from peptic ulcer disease (see Chap. 32).
3. Acalculous cholecystitis—Uncommon, but diagnose with HIDA scan or ultrasound. Treat with antibiotics and either percutaneous drainage or cholecystectomy.

B. OCULAR
1. Keep eyes moist using artificial tears or ointments.
2. Corneal abrasions—Associated with facial burns. Treatment includes topical antibiotics and release and grafting of ectropion.
3. Cataracts (especially with electrical injury)

C. CUTANEOUS
1. Wound contracture—Result of scarring (prevented by massage and pressure garment). May result in cosmetic or functional problems. May limit range of motion, especially if it extends across a joint. Contracture may be released surgically with grafting or Z-plasty. As children grow, contractures will become more pronounced since the scars do not grow; multiple releases may be required.
2. Hypertrophic scar
a. Occurs with wounds that take >2 weeks to heal, but there is an increased incidence with deep burns and extended exposure of ungrafted burn wound, with maximal scarring at 3-6 months after injury
b. Treatment
   (1) Pressure-fitted pressure masks, garments, and massage are used for the first year to reduce scar formation.
   (2) Resurface with graft later.
   (3) Cosmetic treatment is often disappointing.
c. Keloids—Variant of hypertrophic scarring that extend beyond the original wound. Difficult to treat, but steroid injections have been used. Often recur after excision.

16

BURN CARE

D. MISCELLANEOUS
1. Heterotopic calcification
   a. Elbows most common joint
   b. May be related to vigorous OT/PT
2. Chondritis—Secondary to *S. aureus* and *Pseudomonas* spp ear and joint infection
3. Hyperpigmentation—Avoid sun exposure for at least 1 year. Use sun-blocking agents (>15 sun protection factor [SPF]).

Acute Abdomen

Wilson M. Clements, MD

The *acute abdomen* is defined as the rapid onset of abdominal pain, with or without associated symptoms such as nausea and vomiting, in previously well patients. When patients present with signs and symptoms consistent with acute abdomen, the importance of making an *early,* accurate diagnosis cannot be overemphasized. The recovery rate from acute abdominal disease decreases proportionately with delay in diagnosis and treatment.

I. PHYSIOLOGY OF ABDOMINAL PAIN

A. VISCERAL PAIN

The term *visceral* is used to identify diffuse and ill-defined pain. Visceral contraction, spasm, stretching, distention, or chemical irritation results in visceral afferent nerve stimulation. The pain is usually colicky.

1. Visceral pain is usually experienced in the midline, corresponding to the anatomic location of visceral afferent nerve plexuses. The foregut, including stomach, duodenum, pancreas, gallbladder, and liver, has pain transmitted to the celiac plexus, resulting in epigastric pain. The midgut has pain transmitted to the superior mesenteric plexus, causing periumbilical pain. Hindgut pain is transmitted to the inferior mesenteric plexus near the bifurcation of the aorta, characteristically producing pain in the hypogastrium.
2. Pain may be referred to a distant body region, e.g., inflamed gallbladder causes both right upper quadrant pain and shoulder pain. This involves a complicated misinterpretation of visceral afferent impulses that cross the nerve cells of the corresponding somatic dermatome level within the CNS.
3. Visceral efferent fibers control the organ response to the noxious stimulus, both sympathetic and parasympathetic.
   a. Sphincter spasm (sympathetic), decrease in gut motility (parasympathetic), and decrease in organ secretion (parasympathetic)
   b. Responses produce diaphoresis, nausea, emesis, and reflex hypotension.
   c. Severe somatic pain may produce autonomic responses as well.
4. Visceral organs may be burned, crushed, or cut without eliciting pain.

B. PARIETAL PAIN

Parietal pain is abdominal pain secondary to parietal peritoneal irritation, which is perceived through segmental somatic fibers. Reflex involuntary muscle wall rigidity may result from irritation of segmental sensory nerves. Hyperesthesia of the skin may result from ipsilateral peritoneal irritation. This pain manifests as a dull and steady ache.

1. Rebound tenderness elicited by stretching the inflamed parietal peritoneum during examination
2. Does *not* require deep palpation with rapid release; may be elicited with simple percussion or coughing or straining or other subtle change of intra-abdominal pressure

C. GENERALIZED PAIN
Generalized pain is the result of sudden flooding of the peritoneal cavity by pus, blood, or acrid fluid resulting in generalized peritonitis. It may produce somatic as well as autonomic responses.

D. NAUSEA AND VOMITING
1. A nonspecific complaint; its relationship to abdominal pain is important in separating pain of inflammation from mechanical obstruction
2. Severe irritation of the nerves of the peritoneum or mesentery—Ulcer perforation, gangrenous appendicitis, ovarian cyst torsion, pancreatitis (celiac plexus involvement), intestinal strangulation
3. Obstruction of an involuntary muscular tube—Biliary duct, ureter, uterine canal, intestine, appendix; occurs secondary to peristaltic contraction and muscle stretching; hence, colic comes in spasms with vomiting at its peak
a. Character of vomitus may aid in establishing level of intestinal obstruction
4. Action of absorbed toxins on medullary centers—May contribute to vomiting in intestinal obstruction or pancreatitis

II. HISTORY

A. PAIN
1. Location of pain—Localization of pain may give clues to etiology, but abdominal pain may be referred to a site remote from the source of pathology. Diffuse pain suggests two possibilities: visceral pain or uncontained peritonitis.
2. Character of pain—Sharp, dull, burning, constant, intermittent
3. Intensity of pain—Nagging, mild, severe, "worst ever"
4. Onset of pain—Acute vs. insidious
5. Radiation of pain—Back, flank, shoulder, hip, groin
a. Biliary colic—To right scapula
b. Renal colic—To ipsilateral testicle or groin
c. Pancreatitis—To the back
6. Exacerbating or ameliorating factors—Food, medication, activity, deep breathing or coughing, vomiting, defecation, change in position
7. Associated complaints—Respiratory, GI, genitourinary, systemic

B. NAUSEA, VOMITING, AND ANOREXIA
1. Frequency and onset of vomiting—In intestinal obstruction, related to the site of obstruction. The more proximal the obstruction, the more

frequent the vomiting and the earlier the onset. Vomiting may not occur with colonic obstruction, especially if there is a competent ileocecal valve.

2. Character of vomitus
a. Bilious—Nonspecific
b. Food—Upper obstruction
c. Retching—Torsion of viscus
d. Feculent (succus entericus)—Pathognomonic of intestinal obstruction (unusual in colonic obstruction). Feculence is caused by overgrowth of bacteria in stagnant small bowel contents, *not* regurgitation of feces.

3. Relationship of pain to vomiting—In acute appendicitis, nausea and vomiting rarely occur before the onset of pain.

4. Acute appetite loss—Frequently significant, important complaint in acute appendicitis; characteristically precedes onset of pain

C. BOWEL FUNCTION

1. Diarrhea—Gastroenteritis, appendicitis in children, early in partial or complete small bowel obstruction due to evacuation of bowel distal to site of obstruction, acute diverticulitis

2. Constipation or obstipation—Obstruction, paralytic ileus, acute appendicitis

3. Change in stool color
a. Blood and/or mucus—Intussusception in children; colitis, proctitis in adults
b. Acholic stools—Biliary tract obstruction or dysfunction
c. Melenic stools—Upper GI bleed; usually not associated with acute abdominal pain

4. Passage of flatus

D. MENSTRUATION AND SEXUAL HISTORY

In women with acute abdominal pain, rule out ectopic pregnancy, pelvic inflammatory disease, ovarian cysts or torsion, and mittelschmerz, and document the date of the last menses.

E. THOROUGH REVIEW OF SYSTEMS

A comprehensive review can help narrow and refine a differential diagnosis.

1. Cardiopulmonary
a. Pneumonia, emphysema, or myocardial ischemia may often present with severe abdominal complaints.
b. Recent upper respiratory infection symptoms may precede onset of acute mesenteric adenitis, especially in children.

2. Neuromuscular
a. Herpes zoster
b. Fractures, tumors, or osteomyelitis of the spine
c. Tabes dorsalis

17

ACUTE ABDOMEN

3. Genitourinary
   a. Unilateral flank or abdominal pain radiating to the ipsilateral testicle or groin with or without hematuria suggests a renal or ureteral stone.
   b. Pneumaturia—Enterovesical fistula, most commonly due to colonic diverticular disease, frequently associated with pelvic abscess
4. Vascular
   a. Autoimmune diseases or vasculitis
   b. Dissection, rupture, or expansion of abdominal aortic aneurysm
5. Hematologic
   a. Sickle cell crisis or sickle-associated splenic infarct
   b. Lymphoma or leukemia
6. Endocrine/metabolic
   a. Acute diabetic ketoacidosis may present as acute abdomen.
   b. Porphyria
   c. Addisonian crisis
7. Psychiatric

F. PAST MEDICAL HISTORY
The past medical history may suggest the etiology of abdominal pain.
1. Previous abdominal surgeries
2. History of peptic ulcer disease
3. Documented diverticular disease
4. Known gallstones or renal stones
5. Previous episode of similar complaints

G. CURRENT MEDICATIONS
1. Steroids—May mask severity of condition owing to blunted inflammatory response. Patients taking steroids may have intra-abdominal catastrophe with a relatively benign exam.
2. Analgesics, antipyretics, and antibiotics—May mask pain and fever

III. PHYSICAL EXAMINATION

A. GENERAL APPEARANCE
1. Level of discomfort
2. Nutritional status
3. Hydration status

B. ATTITUDE IN BED
1. Still, resists movement, may have knees bent or drawn up—Peritonitis
2. Restless, cannot find comfortable position—Colic
3. Writhing—Consider mesenteric vascular event

C. TEMPERATURE
A subnormal, normal, or elevated temperature can accompany an acute abdomen.

1. 95-96°F (core)—Severe shock of toxemia
2. Normal temperature—Common in noninflammatory process
3. 99-100°F (oral)—Early inflammatory process, usual finding with acute appendicitis
4. 104-105°F—Suspect intra-abdominal abscess or urinary source

D. PULSE
1. Tachycardia is common and may be due to fever, hemorrhage, dehydration, pain, and anxiety.
2. Bradycardia can be seen with advanced sepsis or metabolic disturbances (i.e., hypothyroidism).

E. RESPIRATORY RATE
1. Tachypnea is common.
2. Respiratory alkalosis can be present as an early finding in sepsis.
3. Kussmaul respirations are present with diabetic ketoacidosis.

F. BLOOD PRESSURE
1. Hypertension—May be associated with severe pain
2. Hypotension—Hemorrhage, sepsis, volume depletion

G. CARDIOPULMONARY EXAM
1. Cardiac murmur, rub, or gallops may be significant in cardiac disease presenting as abdominal pain (e.g., myocardial infarction, congestive heart failure, acute rheumatic heart disease, pericarditis).
2. Pulmonary consolidation, effusion, or pleural rub may be significant in pulmonary disease presenting as abdominal pain (e.g., pneumonia, pleuritis, infarct).

H. ABDOMINAL EXAMINATION
1. Observation, inspection
a. Scaphoid, flat, obese, distended
b. Movement with respiration—Note limitation of movement indicating rigidity of the abdominal muscles or diaphragm
c. Have patient indicate the exact point of maximal pain.
d. Inspect all potential sites for hernias, especially the inguinal and femoral region.
2. Auscultation
a. Absent or hypoactive bowel sounds—Peritonitis or ileus
b. High-pitched bowel sounds with rushes, hyperactive—Obstruction
c. Aortic and renal artery bruits—Absence of a bruit never excludes the presence of an aortic aneurysm.
3. Palpation/percussion—Gentleness is essential.
a. Evaluate presence and extent of muscular rigidity.
b. Palpate four quadrants of abdomen and costovertebral angles to assess tenderness (mild, moderate, severe). Palpate for abdominal masses,

17

ACUTE ABDOMEN

abnormal pulsations, and hernial orifices. *Begin away from point of maximal pain.* Conversation or other diversion may be useful in the examination of the anxious patient or young child.

c. Signs of peritoneal irritation
   (1) Percussion ("rebound") tenderness
   (2) Pain with coughing, Valsalva maneuver, or sudden movement
   (3) Rigidity—"Involuntary guarding"
       (a) Pain worsens when rigidity is overcome in abdominal disease.
       (b) Muscular rigidity/resistance may be slight, even in the presence of serious peritonitis with fat, flabby abdominal wall, severe toxemia, and elderly patients.
   (4) Obturator sign—Pain with flexion and internal rotation of the hip indicates inflammation of obturator internus muscle (e.g., appendicitis).
   (5) Psoas sign—Pain on passive extension of hip (stretching the psoas muscle) indicates irritation of the psoas/iliopsoas muscle (retrocecal appendix).
   (6) Rovsing's sign—Pain in the right lower quadrant when pressure is applied to the left lower quadrant; may be present with peritoneal irritation of acute appendicitis
   (7) Cutaneous hyperesthesia—May be tested by pin prick or light touch. Nearly always indicates parietal peritoneal inflammation. Most commonly caused by appendicitis. Occurs in lower abdominal wall.
   (8) Palpation of the flank to detect renal disease (perinephric abscess, inflamed kidney) or retrocecal appendix (both affect quadratus lumborum muscle)
   (9) Liver percussion
       (a) Normal dullness is detected from the 5th rib to the costal margin along the right vertical nipple line and from the 7th to 11th rib in the midaxillary line.
       (b) Loss of liver dullness (with new resonance) occurs with free air in the peritoneum (must be in the absence of abdominal distention).
   (10) Fluid wave
       (a) Indication of free fluid in peritoneal cavity
       (b) Most commonly associated with ascites from liver disease. When a patient with known ascites presents with abdominal pain, fever, and/or leukocytosis, consider spontaneous bacterial peritonitis.

I. EXAMINATION OF THE PELVIC CAVITY

1. Suprapubic palpation and percussion
2. Rectal examination—Extremely important and informative
a. Digital rectal examination to assess localized tenderness, fluctuance, induration, masses, occult or gross blood

b. Digital examination (gentle) of stomas if present
3. Bimanual pelvic examination—Along with the digital rectal exam, this procedure is most helpful and should always be performed by the examining surgeon.
a. Bleeding—Menses, threatened abortion, endometritis, trauma
b. Discharge—Venereal disease, pelvic inflammatory disease
c. Appearance of cervix on speculum exam—Cyanosis of pregnancy, blood from cervical os, purulent discharge
d. Presence of adnexal mass or tenderness—Tubo-ovarian abscess, ectopic pregnancy
e. Uterine size and contour—Consider pregnancy, fibroids
f. Cervical motion tenderness—Classically present in pelvic inflammatory disease, but may be caused by any source of inflammation in the pelvis
4. Check for signs of bladder distention—Percuss bladder size. Catheterize if necessary to ensure empty bladder, especially in elderly patients.

IV. LABORATORY EXAMINATION

A. WHITE BLOOD CELL COUNT
Determine the degree of leukocytosis and the differential.
Note: *The absence of leukocytosis never excludes an inflammatory abdominal diagnosis.*

B. HEMATOCRIT
The hematocrit can indicate anemia, whether chronic (microcytic or macrocytic) or acute. Hemoconcentration may indicate hypovolemia.

C. PLATELET COUNT
Thrombocytopenia is consistent with severe sepsis.

D. ELECTROLYTES
Electrolytes are indicative of volume status and may demonstrate GI losses from diarrhea or protracted vomiting (e.g., hypochloremic hypokalemic metabolic alkalosis or "contraction alkalosis"). Hyperglycemia can be observed in diabetic ketoacidosis or sepsis-induced glucose intolerance.

E. ARTERIAL BLOOD GAS
Arterial blood gases measure metabolic acidosis or alkalosis. Metabolic acidosis in the presence of generalized abdominal pain in the elderly is ischemic colitis until proven otherwise.

F. URINALYSIS
Check for red blood cells, white blood cells, and casts.

17

ACUTE ABDOMEN

G. SERUM β-HUMAN CHORIONIC GONADOTROPIN (HCG)
Determination of serum β-HCG is mandatory in all women of childbearing age to menopause.

H. LIVER FUNCTION TESTS
There are bilirubin (direct and total) and alkaline phosphatase elevations in biliary obstruction and elevated transaminases in hepatocellular injury.

I. AMYLASE ELEVATION
Amylase elevation is seen in pancreatitis, although it is relatively nonspecific. It may be elevated in mesenteric ischemia, perforated duodenal ulcer, ruptured ovarian cyst, and renal failure. The serum lipase determination is more sensitive.

V. RADIOLOGIC EVALUATION

A. UPRIGHT CHEST RADIOGRAPH
Look for pneumonia and free air under the diaphragms; pleural effusion may suggest a subdiaphragmatic inflammatory process.

B. ABDOMINAL FLAT AND UPRIGHT (OR LEFT LATERAL DECUBITUS) RADIOGRAPH
Look for bowel distension and air-fluid levels consistent with ileus or obstruction as well as bowel gas cut-off vs. air through to rectum.
1. Localized ileus ("sentinel loop") may indicate location of inflammatory process (i.e., pancreatitis).
2. Abnormal calcifications—Chronic pancreatitis, 20% of gallstones, 85% of renal calculi
3. Pneumatosis coli and air in the biliary tree (pneumobilia) are ominous signs of dead gut.
4. Mass effect from tumor or abscess
5. Left lateral decubitus may detect free air in patients in whom upright chest radiograph cannot be obtained.

C. ULTRASONOGRAPHY
Ultrasonography is of value in visualizing the hepatobiliary tree, pancreas, vascular structures, kidneys, pelvic organs, and intra-abdominal fluid collections. It is also useful in determining the causes of acute abdominal pain in pediatric patients and gynecologic abnormalities in young women. The focused abdominal sonography in trauma (FAST) is useful and accurate in detecting hemoperitoneum.

D. CT SCAN
CT scan is helpful in cases of acute abdominal pain without clear etiology, but it is most useful in the evaluation of abdominal aortic aneurysm. It provides better definition than ultrasound in the acute evaluation of presumed aortic disease.

E. CONTRAST STUDIES

1. Upper GI studies

a. Water-soluble contrast medium may be helpful in demonstrating a suspected but questionable perforation.

b. Useful in discerning the point of obstruction in small bowel obstruction. Must rule out colonic obstruction first (see section V. E. 2) to avoid inspissated barium above colonic obstruction

2. Lower GI series

a. Useful in discerning the point of obstruction in cases of colonic obstruction

b. Avoid if colonic inflammatory process (i.e., diverticulitis) suspected

c. Air enema is diagnostic and often therapeutic in intussusception in children.

3. IV pyelogram—For diagnosis of ureteral stone or obstruction

4. Angiography—For diagnosis of mesenteric ischemia

VI. OTHER PROCEDURES

A. ENDOSCOPY

1. Upper endoscopy (esophagogastroduodenoscopy)—Primary usefulness in evaluation of GI bleeding, or evaluation of epigastric pain in nonacute setting

2. Sigmoidoscopy or colonoscopy

a. Evaluation of colonic obstruction

b. Diagnosis and potential therapy for nonstrangulated sigmoid volvulus

c. Decompression of severely dilated colon secondary to adynamic ileus

d. Diagnosis of ischemic colitis, pseudomembranous enterocolitis, ulcerative or Crohn's colitis

B. PARACENTESIS AND/OR PERITONEAL LAVAGE

1. Diagnosis of spontaneous bacterial peritonitis in cirrhotic patients; considered diagnostic if absolute neutrophil count ≥500

2. Diagnostic peritoneal lavage may be a useful bedside test in the diagnosis of mesenteric infarction in critically ill patients.

C. CULDOCENTESIS

Culdocentesis is valuable in the diagnosis of ruptured ectopic pregnancy.

D. LAPAROSCOPY

1. Greatest value of laparoscopy is in the diagnosis and treatment of suspected gynecologic causes of acute abdomen.

2. Useful in suspected appendicitis in females of childbearing age (highest negative exploration rate); may also perform appendectomy laparoscopically if appendicitis is found

17

ACUTE ABDOMEN

3. The role of laparoscopy in the evaluation of acute abdomen is changing as laparoscopic instruments and techniques improve.

VII. DIFFERENTIAL DIAGNOSIS OF ACUTE ABDOMEN

A. INFLAMMATORY
1. Perforated viscus
   a. Stomach, duodenum—Ulcer
   b. Bowel—Diverticulum, appendix, carcinoma, traumatic small bowel injury
   c. Gallbladder
2. Primary peritonitis (peritonitis without obvious etiology)
   a. Gram-positive organisms (*Pneumococcus* spp, *Streptococcus* spp) formerly most common; gram-negative infections increasing, especially in females
   b. Tuberculosis—"Doughy" abdomen
   c. Cirrhotic patients with ascites may develop spontaneous bacterial peritonitis and have minimal symptoms.
3. Gastroenteritis, colitis—Viral or bacterial
4. Inflammatory bowel disease
5. Diverticulitis
6. Meckel's diverticulitis
7. Pancreatitis—Alcoholic, biliary, viral, thiazide induced, steroid related, hyperlipidemia, hypercalcemia
8. Hepatitis
   a. Viral—Mimics cholecystitis
   b. Alcoholic
9. Hepatic abscess—Look for other primary septic focus.
10. Splenic abscess
11. Mesenteric lymphadenitis
12. Foreign body perforation of bowel
13. Gynecologic
   a. Pelvic inflammatory disease
   b. Fitz-Hugh–Curtis syndrome (gonococcal perihepatitis)
   c. Endometritis
   d. Toxic shock syndrome
   e. Ruptured ovarian cyst

B. MECHANICAL
1. Intestinal obstruction
   a. Small bowel—Adhesions, hernia, neoplasm, volvulus, intussusception, gallstone ileus, Meckel's band, inflammatory mass
   b. Gastric outlet obstruction—Peptic ulcer disease (pyloric channel), gastric carcinoma
   c. Colon—Neoplasm, hernia, diverticulitis, volvulus
2. Biliary obstruction
   a. Cholelithiasis with impacted or "ball-valve" cystic duct stone

b. Choledocholithiasis

c. Cholangitis
   (1) Neoplasm
   (2) Choledochal cyst
   (3) Choledocholithiasis

3. Solid viscera—Rare

a. Acute splenomegaly—Various hematologic disorders

b. Acute hepatomegaly—Pericarditis, congestive heart failure, Budd-Chiari syndrome

4. Omental torsion—Rare

5. Gynecologic

a. Torsion of ovarian cyst or uterine fibroid

b. Ectopic pregnancy
   (1) Symptoms of early pregnancy—Delayed menses, nausea, vomiting, breast tenderness
   (2) Increased uterine size, but less than anticipated by last menstrual period
   (3) Pain and cramping
   (4) Adnexal mass, cervical motion tenderness
   (5) β-HCG may not be positive.
   (6) Hypovolemic shock due to hemorrhage in 10% of cases

C. VASCULAR

1. Intraperitoneal bleeding

a. Traumatic rupture of liver, spleen, mesentery

b. Delayed splenic rupture

c. Ruptured ectopic pregnancy

d. Ruptured abdominal aortic aneurysm—Sudden onset of new back pain in an individual with atherosclerotic risk factors

e. Ruptured splenic or hepatic aneurysm—Rare

2. Ischemia

a. Mesenteric thrombosis or embolus
   (1) Usually see other signs of peripheral atherosclerosis
   (2) Atrial fibrillation, valvular heart disease, history of myocardial infarction predispose to embolization
   (3) Pain out of proportion to exam
   (4) Metabolic acidosis is a late finding and usually indicates intestinal gangrene
   (5) Short-segment involvement may result in self-limiting episodes and late intestinal stricture formation.

3. Splenic infarction—Common in sickle cell patients

VIII. COMMON CONDITIONS MIMICKING THE ACUTE ABDOMEN

A. ALTERNATIVE CAUSES OF SIGNS AND SYMPTOMS

1. Pneumonia—Pain may be localized in the right or left upper quadrant if the lower lobes are involved.

17

ACUTE ABDOMEN

2. Angina or myocardial infarction—Epigastric pain, heartburn
3. Obstructive uropathy (urethral and prostatic)
4. Acute hepatitis—Right upper quadrant pain, vomiting
5. Sickle cell crisis—Diffuse pain
6. Leukemia—Diffuse pain
7. Radiculopathy—From spinal cord tumors, compression fracture of spine, hip fracture
8. Cystitis—Suprapubic pain and tenderness
9. Prostatitis—Rectal and buttock pain
10. Pyelonephritis—Costovertebral angle tenderness
11. Ureteral obstruction
   a. Calculus or neoplasm
   b. Pain, nausea, vomiting out of proportion to exam

B. **ADDITIONAL ALTERNATIVE CAUSES OF SIGNS AND SYMPTOMS**
   1. Toxins—Lead poisoning, venoms, tetanus, petroleum distillates, aspirin in children
   2. Abdominal wall hematoma—In swimmers, in gymnasts, or following severe effort
   3. Psychogenic—May have ingested foreign body causing psychogenic pain without trauma to the GI tract, or may have true perforation, hemorrhage, or obstruction
   4. Pericarditis
   5. Herpes zoster (shingles)
   6. Diabetic ketoacidosis
   7. Systemic lupus erythematosus
   8. Uremia
   9. Torsion of the testes
   10. Acute intermittent porphyria

IX. INITIAL TREATMENT AND PREOPERATIVE PREPARATION

A. **ASSESSMENT**
Plan on prompt, timely work-up in first 4-6 hours.

B. **DIET**
Keep the patient NPO until the diagnosis is firm and the treatment plan is formulated.

C. **IV FLUIDS**
IV fluid administration should be based on expected fluid losses; large volumes may be required.

D. **HEMODYNAMIC MONITORING**
Hemodynamic monitoring may be required in cases where fluid status and cardiac status are in question or when septic shock is present.

E. NASOGASTRIC INTUBATION
An NG tube should be inserted for bleeding, vomiting, or signs of obstruction or when urgent or emergent laparotomy is planned in a patient who has not been NPO.

F. FOLEY CATHETER
Use a Foley catheter to monitor fluid resuscitation.

G. DECISIONS
1. Immediate surgery
a. If yes, what is the timing of operative intervention (does the patient need time for resuscitation)?
b. What incision should be used?
c. What are the likely findings?
d. Develop a primary operative plan.
e. Consider alternative diagnosis and plans.
f. Use appropriate preoperative antibiotics based on suspected pathology.

2. Admit and observe for possible operation.
a. Serial exams should be performed q 2-4 h during the first 12-24 hours in cases without definite diagnosis. Use narcotics and sedatives minimally to avoid masking physical signs and symptoms (although this is controversial); monitor vital signs frequently.
b. Serial lab exams may be useful; repeat CBC with differential q 4-6 h.

3. No operation—Develop a treatment plan for further diagnostic work-up or nonoperative therapy.

17

ACUTE ABDOMEN

Gynecologic Causes of Acute Abdomen

Kfir Ben-David, MD

Acute abdomen in the female patient is often difficult to define and is associated with a high rate of diagnostic inaccuracies. This is principally related to the fact that abdominal pain in this patient population can arise from a GI, urinary, systemic, or gynecologic source.

I. CAUSES OF ACUTE ABDOMEN IN FEMALES

Approximately 10% of acute abdominal pain in females is attributable to a gynecologic cause. The following represents the incidence of various causes of abdominal pain in females of reproductive age acutely presenting to the emergency department:

Diagnosis	Percentage of Cases
Nonspecific abdominal pain	48
Appendicitis	22
Pelvic inflammatory disease (PID)	14
Urinary tract infection	12
Ovarian cysts	4
Ectopic pregnancy	1

II. DIAGNOSTIC FEATURES OF GYNECOLOGIC DISEASE

A. AGE
The age of the patient can often assist in narrowing the differential diagnosis of acute abdominal pain presentation. The following represents the pathophysiologic incidence of acute abdomen in females relative to the patient's age:

	Incidence (%)			
Diagnosis	*Age <20 Years*	*Age 20-30 Years*	*Age 30-40 Years*	*Age >40 Years*
Appendicitis	50	20	15	15
Pelvic inflammatory disease	34	44	18	14
Ovarian cyst	18	38	14	30
Ectopic pregnancy	4	54	38	4

B. PAIN
The onset, character, location, and duration of abdominal pain all are important parameters in assessing a female patient with an acute abdomen. The location of the pain is influenced by the level of innervation of the pelvic organs, which is as follows.
1. Pain associated with PID, ovarian cysts, and ectopic pregnancies is commonly bilateral.

Origin	Level of Innervation	Location of Pain
Ovary	T10	Lower abdomen
Fallopian tubes	T11-T12	Lower abdomen
Uterus	T10-L1	Lower abdomen
Uterine cervix	T11-S4	Sacrum and buttocks

2. Gynecologic causes of pain do not typically radiate or migrate over time to other sites.

C. ASSOCIATED SYMPTOMS
Gynecologic pathology can often be associated with GI symptoms such as nausea, vomiting, anorexia, or changes in bowel movements. They can also have genitourinary symptoms of frequency, urgency, or dysuria.

III. EVALUATION OF THE FEMALE PATIENT

A. HISTORY
1. Description of the pain—Duration, onset, character, and location
2. Associated symptoms—GI, genitourinary, vaginal discharge, dysmenorrhea, or abnormal vaginal bleeding
3. Gynecologic history
a. Menstrual history—Last menstrual period, regular vs. irregular menses, abnormal flow
b. Sexual history—Safe-sex practice, contraceptive history, history of sexually transmitted diseases or PID
c. Possibility of pregnancy—Nausea, tender breasts, fatigue, frequency
d. Previous gynecologic history—Ectopic pregnancy, ovarian cyst, endometriosis
4. Medical and surgical history

B. PHYSICAL EXAMINATION
1. Vital signs
2. General appearance
3. Abdominal exam—focal vs. diffuse, ± mass, ± peritoneal signs
4. Pelvic exam—Includes manual, speculum, and rectal exam

C. LABORATORY DATA
1. CBC, urinalysis, β-human chorionic gonadotropin (HCG), vaginal prep smear, and Gram stain
2. Radiologic
a. Ultrasound—Pelvic/vaginal ultrasound has become a helpful diagnostic tool in the evaluation of pelvic pathology.
b. Abdominal and pelvic CT scans

D. INVASIVE STUDIES
1. Culdocentesis—Needle aspiration of the posterior cul-de-sac through the posterior vaginal fornix using an 18-gauge spinal needle;

may provide valuable information in evaluating possible intra-abdominal bleeding (e.g., ectopic pregnancy)

2. Laparoscopy—When the diagnosis of an acute abdomen is in question and there is no clear indication for laparotomy, diagnostic laparoscopy may provide a definitive diagnosis and means of treatment.

IV. GYNECOLOGIC CAUSES OF THE ACUTE ABDOMEN

A. PELVIC INFLAMMATORY DISEASE

See Chapter 19 section IV. A.

1. Clinical presentation
a. History—Often patients are asymptomatic. Lower abdominal pain (bilateral) is a frequent complaint (89%) and is described as constant and dull. Other associated symptoms include fever, chills, vaginal discharge, nausea, urethritis, and cervicitis. Most frequent cause is *Neisseria gonorrhoeae* and *Chlamydia* infection. Symptoms present 3-6 days after inoculation.
b. Physical examination—Can vary markedly depending on the extent of disease. Common objective findings are the following.
  (1) Fever
  (2) Bilateral lower abdominal pain
  (3) Vaginal discharge
  (4) Cervical motion tenderness (Chandelier's sign)
  (5) Additional findings—May include bilateral lower abdominal masses or fullness and/or rectal tenderness

2. Right upper quadrant pain or pleuritic pain develops in 5-10% of cases and represents perihepatic inflammation (Fitz-Hugh–Curtis syndrome).

3. Laboratory studies
a. Leukocytosis
b. Negative for β-HCG
c. Gram stain showing *N. gonorrhoeae* and *Chlamydia* sp

4. Pelvic ultrasound—Often useful when the diagnosis is unclear, and particularly useful in the presence of an adnexal mass. Tubo-ovarian abscess is represented by a complex adnexal mass in 94% of cases and cystic mass in 6%.

5. Laparoscopy—If the diagnosis is uncertain, diagnostic laparoscopy may be indicated in selected patients.

6. Treatment—The choice of therapy takes into account the patient's clinical status and suspected diagnosis. The range of therapy from ambulatory treatment to emergent laparotomy is representative of the spectrum of this disease. Because this disease is typically seen during the reproductive years, every effort should be made to minimize the chance of infertility.
a. Outpatient regimens—Reserved for patients who are compliant and likely to follow up. This is frequently associated with a high rate of recurrence.

18

GYNECOLOGIC CAUSES OF ACUTE ABDOMEN

Option 1
1. Ofloxacin 400 mg PO b.i.d. × 14 days *or*
2. Levofloxacin 500 mg PO daily × 14 days with or without
3. Metronidazole 500 mg PO daily × 14 days

Option 2
1. Ceftriaxone 250 mg IM single dose *or*
2. Cefoxitin 2 g IM single dose and probenecid 1 g PO in single dose *and*
3. Metronidazole 500 mg PO b.i.d. × 14 days
b. Inpatient regimens—For patients who are noncompliant, are pregnant, have failed outpatient treatment, are HIV positive, have a pelvic mass, or have a tubo-ovarian abscess

Option 1
1. Cefoxitin 2 g IV q 6 h *or*
2. Cefotetan 2 g IV q 12 h *and*
3. Doxycycline 100 mg PO (preferably) or IV q 12 h

Option 2
1. Clindamycin 900 mg IV q 8 h *and*
2. Gentamicin 2 mg/kg load followed by 1.5 mg/kg IV q 8 h
a. PO therapy can be usually initiated within 24-48 hours of clinical improvement
b. PO therapy should continue to complete 14 days of therapy.

7. Nonpharmacologic treatment
a. Bedrest—Simple elevation of the head of the bed without flexion (White's position)
b. NPO
c. IV fluids

8. Surgical management—Operative intervention is indicated in the following situations.
a. Ruptured tubo-ovarian abscess (5-10% mortality)
b. Septic shock
c. Failure to respond to inpatient therapy
d. The standard surgical therapy in the past was total abdominal hysterectomy/bilateral salpingo-oophorectomy, which carries the lowest morbidity and mortality. The current trend is toward more conservative procedures aimed at preserving reproduction (e.g., unilateral adenectomy).

B. HEMORRHAGE FROM OVARIAN CYSTS

Acute abdominal pain can arise from several benign ovarian pathologic conditions.

1. Corpus luteum cysts
2. Ovarian endometrioma
3. Follicular cysts
4. The pain that is seen with these conditions is frequently due to the expansion of the ovarian capsule or peritoneal irritation secondary to hemorrhage or rupture of these structures. Most follicular and corpus

luteum cysts can be managed expectantly, and most resolve within 4-8 weeks without medical or surgical intervention.

5. Corpus luteum cysts—Formation is following a hemorrhage into the corpus luteum with subsequent resorption of blood. A corpus luteum is termed a *corpus luteum cyst* if it is >3 cm.

a. History—Pain typically begins at or after ovulation. This typically occurs in the lower abdomen and is typically bilateral (unilateral pain may be present). Abnormalities in menstrual cycle may be seen.

b. Physical exam
   (1) Typically febrile
   (2) Bilateral lower abdominal pain
   (3) Adnexal mass may be palpable.
   (4) Diffuse pelvic tenderness
   (5) Rupture with hemoperitoneum is more frequent on the right side (67%). Blood loss may be significant enough to require operative intervention. When bleeding occurs, it may be difficult to differentiate from ectopic pregnancy.

c. Laboratory test—A pregnancy test in this group of patients is helpful in differentiating from ectopic pregnancy. A negative β-HCG test in an ovulating female with blood in the pelvis is highly suggestive of a ruptured corpus luteum cyst.

d. Pelvic ultrasound—When the patient is stable, a pelvic ultrasound may be valuable. Classic findings include the following.
   (1) Free fluid in the cul-de-sac
   (2) Presence of complex or cystic adnexal mass
   (3) Presence of an intrauterine gestational sac rules out ectopic pregnancy

e. Management—Most functional cysts resolve spontaneously within 4-8 weeks and hence are best managed conservatively. In the absence of hemorrhage or torsion, an interval ultrasound in 4-6 weeks is all that is needed to assess for cyst regression. When significant hemorrhage or torsion is present, operative intervention is indicated. After confirmation that the bleeding is secondary to an ovarian cyst, cystectomy is the operative treatment of choice.

C. OVARIAN ENDOMETRIOMA

Acute abdominal pain can result from rupture or leakage from an ovarian endometrioma that can cause an intense chemical peritonitis often associated with a low-grade fever. Contents of the endometrioma may pool in the cul-de-sac and cause rectal discomfort with defecation. This condition is typically associated with pelvic endometriosis and history of pelvic pain with menstrual cycle.

D. ECTOPIC PREGNANCY

Ectopic pregnancy is defined as an implantation of a fertilized ovum outside the uterine cavity. Extrauterine sites include the fallopian tubes (≈99%), ovary (≈1%), uterine cervix, and abdominal cavity. The incidence has been

18

GYNECOLOGIC CAUSES OF ACUTE ABDOMEN

increasing since the 1970s and parallels the rise in PID. Approximately 3% of pregnancies are ectopic, which makes this type of pregnancy the leading cause of maternal mortality. The arterial supply to the fallopian tube is derived from the ovarian and uterine artery, which provides a rich blood supply that can result in significant hemorrhage with a tubal pregnancy.

1. Risk factors include a history of PID, presence of intrauterine device, previous pelvic surgery, previous ectopic pregnancy, prior tubal ligation, history of infertility, and use of progestin-only contraceptives.
2. History—Presenting complaints
a. Abdominal pain (usually unilateral; 90-100%)
b. Amenorrhea or abnormal uterine bleeding (50-80%)
c. Symptoms of early pregnancy (10-25%)
d. Shoulder pain occurs in 25% of women with ectopic pregnancies as a result of diaphragmatic irritation from hemoperitoneum.
3. Physical examination—May be nonspecific and as a result a high index of suspicion is required. Pelvic exam reveals adnexal mass in $\frac{1}{3}$ of patients and is typically tender. The uterus is slightly enlarged in $\frac{1}{3}$ of cases.
4. Diagnostic studies
a. Pregnancy test—Ectopic pregnancies produce low levels of HCG and require a sensitive test for detection. Currently the enzyme-linked immunoassay urine pregnancy test (ICON) is used. Serial pregnancy tests may be useful.
b. Culdocentesis—A simple test that can diagnose intraperitoneal bleeding. A positive test result is >0.5 mL of nonclotting blood with a hematocrit >15%.
c. Ultrasound—Transvaginal ultrasound can identify intrauterine pregnancies and effectively rule out ectopic pregnancies. Fetal heart activity outside the uterus is diagnostic of ectopic pregnancy. Free fluid in the cul-de-sac is not uncommon.
d. Laparoscopy—Helpful if the diagnosis is uncertain after the other diagnostic tests in this section
5. Management—Surgery is the mainstay of therapy for diagnosed or suspected ectopic pregnancy. The stability of the patient, the size of the ectopic pregnancy, and the patient's desire for future fertility affect the therapeutic approach.
a. Hemodynamically unstable—Immediate exploratory laparotomy
b. Hemodynamically stable—Exploratory laparoscopy
6. Surgical options—Partial or complete salpingectomy or salpingostomy with removal of the ectopic pregnancy and preservation of the tube. Serum HCG must be followed to zero if the involved fallopian tube is left in place.
7. Medical options—Methotrexate has been used as an alternative to surgical therapy in selected patients with success. These patients include those with the following: ectopic <3 cm, intact tubal serosa, desire for future fertility, no active bleeding, stable or rising HCG, and no hepatic or renal dysfunction.

E. OVARIAN TORSION

Ovarian torsion is an unusual but important cause of acute abdominal pain. It occurs most commonly during the reproductive years but may happen at any age. Occasionally, torsion may be intermittent, with spontaneous resolution. Frequently it occurs on the right. Most cases of ovarian torsion are due to ovarian enlargement caused by a functional cyst or neoplasm (50-60% of cases). The most common neoplasm leading to torsion is the benign cystic teratoma and fibroma.

1. History—Acute onset of unilateral lower quadrant abdominal pain. Associated nausea and vomiting in $^2/_3$ of patients. Intermittent pain may precede the event.
2. Physical exam—± Low-grade fever, tenderness to palpation, peritoneal signs are uncommon. Pelvic exam reveals unilateral tenderness. Mass may or may not be present. Interval pelvic exam may reveal ovarian or adnexal swelling secondary to developing edema.
3. Diagnostic studies
a. Negative β-HCG test results
b. Pelvic ultrasound—Typically shows an enlarged ovary that is uniformly echogenic
c. Diagnostic laparoscopy—Indicated if the diagnosis is uncertain and there is a high degree of suspicion for torsion
4. Management—The key to successful management of torsion is early diagnosis to prevent infarction of the ovary or adnexa. Hence, surgical treatment of ovarian torsion is based on the presence or absence of infarction.
a. Infarction present—Salpingo-oophorectomy
b. No infarction
   (1) Untwist the pedicle.
   (2) Perform cystectomy.
   (3) Stabilize the ovary.

F. MIDCYCLE OVULATORY PAIN (MITTELSCHMERZ)

Midcycle ovulatory pain is associated with intraperitoneal bleeding related to ovulation. The pain is highly variable. Pain is described as sharp and sudden, and it localizes to one quadrant. Pain usually subsides over several hours. Ovulatory pain in the anticoagulated patient may be more severe because of increased bleeding from the follicle.

18

GYNECOLOGIC CAUSES OF ACUTE ABDOMEN

The Surgical Abdomen During Pregnancy

Kfir Ben-David, MD

I. PHYSIOLOGIC ALTERATIONS DURING PREGNANCY

A. CARDIOVASCULAR
1. Total blood volume is increased 25-40%.
2. Plasma volume is increased 50%.
3. Red blood cell mass remains unchanged or may increase up to 15%.
4. These changes lead to the physiologic anemia of pregnancy.
5. Cardiac output is increased by 30-50%.
6. Blood flow is redistributed to the placenta, uterus, skin, kidneys, and mammary glands.
7. Progesterone and prostacyclin reduce systemic vascular resistance.

B. PULMONARY
1. Functional residual capacity is decreased 20%.
2. Oxygen consumption is increased 15%.

C. HEMATOLOGIC
1. The pregnant patient is hypercoagulable with a fivefold to sixfold increased incidence of deep venous thrombosis.
2. Increased levels of factors VII, VIII, X, and fibrinogen
3. Fibrinolytic activity of the plasma is depressed.
4. Reduction in the velocity of venous blood returning from the lower extremities and a rise in venous pressure in the lower extremities

D. RENAL
1. The glomerular filtration rate and renal plasma flow are increased by 30-50%.
2. Blood urea nitrogen and creatinine are 25% lower than for nongravid females.
3. The renal calices, pelves, and ureters dilate.
4. Urinary stasis in gravid women may explain why a higher incidence of pyelonephritis is associated with bacteriuria in them than in nonpregnant women.

E. FETAL HEMOGLOBIN
1. Fetal hemoglobin is oxygen avid.
2. A maternal Pao_2 of 60 mm Hg saturates fetal hemoglobin 100%.
3. Raising maternal Pao_2 higher than this does not provide more oxygen to the fetus.
4. If maternal Pao_2 falls below 60 mm Hg, fetal hemoglobin saturation falls dramatically.

19

5. Fetal Pao_2 is 10-33 mm Hg and depends on uterine blood flow provided maternal Pao_2 is >60 mm Hg.

II. RADIOGRAPHS AND THE PREGNANT PATIENT

The maternal and fetal mortality of surgical disease is related to diagnostic and therapeutic delay. In general, radiographic studies that are deemed necessary to document a life-threatening condition in the pregnant patient should be performed without delay. Many studies have shown no increase in the incidence of abortions or malformations with exposures <0.05 Gy delivered at any time during pregnancy (Tables 19-1 and 19-2).

III. COMPLICATIONS OF PREGNANCY

The incidence of nonobstetric surgery in pregnant patients is approximately 1:500 deliveries. Pregnancy-specific causes of abdominal pain occur in 1:100-300 deliveries and are thus far more common than general surgical causes of abdominal pain.

A. ECTOPIC PREGNANCY

Ectopic pregnancy is defined as implantation of a fertilized ovum outside the uterine cavity.

1. Extrauterine sites include the fallopian tubes (99%), ovary (1%), uterine cervix, and abdominal cavity. The incidence has been increasing since the 1970s and parallels the rise in pelvic inflammatory disease (PID).
2. ≈3% of pregnancies are ectopic and are the leading cause of maternal mortality.
3. Risk factors include a history of PID, presence of intrauterine device, previous pelvic surgery, previous ectopic pregnancy, prior tubal ligation, history of infertility, and use of progestin-only contraceptives.
4. History—Abdominal pain, amenorrhea or abnormal uterine bleeding, and symptoms of early pregnancy
5. Physical examination—Adnexal mass in $1/3$ of patients and is typically tender. The uterus is slightly enlarged in $1/3$ of cases.
6. Diagnostic studies
a. Pregnancy test
b. Culdocentesis

TABLE 19-1		
ACCEPTABLE LEVELS OF FETAL RADIATION EXPOSURE		
Pregnancy Trimester	Acceptable Exposure (Gy)	Overexposure Malformations
Implantation	<0.1	>0.1 Gy—abortion likely
First	<0.1	Retardation, microcephaly, retinal degeneration
Second	<0.15	Stunted growth, microcephaly, mental retardation
Third	<0.15	Dermal and hematologic cancer

TABLE 19-2

AVERAGE RADIATION EXPOSURE OF SELECTED STUDIES

Study	Exposure (Gy)
Chest radiograph PA and lateral	0.0001-0.0003
KUB flat and upright	0.0001-0.0004
IV pyelogram	0.004-0.1
Voiding cystourethrogram	0.004-0.008
Barium enema	0.003-0.005
Upper GI	0.003-0.005
Small bowel follow-through	0.004-0.006
CT abdomen	0.02-0.03
CT chest	0.02-0.03
HIDA scan	0.005-0.007
Nuclear bleeding scan	0.001-0.005
Feeding tube placement	0.001-0.01
V̇/Q̇ scan	0.0002
ERCP	0.0004-0.0004

PA = posteroanterior; KUB = kidney, ureter, bladder; V̇/Q̇ = ventilation/perfusion;
ERCP = endoscopic retrograde cholangiopancreatography.

    c. Ultrasound

    d. Laparoscopy

  7. Management—Surgery is the mainstay of therapy for diagnosed or suspected ectopic pregnancy.

B. RUPTURED OVARIAN CYSTS

1. May present early in pregnancy
2. Ill-defined, bilateral lower abdominal pain
3. GI symptoms are not prominent.
4. Pelvic ultrasound reveals pelvic fluid.
5. Intrauterine gestation sac excludes ectopic pregnancy.
6. When hemorrhage necessitates ovary resection, progesterone replacement may be tried, with variable fetal salvage.

IV. NONOBSTETRIC GYNECOLOGIC DISEASE

Sexually transmitted diseases (STDs) can have profound effects on maternal and neonatal outcome. PID must be considered in every woman of reproductive age with low abdominal pain.

A. PELVIC INFLAMMATORY DISEASE (see Chap. 18 section IV. A)

1. History—Asymptomatic, lower abdominal pain (bilateral), fever, chills, vaginal discharge, nausea, urethritis, cervicitis
2. Most frequent cause is *Neisseria gonorrhoeae* and *Chlamydia* sp infection. Symptoms present 3-6 days after inoculation.

  a. *N. gonorrhoeae*

    (1) A strong association between gonococcal infection and septic spontaneous abortion

b. *Chlamydia trachomatis*
   (1) Cultured from 2-24% of gravidas
   (2) The most common bacterial STD in women—Urethritis, cervicitis, salpingitis
   (3) Causes neonatal conjunctivitis and pneumonias
3. Physical examination—Fever, bilateral lower abdominal pain, vaginal discharge, cervical motion tenderness (Chandelier's sign), rectal tenderness
4. Studies—Leukocytosis, negative β-human chorionic gonadotropin, Gram stain showing *N. gonorrhoeae and Chlamydia* sp, pelvic ultrasound
5. Treatment
a. Outpatient regimens
Option 1
1. Ofloxacin 400 mg PO b.i.d. × 14 days *or*
2. Levofloxacin 500 mg PO daily × 14 days *with or without*
3. Metronidazole 500 mg PO b.i.d. × 14 days
Option 2
1. Ceftriaxone 250 mg IM single dose *or*
2. Cefoxitin 2 g IM single dose and probenecid 1 g PO in single dose *and*
3. Metronidazole 500 mg PO b.i.d. × 14 days
b. Inpatient regimens
Option 1
1. Cefoxitin 2 g IV q 6 h *or*
2. Cefotetan 2 g IV q 12 h *and*
3. Doxycycline 100 mg PO q 12 h
Option 2
1. Clindamycin 900 mg IV q 8 h *and*
2. Gentamicin 2 mg/kg load followed by I.5 mg/kg IV q 8 h

B. TUBO-OVARIAN ABSCESS
1. A frequent complication of acute salpingitis
2. The abscess may be confined to the tube but more commonly involves the entire tube and ovary complex.
3. Unilateral in 70% of cases
4. Polymicrobial in almost 100% of cases
a. *Bacteroides* sp (48%)
b. *Escherichia coli* (37%)
c. *Streptococcus* sp (18%)
d. *Peptostreptococcus* sp (18%)
e. *Haemophilus influenzae* (11%)
5. *C. trachomatis* and *N. gonorrhoeae* are usually not present in the abscess but can be recovered from the cervix in 30% of cases.
6. Pelvic and cervical motion tenderness are present in 90%.
7. Nausea and vomiting occur in up to 40% of cases.

8. Pelvic ultrasound shows a complex adnexal mass in 95%.
9. Unruptured abscess should be treated with clindamycin and cefotaxime (Claforan).
10. 25% of patients fail antibiotic therapy, and most lose their pregnancy, except patients in the first trimester who have the corpus luteum–containing ovary resected.

C. LEIOMYOMA
1. Most common benign tumor in the female pelvis
2. Can degenerate, bleed, and torse during pregnancy
3. Abnormal vaginal bleeding
4. Exquisite pain and tenderness
5. The patient may be in labor.
6. White blood cell (WBC) count is often elevated.
7. Ultrasound can show the leiomyoma but may not differentiate infarcted or torsed leiomyomas from nonpathologic ones.

D. OVARIAN TORSION
1. Usually the ovary is enlarged by a cyst or neoplasm.
2. Can be intermittent with periods of symptomatic remission
3. The pain may be colicky, constant, or progressive.
4. Persistent fever is not prominent; if present, reconsider the differential diagnosis.
5. Ultrasound usually can demonstrate the torsion.
6. Operation may allow salvage of the ovary and pregnancy.

E. OVARIAN CANCER
1. Occurs in 1:18,000-20,000 pregnancies
2. Most are epithelial carcinomas followed by germ cell tumors.
3. Symptomatic during the first trimester as a result of ovarian torsion. When symptomatic late in pregnancy, it is usually due to rupture or hemorrhage of the tumor.
4. Large tumors can obstruct delivery and may make cesarean section necessary.
5. When >5 cm and persistent into the second trimester, surgical exploration is mandatory.
6. 2-5% of ovarian tumors discovered during pregnancy are malignant compared to 20% in nonpregnant patients.
7. Pregnancy does not adversely affect the maternal prognosis.

V. GENERAL SURGICAL DISEASE DURING PREGNANCY

A. ACUTE APPENDICITIS
Acute appendicitis occurs in 1:200 pregnancies.
1. The most common extrauterine complication that requires surgical treatment

19

THE SURGICAL ABDOMEN DURING PREGNANCY

2. Most common in the first two trimesters, but can occur in the third trimester
3. Anorexia, which is present in >90% of people with appendicitis between 15-60 years of age, is present in only 60% of pregnant patients with appendicitis.
4. Nausea and vomiting are variable.
5. Right-sided abdominal pain is the only constant finding.
6. Rebound and guarding become less prevalent in the second and third trimesters and may be present in only 50-60% of patients in the first trimester.
7. Temperature <100°F in 25-50% of patients
8. Tachycardia in <25%
9. WBC count during pregnancy is 15,000-20,000/mL blood. >90% of pregnant women with appendicitis are often within this range. However, predominance of polymorphonuclear cells are usually present.
10. If appendicitis cannot be ruled out in the gravid female, the patient should undergo appendectomy.
11. Fetal mortality increases by fourfold from 5% with early appendicitis to 20% with perforated appendix.
12. Premature labor is 15% and is similar to both a negative laparotomy and simple appendectomy (nonperforated).
13. Laparoscopy may be indicated in equivocal cases, especially early in pregnancy.
14. In the second and third trimesters, a muscle-splitting incision should be made over the point of maximal tenderness.
15. A surgical abdominal incision is not contraindication to labor, and dehiscence is rare.

B. ACUTE CHOLECYSTITIS
Acute cholecystitis occurs in roughly 1:2000 pregnancies.
1. Occurs during pregnancy.
   a. Resting volume of the gallbladder increases.
   b. Residual volume after emptying increases.
   c. Content of cholesterol in bile increases.
   d. Circulating bile salt pool decreases.
2. Nausea and vomiting are variable.
3. Right upper quadrant pain is invariably present.
4. Murphy's sign is present in only 5% of pregnant females.
5. Laboratory evaluation is seldom helpful.
6. Jaundice occurring during pregnancy is due to hepatitis in 45% of cases, benign cholestasis of pregnancy in 20%, and common bile duct stones in only 7% of cases.
7. Ultrasonic evaluation retains 95% sensitivity.
8. Management should be conservative and is successful in 85% of patients.

9. Surgical treatment should be considered when clinical condition does not respond to antibiotics.
10. Fetal loss from surgical treatment of acute cholecystitis is ≈15% during the first trimester and 5% during the latter trimesters.
11. If gangrene or perforation occurs, maternal and fetal mortality approach 15% and 60%, respectively.
12. Endoscopic retrograde cholangiopancreatography and sphincterotomy can be performed for obstructing common bile duct stones. Radiation exposure to the fetus can be limited to <0.0004 Gy by lead apron.

C. PANCREATITIS
Pancreatitis occurs in 1:3000 pregnancies.
1. Usually due to gallstones
2. Alcoholic pancreatitis is rare.
3. Management is conservative—>90% of cases resolve within 3 days.
4. When unresponsive, most would opt for endoscopic sphincterotomy, which will be successful in >90% of patients.
5. Definitive cholecystectomy can then be performed after delivery or, if necessary, during the second trimester.

D. BOWEL OBSTRUCTION
Bowel obstruction occurs in 1:4000 pregnancies.
1. Causes
a. 60% are due to adhesions.
b. 25% are due to volvulus.
c. 5% are due to intussusception.
d. 3% are due to hernias.
e. <1% are due to neoplasms.
2. Greater risk during their first pregnancy following abdominal surgery
3. Three periods of greatest risk
a. In the 4th and 5th months, when the uterus changes from a pelvic to an abdominal organ, leading to traction on previously formed adhesions
b. In the 8th and 9th months, when the fetal head descends into the pelvis
c. During delivery, when a sudden change in the intra-abdominal anatomy occurs
4. Abdominal pain, vomiting, and obstipation in nonpregnant patients with small bowel obstruction is unchanged by pregnancy.
5. Obstruction presents with acute onset of pain in 85% of patients.
6. Vomiting may be present in as few as 25%.
7. Diarrhea may occur in up to 20%.
8. Distention can be difficult to assess, and bowel sounds may be normal.
9. 60% have a leukocyte count within the normal range.
10. Fever, tachycardia, oliguria, and hypotension occur late in the presentation and usually signify compromised bowel that portends near 100% fetal mortality.

11. Maternal hypovolemia and hypoxia are most often responsible for fetal death.
12. Early surgery should be the rule.
13. The incision should be vertical and sufficient to afford good exposure without undue manipulation of the uterus.
14. Only sigmoid volvulus should be managed nonoperatively with colonoscopic detorsion with or without rectal tube as a temporizing measure. Recurrence rates are high, so definitive therapy should be planned.
15. Maternal mortality for bowel obstruction is 10-15%; fetal mortality is 33-50%.

E. PEPTIC ULCER
Peptic ulcer is rare in pregnancy.
1. Most bleeding ulcers can be managed endoscopically to completion of pregnancy, then the appropriate surgical therapy can be undertaken.
2. When perforation occurs, management should be the same as for nonpregnant patients.
3. Consideration should be given to the length of the procedure, because limiting general anesthetic time decreases the chances of premature labor.
4. Vagotomy and pyloroplasty or Graham patch seem the best choices.
5. Hypotension with bleeding episodes requires aggressive surgical resuscitation. The uterus cannot autoregulate during hypotensive episodes resulting in fetal hypoxia. Episodes of hypoxemia certainly are of greater risk to the fetus than a single general anesthetic for definitive surgical therapy.

F. COLORECTAL CANCER
Colorectal cancer occurs in 1:50,000-1000,000 pregnancies.
1. Delay in diagnosis is common because pregnancy may mimic some of the early signs of colon cancer (distention, constipation, and anorexia).
2. 75% of these cancers are discovered because of rectal exam done during pregnancy or at the time of delivery.
3. Management should be as for nonpregnant patients. Severe constipation, weight loss, anorexia, abdominal pain, distention, rectal bleeding, and occult fecal blood can and should be evaluated in the pregnant patient by colonoscopy.
4. Carcinoembryonic antigen is of little use during pregnancy.
5. Resectable lesions should be operated expeditiously unless fetal maturity is shortly forthcoming.
6. With metastatic disease, surgery should be delayed until after delivery.
7. Cesarean section may be indicated for large lesions occurring below the pelvic brim; otherwise, the type of delivery is dictated by the usual obstetric indications.
8. Pregnancy does not seem to affect long-term maternal outcome.

VI. UROLOGIC DISEASE

A. BACTERURIA
Bacteruria occurs in 4-7% of gravidas.
1. Usually asymptomatic
2. 20-40% of pregnant patients with bacteruria develop pyelonephritis.
3. Gravidas should receive 7-10 days of antibiotics for bacteruria.

B. UROLITHIASIS
Urolithiasis occurs in approximately 1:1500 pregnancies.
1. Most prevalent during the 2nd and 3rd trimesters
2. Ultrasound is diagnostic in ≈50% of cases.
3. Initial management should be conservative, because 50-80% of stones pass spontaneously.
4. If conservative management fails, internal urinary stents can be placed under ultrasonic guidance. If stents cannot be passed from below, ultrasound-guided percutaneous nephrostomy tube placement under local anesthesia should be considered. Internal stents should be changed q 8 weeks.
5. Nephrolithotomy should not be undertaken because of prolonged anesthetic requirements and ionizing radiation exposure.
6. Extracorporeal shockwave lithotripsy has not been approved for use during pregnancy.

19

THE SURGICAL ABDOMEN DURING PREGNANCY

GI Bleeding

David R. Fischer, MD

I. HISTORY

A history and physical exam can often elucidate the cause of GI bleeding. In addition to the routine questions, particular attention should be paid to the following areas.

A. INITIAL PRESENTATION OF BLEEDING

This initial assessment includes the type of bleeding and an estimation of the volume of blood loss.

1. Hematemesis (bright red or coffee-ground emesis)—Usually indicates an upper GI source proximal to the ligament of Treitz. Massive pulmonary, upper airway, or nasopharyngeal hemorrhage may be mistaken for GI bleeding.
2. Hematochezia (bloody stool)—Often a lower GI source, but may also occur with brisk upper GI bleeding
3. Melena (black tarry stool)—Frequently an upper GI source
4. Occult blood may be either an upper or a lower GI source.

B. BOWEL HABITS

Note any recent changes in bowel habits (new onset of constipation or diarrhea) and in stool color, consistency, or size.

C. ASSOCIATED ABDOMINAL PAIN

1. Painless bleeding may occur with varices, angiodysplasia, diverticulosis, or carcinoma.
2. Epigastric pain at presentation or a history of epigastric pain may be associated with ulcer disease, gastritis, or esophagitis.
3. Crampy abdominal pain associated with diverticulitis, inflammatory bowel disease, partially obstructing colon cancer, or colitis
4. Pain out of proportion to abdominal tenderness and associated with lower GI bleeding is the hallmark of bowel ischemia.
5. Severe, acute, sudden onset of pain usually indicates a perforated viscus.

D. RISKS AND PRECIPITATING FACTORS

1. Ulcerogenic agents—Steroids, aspirin or salicylates, nonsteroidal anti-inflammatory agents, alcohol and tobacco use
2. Severe stress—Major trauma or massive burns (Curling's ulcer), intracranial pathology (Cushing's ulcer)
3. GI instrumentation—Nasogastric (NG) intubation, colonoscopy, esophagogastroduodenoscopy (EGD)
4. Severe vomiting or retching (Mallory-Weiss tear of the gastroesophageal junction)
5. Blunt or penetrating trauma

E. SYSTEMIC COMPLAINTS
1. Fevers and chills—Inflammatory or infectious etiology
2. Weight loss, anorexia, and fatigue—Common symptoms associated with malignancies
3. Dizziness, orthostatic symptoms—Indicate large acute volume loss or severe anemia

F. PAST HISTORY
1. Prior episodes of GI bleeding—Including severity (how much blood was transfused), frequency, diagnostic and therapeutic interventions performed
2. Prior surgeries—GI; vascular; ear, nose, throat
3. Prior GI complaints
4. Significant medical history—Cardiac, vascular, pulmonary, diabetes, cirrhosis, anticoagulation therapy, blood dyscrasias

G. SOCIAL HISTORY
Note any drug and alcohol use.

II. PHYSICAL EXAMINATION

A. GENERAL APPEARANCE
Note the patient's appearance, which may be pale, diaphoretic, or anxious, with moderate to severe hemorrhage.

B. VITAL SIGNS
1. Blood pressure—Watch for hypotension or orthostatic changes (postural drop in systolic blood pressure >20 mm Hg).
2. Pulse—Tachycardia or orthostatic changes (postural increase of >20 beats/min)
3. Temperature—May be elevated with infection or falsely low or normal with dehydration
4. Respirations—May be shallow and rapid with significant blood loss

C. SKIN
Note the appearance of the patient's skin. Jaundice, palmar erythema, and spider angiomata associated with cirrhosis and portal hypertension are commonly seen with variceal bleeding. (Other signs of portal hypertension include gynecomastia, atrophic testicles, and asterixis.) Significant ecchymosis or petechiae may be noted if there is a contributory coagulopathy or thrombocytopenia.

D. HEAD AND NECK
Inspection may reveal an oropharyngeal source or scleral icterus.

E. ABDOMEN
1. Distention, caput medusae, scars
2. Bowel sounds—Usually increased with upper GI bleeding
3. Localization of abdominal tenderness
4. Palpation of masses, ascites, hepatosplenomegaly

F. RECTAL EXAM
Include the stool guaiac and any hemorrhoids, rectal mass, anal fissure or fistula.

III. LABORATORY EVALUATION

A. TYPE AND CROSSMATCH
Have available 6 units of packed red blood cells. This should be done immediately and should be available at all times.

B. HEMOGLOBIN/HEMATOCRIT
Hemoglobin and hematocrit determinations underestimate the volume of acute blood loss prior to resuscitation because equilibration has not occurred. Hypochromia and microcytosis suggest chronic blood loss. Megaloblastosis suggests nutritional abnormalities due to alcohol abuse.

C. PLATELET COUNT
Thrombocytopenia is the usual defect present in coagulopathies secondary to massive hemorrhage. This condition is also found in cirrhotic patients owing to hypersplenism.

D. PROTHROMBIN AND PARTIAL THROMBOPLASTIN TIMES
Screen for coagulation defects. Check fibrinogen and fibrin split products to identify a dilutional coagulopathy after massive transfusion.

E. RENAL PROFILE
Renal failure and electrolyte disturbances secondary to volume loss or emesis may be identified. Increased BUN can be due to the increased protein absorbed from blood in the GI tract as well as a state of dehydration.

F. LIVER FUNCTION STUDIES
The liver function studies provide an assessment of hepatic dysfunction.

G. CHEST RADIOGRAPH AND ABDOMINAL FILMS
Chest radiographs and abdominal films identify free air, pulmonary infiltrate, and splenic or hepatic enlargement.

20

GI BLEEDING

IV. INITIAL MANAGEMENT

A. ASSESSING MAGNITUDE OF HEMORRHAGE

B. STABILIZING HEMODYNAMIC STATUS
1. Two large-bore IVs (14-16 gauge if possible)
2. Begin resuscitation with crystalloid (lactated Ringer's solution).
3. Type-specific blood used if further resuscitation is required after 2 L of crystalloid.
4. Place Foley catheter.
5. Place NG tube—This helps differentiate an upper from a lower GI source. Saline lavage should be used to remove blood from the stomach until the fluid returning is clear. An upper GI source can be present with clear NG return in up to 20%. Return of bilious fluid without blood suggests a bleeding site beyond the ligament of Treitz (i.e., return of nonbilious fluid does not necessarily rule out a duodenal source of bleeding).

C. MONITORING FOR CONTINUED BLOOD LOSS
1. Frequent vital signs, hourly urine output
2. Frequent lab studies to assess the adequacy of transfusion and correction of coagulopathy. The hematocrit should be maintained >28-30 mL/dL, especially in elderly patients with cardiovascular disease.
3. Central venous pressure or pulmonary artery monitoring in unstable patient
4. Generally, an ICU setting is required.

V. DIAGNOSTIC PROCEDURES

A. NASOGASTRIC TUBE (see section IV. B. 5)

B. ENDOSCOPY
Endoscopy is most useful in localizing sources of bleeding; therapeutic interventions may also be instituted at the same time.
1. EGD—For upper GI source, has 95% diagnostic accuracy if used within the first 24 hours. Esophagitis, varices, Mallory-Weiss tears, gastritis, and peptic ulcer disease can be identified. The stomach must first be lavaged clear if possible. EGD may be used for sclerotherapy of varices or cauterization of bleeding vessels.
2. Anoscopy/sigmoidoscopy/colonoscopy—Diverticular disease, angiodysplasia, and carcinoma may be found if bleeding permits an accurate exam. Lack of adequate bowel prep often renders these tests inconclusive, but at a minimum rigid sigmoidoscopy can exclude a rectal source of bleeding.

C. ANGIOGRAPHY
1. Requires brisk bleeding (>0.5 mL/min) to identify the source
2. Can be used for therapeutic interventions such as selective vasopressin or embolization

D. TECHNETIUM-LABELED RED BLOOD CELL SCAN
1. Very sensitive (requires 0.1 mL/min bleeding) and less invasive than angiography, but far less specific
2. May identify the location of bleeding but not the source
3. Usually performed prior to angiography and may be the first test of choice for lower GI bleeding

E. RADIOGRAPHIC CONTRAST STUDIES
Radiographic contrast studies are rarely useful and interfere with other diagnostic procedures.

VI. NONSURGICAL TREATMENT

A. SCLEROTHERAPY
Sclerotherapy is used for bleeding varices during EGD.

B. ELECTROCAUTERY
Electrocautery of bleeding vessels is used in peptic ulcer disease. This is useful in high-risk patients and can be performed at the time of the diagnostic study.

C. VASOPRESSIN INFUSION
1. Can be given systemically or by selective arterial infusion
2. Selective infusion may be initiated at the time of the diagnostic angiogram and may minimize the systemic effects of the drug.
3. Recent myocardial infarction or significant coronary artery disease are relative contraindications to this form of therapy. Simultaneous infusion of nitroglycerin may also help reduce risks of infarction.
4. Dosage
a. Loading—20 units over 20-30 minutes
b. Infusion—0.2-0.4 units/min

D. EMBOLIZATION
Embolization is usually reserved for upper GI sources of bleeding, because there is a high risk of ischemia with infarction or perforation with colonic embolization.

VII. DISEASE-SPECIFIC THERAPY

A. GASTRITIS
1. Prophylaxis (antacids, H_2 receptor antagonists, proton-pump inhibitors, cytoprotective agents)

20

GI BLEEDING

2. Prompt resuscitation of shock
3. Usually stops spontaneously after lavage
4. Operation may be required if the patient remains unstable or with continued blood loss.

B. PEPTIC ULCER DISEASE

1. Conservative measures
2. NG suctioning and prophylactic measures to keep gastric pH >5—H_2 receptor blockers, antacids, cytoprotective agents
3. Therapeutic EGD
4. Surgery should be performed if there is an ongoing need for transfusion, or if there is rebleeding on maximal medical therapy.
5. Giant duodenal ulcer (ulcer >2 cm) is more likely to require surgical intervention.
6. For gastric ulcer, biopsy should always be done at operation or endoscopy to rule out malignancy.

C. ESOPHAGOGASTRIC VARICES

1. Lactulose, neomycin for prophylaxis of encephalopathy
2. Endoscopy (banding, sclerotherapy)
3. Vasopressin
4. Sengstaken-Blakemore tube if bleeding continues
5. Operation
a. Nonshunting (esophagogastric devascularization)
b. Shunting
   (1) Nonselective (e.g., portacaval shunt)
   (2) Selective (e.g., distal splenorenal)
6. Orthotopic liver transplant has become an alternative in select patients with severe hepatic dysfunction.

D. MALLORY-WEISS TEAR

Mallory-Weiss tear is a mucosal tear at the gastroesophageal junction. It occurs after violent retching or emesis, and most heal spontaneously with supportive measures alone. Occasionally operative treatment with oversewing of the lesion is required.

E. ESOPHAGITIS

Medical management or operation for intractable disease is required in esophagitis.

F. DIEULAFOY LESION

Endoscopic measures should be attempted first in Dieulafoy lesions. Operative treatment may be required if this fails (resection of lesion vs. ligature of vessel).

G. GASTRIC CANCER
Operation may be required for gastric cancer. In advanced cancer, operation may still be required for control of hemorrhage.

H. DIVERTICULOSIS
1. 70% of lower GI bleeding can occur anywhere.
2. Surgery for a blood loss exceeding 5 units in 24 hours
3. 60% stop spontaneously; 25% rebleed.
4. Surgical options should be considered after the second significant bleed. For persistent hemorrhage, resect the segment of colon involved with diverticula. If question exists, subtotal colectomy with ileoproctostomy is the procedure of choice. Preoperative localization should be attempted to minimize the extent of necessary resection.

I. ANGIODYSPLASIA
1. Occurs throughout GI tract, commonly in the right colon
2. Surgical treatment for massive acute bleeding or chronic intermittent bleeding
3. Segmental resection of localized segment is preferred.

J. CARCINOMA
In carcinoma, elective surgery following adequate bowel prep is preferred.

K. MECKEL'S DIVERTICULUM
Ileal ulceration secondary to a Meckel's diverticulum containing gastric mucosa is treated with segmental resection and end-to-end anastomosis or wedge resection. The lesion can be localized preoperatively using a nuclear medicine scan.

20

GI BLEEDING

RECOMMENDED READINGS

Nyhus L, Baker R, Fischer J (eds): Mastery of Surgery, 3rd ed. Boston, Little, Brown, 1997, pp 1285-1339.

Sabiston DC (ed): Textbook of Surgery: The Biological Basis of Modern Surgical Practice, 15th ed. Philadelphia, WB Saunders, 1997, pp 859, 878-882.

Zuidema G, Yeo C (eds): Shackelford's Surgery of the Alimentary Tract, 5th ed. Philadelphia, WB Saunders, 2002, pp 57-101, 117-140.

Intestinal Obstruction

David R. Fischer, MD

I. DEFINITIONS

A. ILEUS
Ileus is a mechanical or functional intestinal obstruction; the most common usage of the word is to connote failure of aboral passage of bowel contents due to dysfunctional motility of the bowel, as in *adynamic* or *paralytic ileus*.

B. MECHANICAL OBSTRUCTION
Mechanical obstruction is complete or partial physical blockage of the intestinal lumen (85% small bowel, 15% large bowel).

C. SIMPLE OBSTRUCTION
Simple obstruction has one obstructing point.

D. CLOSED-LOOP OBSTRUCTION
In closed-loop obstruction, both the afferent and efferent limbs of bowel are occluded, as in volvulus; it may be accompanied by strangulation.

E. STRANGULATED
In strangulation, circulation to the obstructed intestine is impaired. It is more likely in closed-loop than simple obstruction secondary to sustained increased intraluminal pressure.

II. ETIOLOGY

A. SMALL BOWEL OBSTRUCTION
1. Adhesions—The most common cause of small bowel obstruction (SBO). ≈80-90% of SBOs in patients with prior abdominal surgery are due to adhesions or internal herniation through a surgically created defect.
2. Hernias—The second most common cause of obstruction overall, but the most common cause in patients without prior abdominal surgery. This includes hernias of any type (i.e., inguinal, umbilical, incisional, obturator).
3. Other causes of SBO
a. Extrinsic
    (1) Carcinomatosis or tumor encasement from non-small bowel source
    (2) Intra-abdominal abscess
    (3) Hematoma
    (4) Malrotation with Ladd's bands or midgut volvulus
    (5) Annular pancreas (duodenal obstruction)
    (6) Endometriosis

       (7) Superior mesenteric artery (SMA) syndrome—Compression of third portion of the duodenum by the SMA in thin patients with severe acute weight loss

       (8) Intussusception

       (9) Atresias

  b. Intrinsic

       (1) Small bowel neoplasms

       (2) Congenital lesions

          (a) Small bowel atresia, stenosis, or webs

          (b) Small bowel duplications or mesenteric cysts

          (c) Meckel's diverticulum or other remnants of the omphalomesenteric duct

       (3) Inflammatory lesions

          (a) Regional enteritis, Crohn's disease

          (b) Radiation enteritis, stricture

  c. Intraluminal obstruction

       (1) Meconium ileus

       (2) Gallstone ileus—More common in elderly

       (3) Intussusception

       (4) Foreign bodies—Bezoars, barium, worms

4. Other conditions that mimic the clinical picture of SBO

a. Colonic obstruction—Right colonic obstruction near the ileocecal valve may be indistinguishable from SBO.

b. Adynamic ileus (see section II. C)

c. Vascular insufficiency

       (1) Mesenteric embolism

       (2) Nonocclusive mesenteric ischemia

       (3) Mesenteric thrombosis—Due to severe dehydration, disseminated intravascular coagulation, polycythemia, atherosclerosis

d. Hirschsprung's disease involving small bowel

B. COLONIC OBSTRUCTION

In general, colon obstruction produces less fluid and electrolyte disturbance than mechanical SBO.

1. Extrinsic

a. Volvulus—Sigmoid, 60-80%; cecal, 20-40%

b. Adhesions

c. Hernia—Particularly sliding type

d. Endometriosis

2. Intrinsic

a. Carcinoma of the colon—Most common cause (60%) of colonic obstruction

b. Inflammatory lesions

       (1) Ulcerative colitis

       (2) Diverticulitis

       (3) Radiation enteritis

c. Congenital lesions—Imperforate anus
3. Intraluminal obstruction
a. Meconium ileus
b. Intussusception
c. Fecal impaction, foreign bodies, barium
4. Other conditions that may mimic colonic obstruction
a. Adynamic ileus—See section II. C
b. Hirschsprung's disease
c. Focal ischemic colitis

C. ADYNAMIC ILEUS
1. Metabolic
a. Hypokalemia
b. Hypomagnesemia
c. Hyponatremia
d. Ketoacidosis
e. Uremia
f. Porphyria
g. Heavy metal poisoning
2. Response to localized inflammatory process within or adjacent to the peritoneal cavity—Appendicitis, cholecystitis, diverticulitis, abscess, pyelonephritis
3. Sepsis
4. Diffuse peritonitis—Bacterial or chemical
5. Retroperitoneal process
a. Retroperitoneal hematoma
b. Pancreatitis
c. Spinal or pelvic fracture
6. Drugs
a. Narcotics
b. Antipsychotics
c. Anticholinergic
d. Ganglionic blockers
e. Agents used to treat Parkinson's disease
7. Neuropathic disorders
a. Diabetes
b. Multiple sclerosis
c. Scleroderma
d. Lupus erythematosus
e. Hirschsprung's disease
8. Postoperative ileus following intra-abdominal surgery
a. Small bowel motility usually returns within 24-48 hours.
b. Gastric motility usually returns by 48 hours.
c. Return of colonic motility may take 3-5 days.
9. Ogilvie's syndrome
a. Colonic pseudo-obstruction of uncertain etiology

21

INTESTINAL OBSTRUCTION

b. Associated with pelvic retroperitoneal processes, long-term debilitation, chronic disease, immobility, narcotics, prolonged bedrest, laxative abuse, and polypharmacy
c. Usually manifested by moderate to marked cecal dilation. Cecal diameter >12 cm significantly increases the risk of perforation according to Laplace's law.
d. Treatment of choice is decompression with gentle enemas. If this is unsuccessful or if marked cecal dilation is already present, colonoscopic decompression is indicated. Rarely, cecostomy or right hemicolectomy is needed for perforation, ischemia, or unsuccessful colonoscopic decompression.

III. DIAGNOSIS OF INTESTINAL OBSTRUCTION

A. History
1. Age
a. Neonate—Consider meconium ileus, Hirschsprung's disease, malrotation, intestinal atresias
b. 2-24 months—Consider intussusception, Hirschsprung's disease
c. Young adults—Consider hernia, inflammatory bowel disease
d. Adults—Consider hernia, neoplasms, diverticular disease
e. Elderly—Consider neoplasms, diverticular disease, hernia, Ogilvie's syndrome
2. Nausea, vomiting, obstipation—In proximal obstruction, bilious vomiting may occur early and patients may have little abdominal distention. They may continue to pass stool and flatus as the bowel distal to the obstruction is evacuated. In distal bowel obstruction, patients may initially complain of obstipation and distention prior to the onset of vomiting feculent material (secondary to bacterial overgrowth of small bowel contents). Blood in the vomitus suggests strangulation or associated lesion. Obstipation and failure to pass gas from the rectum are characteristic of complete obstruction. These are evident only after bowel distal to the obstruction has been evacuated.
3. Pain—In proximal obstruction, pain is typically crampy and referred primarily to the periumbilical region. It is due to distention of the bowel lumen secondary to continued peristalsis against the obstruction and may subside after a long period secondary to inhibited bowel motility. In distal obstruction, pain is usually referred to the lower abdomen. When crampy abdominal pain is succeeded by continuous severe pain, strangulation and peritonitis should be suspected. If there is immediate torsion and vascular compromise of a bowel segment, obstruction and ischemia can occur early.
4. Past surgical history—Prior operative procedures, particularly pelvic and lower abdominal, implicate adhesions or internal herniation as the cause of the obstruction. Sudden cessation of colostomy or ileostomy output signals mechanical obstruction.

5. Past medical history

a. History of severe atherosclerosis, cardiac arrhythmias, prior myocardial infarction, chronic congestive heart failure, and atrial fibrillation may suggest intestinal ischemia.

b. Previous history of inflammatory bowel disease or diverticulitis may suggest mechanical obstruction.

c. Gallstone ileus should be considered in a patient with known gallstones or history of recurrent biliary colic, especially in patients >70 years of age.

6. Medications

a. Digitalis—Possible intestinal ischemia

b. Narcotics—Adynamic ileus

c. Anticholinergics, ganglion blockers, antipsychotics, drugs for Parkinson's disease suggest adynamic ileus

d. Diuretics—Consider hypokalemia as the source of adynamic ileus.

e. Polypharmacy—Consider Ogilvie's syndrome (see section II. C. 9).

7. Review of systems

a. Recent weight loss—Consider neoplasm first, then chronic intestinal ischemia.

b. If severe acute weight loss from other cause, consider SMA syndrome (see section II. A. 3. a).

B. PHYSICAL EXAM

1. Vital signs

a. Fever—Usually absent in uncomplicated obstruction. If present, consider inflammatory process or strangulation.

b. Tachycardia—May be secondary to dehydration and hypovolemia. However, if associated with leukocytosis and localized tenderness, it is one of the cardinal signs of strangulation.

c. Orthostatic hypotension—Often associated with dehydration and third-space losses because fluid is sequestered in obstructed bowel.

2. Abdominal exam

a. Distention—Minimal in proximal obstruction, but marked in prolonged distal obstruction

b. The presence of surgical scars from prior operations should always be noted.

c. Mild tenderness is common; however, localized tenderness and guarding suggest peritonitis and the likelihood of strangulation or perforation.

d. Mass—May be palpable due to a fixed distended loop of bowel or due to a carcinoma or inflammatory mass that is the cause of the obstruction. A careful exam for the presence of inguinal, femoral, umbilical, or incisional hernia is mandatory.

e. Bowel sounds—Initially active with intermittent rushes and borborygmus, but decrease with time. In adynamic ileus, bowel sounds are usually absent.

3. Rectal exam

a. Rectal vault is usually empty with established obstruction.

21

INTESTINAL OBSTRUCTION

b. Fecal impaction can be ruled out.

c. Guaiac-positive stool suggests an alimentary mucosal lesion, as may occur with cancer, intussusception, or mesenteric infarction.

d. Extrinsic pelvic masses as well as intrinsic colon lesions can be diagnosed.

C. LABORATORY EVALUATION

1. White blood cell (WBC) count—Usually normal in uncomplicated SBO. Elevated with strangulation or if the source of obstruction is inflammatory.Markedly elevated late with mesenteric infarction.

2. Hematocrit—Is often increased due to hemoconcentration. Anemia in the presence of clinical low SBO or colonic obstruction often is characteristic of colon carcinoma.

3. Electrolyte abnormalities—Especially hypokalemia

4. Alkalosis—Usually develops in proximal SBO or pyloric obstruction because vomiting results in loss of hydrogen and chloride via gastric acid and fluid

5. Acidosis—Usually occurs late in the course of bowel infarction. A normal pH does not rule out bowel infarction.

6. Amylase—May or may not be elevated in SBO

D. RADIOGRAPHS

Radiographs are essential to confirm clinical diagnosis and define more accurately the site of obstruction.

1. Upright chest radiograph—Sensitive for detection of free air under the diaphragm

2. Abdominal flat and upright (left lateral decubitus if the patient is unable to stand)—Characteristic features of intestinal obstruction are dilated bowel loops usually containing air-fluid levels proximal to the point of obstruction with little or no gas distally. Air-fluid levels are not normally seen in an upright radiograph of the abdomen in persons with normal bowel motility. Gas may still be visualized distally with partial obstruction, early in the course of complete obstruction, or if air has been introduced from below during rectal exam or enema.

a. Small bowel can be distinguished from large bowel by the presence of valvulae conniventes (also known as *plicae circulares*), which traverse the entire diameter of the bowel, as opposed to haustral markings of the colon, which extend only $1/2$ to $2/3$ the diameter of the bowel.

b. Air-fluid levels in the upright projection can be seen with both ileus and obstruction. In obstruction they are usually more pronounced and a step-ladder pattern is often seen progressing down the abdomen.

c. Fluid-filled loops of bowel appear as areas of increased density without gas and can easily be overlooked.

d. In colonic obstruction or ileus, if the cecal diameter is >12 cm, the patient is at increased risk for perforation; emergency decompression of the colon should be considered. When the cecum is acutely dilated to 12-14 cm, the wall tension exceeds perfusion pressure, and focal areas of necrosis may occur. These may progress even though the cecum is decompressed by nonoperative means.

e. Sigmoid volvulus—Appears as a large dilated loop of bowel that resembles a "bent inner tube" with the apex in the left lower quadrant and the convexity in the right upper quadrant

f. Cecal volvulus—A large, dilated, ovoid, air-filled cecum is usually visualized in the upper abdomen as the hypermobile cecum has rotated upward and to the left around ileocolic vessels.

g. In "high" intestinal obstruction, the number of dilated loops is usually small relative to that number in distal SBO.

3. **Contrast enema—Most commonly used to rule out obstruction of the colon**

a. Useful when the diagnosis is uncertain

b. Must be done with low pressure. The objective is identifying the site of obstruction, not defining mucosal detail. Free barium in the peritoneum from perforation of the colon has a high mortality. If any question of a perforation exists, use water-soluble contrast medium.

c. Will show the point of colonic obstruction, but care must be taken not to force barium beyond a partial obstruction and thereby create complete obstruction (controversial)

d. In unclear cases of suspected distal SBO, barium enema should be done prior to upper GI series.
   (1) To rule out colonic obstruction with fluid-filled proximal colon indistinguishable from SBO on plain radiographs
   (2) Reflux through the ileocecal valve often visualizes a collapsed terminal ileum, confirming the diagnosis of SBO.

e. Hydrostatic or air contrast barium enema may be used if intussusception is suspected to make the diagnosis and to attempt a reduction. Up to 60-70% of children with intussusception reduce with enema alone. Hydrostatic reduction should not be attempted in adults because of the high frequency of underlying mucosal lesions as the lead point for the intussusception.

f. In sigmoid or cecal volvulus, a "bird's beak" pattern is demonstrated at the site of the volvulus.

4. **Upper GI series with small bowel follow-through**

a. Useful if the diagnosis is uncertain or for demonstrating a partially obstructing lesion

b. In cases of uncertain diagnosis, barium enema should be done *first* to rule out colonic obstruction.

c. This is considered the study of choice when ruling out malrotation in the pediatric population and the occasional adult.

5. **CT scan—May define a transition point and give information regarding etiology**

21

INTESTINAL OBSTRUCTION

IV. TREATMENT

A. RESUSCITATION
1. Rehydration—Rapid volume repletion with normal saline until adequate urine output (0.5 mL/kg body weight per hour) is established
2. Correction of electrolyte abnormalities—Patients often have hypochloremic, hypokalemic metabolic alkalosis, and normal saline with added potassium is the fluid of choice. (KCl is added only after urine output is established.)
3. Foley catheter to monitor urine output

B. NASOGASTRIC SUCTION
Use nasogastric (NG) suction to prevent vomiting with aspiration.
1. Prevents further gaseous distention from swallowed air and partially decompresses the bowel
2. The stomach must be empty in preparation for and during induction of anesthesia. Anesthesia relaxes the esophageal sphincters, allowing free regurgitation of both gastric and small bowel contents (which may rapidly refill the stomach).

C. SMALL BOWEL INTUBATION
This section discusses small bowel intubation with a long (i.e., Miller-Abbott or Cantor) tube. Use of a long tube as therapy for mechanical intestinal obstruction is generally inappropriate, because it may delay operation for a complete mechanical obstruction. The only major indications for long-tube therapy are the following.
1. Resolving partial obstruction
2. Partial obstruction in the immediate postoperative period. About 50-60% of cases resolve with a long tube.
3. Partial SBO or obstruction due to inflammation that is expected to resolve with nonoperative therapy or due to carcinomatosis or radiation enteritis. These seldom strangulate and are often difficult operative procedures, with high complication and recurrence rates.

D. PERIOPERATIVE ANTIBIOTICS
Coverage of gram-negative aerobes and anaerobes is indicated because of bacterial overgrowth in the obstructed lumen and the possibility of small or large bowel resection. If necrotic bowel or abscess is found, a full treatment course rather than perioperative prophylaxis is given.

E. OPERATIVE TREATMENT OF SBO
SBO is a surgical emergency and should be treated by laparotomy with few exceptions. When obtaining informed consent, one should usually include the possibility of an enterocutaneous stoma. A stoma site may be marked preoperatively but should not delay operation.

1. Patients with localized peritoneal signs, leukocytosis, fever, and tachycardia with SBO should be assumed to have ischemic or necrotic bowel and should be taken to the OR as soon as they are hemodynamically stable. Generally, a midline incision should be used, although variations may be necessary in patients with extensive scar tissue.

2. Patients with complete obstruction but without signs of vascular compromise should be resuscitated and operated on urgently (as soon as possible within 6-8 hours of admission).

3. Patients with an uncertain diagnosis or those who continue to pass flatus or stool, indicating either a very early complete obstruction or a partial obstruction, can be treated conservatively while a diagnostic evaluation is in progress. Intestinal obstruction due to an acute exacerbation of Crohn's disease treated conservatively may permit resolution of the obstruction.

4. Lysis of all adhesions or resection of the involved segment of bowel is recommended. Intestinal bypass may be necessary in cases of advanced malignancy.

5. In obstruction due to radiation injury, lysis of adhesions should be limited. Radiation-injured bowel may be "revascularized" through adhesions.

6. In cases of extreme bowel distention preventing easy abdominal closure, the intraluminal fluids can be carefully milked back into the stomach. A long intestinal tube is useful if it has passed through the ligament of Treitz prior to surgery; otherwise it is difficult to manipulate through the duodenum. Intentional enterotomy is not recommended due to a high likelihood of fecal contamination, late leakage, abscess, or fistula.

7. It is important to determine whether a segment of bowel is viable. The general criteria are color, motility, and arterial pulsation. If in question, the bowel segment should be completely released and placed in a warm saline-moistened sponge for 15-20 minutes and then re-examined. If normal color and peristalsis are evident, the bowel may be returned safely. Any nonviable bowel should be resected. IIV fluorescein and a Wood's lamp can be helpful in determining viability, as can Doppler examination of the involved segment. If there is any question of bowel viability, a second-look laparotomy can be performed at 24-48 hours.

8. Anastomosis may be difficult if there is size disparity between the proximal and distal ends. There are numerous options for dealing with this situation (i.e., enterocutaneous stoma, end-to-side anastomosis, tapered anastomosis).

F. OPERATIVE TREATMENT OF COLONIC OBSTRUCTION

1. Obstructing carcinoma

a. Right colonic obstruction—Usually treated by resection and primary anastomosis when there is no gross contamination, massive edema, shock, or long-standing peritonitis; otherwise should have decompressive ileostomy and mucous fistula

b. Left colonic obstruction

(1) Primary resection with creation of a colostomy and mucous fistula or rectal pouch (two-stage procedure) is usually indicated. In extremely debilitated or unstable patients without perforation or abscess, an initial diverting colostomy allows decompression and stabilization prior to resection and colostomy closure later (three-stage procedure). (*Mucous fistula* is the term used to describe a stoma created from the proximal end of the remaining distal bowel after a segment has been resected. A rectal pouch is created by leaving the distal divided end of rectosigmoid colon within the abdomen after sigmoid resection. This procedure is done if there is insufficient length to bring the bowel to the abdominal wall as a mucous fistula.)

(2) There are data that support resection with primary anastomosis using on-table bowel preparation, but this is controversial.

c. Ischemic colon—Patients with peritonitis secondary to an ischemic colon should be treated with resection of the involved bowel, end colostomy, and mucous fistula or rectal pouch.

d. Rectal obstruction—Colostomy with mucous fistula and later resection versus primary resection

2. Obstructing diverticulitis—See Chapter 36

3. Sigmoid volvulus

a. Initial treatment—Nonoperative decompression via sigmoidoscopy and placement of a long, soft, well-lubricated rectal tube past the point of obstruction. In 80% of cases, this results in reduction of the volvulus with immediate passage of stool and flatus. Mucosal inspection is then done to evaluate bowel viability.

b. Because of the high incidence of recurrence (>50% in first year), many authors recommend elective sigmoid resection after the first episode if the patient is a reasonable operative risk.

c. If volvulus cannot be reduced, strangulation should be suspected and immediate resection carried out.

4. Cecal volvulus—Always treated operatively. Resection is indicated for vascular compromise, but cecopexy or cecostomy is adequate in remaining cases.

5. Closed-loop obstruction—A competent ileocecal valve or any closed loop generally makes treatment more emergent because the bowel cannot decompress proximally.

G. PARALYTIC ILEUS

Paralytic ileus is treated by NG suction and IV fluids. Electrolyte imbalances, especially hypokalemia, are corrected. Long tubes or colonoscopic decompression should be employed for extreme distention. It most commonly occurs after surgery and is transient (2-3 days). If persistent and without obvious etiology, mechanical obstruction or an extrinsic process must be excluded. The underlying etiology must be treated.

H. POSTOPERATIVE CARE
1. NG decompression until bowel activity is re-established
2. If the postoperative course is prolonged (>5 days), parenteral nutrition should be considered.
3. Attention should be paid to correcting electrolyte imbalances.

V. RESULTS OF SURGICAL TREATMENT OF BOWEL OBSTRUCTION

A. RECURRENT SBO
Recurrent SBO occurs in 10% of patients treated by enterolysis, and this incidence increases with each subsequent enterolysis.

B. MULTIPLE ADHESIVE SBO
Patients who have had multiple adhesive SBOs requiring enterolysis may benefit from plication of the bowel in an organized position to promote the formation of adhesions in a nonobstructed pattern.
1. Transmesenteric plication—Seromuscular stitches are used to plicate adjacent bowel loops.
2. Intraoperative oral placement of a Leonard tube or a Baker tube through a gastrostomy or high jejunostomy. The tube is left in place 12-14 days to maintain an adequate intestinal lumen while healing occurs.

C. MORTALITY OF OPERATION
1. SBO—0-5% (4.5-31% if gangrene has occurred)
2. Colonic obstruction
a. 1-5% in diverticulitis
b. 5-10% in carcinoma
c. 40-50% if bowel necrosis has occurred with volvulus

RECOMMENDED READINGS
Holzheimer R, Mannick J (eds): Surgical Treatment: Evidence Based and Problem Oriented. Munchen, W. Zuckschwerdt Verlag, 2001, pp 102-113, 190-192.
Nyhus L, Baker R, Fischer J (eds): Mastery of Surgery, 3rd ed. Boston, Little, Brown, 1997, pp 1343-1349.
Schwartz SI, Shires GT, Spencer FC, et al (eds): Principles of Surgery, 7th ed. New York, McGraw-Hill, 1999, pp 1054-1061.

INTESTINAL OBSTRUCTION 21

Neurosurgical Emergencies

Jeffrey Larson, MD, PhD

Neurosurgical emergencies represent clinical conditions in which rapid evaluation and appropriate intervention may significantly decrease morbidity and mortality. Early assessment of altered level of consciousness and any focal neurologic deficit, as well as prompt initial management, ensures the best possible outcome, particularly in the head-injured patient.

It must be stressed that conditions leading to central, uncal, upward cerebellar, and tonsillar herniation syndromes can be fatal within a few minutes. This chapter provides the basic principles necessary for the early care of the patient with an acute neurosurgical problem.

22

I. APPROACH TO THE UNCONSCIOUS PATIENT

A. UNCONSCIOUSNESS
The state of unconsciousness implies bilateral hemispheric dysfunction, depression of the reticular activating system (RAS) in the upper brain stem, or both.

B. ETIOLOGIES
1. Structural causes of coma—May originate for multiple reasons, including traumatic, vascular (both ischemic and hemorrhagic), neoplastic, infectious, congenital, and inflammatory factors
a. Supratentorial mass—Leads to compression of the diencephalon and eventually the brain stem. Initial depression of level of consciousness followed by rostral-to-caudal deterioration is characteristic. Symmetrical deterioration suggests central herniation, whereas asymmetrical decline suggests uncal herniation.
b. Infratentorial mass—Leads to direct compression of RAS and characterized by extremely sudden onset of coma. Deterioration is typically caudal to rostral with hemodynamic instability, abnormal respiratory pattern, and cranial nerve palsies common.
2. Toxic and metabolic causes of coma—May be due to electrolyte or endocrine imbalance; self-induced, accidental, or iatrogenic intoxication; CNS or systemic infection; nutritional deficiencies; inherited metabolic disorders; global hypoxia or ischemia; seizure (e.g., postictal state or nonconvulsive status epilepticus); or organ failure (e.g., uremic and hepatic encephalopathy). Note that onset of coma is more gradual, with a symmetrical neurologic exam and preserved pupillary responses. Look for asterixis, tremor, myoclonus, and acid-base disturbances that are characteristic of toxic and metabolic causes.
3. Pseudocoma—Includes psychiatric causes, such as catatonia and conversion reaction, as well as "locked-in" syndrome due to ventral pontine infarction. Note that in psychiatric causes, objective findings

are absent and one will detect active lid closing, normal pupillary response, physiologic reflexes, and normal motor tone and responses.

C. HISTORY

1. Important features include abrupt vs. subacute vs. insidious onset; presence of lucid interval; recent neurologic complaints; and spatial progression of neurologic deficits.
2. Look for factors in past medical and surgical histories, allergies, social and sexual habits, occupational exposure, and travel that could explain decline.
3. A medication history is essential, especially history of use of psychotropics, sedatives, and opiates.

D. PHYSICAL EXAM

1. General
a. Vital signs
b. Respiratory pattern
c. External evidence of trauma or IV drug abuse
d. Nuchal rigidity
2. Level of consciousness
a. Awake and alert—Eyes open, responsive to verbal stimuli
b. Lethargic—Sleepy, but easily arousable to full waking state
c. Obtunded—Sleeps unless continually stimulated but can be fully aroused with effort
d. Stupor—Responds to vigorous physical stimuli but cannot be fully aroused to waking state
e. Coma—Totally unarousable
3. Glasgow Coma Scale (GCS)
a. Scores ranges from 3 to 15
b. Best suited for trauma
c. Is not a neurologic examination but a reproducible measure of level of consciousness

Best Eye Opening	Best Verbal	Best Motor	Points
—	—	Obeys	6
—	Oriented	Localizes	5
Spontaneous	Confused	Withdraws to pain	4
To speech	Inappropriate	Decorticate	3
To pain	Incomprehensible	Decerebrate	2
None	None	None	1

4. Children's Coma Scale
a. For age <4 years
b. Ranges from 3 to 15

Best Eye Opening	Best Verbal		Best Motor	Points
—	—		Obeys	6
—	Smiles, oriented to sound, follows objects, interacts		Localizes	5
	Crying	*Interaction*		
Spontaneous	Consolable	Inappropriate	Withdraws to pain	4
To speech	Inconsistently consolable	Moaning	Decorticate	3
To pain	Inconsolable	Restless	Decerebrate	2
None	None	None	None	1

5. Evaluation of brain stem
a. Response to visual threat—Cranial nerves II, VII
b. Pupillary responses—Cranial nerves II, III
c. Corneal reflexes—Cranial nerves V, VII
d. Extraocular movements—Cranial nerves III, IV, VI. Look for conjugate vs. dysconjugate gaze, gaze deviation, and roving eye movements.
e. Oculocephalic reflex—Cranial nerves VI, VIII. Known as doll's eyes reflex. Test only if the cervical spine is cleared.
f. Oculovestibular reflex—Cranial nerves VI, VIII. Known as cold calorics test (see section IV. F).
g. Gag reflex—Cranial nerves IX, X
h. Response to central pain using supraorbital or sternal pressure—Tests general integrity of motor and sensory tracts in brain stem. Use only if the patient is not obeying commands.

6. Motor examination
a. Check tone and bulk.
b. Test strength, if possible.
c. Decorticate posturing—Indicates level of lesion above red nucleus
d. Decerebrate posturing—Indicates levels of lesion above lateral vestibular nucleus but below red nucleus

7. Sensory examination
a. Difficult to assess in unconscious patient
b. Check if patient withdraws to pin prick or nail bed pressure.

8. Reflexes
a. Check superficial and deep tendon reflexes.
b. Check the presence or absence of pathologic reflexes.
c. Check sphincter tone and check for clonus.

E. INITIAL MANAGEMENT OF COMA
1. Airway—Intubate for airway protection if necessary, supplemental O_2 for any hypoxemia
2. Breathing—Hyperventilate if elevated intracranial pressure (ICP) is suspected.
3. Circulation—Optimize hemodynamic status with fluids and vasopressors, if necessary. Brain injury rostral to the medulla is rarely a primary cause of systemic hypotension, except in very young children.

22

NEUROSURGICAL EMERGENCIES

4. Treat remediable causes of coma immediately.
   a. Hypoglycemia—25 g glucose IV piggyback (50 mL of D-50). Always give unless it is certain that the glucose level is normal.
   b. Opiate intoxication—Naloxone 1 ampule (0.4 mg) IV piggyback
   c. Give also thiamine 100 mg IV piggyback to prevent Wernicke-Korsakoff syndrome, which can be caused by a large infusion of glucose.

5. Laboratory studies
   a. CBC, renal profile, Ca^{2+}, Mg^{2+}, PO_4, arterial blood gas, osmolarity, coagulation profile, toxicology screen, ethyl alcohol level, type and screen, urinalysis
   b. Consider hepatic profile, ammonia level, thyroid function tests, endocrine panel, blood cultures if febrile

6. Control ICP.
   a. Elevate head of bed to 30 degrees if blood pressure permits.
   b. Maintain head in a neutral position to prevent jugular venous obstruction.
   c. Hyperventilate to $Paco_2$ of 25-30 mm Hg in adults, 22-26 mm Hg in children.
   d. Consider 1 g/kg IV bolus of mannitol.
   e. Consider steroids—Quite useful for edema secondary to brain tumors, but of questionable value in trauma, hemorrhage, or infarction

7. Control seizures, if necessary.
   a. Lorazepam 1.5-2 mg or diazepam 5-10 mg IV piggyback. Also load with longer-acting phenytoin.
   b. For management of status epilepticus, see section IV. D.
   c. Consider electroencephalogram (EEG) if nonconvulsive status epilepticus is suspected.

8. Obtain head CT scan as soon as possible. Contrast agent is generally not necessary, unless one suspects tumor, abscess, or encephalitis. MRI generally is not useful in the acute setting and may not be possible in artificially ventilated patients.

9. Pan-culture if febrile
   a. Consider lumbar puncture if there is no evidence of increased ICP (Table 22-1).
   b. Consider empiric treatment of infections.

10. Normalize pH if necessary.

11. Normalize temperature if necessary.

12. Protect eyes with Lacri-Lube or artificial tears.

13. Use sedation as needed for agitation. Try to use reversible agents such as fentanyl if possible to preserve an ability to evaluate the patient neurologically. Avoid using benzodiazepines and paralytics if possible.

II. HEAD TRAUMA (Fig. 22-1)

A. GENERAL CATEGORIES OF HEAD TRAUMA

1. Mild—GCS score 13-15. Patient often asymptomatic but may have headache, dizziness, mild memory loss, scalp lacerations, or

TABLE 22-1

CSF FINDINGS IN VARIOUS PATHOLOGIC CONDITIONS (ADULT VALUES)

Condition	Opening Pressure (cm H₂O)	Appearance	Cells (per mm³)	Protein (mg/dL)	Glucose (% serum)	Miscellaneous
Normal	7-18	Clear, colorless	0 PMN, 0 RBC, 0 mono	15-45	50	—
Acute purulent meningitis	Frequently increased	Turbid	Few-20,000 (WBCs, mostly PMN)	100-1000	<20	Few cells early or if treated
Viral meningitis and encephalitis	Normal	Normal	Few-350 (WBCs mostly monos)	40-100	Normal	PMNs early
Guillain-Barré syndrome	Normal	Normal	Normal	50-1000	Normal	Protein ↑, frequently IgG
Polio	Normal	Normal	50-250 (monos)	40-100	Normal	—
Tuberculosis meningitis	Frequently increased	Opal, yellow, fibrin clot	50-500 (monos)	60-700	<20	PMN early, positive AFB culture, positive Ziehl-Neelsen stain
Fungal meningitis	Frequently increased	Opalescent	30-300 (monos)	100-700	<30	Positive India ink for *Cryptococcus*
Traumatic (bloody) tap	Normal	Bloody, supernatant colorless	RBC:WBC as in peripheral	Slight ↑	Normal	Blood ↓ in succeeding tubes, xanthochromia takes hours
Subarachnoid hemorrhage	Increased	Bloody Supernatant xanthochromic	Early ↑ RBCs Late ↑ WBCs	50-400 100-800	Normal	RBCs disappear in 2 weeks; xanthochromia may persist for weeks
Multiple sclerosis	Normal	Normal	5-50 (monos)	Normal—800	Normal	Usually ↑ gamma globulins (oligoclonal)

CSF = cerebrospinal fluid; RBC = red blood cell; WBC = white blood cell count; PMN = polymorphonuclear leukocyte; mono = monocyte; AFB = acid-fast bacilli.

NEUROSURGICAL EMERGENCIES

22

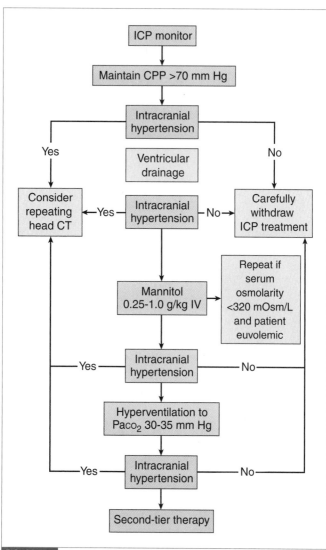

FIG. 22-1

Treatment protocol for intracranial hypertension after a severe head injury, based on guidelines of the Brain Trauma Foundation. ICP = intracranial hypertension; CPP = cerebral perfusion pressure.

mild contusions. Requires short-term observation for neurologic change.

2. Moderate—GCS score 8-12. Associated with slightly depressed level of consciousness and usually amnestic of event. Can also be associated with basilar skull fractures and severe facial or multiple traumatic injuries. If the patient is hemodynamically stable but needs to go to the OR urgently, obtain a head CT to rule out a mass lesion.

3. Severe—GCS score <7. Extremely depressed level of consciousness. Patient often has focal neurologic deficit. Many patients have mass lesions, hemorrhagic contusions, diffuse cerebral edema, diffuse axonal injury, depressed skull fracture, or penetrating head injury. 50-60% have multisystem trauma, 5% have simultaneous spinal injury.

B. INDICATIONS FOR MANNITOL THERAPY IN THE EMERGENCY DEPARTMENT

1. Clinical evidence of mass effect or herniation
2. Sudden deterioration prior to CT scan
3. After CT, if the following are present.
a. Lesion found is associated with increased ICP.
b. Lesion found on CT requires surgical intervention.
4. To assess "salvageability" of patients without brain stem function by looking for return of reflexes
5. Mannitol is *contraindicated* if hypotension is present.

C. INDICATIONS FOR TEMPORAL BURR HOLES IN THE EMERGENCY DEPARTMENT WITHOUT OBTAINING A CT SCAN

1. A patient dying from acute uncal herniation whose deterioration has been witnessed by reliable observers, either in transit or in the emergency department
2. While preparations are being made to perform a burr hole, the patient should be intubated, hyperventilated, and given mannitol.
3. Should be performed by most qualified available physician
4. Even if indications are correct, a positive finding (i.e., epidural or subdural hematoma) is present only approximately 50-55% of time.

D. INCREASED INTRACRANIAL PRESSURE

1. Clinical manifestations
a. Classic signs of headache, oculomotor palsies, Cushing's triad (hypertension, bradycardia, respiratory irregularities), and papilledema are often not seen in trauma patients.
b. Suspect elevated ICP if there is a deterioration in neurologic exam, drop in GCS, or progression of focal neurologic deficit.
c. Upper limits of normal ICP = 10-15 cm H_2O. Treatment is indicated if ICP >16 cm H_2O for >5 minutes. Sustained ICP at 25-30 cm H_2O increases mortality.

22

NEUROSURGICAL EMERGENCIES

2. Indications for ICP monitoring (intraventricular, intraparenchymal, or subarachnoid monitor)

a. Any motor exam <4 at initial presentation. A monitor may be placed in the OR if the patient is undergoing other procedures or is in the ICU.

b. GCS scale <8 if not improved after 6 hours of empiric therapy

c. Multisystem trauma in which other therapies may have adverse effect on ICP or ability to follow neurologic examination (e.g., paralytics, heavy sedation)

d. The presence of coagulopathy is a relative contraindication. If absolutely needed, subarachnoid bolt or epidural monitor (not intraventricular or intraparenchymal monitor) can be used after coagulopathy is corrected.

e. Placement of a monitor has never been shown to improve outcome in head injury if all usual measures are being taken. It does allow more precise titration of therapy.

3. Management of elevated ICP

a. Postural—Elevate head of bed to 30-45 degrees and maintain neck in neutral position to facilitate venous return and avoid obstruction of jugular veins.

b. Hyperventilation—Increase rate on the ventilator so that $Paco_2$ is 25-30 mm Hg.

   (1) Hypocarbia results in arteriolar constriction in the cerebral circulation.

   (2) Duration of effectiveness is controversial but hyperventilation probably not effective after 48-72 hours

   (3) A rapid rise in $Paco_2$ even after that time could result in a rebound elevation of ICP, so hyperventilation should always be slowly weaned.

   (4) Degree of hyperventilation can be titrated by monitoring jugular venous O_2 saturation via a jugular bulb catheter.

c. Osmotic therapy

   (1) Mannitol—Use lowest possible effective dose, usually 0.25 g/kg IV piggyback q 6 h or 25 g IV piggyback q 6 h. In emergent situations, may bolus with up to 1 g/kg.

   (2) Furosemide (Lasix)—20-40 mg IV piggyback q 6 h on alternating schedule with mannitol; has synergistic effect with mannitol; is also thought to decrease cerebrospinal fluid (CSF) production

   (3) Follow renal profile and measured serum osmolarity q 6 h. Hold diuretics for serum osmolarity >310 mOsm/L.

   (4) The goal is not to dehydrate the patient, but to attain a euvolemic, hyperosmotic state. May also need to measure pulmonary capillary wedge pressure with Swan-Ganz catheter during osmotic therapy.

d. Hypertension control—Do not overtreat, because an increase in blood pressure is one way an injured brain attempts to perfuse itself.

e. Control agitation—Boluses of short-acting agents are preferable (fentanyl 50 μg IV piggyback q 30-60 min or pentobarbital 2-5 mg/kg IV piggyback q 4 h). Avoid benzodiazepine or fentanyl drips if possible.

f. IV fluids—Remember that the goal is euvolemia. Isotonic fluids are preferable, but other injuries may dictate fluid management.

g. Steroids—Use of dexamethasone is controversial in head injury and is not currently used at this institution. Whether or not steroids are used, head-injured patients require aggressive stress ulcer prophylaxis with antacids, H_2 blockers, or sucralfate.

h. CSF drainage—Via intraventricular catheter. In the noncompliant brain with elevated ICP, removal of a small amount of CSF can significantly lower ICP.

i. Pentobarbital coma—Reserved for young patients with reasonably good neurologic exams who deteriorate secondary to cerebral edema, not mass lesions. Does not improve but maintains neurologic status at time of induction.

j. Surgical techniques—Used in most extreme cases as a last resort; involves resection of "silent" areas of brain (e.g., right anterior temporal lobe, right frontal lobe), areas of contused brain, or decompressive craniectomy with dural augmentation

E. EPIDURAL HEMATOMA

1. Seen in ≈1% of head trauma patients
2. Classic presentation is brief loss of consciousness, followed by lucid interval, then progressive obtundation, ipsilateral pupillary dilation, and contralateral hemiparesis (seen in 60%). Other presentations include headache, nausea, vomiting, seizure, unilateral hyperreflexia, and Babinski's sign.
3. Usual etiology is laceration of middle meningeal artery by fracture of squamous portion of temporal bone, but can also be produced by a dural sinus tear
4. On CT scan, seen as lenticular, biconcave mass overlying brain with high attenuation
5. Optimally treated, has a 5-10% mortality

F. SUBDURAL HEMATOMA

1. Twice as common as epidural hematomas
2. Source of bleeding usually venous, but can also be arterial
3. Two types are described.

a. Tearing of bridging veins from acceleration/deceleration; often presents with a lucid interval followed by later deterioration secondary to mass effect

b. Laceration of parenchyma and cortical vessels; usually presents with coma, localizing signs, and severe underlying brain injury

4. On CT scan, seen as crescent-shaped mass overlying convexities with high density; usually less dense than epidural hematoma due to dilution of blood in CSF
5. Classified as acute from 0-48 hours, subacute from 2 days-3 weeks, and chronic after 3 weeks

22

NEUROSURGICAL EMERGENCIES

6. If evacuated in OR in <4 hours, 30% mortality. If >4 hours elapses, 90% mortality. Also much worse outcome if postoperative ICP >20 cm H_2O.

G. HEMORRHAGIC CONTUSIONS
1. Most commonly found in temporal, frontal, and occipital lobes
2. Will typically "blossom" with continued hemorrhage and edema 24-72 hours after presentation
3. Generally managed medically with usual maneuvers to lower ICP, but if medical therapy fails, region of contused brain can be resected depending on its location
4. Patients with an isolated temporal lobe contusion can undergo brain herniation and die without evidence of increased ICP because of local temporal swelling.

H. DIFFUSE AXONAL INJURIES
1. Result from "shearing" of white matter tracts from rotational forces at time of impact
2. Can be visualized on MRI or CT scan as puncture hemorrhages in centrum semiovale, corpus callosum, or brain stem
3. Generally not associated with elevations in ICP
4. If brain stem is affected, the prognosis for functional neurologic recovery is extremely poor.

I. SKULL FRACTURES
1. Can be open, closed, linear, compound, or depressed
2. "Raccoon's eyes" diagnostic of fracture of floor of anterior fossa
3. Basilar skull fracture usually diagnosed clinically without benefit of CT, in presence of Battle's sign (retroauricular hematoma), CSF otorrhea, or CSF rhinorrhea
4. Criteria to elevate depressed skull fracture
a. >8-10 mm depression
b. Deficit related to underlying brain
c. CSF leakage secondary to dural laceration
d. Open, depressed skull fractures

III. SPINE AND SPINAL CORD INJURIES

A. GENERAL CONSIDERATIONS
1. These injuries are usually due to severe cervical spine fractures and/or subluxations. Because of its greater mass and greater inherent stability, the thoracolumbar spine is not as frequently affected.
2. Not all spine injuries are associated with paralysis. More than half of patients with spinal injuries have a normal motor, sensory, and reflex examination.

3. Any patient sustaining an injury above the clavicle or a head injury resulting in unconsciousness should be suspected of having an associated cervical spine injury unless proven otherwise.

B. ASSESSMENT

1. General assessment

a. Examination must be carried out with patient in a neutral position on a backboard and cervical spine immobilized.

b. Other associated injuries must be ruled out, including head injury.

c. The paralyzed patient's abdominal exam is unreliable, so a diagnostic peritoneal lavage is generally required.

2. Mechanical assessment

a. Log-roll patient, so entire spine can be visualized.

b. Look for any open wounds, step-off deformities, and prominence of spinous processes.

c. Palpate for any regions of tenderness.

3. Neurologic assessment

a. Complete vs. incomplete spinal cord lesion

  (1) If patient has any neurologic deficit, this is most important part of assessment.

  (2) Distinction between complete and incomplete injury determines the prognosis and the urgency of subsequent treatment.

  (3) Any preservation of motor or sensory function below the level of injury indicates incomplete injury. Sparing of pin-prick and fine-touch sensation in sacral dermatomes indicates incomplete injury ("sacral sparing"). Preservation of any voluntary control of sphincter tone also indicates sacral sparing, thus incomplete injury.

  (4) Preservation of anal wink and bulbocavernosus reflexes alone does not constitute sacral sparing.

b. Sensory and motor function

  (1) Determine level of lesion by assessing sensory and motor function.

  (2) See motor chart (Table 22-2) and sensory dermatome diagram (Fig. 22-2).

  (3) Check sphincter tone and the presence or absence of superficial, deep tendon, and pathologic reflexes.

  (4) Injuries at C4 or higher have impairment of ventilation, and the patient requires blind or fiberoptic-guided nasal intubation.

4. Spinal shock

a. May occur immediately after spinal cord injury, particularly complete injury

b. Due to abrupt loss of sympathetic tone

c. Characterized hemodynamically by hypotension and bradycardia; extremities warm due to dilated peripheral vessels ("cold nose, warm feet")

d. Characterized neurologically by flaccid paralysis, absent sensory function, flaccid sphincter, absent pathologic and normal reflexes

e. Usually responds to fluid resuscitation, but vasopressors (e.g., Neo-Synephrine) are occasionally needed

22

NEUROSURGICAL EMERGENCIES

TABLE 22-2

MOTOR LEVEL ASSESSMENT

Segment	Muscle	Action to Test	Reflex
C1-C3	Neck muscles	—	—
C4	Diaphragm, trapezius	Inspiration	—
C5	Deltoid	—	—
C5-C6	Biceps	Elbow flex	Biceps
C6	Extensor carpi radialis	Wrist extension	Supinator
C7	Triceps, extensor digitorum	Elbow extension	Triceps
C8	Flexor digitorum	Hand grasp	—
T1	Hand intrinsics	—	—
T2-T12	Intercostals	—	—
T7-L1	Abdominals	—	Abdominal cutaneous
L2	Iliopsoas, adductors	Hip adduction	—
L3-4	Quadriceps	Knee extension	Quadriceps
L4-5	Medial hamstrings, tibialis anterior	Ankle dorsiflex	Medial hamstrings
L5	Lateral hamstrings, posterior tibialis, peroneals	Knee flexion	—
L5-S1	Extensor digitorum, extensor hallucis longus	Great toe extension	—
S1-S2	Gastrocnemius, soleus	Ankle plantarflex	Ankle jerk
S2	Flexor digitorum, flexor hallucis	—	—
S2-S4	Bladder, lower bowel	—	Anal wink and bulbocavernosus

5. Radiographic evaluation

a. Cervical spine

   (1) Lateral cervical spine—All 7 cervical vertebrae and C7-T1 interspace must be seen. Best obtained while pulling down on shoulders. "Swimmer's view" may be necessary.

   (2) Assess alignment, presence of fractures, and soft tissue swelling.

   (3) Anteroposterior cervical and odontoid views are needed to fully clear the cervical spine. These views should be obtained only once the patient is stabilized.

   (4) Tomograms, oblique views, lateral flexion/extension films, CT, MRI, or myelography may be needed to completely clear the cervical spine.

   (5) Lateral flexion/extension films should be obtained in patients with posterior neck pain only (i.e., with no neurologic deficit) to rule out ligamentous instability.

b. Thoracolumbar spine

   (1) Anteroposterior and lateral views needed

   (2) Assess alignment and presence of fractures.

   (3) Spine must be cleared before removing backboard and allowing flexion at waist

c. Emergency MRI or CT myelogram mandatory in patient with *incomplete injury* whose examination cannot be explained by plain CT or plain radiographs alone. Soft tissue injury, e.g., epidural hematoma and traumatic herniated disc, must be ruled out. These patients would be taken to surgery emergently to decompress cord and preserve or improve neurologic function. Patients with *complete* injury do not need emergent surgery.

C. TREATMENT
1. Neurosurgical consultation is mandatory.
2. Immobilization
a. Semirigid cervical (Philadelphia) collar and spine board are sufficient for prehospital care and initial evaluation.
b. Every attempt should be made to clear the thoracic, lumbar, and sacral spines as soon as possible so the backboard can be removed, thus preventing pressure sores.
3. Realignment
a. Every effort is made to achieve realignment and closed reduction as soon as possible in the cervical spine with Gardner-Wells tongs and weight in both complete and incomplete injuries, as well as in intact patients.
b. If a closed reduction is not possible in an incomplete injury, emergent open reduction is necessary to decompress the cord and/or roots. An emergent open reduction in a complete injury is not necessary.
4. Stabilization
a. Generally is not necessary emergently, but is done as expediently as possible to minimize medical complications of recumbency
b. Stabilizing devices may be external (e.g., halo, SOMI brace, hip spica cast) or internal (e.g., plates, screws, rods).
c. The choice of which devices to use depends on type of injury, location of instability, and medical condition of patient.
5. Medications—Immediate treatment with high-dose methylprednisolone (i.e., 30 mg/kg bolus at presentation, followed by 23-hour drip at 5.3 mg/kg/h) is now standard of care.
6. IV fluids—Limit to maintenance fluids unless more needed for spinal shock
7. Airway—Nasal intubation or tracheostomy often is required for high cervical injuries.
8. Effective nursing care with attention to skin, bowel training, and bladder training is absolutely essential in long-term care of these patients.
9. Every attempt should be made to start rehabilitation as soon as possible.

IV. OTHER NEUROSURGICAL EMERGENCIES

A. SUBARACHNOID HEMORRHAGE
1. Characterized by sudden onset of "the worst headache of my life," nuchal rigidity, photophobia, and sometimes loss of consciousness

22

NEUROSURGICAL EMERGENCIES

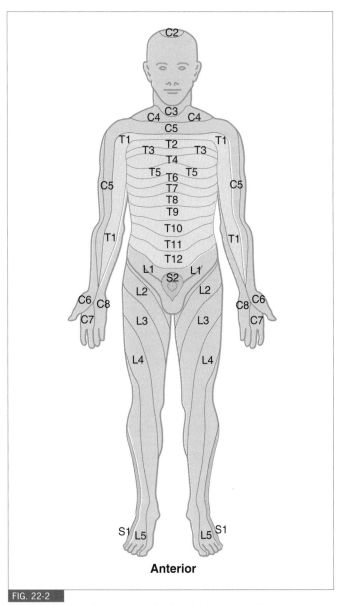

Anterior

FIG. 22-2

Arrangement of dermatomes: anterior (front) and posterior (back) views.

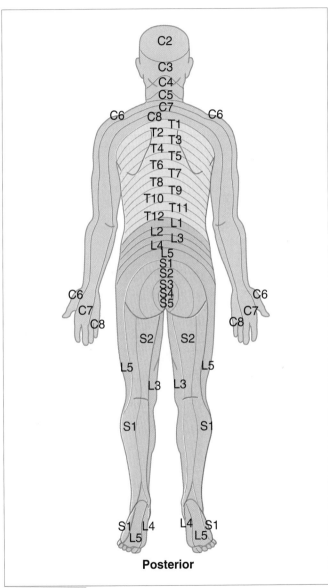

Posterior

C2
C3
C4
C5
C7
C6   C8   C6
T1
T2 T3
T4 T5
T6
T7
T8 T9
T10
T11
T12 L1
L2 L3
L4
L5
S1
S2
S3
S4
S5
C6   C6
C7   C7
C8   C8
S2   S2
L5   L5
L3   L3
S1   S1
S1 L4   L4 S1
L5   L5

22

NEUROSURGICAL EMERGENCIES

FIG. 22-2—Cont'd

2. Seen on noncontrast CT scan in ≈90% of cases if scanned within 48 hours. Regions of high density found in subarachnoid spaces, particularly around basilar cisterns. Often accompanied by acute hydrocephalus.

3. Etiologies
   a. Trauma—Most common cause of subarachnoid hemorrhage (SAH)
   b. Aneurysm—75-80% of cases of spontaneous SAH
   c. Arteriovenous malformation—≈5% of cases of spontaneous SAH
   d. Unknown etiology—≈15% of cases of spontaneous SAH

4. If CT scan is negative in cases in which the index of suspicion is high, lumbar puncture is obligatory to look for red blood cells in CSF and xanthochromia.

5. Initial medical management
   a. Control of blood pressure. Should use IV labetalol, esmolol, or sodium nitroprusside. Hypertension can contribute to rebleeding.
   b. Avoid overtreatment of blood pressure if patient's baseline is hypertension.
   c. Prophylaxis for seizures with anticonvulsant such as phenytoin
   d. Prevention of vasospasm with nimodipine, a calcium channel blocker
   e. CSF drainage with intraventricular catheter if patient develops acute hydrocephalus
   f. Intubate if patient becomes lethargic
   g. Treat elevated ICP, if necessary, with hyperventilation, osmotic diuretics, and CSF drainage.
   h. Consider steroids (controversial).
   i. Cerebral angiogram (four-vessel) is obligatory to rule out aneurysm. In patients with aneurysm, 20% have multiple aneurysms.
   j. MRI scan is useful for subacute SAH and in those cases in which angiogram is negative.

6. Surgical management
   a. For most ruptured aneurysms, direct clipping is the procedure of choice.
   b. Endovascular balloon occlusion is becoming a more accepted form of therapy for difficult aneurysms.
   c. Early surgery (within 48-72 hours after SAH) is favored in patients in good medical and neurologic condition, with large amounts of subarachnoid blood, and with intracerebral hemorrhage (ICH) with mass effect.
   d. Delayed surgery (10-14 days after SAH) is favored in patients in poor medical and neurologic condition and those experiencing the effects of vasospasm.

B. INTRACEREBRAL HEMORRHAGE

1. ICH is defined as hemorrhage within the brain matter itself. ICH accounts for approximately 10% of all strokes, both ischemic and hemorrhagic.

2. Seen easily on noncontrast CT scan as region of high density within brain parenchyma

3. Location of hemorrhage on CT often suggests etiology of bleed. For example, basal ganglia, thalamic, pontine, and cerebellar ICHs are likely hypertensive in origin.
4. Etiologies
a. Hypertension
b. Arteriovenous malformation
c. Aneurysm
d. Hemorrhage into brain tumor, either primary or metastatic
e. Arteriopathies such as amyloid angiopathy, fibrinoid necrosis, or lipohyalinosis
f. Coagulation or clotting disorders, either as result of primary illness or iatrogenic (e.g., as complication of use of warfarin [Coumadin], thrombolytic agents, or aspirin)
g. Trauma (unusual)
h. Hemorrhage into infarct
i. Sympathomimetic abuse (e.g., cocaine)
j. Other vascular malformations, such as venous angioma, cavernous malformation, or capillary telangiectasia
5. Initial medical management is similar to that of SAH.
6. Surgical management
a. Advisability of surgery depends on etiology, patient's neurologic condition, and location of hemorrhage.
b. Aneurysms should generally be clipped; arteriovenous malformations can be either surgically resected or embolized.
c. Hypertensive hemorrhages can generally be managed medically, but if the patient begins to deteriorate, they can be evacuated stereotactically, endoscopically, or through an open procedure.

C. CAROTID DISSECTION

1. Often seen in setting of trauma but can also be spontaneous
2. Suspect in those cases in which a lateralizing sign (e.g., hemiparesis) cannot be explained by an intracranial CT finding.
3. Diagnosed by angiography. Characterized by "string sign" or "double-lumen sign." Can be bilateral.
4. Most dissections heal with recanalization and so are treated with anticoagulation (IV heparin followed by warfarin) to prevent clot propagation and emboli.
5. Medical failures can be managed by direct repair with interposition vein graft or carotid ligation with or without extracranial-intracranial bypass.

D. STATUS EPILEPTICUS

1. Defined as recurrent seizures occurring too frequently for consciousness to be regained between seizures or any seizure that lasts >30 minutes
2. Most common scenario is a patient with known seizure disorder with low anticonvulsant levels for any reason.

3. Permanent CNS injury results if seizures are not controlled within 60 minutes; can be fatal
4. Management involves control of seizures as follows.
a. Intubate if airway compromised or if seizures persist unabated.
b. Lorazepam 0.02 mg/kg (1.4 mg/70 kg) IV piggyback over 2 minutes. Repeat if ineffective q 2-3 min for three doses total. Alternatively, may use diazepam 10 mg IV piggyback (at rate of <2 mg/min) q 20 min if necessary for three doses total.
c. Simultaneous loading with phenytoin
    (1) If patient not on phenytoin, give phenytoin 18 mg/kg (1200 mg/70 kg) IV at rate <50 mg/min
    (2) If patient on phenytoin, give phenytoin 500 mg IV at rate <50 mg/min
d. If seizure activity persists
    (1) Continue phenytoin 8 mg/kg at rate <50 mg/min.
    (2) Then
        (a) Phenobarbital drip at 100 mg/min up to 20 mg/kg (1400 mg/70 kg), *or*
        (b) Diazepam infusion of 100 mg in 500 mL of D-5-W at 40 mL/min
    (3) If seizures still continue
        (a) Initiate induction of pentobarbital coma with IV dose of 10-15 mg/kg followed by maintenance drip of 1 mg/kg/h.
        (b) Consider calling the anesthesiologist and placing the patient under general inhalation anesthesia and neuromuscular junction blockade.
        (c) As a temporizing measure, may give paraldehyde 5 mL in 500 mL of D-5-W at 50 mL/h and titrating to stop seizures or lidocaine 2-3 mg/kg IV piggyback at <50 mg/min, followed by infusion of 100 mg in 250 mL of D-5-W at 1-2 mg/min

E. COMPRESSIVE SPINAL EPIDURAL METASTASES

1. Spinal epidural metastases present in up to 10% of all cancer patients at some time during disease; 5-10% of malignancies present with cord, conus, or cauda equina compression.
2. Usual route of spread is hematogenous via spinal epidural veins (Batson's plexus), but can be arterial or perineural.
3. Usual location is epidural, but can be intradural (2-4%) and even intramedullary (1-2%).
4. Back pain is usually the first symptom. Radicular pattern of pain, paresthesia, and weakness often follows. Symptoms are exacerbated by recumbency, movement, neck flexion, straight-leg raising, coughing, sneezing, or straining.
5. If cord compression develops, patient experiences quadriplegia or paraplegia, sensory loss (manifested as a sensory level on exam), loss of reflexes acutely, and bowel or bladder dysfunction.
6. If symptoms involve the perineum and lower extremities symmetrically, a conus medullaris lesion is most likely. If the perineum and lower

extremities are involved asymmetrically, a cauda equina lesion more likely.

7. Patients presenting with acute neurologic deterioration should be given dexamethasone (100 mg IV piggyback) stat, and plain films of the entire spine should be obtained. An emergency MRI or CT-myelogram should also be obtained. Neurosurgical consultation is mandatory.

8. Most patients are treated initially with local radiation therapy. Surgery is indicated if local radiation therapy fails, for tissue diagnosis, for unstable spine, or if compression due to bone rather than tumor.

9. A key point is that back pain in cancer patients represents metastatic disease until proven otherwise.

F. BRAIN DEATH

1. Criteria established by Cincinnati Society of Neurologists and Neurosurgeons. These may vary in different locations.

a. Absence of brain stem function

(1) Pupillary light reflex absent

(2) Corneal reflex absent

(3) Oculocephalic (doll's eyes) reflex absent

(4) Oculovestibular (cold water calorics) reflex absent

(a) With head of bed at 30 degrees, 60 mL of ice water flushed into each ear with eyes held open

(b) Intact response is slow deviation of eyes toward flushed ear and fast nystagmus toward opposite ear. Remember the mnemonic COWS—cold: *opposite/warm: same*—which indicates direction of fast nystagmus depending on the temperature of water used.

(5) Oropharyngeal (gag) reflex absent

(6) No spontaneous respirations for 3 minutes in normocarbic state

b. No response to central pain stimulation (supraorbital notch pressure)

c. The presence of monosynaptic spinal withdrawal reflexes does not rule out brain death.

2. The following conditions must be ruled out.

a. Hypothermia as cause of coma

b. Remediable endogenous or exogenous intoxication, especially metabolic factors, barbiturates, paralytics, benzodiazepines

c. Hypotension

d. Nonconvulsive status epilepticus

3. Two clinical examinations 6 hours apart meeting criteria of section IV. F. 1 and 2 confirm brain death. The brain death examination is not reliable in setting of hypoxic or ischemic brain damage for 24-48 hours after correction of insult, because brain stem dysfunction as result of hypoxia or ischemia often resolves during this period.

4. At this institution, no further laboratory tests, including angiography, EEG, or cerebral blood flow studies, are mandatory.

Malignant Skin Lesions

Robert M. Cavagnol, MD

I. PREMALIGNANT LESIONS

A. ACTINIC KERATOSIS
1. Develops on sun-exposed areas, mostly the face and hands
2. ≈20% evolve into squamous cell carcinoma.
3. Treatment is local excision or topical 5-fluorouracil.

B. BOWEN'S DISEASE
1. Squamous cell carcinoma in situ
2. Erythematous, irregular border lesion with crusting center
3. ≈5% become invasive carcinoma.
4. Treatment is wide local excision.

23

II. CARCINOMA

A. BASAL CELL CARCINOMA (BCC)
1. General
a. Most common human malignancy
b. Associated with excessive sun exposure and immunosuppression
2. Clinical presentation
a. Most common in elderly white men
b. Lesion classically described as a "pink, pearly, papule"; may have a central ulcer
c. May present as a superficial erythematous patch or plaque
d. Slow growing, locally invasive but rarely associated with metastatic spread
3. Diagnosis
a. Punch biopsy on the edge of the lesion to include small portion of normal skin
b. Local excision for smaller lesions
c. Incisional biopsy for larger lesions or those in delicate areas

B. SQUAMOUS CELL CARCINOMA (SCC)
1. General
a. The most serious risk factor is ultraviolet radiation.
b. Also may arise in areas of chronic ulcers, old burn scars, or areas exposed to irradiation
c. Rate of metastasis about 2-3% in sun-exposed skin, much higher in chronic wounds
d. Marjolin's ulcer—Refers to SCC arising in a burn scar
2. Clinical presentation
a. Typical sun-exposed areas (face, neck, trunk, arms)

b. May present as an erythematous plaque, exophytic ulcerated mass, or firm keratotic nodule

3. Diagnosis—Punch biopsy or wide local excision

4. Treatment

a. Surgical excision with 5-10 mm margin depending on size, cellular differentiation, and depth of tumor

b. Regional lymph node dissection indicated in cases of clinically palpable nodes, tumor >2 cm in diameter or 4 mm in depth, perineural invasion, or those arising in chronic wounds

C. SYNDROMES ASSOCIATED WITH BCC AND SCC

1. Xeroderma pigmentosum
a. Autosomal recessive
b. Intolerance to ultraviolet radiation
c. Skin cancer 1000 times more common and appears at a young age

2. Gorlin's syndrome
a. Autosomal dominant
b. Characterized by multiple BCC in second and third decades of life

III. MALIGNANT MELANOMA

A. GENERAL

1. Has the fastest increasing incidence of any malignancy
2. Associated with ultraviolet radiation

B. RISK FACTORS

1. Previous melanoma—Person has a 3-5% risk of developing second melanoma
2. Fair complexion—Light-colored skin and eyes, easily sunburned
3. Excessive sunlight exposure, especially with a history of severe sunburn
4. Large number of benign nevi
5. Genetics—Strong family history may increase risk up to 5-10% for development of melanoma
6. Dysplastic nevus syndrome—Patients have large numbers of atypical nevi that can be precursors to malignant melanoma.

C. CLINICAL PRESENTATION

1. "ABCDs" of melanoma
   A—Asymmetrical lesion
   B—Border irregularity
   C—Color variegation
   D—Diameter >6 mm

D. DIAGNOSIS

1. Thickness of the lesion is the single most important prognostic feature.
2. Shave biopsy is absolutely contraindicated, because thickness cannot be measured.

3. Biopsy should be taken of the thickest appearing portion of the lesion.
a. Excisional biopsy with a narrow margin
b. Punch biopsy to include some normal skin
c. Incisional biopsy for large lesions

E. TYPES OF MELANOMA
1. Superficial spreading
a. Most common type (≈70%), usually on upper back or lower extremities
b. Horizontal growth pattern
2. Nodular
a. Second most common type
b. All are in the vertical growth phase at diagnosis.
c. 5% are amelanotic.
d. More aggressive lesion
3. Lentigo maligna
a. Most occur on the neck, face, and back.
b. Best prognosis, low propensity for metastasis
4. Acral lentiginous
a. Occurs on the palms, soles, or nail beds
b. Accounts for a higher percentage in dark-skinned people
c. Subungual are blue-black lesions, most commonly on the great toe or thumb
d. Most aggressive type

F. PROGNOSTIC FACTORS AND STAGING
1. Tumor thickness, rather than level of tissue invasion, is accepted as the most important tumor characteristic in determining prognosis.
2. TNM classification
a. Primary tumor (T)
  T1: ≤1.0 mm
  T2: 1.01-2.0 mm
  T3: 2.01-4.0 mm
  T4: >4.0 mm
b. Regional lymph nodes (N)
  N1: 1 node
  N2: 2-3 nodes
  N3: ≥4 nodes, in-transit lesions
c. Distant metastases (M)
  M0: no evidence of metastatic disease
  M1: metastatic disease
3. Staging
  Stage I: T1 or T2 N0 M0
  Stage II: T3 or T4 N0 M0
  Stage III: any T N1-3 M0
  Stage IV: any T, any N, M1

23

MALIGNANT SKIN LESIONS

G. TREATMENT

1. Primary therapy is wide local excision to the deep fascia with appropriate margin of normal appearing tissue.
   a. T1 lesion requires a 1-cm margin.
   b. T2 or T3 lesion requires a 2-cm margin.
   c. T4 lesion requires at least a 2-cm margin, although some surgeons use a 3-cm margin for larger lesions.
2. Regional lymph nodes
   a. Most common site of metastatic disease
   b. All patients with clinically palpable regional lymph nodes should undergo therapeutic lymph node dissection.
      (1) Therapeutic lymph node dissection removes all nodes in a specific region.
      (2) Any positive nodes left behind will lead to recurrent disease.
   c. Patients with clinically negative nodes can be offered a sentinel lymph node biopsy, although this is controversial for early-stage lesions.
      (1) Sentinel lymph node biopsy involves the injection of radiolabeled sulfur colloid around the tumor with subsequent nuclear scanning (lymphoscintigraphy) to identify the sentinel nodes preoperatively.
      (2) Intraoperatively, isosulfan blue is injected around the tumor prior to excision. The blue dye migrates to the regional lymph nodes and highlights the sentinel node for excision. A gamma probe is also used intraoperatively to detect the radiation from the radiolabeled sulfur colloid.
      (3) A positive sentinel node biopsy requires a follow-up therapeutic lymph node dissection.
3. Metastatic disease
   a. Sites of metastases in decreasing order of frequency: lymph nodes, skin and subcutaneous tissue, lung, liver, brain, GI tract
   b. Isolated lung or brain metastases can be surgically excised.
   c. Chemotherapy has limited effectiveness.
   d. High-dose interferon-alfa 2b can be used as an adjunctive therapy for patients with stage III disease or as a primary treatment in those with stage IV disease.

Head and Neck Malignancy

Melissa McCarty Statham, MD

Approximately 60,000 head and neck cancers are diagnosed in the United States annually, representing nearly 5% of cancers diagnosed in North America and 1-2% of all cancer deaths. The male-to-female ratio is 3:1, and the average age of onset is in the sixth decade. Risk factors include tobacco and alcohol abuse, exposure to human papillomavirus, and poor oral hygiene. Ninety percent of head and neck cancers are squamous cell carcinoma (SCC). These lesions most commonly metastasize to locoregional lymph node basins, and distant metastases occur late in the course of disease.

Common symptoms include painless neck mass, nonhealing lesions, hoarseness, dysphagia, odynophagia, hemoptysis, persistent otalgia, and epistaxis. Evaluation includes a thorough physical exam of the neck, oral cavity, base of tongue, and nasopharynx. Indirect laryngoscopy and endoscopic nasolaryngoscopy aid in the visualization of the oropharynx, hypopharynx, and larynx. Radiographic modalities such as ultrasonography, CT, or MRI are useful in the evaluation of a mass or for staging purposes. In well-trained hands, ultrasound-guided fine-needle aspirate (FNA) is a sensitive and specific means of biopsying a mass—a mass after 2 weeks of antibiotics should be evaluated by FNA. Poor prognosis is associated with an extracapsular invasion of lymph nodes and bilateral lymph node metastases. Patients with a known primary head and neck cancer or known neck metastasis without a known primary lesion should undergo a staging "quadscope," which involves nasopharyngoscopy, laryngoscopy, bronchoscopy, and esophagoscopy, with necessary biopsies performed under general anesthesia.

24

I. NECK DISSECTION

A. LYMPH NODE GROUPS
Level I: submental and submandibular nodes
Level II: upper jugular nodes
Level III: middle jugular nodes
Level IV: lower jugular and supraclavicular nodes
Level V: posterior triangle nodes (postauricular, occipital, spinal accessory chain)
Level VI: anterior nodes (pretracheal and paratracheal nodes, Delphian node)

B. RADICAL NECK DISSECTION
1. Classically described by Cline as the en bloc resection of all nodal tissue in levels I-V, including sacrifice of the sternocleidomastoid (SCM) muscle, the internal jugular (IJ) vein, spinal accessory nerve, and the submandibular gland. Dissection extends to the deep layer of deep cervical fascia investing the scalene muscles and the levator

scapulae muscle. Remaining structures include the carotid arteries, vagus nerve, hypoglossal nerve, brachial plexus, and phrenic nerve.

2. Indications
a. Nodal metastases in multiple nodal levels, particularly level V
b. Nodal metastases with extracapsular extension with close proximity to the SCM, the IJ vein, or the accessory nerve
c. When bilateral radical neck dissections are called for, one IJ vein should be spared if at all possible.

3. Complications
a. Facial edema from sacrifice of IJ vein
b. Shoulder immobility from resection of accessory nerve
c. Cranial nerves X and XI injury
d. Thyroglossal duct injury
e. Risk of cerebrovascular accident from carotid manipulation

C. MODIFIED RADICAL NECK DISSECTION

1. Rationale—Lymphatics in the neck are fibroadipose tissue contained within a complex system of aponeurotic partitions that are separate from the SCM and IJ vein.
2. Resection en bloc of lymph nodes in levels I-V, sparing one or all of the following
a. SCM
b. IJ vein
c. Spinal accessory nerve
3. Equally effective oncologic resection without the morbidity of shoulder immobility from sacrifice of cranial nerve XI and less physically deforming from loss of the SCM or facial edema from resection of the IJ vein

D. SELECTIVE NECK DISSECTION

1. Rationale—Based on the location of the primary tumor and its known patter of spread
2. Consists of an en bloc removal of one or more lymph node basins at risk of harboring metastatic lesions
a. Supraomohyoid dissection—Levels I-III
b. Extended supraomohyoid dissection—Levels I-IV
c. Lateral neck dissection—Levels II-IV
d. Posterolateral neck dissection—Levels II-V
e. Anterior compartment neck dissection—Level VI
3. Indication—Performed in the clinically N0 neck

II. CARCINOMA OF ORAL CAVITY AND LIP

A. PHYSICAL FINDINGS SUSPICIOUS FOR MALIGNANCY

Physical findings suspicious for malignancy include nonhealing mucosal ulceration; violaceous mucosa; pain, bleeding, or friability of mucosa; and erythroplakia.

B. TONGUE
1. Exophytic—Plaque-like tumor grows off tongue mucosa
2. Infiltrative—Have large submucosal extension and ulcerate late in course
3. Early lesions—Partial glossectomy with extended supraomohyoid neck dissection with more extensive neck dissection based on nodal status
4. Late lesions—Total glossectomy with extended supraomohyoid neck dissection
5. Midline lesions—Bilateral neck should be dissected

C. LIP
1. Most commonly SCC
2. Early lesions—Local excision
3. Late lesions—Tumor resection with supraomohyoid neck dissection

III. OROPHARYNGEAL CARCINOMA

A. TONSILLAR CARCINOMA
The tonsils are the most common site of SCC in the oropharynx.
1. ≈70% of patients present with nodal metastases.
2. Early lesions—Radiation
3. Advanced lesions—Resection with selective lateral neck dissection, postoperative radiation

B. TONGUE BASE CARCINOMA
1. Frequently present late, 80% with nodal metastases
2. Treatment—Resection of tumor with near-total glossectomy, laryngectomy for more advanced lesions, with extended supraomohyoid neck dissection and postoperative radiation; midline tongue lesions call for bilateral dissections

IV. NASOPHARYNGEAL CARCINOMA

A. GENERAL
1. Rare in the United States, but common in China
2. Associated with Ebstein-Barr virus and nickel exposure
3. Pathology—70% are SCC

B. SYMPTOMS
1. Nasal tumors present early with painless neck mass, nasal obstructive symptoms, epistaxis, and chronic otitis media from eustachian tube obstruction.
2. As tumors enlarge, adjacent cranial nerves may become involved.

C. TREATMENT
1. Radiation is the mainstay of treatment.
2. Surgical resection of value as salvage therapy after radiation failure

24

HEAD AND NECK MALIGNANCY

V. SALIVARY TUMORS

A. PATHOLOGY
1. Benign
a. Presentation—Slowly enlarging, painless mass in the area of the involved gland
b. Pleomorphic adenoma
   (1) Incidence—85% occur in the parotid.
   (2) Recurrence rate 2% after surgical treatment
c. Warthin's tumor (papillary cystadenoma lymphomatosum)
   (1) Very slow-growing mass
   (2) Appear almost exclusively in tail of parotid
   (3) Observation may be indicated in asymptomatic elderly patients.
2. Malignant
a. Presentation—Typically present as slow-growing painless mass but later display pain or palsy from neural involvement
b. Correlation with previous radiation exposure
c. Mucoepidermoid carcinoma—Most common parotid malignancy
d. Malignant mixed tumor
   (1) Malignancy arising from preexisting pleomorphic adenoma
   (2) Predominantly involve parotid gland

B. PAROTID TUMORS
1. Incidence—80% of neoplasms occur in the parotid.
2. Treatment
a. Parotidectomy with facial nerve preservation unless nerve invaded, then nerve sacrificed
b. With malignant tumors, radical neck dissection performed for N+ disease, postoperative radiation
c. Observation recommended in elderly patients with recent history of rapid tumor growth and without evidence of malignancy on FNA

C. SUBMANDIBULAR GLAND TUMORS AND MINOR SALIVARY GLAND TUMORS
1. ≈10% of neoplasms
2. 50% of tumors are malignant.
3. Adenoid cystic carcinoma the most common malignancy—Often presents with distant metastases
4. Treatment—Excision of gland, neck dissection performed for N+ disease, postoperative radiation

D. SUBLINGUAL GLAND TUMORS
1. <1% of all salivary gland tumors
2. ≈90% tumors are malignant.
3. Treatment—Gland excision with neck dissection for N+ disease, postoperative radiation

VI. HYPOPHARYNGEAL CARCINOMA

A. PIRIFORM SINUS
The piriform sinus is located in the most inferior extent of the hypopharynx just before it becomes the cervical esophagus.
1. Highly infiltrative, invades the larynx medially, thyroid cartilage, or pharyngeal wall laterally, high incidence of nodal invasion
2. Often present late as neck mass with referred otalgia
3. 3-year survival with combined surgery and radiation is 40%.
4. Treatment
a. En bloc resection of tumor, total laryngectomy, lateral neck dissection, postoperative radiation, and reconstruction via jejunal free flap
b. When extends into esophagus and inferiorly to the thoracic inlet, must perform laryngopharyngoesophagectomy, modified radical neck dissection, and reconstruction via jejunal free flap

VII. LARYNGEAL CARCINOMA

A. GENERAL
1. Pathology—95% are SCC.
2. Incidence—Male-to-female ratio is 4:1.

B. SYMPTOMS
1. Commonly presents with hoarseness, as well as dysphagia, odynophagia, otalgia
2. Stridor and hemoptysis are more rare, late findings.

C. STAGING
Staging is by site of involvement; with more advanced stage, tumor fixes the cords, extends throughout the larynx, and invades surrounding structures.

D. SUPRAGLOTTIC
1. Extends from epiglottis to the ventricular fold
2. Represents ≈30% of laryngeal tumors
3. Has extensive lymphatics that feed neck bilaterally—Commonly drain to levels II and III, and up to 35% metastases are bilateral
4. Treatment
a. Early lesions—Radiation or partial laryngectomy with bilateral selective neck dissections
b. Later lesions—Total laryngectomy with bilateral selective lateral neck dissections, ± radiation

E. GLOTTIC
1. Begins at ventricular fold and extends 1 cm below true vocal cord
2. Represents 67% of laryngeal tumors

3. Has limited lymphatic drainage—<10% metastasize to neck lymph nodes
4. Treatment
a. Early lesions—Radiation or less invasive surgical procedures
b. Advanced disease—Total laryngectomy with neck dissections, ± radiation

F. SUBGLOTTIC
1. Begins 1 cm below true vocal cord and extends to inferior cricoid cartilage
2. Represents <5% of laryngeal tumors
3. Tends to invade cricoid cartilage and involve level VI nodes
4. Treatment—Total laryngectomy with selective anterior compartment neck dissection, with larger dissection with more extensive node disease, ± radiation

VIII. CUTANEOUS MALIGNANCY OF THE HEAD AND NECK
For further explanation, see Chapter 23.

A. GENERAL
1. >800,000 cases of skin cancer in the United States annually
2. >80% of these occur in the head and neck

B. CHARACTERISTICS
1. Those areas of the head and neck that correlate with embryonic fusion planes have a higher risk of recurrence.
2. Combine to form an H-shaped zone on the face
a. Medial canthi, the periorbital lower eyelids
b. Periauricular region extending to the temple
c. Nasolabial-alar junction, the nasal septum, the nasal ala

C. BASAL CELL CARCINOMA (BCC)
1. 85% of all skin cancers
2. Slowly growing malignant neoplasm originating in the epidermis
3. Rarely metastasizes but is capable of extensive local destruction
4. Metastatic lesions tend to be large, locally aggressive, and neglected lesions that have recurred.

D. SQUAMOUS CELL CARCINOMA (SCC)
1. Presentation—Crusting, erythematous, ulcerated lesion with a friable base; less commonly, as a nodular or exophytic lesion; may present as areas of persistent ulceration in the site of previous trauma, burns, or an old scar (Marjolin's ulcer)
2. Premalignant lesions are actinic keratoses or Bowen's disease.
3. Aggressive tumors—Undifferentiated histology, extension into and beyond the subcutaneous fat, invasion of neural and lymphatic tissue

E. TREATMENT FOR BCC AND SCC IN THE HEAD AND NECK

1. Surgical excision—Treatment of choice; wide local excision or by Mohs' excision

a. Indications for Mohs' excision

   (1) Recurrent lesion, histologically aggressive skin cancer, lesion in previously irradiated area, large lesion, or those with ill-defined margins

   (2) Lesion in difficult anatomic or cosmetically important area—Ears, periauricular region, temporal region, periocular region, nasal tip ala, melolabial sulcus, upper lip

2. Repair with primary closure, skin grafts, and flaps

3. Lymphadenectomy—Indicated with advanced tumors that invade muscle, bone, cartilage or nerves, larger SCC (>2 cm), recurrent tumors, Marjolin's ulcer, and clinically positive nodal disease

a. Dissection dependent on primary tumor location

b. Lips, nasal vestibule and chin—Supraomohyoid neck dissection

c. Anterior parietal scalp, forehead, temple, ear, eyelid, zygoma, nasal ala—Parotidectomy and lateral neck dissection

d. Posterior parietal scalp, ear and mastoid—Level V or posterolateral neck dissection

4. Postoperative radiation for multiple positive nodes, extracapsular spread and lymphovascular invasion

F. MALIGNANT MELANOMA

1. Prevalence—Sixth most common cancer in the United States

2. Incidence—Head and neck melanoma accounts for nearly 25-30% of all melanomas.

3. Staging—2002 American Joint Committee on Cancer guidelines deem Breslow measurements to be the most reliable for staging purposes, and the most powerful indicator of prognosis is regional nodal metastasis.

a. Stage I (<0.75 mm)—Wide local excision (WLE) with margins of 1 cm is acceptable.

b. Stage II lesions (0.75-1.5 mm)—WLE with 2-cm margins; if 2-cm margins cannot be obtained due to location, then combined surgery and radiation therapy

   (1) Significant percentage present with nodal metastasis, so adjuvant elective neck dissection, elective radiation, or sentinel lymph node biopsy considered

c. Stage III (1.5-4.0 mm)—Excision with 2-cm margins

   (1) Commonly harbor in-transit nodal disease—If a node is present distant to a lesion, all in-transit node basins should be resected and postoperative radiation done.

d. Stage IV (>4.0 mm)—Excision with 2-cm margins

   (1) Radiation therapy for local control

   (2) Chemotherapy for palliation should be considered.

4. Treatment
a. WLE
b. Elective lymph node dissection based on known drainage patterns of site of primary tumor, depending on stage
   (1) Forehead, anterior scalp—Parotidectomy, lateral neck dissection
   (2) Facial lesions—Supraomohyoid neck dissection
   (3) Occiput, posterior scalp, posterior ear—Posterolateral neck dissection
c. Sentinel lymph node biopsy—If positive node, then a completion neck dissection should be performed based on location of lesion as outlined in section VIII. E. 3. a–d.
   (1) Controversial in the head and neck
      (a) Complex lymphatic drainage patterns many times require biopsy of multiple nodes within the neck, with dissection into deep neck, rendering this a morbid procedure as well.
      (b) Frequently need to remove sentinel lymph nodes from the parotid gland, thus placing the facial nerve at risk
      (c) However, primary lymphatic drainage basins for melanoma in the head and neck are often unpredictable and often bilateral, rendering the sentinel lymph node biopsy a good method to address the N0 neck.
d. Radiation to lymphatic basins results in a significant local and regional control in stages II-IV lesions and recurrent melanoma of the head and neck; however, no statistical significance in survival has been proven in any of the groups.
e. Chemotherapy
   (1) Reserved for proven distant disease
   (2) Several regimens exist for stage IV melanoma, but none have shown any significant improvement in outcomes and are considered experimental.

Diseases of the Breast

Joshua M. V. Mammen, MD

I. ANATOMIC AND PHYSIOLOGIC CONSIDERATIONS

A. RELEVANT ANATOMY
1. Modified sweat gland of ectodermal origin that lies cushioned in fat and enveloped by superficial and deep layers of superficial fascia of the anterior chest wall
2. Each mammary gland consists of 15-20 lobules that are drained by lactiferous ducts that open separately on the nipple.
3. Fibrous septa (Cooper's ligaments) interdigitate the mammary parenchyma and extend from the deep pectoral fascia to the superficial layer of fascia within the dermis. These provide structural support to the breast.
4. Base of breast extends from the 2nd to the 6th rib. Medial border = lateral margin of sternum. Lateral border = midaxillary line. Axillary tail of Spence pierces deep fascia and enters axilla.
5. Divided into four quadrants—Upper outer, lower outer, upper inner, and lower inner

B. LYMPHATIC DRAINAGE
Lymphatic drainage is of importance during mastectomy and axillary node dissection.
1. Axillary nodes—75% of drainage from ipsilateral breast; contains about 40-50 nodes. Axillary nodes secondarily drain to supraclavicular and jugular nodes.
2. Levels of axillary nodes
   Level I: lateral to pectoralis minor. Includes external mammary, subscapular, axillary vein, and central nodal groups.
   Level II: deep to insertion of pectoralis minor muscle on the coracoid process. Includes central nodal groups; borders of levels I and II axillary nodes include the latissimus dorsi muscle laterally, the axillary vein superiorly, and the pectoralis minor muscle medially.
   Level III: medial to pectoralis minor and extending up to apex of axilla. Includes central nodal groups.
3. Internal mammary nodes—Account for 20% of drainage; contains about four nodes per side, with one node in each of first three interspaces and another in the 5th or 6th interspace; drains upper and lower inner quadrants
4. Interpectoral (Rotter's) nodes—Lie between pectoralis major and pectoralis minor muscles
5. Abdominal and paravertebral nodes—Account for 5% of drainage

25

C. ASSOCIATED NERVES (OF SURGICAL IMPORTANCE)

1. Intercostobrachial nerve—Traverses the axilla from chest wall to supply cutaneous sensation to upper medial arm. Sacrificing this nerve results in hypoesthesia or anesthesia of upper medial arm.
2. Long thoracic nerve (of Bell)—Arises from roots of C5, C6, and C7. Courses close to chest wall along medial border of axilla to innervate serratus anterior muscle. Injury results in a "winged" scapular deformity.
3. Thoracodorsal nerve—Arises from posterior cord of brachial plexus (C5, C6, C7). Courses along lateral border of axilla to innervate latissimus dorsi muscle. Loss does not lead to significant functional or cosmetic loss.
4. Lateral pectoral nerve—Arises from lateral cord of brachial plexus. Innervates both pectoralis major and minor muscles.
5. Medial pectoral nerve—Arises from the medial cord of the brachial plexus. Innervates the pectoralis minor muscle.

D. RELEVANT PHYSIOLOGY

1. Phases of breast development are dependent on mammotropic effects of pituitary and ovarian hormones.
a. Estrogen—Promotes ductal development and fat deposition in preparation for lactation
b. Progesterone—Promotes lobular-alveolar development and prepares breast for lactation
c. Prolactin—Involved in milk production
d. Oxytocin—Involved in milk ejection
2. Menopause—Cessation of ovarian hormonal stimulation results in involution of breast tissue with atrophy of lobules, loss of stroma, and replacement with fatty tissue.

II. HISTORY

A. AGE

1. Fibroadenoma is most common breast lesion in women <30 years of age.
2. Risk for breast cancer increases with increasing age—Rare in patients <30 years of age (<1%). >70% of all cases occur in patients >50 years of age.

B. MASS

Determine when the mass was first noted, how it was first noted, whether it is tender or nontender, and any change in size over time and in relation to the menstrual cycle.

C. NIPPLE DISCHARGE

Determine the nature of the discharge—whether it is serous, serosanguineous, or bloody; whether it is unilateral or bilateral; whether it is from single or multiple duct orifices; whether it is spontaneous or induced; and whether it is associated with mass, frequency, and duration.

1. Bloody—Intraductal papilloma or invasive papillary cancer. Discharge should be sent for cytology.
2. Milky (galactorrhea)—Pregnancy, lactation, pituitary adenoma, acromegaly, hypothyroidism, stress, drugs (oral contraceptives, antihypertensives, certain psychotropic drugs). Evaluation may include urine or serum pregnancy tests and prolactin levels.
3. Serous—Normal menses, oral contraceptives, fibrocystic change, early pregnancy
4. Yellow—Fibrocystic change, galactocele
5. Purulent—Superficial or central breast abscess

D. BREAST PAIN
Breast pain may be associated with menstrual irregularity, may be a premenstrual symptom, may be related to administration of exogenous ovarian hormones during or after menopause, or may be associated with fibrocystic change. Rarely is it a symptom of breast cancer. Query regarding its type, relation to menses, duration, and location.

E. GYNECOLOGIC HISTORY (see section VII)
Include the woman's age at the birth of her first child, age of menarche, age at menopause, oral contraceptive and estrogen replacement use, and induced abortions.

F. PAST MEDICAL HISTORY
Include any prior history of benign breast disease (i.e., fibrocystic change), breast cancer, and radiation therapy to the breast or axilla.

G. PAST SURGICAL HISTORY
Include any prior history of breast biopsy, lumpectomy, mastectomy, axillary node dissection, hysterectomy, oophorectomy, and adrenalectomy.

H. FAMILY HISTORY OF BREAST DISEASE
Note any family history of breast disease, especially in mother, sisters, or daughters.

I. CONSTITUTIONAL SYMPTOMS
Constitutional symptoms include anorexia, weight loss, dyspnea, cough, chest pain, hemoptysis, and bony pain.

III. PHYSICAL EXAMINATION

A. INSPECTION
Examine with the patient seated with her arms at her side; seated with her arms raised over her head; seated with her hands on her hips; and supine.

25

DISEASES OF THE BREAST

Note breast size, shape, contour, and symmetry; skin coloration, skin dimpling, edema, erythema, peau d'orange, and excoriation; or nipple inversion, retraction, symmetry, or discharge.

B. PALPATION

1. With the patient in the sitting position, support the patient's arm and palpate each axilla to detect axillary adenopathy. The supraclavicular fossae and cervical region should also be palpated. Note node size, character, and mobility.
2. Palpation of the breast is performed with the patient in the supine position with the arms stretched above the head and with the arms at her sides. Identify any masses, noting location, size, shape, consistency, tenderness, skin dimpling, and mobility. 4 Ds to distinguish a true lump from a lumpy area—*d*ominant, *d*iscrete, *d*ense, and *d*ifferent. Carcinoma is typically firm, nontender, poorly circumscribed, and relatively immobile. The flat portion of one's fingers should be used for the exam.
3. Nipples should be palpated to identify any discharge.

C. EMPHASIZE BREAST SELF-EXAMINATION (BSE)

BSE should be performed ≈5 days after completion of menses in the premenopausal woman and monthly in the postmenopausal woman.

D. RECOMMENDED FOLLOW-UP

1. BSE on monthly basis beginning at 20-25 years of age. Most breast masses are found by patients themselves.
2. Physician exam every 1-3 years depending on risk factors. In general, q 3 yr beginning at age 18 and annually beginning at age 40.

IV. RADIOGRAPHIC STUDIES

A. INDICATIONS FOR MAMMOGRAPHY

1. Screening (current American Cancer Society recommendations)
a. Baseline mammogram for women by age 40 years or earlier if risk factors are present
b. Mammogram yearly thereafter
2. Metastatic adenocarcinoma without known primary
3. Nipple discharge without palpable mass

B. MAMMOGRAPHIC FINDINGS SUGGESTIVE OF MALIGNANCY

1. Irregularly marginated stellate or spiculated mass
2. Architectural distortion with retraction and spiculation
3. Asymmetrical localized fibrosis
4. Fine pleomorphic microcalcifications with a linear, branched, or rodlike pattern, especially when focal or clustered. Increased likelihood of cancer with increased number of microcalcifications.

5. Increased vascularity
6. Altered subareolar duct pattern
7. Unclear border with the rest of breast tissue

C. ULTRASONOGRAPHY
Ultrasonography is useful for distinguishing between cystic and solid masses. It is effective for lesions >0.5 cm in diameter. The value of ultrasonography is limited, however, because needle aspiration provides both diagnosis and treatment for most cystic masses.

V. EVALUATION OF BREAST MASS

A. PALPABLE LESIONS
1. Cystic—Suspect it is cystic if it fluctuates with the menstrual cycle, is well demarcated, is mobile, and is firm. Most common in women in their 40s. Perform fine-needle aspiration (FNA). If the woman is premenopausal, the fluid is nonbloody, and the mass disappears, no further work-up required. If the fluid is bloody, the mass remains, or the cyst recurs multiple times, proceed to excision biopsy.
In postmenopausal women, the area needs to be re-examined in 4-6 weeks for recurrence. If an ultrasound is performed and a simple cyst is noted, no further work-up is required.
2. Solid—Two options are present.
a. Proceed immediately to excisional biopsy (only 20% reveal malignancy).
b. Triple-diagnosis strategy—Serial clinical breast examinations, mammography, and FNA; monitor the mass for at least 1 year in 3-6 month intervals.

B. FINE-NEEDLE ASPIRATION BIOPSY
Fix the area of interest between the fingers of the nondominant hand. Infiltrate lidocaine intradermally with a 25-gauge needle. Make multiple passes at different angles through the mass while aspirating on syringe. Repeat these steps two or three times. Immediately fix the sample in 95% ethanol. Accuracy rates approach 90%.
1. Nondiagnostic cytology—Excisional biopsy
2. Diagnostic cytology—Discuss cancer treatment options.

C. CORE NEEDLE BIOPSY
Core needle biopsy usually is used for palpable masses; it involves making a small nick in the skin after infiltrating with local anesthetic. Make multiple passes with a Tru-Cut needle. Five passes are required for stereotactic biopsies.

D. EXCISIONAL BIOPSY
Excisional biopsy is a *definitive* method for tissue diagnosis. The majority of procedures are performed on outpatients, usually under local anesthesia.

1. Nonpalpable lesion—Requires prior mammographic localization with a needle or hook wire. The wire tip should be located within 0.5 cm of the lesion. The location of the lesion can be appreciated by palpating the breast and observing movement of the wire. Postbiopsy radiograph of the specimen should be obtained to confirm the adequacy of the biopsy. Perform a postbiopsy mammogram in 6-8 weeks to confirm removal of the lesion.

2. Biopsy incisions should be placed with deliberation—Transversely oriented, curvilinear incisions in the upper hemisphere of the breast; radial incisions in the lower hemisphere of the breast, and circumareolar incisions to be used only for masses just beneath the areola. Incision should be made so that subsequent mastectomy can incorporate biopsy site. *All* breast biopsies should be performed with the assumption that the lesion is malignant. Plan incision with regard to natural skin tension lines while the patient is sitting.

3. Sharp dissection should be used with little or no electrocautery because steroid hormone receptors are heat labile.

4. The entire mass and a surrounding 1-cm rim of normal tissue should be excised to fulfill requirements for lumpectomy, thus avoiding the need for re-excision if pathology reveals malignancy. The specimen should be properly oriented, labeled, and sent fresh (unfixed) on ice for pathology. The specimen should be processed for hormone receptor analysis and flow cytometry.

5. Deep parenchymal sutures to close dead space should be avoided because they act as a nidus for infection and distort breast architecture, yielding a poorer cosmetic result. Fibrin quickly fills dead space and restores normal breast contour. A simple subcuticular closure of skin is all that is necessary.

VI. BENIGN BREAST DISEASE

A. FIBROCYSTIC CHANGE
Fibrocystic changes encompass a wide spectrum of clinical and histologic findings, including cyst formation, breast nodularity, stromal proliferation, and epithelial hyperplasia. They may represent an exaggerated response of normal breast stroma and epithelium to circulating and locally produced hormones and growth factors. The changes are more accurately described as nonproliferative lesions.

1. Incidence greatest around age 30-40 years, but may persist into 8th decade

2. Usually presents with breast pain, swelling, and tenderness that may be associated with focal areas of nodularity, induration, or gross cysts. Frequently bilateral. Varies with menstrual cycle. Sustained symptoms may reflect anovulatory cycles.

3. Not associated with an increased risk of breast cancer unless there is a combination of gross cysts with family history of breast cancer

4. Treatment
a. Rule out carcinoma by aspiration or excisional biopsy of any discrete mass that persists without change over several menstrual cycles.
b. Frequent breast examinations (BSE and physician)
c. Baseline mammogram for ages 35-39 years and annual mammogram for age >40 years to identify any new or changing lesions
d. Patient should avoid xanthine-containing products (coffee, tea, chocolate, cola drinks) and nicotine.
e. Danazol, a weak androgen, 50-200 mg PO b.i.d. for severe symptoms—Must be continued for 2-3 months to see a potential effect. 50% recurrence within 1 year of discontinuing drug. Side effects include amenorrhea, body fat redistribution, weight gain, hirsutism, deepening of the voice, acne, and liver dysfunction.
f. Tamoxifen 20 mg PO q.d. for severe symptoms—Antiestrogenic. Binds estrogen receptors. Administer for a 4-6 week course, then discontinue to assess for continued symptoms.

B. FIBROADENOMA

1. Most common breast lesion in women <30 years of age. Present in 9-10% of women. Comprises 50% of breast biopsies and 75% of those in women <20 years of age.
2. Round, well-circumscribed, firm, rubbery, mobile, nontender mass 1-5 cm in diameter that is usually solitary. Lesions >5 cm referred to as *giant fibroadenomas*, which must be differentiated from cystosarcoma phyllodes. Usually solitary, but may be multiple and bilateral. Hormonally dependent; may increase in size with normal menses, pregnancy, lactation, and use of oral contraceptives.
3. Increases risk of breast cancer, especially if a family history of breast cancer present
4. Treatment—Excisional biopsy to remove the tumor and establish the diagnosis, or combination of physical exams, ultrasonography, and FNA

C. CYSTOSARCOMA PHYLLODES (PHYLLODES TUMOR)

Cystosarcoma phyllodes (phyllodes tumor) is a rare variant of fibroadenoma.
1. May occur at any age, but mean patient age is 30-40 years.
2. Presents as a smooth, rounded, multinodular, painless mass; overlying skin is red, warm, and shiny, with venous engorgement. The tumor itself is smooth, well-circumscribed, and freely mobile, with a median size of 4-5 cm; is characterized by rapid growth. Absence of suspicious axillary lymphadenopathy.
3. May be considered a low-grade malignancy. Contains both mesenchymal and stromal components. Most are benign, but a few develop true sarcomatous potential. Metastases are infrequent.
4. High rate of local recurrence after simple excision or enucleation
5. Treatment—Wide local excision (WLE) with at least 1-cm margins for smaller tumors; simple mastectomy for larger tumors.

25

DISEASES OF THE BREAST

D. INTRADUCTAL PAPILLOMA

Intraductal papilloma is a benign, solitary polypoid lesion involving epithelium-lined major subareolar ducts.

1. Presents as bloody nipple discharge in premenopausal women. Fluid should be sent for cytology. Most common lesion to cause serous or serosanguineous discharge.
2. Major differential diagnosis is between intraductal papilloma and invasive papillary carcinoma
3. Treatment—Excision of involved duct after localization by physical examination

E. FAT NECROSIS

1. Presents as an ecchymotic, tender, firm, ill-defined mass, often accompanied by skin or nipple retraction, which is almost impossible to differentiate from carcinoma by physical exam or mammography; usually located in superficial breast tissue and averages only 2 cm in diameter; more common in overweight women or those with pendulous breasts
2. History of antecedent trauma may be elicited in about 65% of patients; can also be caused by surgery, infection, duct ectasia, aseptic saponification
3. Treatment—If a clear history of trauma, observe. Otherwise, need to excise to rule out malignancy.

F. MAMMARY DUCT ECTASIA (PLASMA CELL MASTITIS)

1. Subacute inflammation of ductal system characterized by dilated mammary ducts with inspissated secretions and marked periductal inflammation, and infiltration of plasma cells causing yellowish white viscous nipple discharge
2. Occurs at or after menopause. History of difficult nursing may be elicited.
3. Presenting symptoms include noncyclical breast pain (mastodynia) associated with nipple retraction or discharge and subareolar masses.
4. A benign lesion that is difficult to differentiate from carcinoma clinically or radiographically. Excisional biopsy is indicated to rule out carcinoma. Multiple biopsies may be required due to the diffuse nature of the lesion. Curative treatment usually requires subareolar duct excision.

G. GALACTOCELE

1. Occurs after cessation of lactation secondary to an obstructed lactiferous duct filled with inspissated milk and desquamated epithelial cells
2. Presents as round, well-circumscribed, mobile, tender subareolar mass associated with milky yellow or greenish-yellow nipple discharge
3. Treatment—Needle aspiration; excision indicated if cyst cannot be aspirated or cyst becomes infected

H. MASTITIS AND BREAST ABSCESS

1. Common in lactating women after the third week, possibly due to inspissation of milk, obstruction, and secondary infection. May develop generalized cellulitis of breast tissue (mastitis) or abscess.
2. Patients present febrile and with a hard, painful, erythematous breast.
3. Progression from mastitis to abscess formation occurs in 5-10% of cases.
4. Most common etiologic organisms in lactating women are *Staphylococcus aureus* and *Staphylococcus epidermidis*; less commonly are *Streptococcus* and diphtheroid organisms.
5. Most common etiologic organisms in nonlactating women are *S. aureus* and anaerobes such as *Bacteroides* and *Peptostreptococcus.*
6. Treatment
   a. Culture breast milk, begin broad-spectrum antibiotics, and cease breastfeeding to prevent reinfection.
   b. Incision and drainage if fluctuant and not improved with appropriate antibiotic therapy
   c. Recurrent infection best treated by excision of diseased subareolar ducts
7. Differential diagnosis of mastitis includes inflammatory carcinoma. When incision and drainage is performed, biopsies of abscess cavity should be sent in all patients.

I. MONDOR'S DISEASE (THROMBOPHLEBITIS OF LATERAL THORACIC VEIN OR ITS BRANCH)

1. Presents as local pain associated with a tender, palpable, subcutaneous area or linear skin dimpling
2. Finding of palpable cord is diagnostic.
3. Treatment—Resolves spontaneously, but nonsteroidal anti-inflammatory drugs alleviate pain. Need a mammogram if the patient is >35 years of age.

J. GYNECOMASTIA

1. Physiologic
   a. Benign proliferation of male breast glandular tissue; prevalence of 34-65%
   b. Newborns—Due to exposure to maternal estrogens
   c. Pubertal (ages 13-17 years)—May be bilateral or unilateral; highest prevalence in adolescence beginning at 10-12 years of age with complete involution by age 16 or 17 years; treated with reassurance
   d. Senescent (>age 50 years)—Due to male "menopause" with relative estrogen increase; frequently unilateral; breast tissue is enlarged, firm, and tender; usually regresses spontaneously within 6-12 months
2. Drug induced (10-20%)—Associated with use of estrogens, digoxin, thiazides, phenothiazines, phenytoin, theophylline, cimetidine, antihypertensives (reserpine, spironolactone, methyldopa), diazepam, tricyclics, antineoplastic drugs, marijuana. Treatment is discontinuation of offending drug.

3. Pathologic—Associated with cirrhosis, renal failure, malnutrition, hyperthyroidism, adrenal dysfunction, testicular tumors, hermaphroditism, hypogonadism (e.g., Klinefelter's syndrome)
4. Any dominant or suspicious mass should be biopsied to rule out carcinoma, especially in the senescent male.

VII. BREAST CANCER

A. EPIDEMIOLOGY
1. Most common nonskin cancer in U.S. women—12% ($\approx$1:8 or 180,000 U.S. women each year) will develop breast cancer during their lifetime and 3.5% (44,000 U.S. women each year) will die of the disease; constitutes 30% of cancers diagnosed in women
2. Incidence increases with increasing age.
3. Leading cause of death in U.S. women 40-55 years of age
4. Age-adjusted incidence appears to be increasing while age-adjusted death rate appears to be decreasing—May be related to earlier detection and/or improved therapy

B. RISK FACTORS
1. Sex—Female-to-male ratio for breast cancer is 100-150:1.
2. Age—Risk increases with increasing age. The risk that breast cancer will develop in a white American female in a single year increases from 1:5900 at age 30 years to 1:290 at age 80 years.
3. Mother and/or sister(s) (first-degree relative) with breast cancer— Two or three times increased risk. Risk decreases with more distant affected relatives. Overall risk depends on number of first-degree relatives with breast cancer, their ages at diagnosis, and whether the disease was unilateral or bilateral.
   a. If woman is premenopausal with unilateral breast cancer—20-30% risk of development
   b. If woman is premenopausal with bilateral breast cancer—50% risk of development
4. Genetic predisposition—Accounts for <3% of all breast cancers. Breast cancer invariably develops in patients with Li-Fraumeni syndrome, a rare disorder involving a germline mutation in the tumor suppressor gene *P53*. The *BRCA1* gene, located on chromosome 17q, may be responsible for early-onset (familial) breast cancer.
5. Prior history of breast cancer—Five times increased risk in contralateral breast
6. History of breast biopsy regardless of underlying pathology
7. Atypical ductal or lobular hyperplasia identified on breast biopsy— $\approx$five times increased risk
8. Coexistence of positive family history of breast cancer and atypical ductal or lobular hyperplasia on biopsy—Nine times increased risk

9. Noninvasive carcinoma (ductal carcinoma in situ [DCIS] or lobular carcinoma in situ [LCIS])
10. Early menarche (<12 years of age) or late menopause (>55 years of age)
11. Cumulative duration of menstruation. Risk is increased for women that menstruate for >30 years.
12. Nulliparity or age >30 years at first delivery
13. Exogenous hormone use—Use of postmenopausal estrogen replacement increases risk of breast cancer by ≈40%.
14. Oral contraceptives
15. Exposure to low-dose ionizing radiation between 13 and 30 years of age
16. Alcohol consumption, especially before 30 years of age
17. Induced abortion (conflicting studies)

C. **CLINICAL PRESENTATION**
1. Nonpalpable, suspicious lesion on mammogram—Requires needle localization biopsy or stereotactic FNA biopsy for diagnosis
2. Palpable mass—Most common presentation; most detected by patient on routine self-exam; typically nontender, firm, irregular, relatively immobile, most commonly located in upper outer quadrant of breast (≈50%); may be multifocal, multicentric, or bilateral
3. Skin changes—Skin dimpling (tethering of Cooper's ligaments), nipple retraction or inversion, erythema, warmth, edema, peau d'orange (dermal lymphatic invasion), ulceration, eczema or excoriation of superficial epidermis of nipple (as in Paget's disease)
4. Nipple discharge—Bloody; most commonly due to intraductal papilloma, but invasive papillary carcinoma must be ruled out
5. Metastatic spread—To lungs, bone, brain, liver, and lymph nodes; may present with anorexia, weight loss, cachexia, dyspnea, cough, hemoptysis, bony pain (especially vertebral), pathologic fractures

D. **TNM CLASSIFICATION**
1. Primary tumor (T)
   - T0: No evidence of primary tumor
   - TIS: Carcinoma in situ—ductal or lobular, or Paget's disease of nipple without tumor
   - T1: Tumor 2.0 cm or smaller
   - T2: Tumor >2.0 cm but <5.0 cm
   - T3: Tumor >5.0 cm
   - T4: Tumor of any size with direct extension to chest wall or skin
   - T4a: Extension to chest wall
   - T4b: Edema (including peau d'orange), ulceration of skin of breast, or satellite skin nodules confined to same breast
   - T4c: Both T4a and T4b

DISEASES OF THE BREAST 25

T4d: Inflammatory carcinoma—characterized by diffuse, brawny induration of skin, with erysipeloid edge, usually without underlying palpable mass

2. Regional lymph nodes (N)

N0: No regional lymph node metastases

N1: Metastases to moveable ipsilateral axillary lymph nodes

N2: Metastases to ipsilateral axillary lymph nodes fixed to one another or to other structures

N3: Metastases to ipsilateral internal mammary lymph nodes

3. Distant metastases (M)

M0: No distant metastasis

M1: Distant metastasis—includes supraclavicular, cervical, or contralateral internal mammary lymph nodes

E. STAGING

Stage 0: Tis N0 M0

Stage I: T1 N0 M0

Stage IIa: T0 N1 M0, T1 N1 M0, T2 N0 M0

Stage IIb: T2 N1 M0, T3 N0 M0

Stage IIIa: T0 N2 M0, T1 N2 M0, T2 N2 M0, T3 N1,2 M0

Stage IIIb: T4 any N M0, any T N3 M0

Stage IV: any T, any N, M1

F. PATHOLOGY

1. Growth patterns

a. May be broadly divided into epithelial tumors arising from cells lining ducts or lobules vs. nonepithelial tumors arising from supporting stroma (i.e., angiosarcoma, malignant cystosarcoma phyllodes, primary stromal sarcomas). Nonepithelial tumors are much less common.

b. May be noninvasive (DCIS or LCIS) or invasive (infiltrating ductal or lobular carcinoma). *Noninvasive* refers to the absence of invasion of the basement membrane.

c. May be multifocal (disease within same quadrant as dominant lesion), multicentric (disease in distant quadrant within the same breast), or bilateral (disease in both breasts)

2. Common histologic types of breast cancer

a. Noninvasive

(1) DCIS—Proliferation of malignant epithelial cells completely contained within breast ducts; more common than LCIS; average age at diagnosis is mid-50s; ≈80% of DCIS lesions are nonpalpable and detected by screening mammography; occasionally may present with palpable mass; clustered microcalcifications may be seen on mammography; tends to be multicentric (35%); occult invasive carcinoma may coexist with in situ lesion in 11-21% of cases; risk for subsequent invasive ductal carcinoma is ≈25-30% and usually occurs within 10 years of diagnosis; size and extent of DCIS appear

to correlate with incidence of multicentricity and synchronous invasive foci as well as risk for progression to invasive carcinoma; considered a premalignant lesion

(2) LCIS—Proliferation of malignant epithelial cells completely contained within breast lobules; the mean age of diagnosis is 44-46 years with 80-90% of cases in premenopausal women; estrogens are hypothesized to play an important role in the pathogenesis of LCIS; does not form a palpable mass; no mammographic findings; usually discovered incidentally on biopsy for another abnormality; identified in ≈4% of biopsy specimens obtained for benign disease; tends to be bilateral and multicentric (60-80% of cases); LCIS identified in contralateral breast in 25% of cases; risk for subsequent invasive carcinoma (usually ductal) is increased 7-10 times in the ipsilateral breast and about the same in the contralateral breast; 1% risk of breast cancer development per year; invasive carcinoma usually occurs >15 years after diagnosis; considered a marker for increased risk of invasive disease

b. Invasive

(1) Infiltrating ductal carcinoma—Most common breast malignancy (80%); originates from ductal epithelium and infiltrates supporting stroma; less common forms include medullary carcinoma, colloid carcinoma, tubular carcinoma, and papillary carcinoma; most commonly presents as a palpable mass or mammographic abnormality

(2) Invasive lobular carcinoma—Accounts for 5-10% of all invasive breast malignancies; originates from lobular epithelium and infiltrates supporting stroma; does not form microcalcifications; more apt to be bilateral; similar prognosis to invasive ductal carcinoma; presents as a palpable mass or mammographic abnormality

(3) Paget's disease of the nipple—Accounts for 1-3% of all breast malignancies; is usually associated with intraductal carcinoma (DCIS) or invasive carcinoma just beneath the nipple; malignant cells invade across epithelial-epidermal junction and enter epidermis of the nipple; presents initially as erythema and mild eczematous changes that become erosions and ulcerations; rapid and lethal malignancy; diagnosis by scrape cytology, shave biopsy, punch biopsy, or nipple excision; treatment: mastectomy or excision of nipple-areolar complex if limited to retroareolar area

(4) Inflammatory breast carcinoma—Accounts for 1-4% of all breast malignancies; most rapidly lethal malignancy of the breast; poorly differentiated; characterized by dermal lymphatic invasion on pathologic exam; presents as diffuse induration, erythema, warmth, edema, peau d'orange of the skin of the breast with or without palpable mass; axillary lymphadenopathy is almost always present; distant metastases common at time of diagnosis (17-36%); rapid and lethal malignancy; induction chemotherapy led to increased

25

DISEASES OF THE BREAST

survival with combined-modality therapy leading to a 40-70%
3-year survival
c. Staging is more important than histology in determining prognosis.
d. Other prognostic indicators include nuclear and histologic grade,
presence or absence of estrogen and progesterone receptors, DNA
content and proliferative fraction (S-phase). Aneuploid tumors with high
S-phase fraction tend to be more aggressive and carry poorer prognosis
than diploid tumors with low S-phase fraction.

G. SURGICAL TREATMENT OPTIONS
1. WLE, lumpectomy, and segmental mastectomy
a. Breast-conserving therapy
b. Two major objectives
    (1) Complete excision of tumor with tumor-free margins
    (2) Good cosmetic result
c. Usually accompanied by axillary node dissection (through a separate
incision) and radiation therapy to the whole breast ($\approx$50 Gy over
5-week period beginning 2-4 weeks after surgery), often with "boost" of
radiation to tumor bed
d. Eligibility criteria include the following.
    (1) Tumor size $\leq$4 cm
    (2) Appropriate tumor size–to–breast size ratio
    (3) No fixation of tumor to underlying muscle or chest wall
    (4) No involvement of overlying skin
    (5) No multicentric cancer (unless immediately juxtaposed)
    (6) No fixed or matted axillary nodes
e. For best cosmetic results, curvilinear incisions should be used in the upper
quadrants, and radial incisions should be used in the lower quadrants.
2. Subcutaneous mastectomy
a. Removes breast tissue only, sparing nipple-areolar complex, skin, and
nodes
b. Not a cancer operation—Leaves 1-2% of breast tissue behind; rarely,
if ever, indicated
3. Simple mastectomy (total mastectomy)
a. Removes breast tissue, nipple-areolar complex, and skin
b. No axillary node dissection is performed.
c. Often performed for DCIS or LCIS
4. Modified radical mastectomy (MRM)—Removes breast tissue, pectoralis fascia, nipple-areolar complex, skin, and axillary lymph nodes in continuity. Spares pectoralis major muscle.
a. Patey modification—Preserves pectoralis major, but sacrifices the
pectoralis minor to remove levels I-III axillary lymph nodes
b. Auchincloss modification—Preserves both pectoralis major and pectoralis
minor. Preservation of pectoralis minor limits high axillary node
dissection (level III), but this does not appear to be clinically significant
in most cases.

5. Radical mastectomy (Halsted)

a. Removes breast tissue, nipple-areolar complex, skin, pectoralis major and minor, and axillary lymph nodes in continuity

b. Leaves bare chest wall with significant cosmetic and functional deformity

c. Of historical interest only. Clinical trials comparing MRM with radical mastectomy reveal no significant difference in disease-free survival, distant disease-free survival, or overall survival.

6. Contraindications to breast conservation surgery

a. Absolute

    (1) ≥2 primary tumors in separate quadrant

    (2) Diffuse malignancy with minicalcifications

    (3) History of breast irradiation causing excessive total dosage

    (4) Pregnancy

    (5) Persistent positive surgical margins

b. Relative

    (1) Collagen vascular disease

    (2) Tumors >4 cm in diameter

    (3) Multiple tumors in the same quadrant

    (4) Large breast size

H. SURGICAL TREATMENT BY STAGE

1. Stage 0

a. DCIS—Total ipsilateral mastectomy vs. WLE + radiation therapy. General agreement that axillary node dissection is not required for DCIS. Overall 5-year survival rate of 95-100% independent of whether treated by total mastectomy or WLE + radiation therapy.

b. LCIS—Bilateral total mastectomy vs. tamoxifen 20 mg daily for 5 years coupled with close observation. Axillary node dissection is not required.

c. Clinically occult invasive carcinoma—MRM vs. WLE with axillary node dissection + radiation therapy

d. Paget's disease—Total mastectomy vs. MRM

2. Stages I and II—Represent ≈85% of breast cancers

a. Current treatment recommendations—MRM vs. WLE with axillary node dissection + radiation therapy

b. Clinical trials have shown WLE with axillary node dissection + radiation therapy to be equivalent to MRM in terms of disease-free survival, distant disease-free survival, and overall survival.

c. WLE with axillary node dissection + radiation therapy offers breast conservation with clinical outcome equivalent to MRM.

d. Tumor-free margins are essential when WLE is performed.

e. Addition of radiation therapy to WLE with axillary node dissection improves disease-free survival (e.g., decreased locoregional recurrence) but does not improve distant disease-free survival or overall survival in node-negative patients.

    f. Adjuvant chemotherapy is indicated for node-positive patients and high-risk node-negative patients. Preoperative chemotherapy may have a role in converting tumors to make breast conservation surgery possible.

    g. Factors associated with high risk of recurrence
      (1) Age <35 years
      (2) Tumor size >2 cm
      (3) Poor histologic and nuclear grade
      (4) Absence of estrogen and progesterone receptors
      (5) Aneuploid DNA content
      (6) High-proliferative fraction (S-phase)
      (7) Overexpression of epidermal growth factor receptor II
      (8) Presence of cathepsin D
      (9) Amplification of c-*erb*-b2 oncogene

    h. Lobular carcinoma—Use of mirror-image biopsy or total mastectomy for the contralateral breast is controversial.

    i. 5-year survival rates for stages I and II breast cancer are ≈80% and 60%, respectively.

3. Stages III and IV

    a. Multimodality therapy including surgery, radiation therapy, and systemic therapy is usually employed.

    b. Surgical therapy must be individualized based on extent of tumor and technical ease of resection. Role of breast conservation has not been specifically defined. Mastectomy (total or MRM) remains the mainstay of surgical therapy.

    c. Preoperative chemotherapy and local radiation therapy is currently under investigation as potential treatment for inflammatory breast carcinoma.

    d. Goal of multimodality therapy is control of locoregional and distant disease. However, even with aggressive therapy, most of these patients die due to distant metastatic disease.

    e. 5-year survival rates for stages III and IV breast cancer are ≈20% and 0%, respectively.

I. CHEMOTHERAPY AND HORMONAL THERAPY

1. Surgery and radiation therapy are used to achieve locoregional control, whereas chemotherapy and hormonal therapy are used to achieve systemic control.

2. Adjuvant therapy

    a. Palliation for metastatic disease

Nodes	ER Status	Therapy
Positive	Positive	Tamoxifen or chemo + tamoxifen
	Negative	Chemo
Negative	Low risk (irrespective of ER)	None
	Positive	Tamoxifen or chemo + tamoxifen
	Negative	Chemo

Chemo = chemotherapy; ER = estrogen receptor.

(1) Decision to offer systemic therapy for metastatic disease should be based on the extent and rate of progression of metastatic disease, hormone receptor status, degree and progression of symptoms, and the patient's ability to tolerate therapy without significant toxicity.

(2) Chemotherapy tends to have a shorter time to response (4-6 weeks vs. 8-12 weeks), better overall response rate (40-60% vs. 25-35%), shorter mean duration of action (8-12 months vs. 14-18 months), and increased toxicity compared to hormonal therapy.

(3) Chemotherapy should be considered for patients with hormone receptor–negative tumors, aggressive metastatic disease, and the ability to tolerate side effects of cytotoxic drugs.

(4) Hormonal therapy should be considered for patients with hormone receptor–positive tumors and relatively indolent metastatic disease. Tamoxifen is the treatment of choice for most of these patients.

3. Cytotoxic chemotherapy

a. Combination chemotherapy is more effective than single-agent chemotherapy.

b. Associated with higher toxicity than hormonal therapy; may be poorly tolerated by elderly or debilitated patients

c. Premenopausal patients tend to have better response to cytotoxic chemotherapy, whereas postmenopausal patients tend to have better response to hormonal therapy. Difference in response is based on more aggressive nature of tumors in premenopausal patients (i.e., hormone receptor–negative, aneuploid, high S-phase fraction), which increases the likelihood of response to cytotoxic agents.

4. Hormonal therapy

a. Indications

(1) Adjuvant therapy for hormone receptor–positive, premenopausal or postmenopausal, node-positive or high-risk node-negative patients

(2) Palliative therapy for relatively indolent metastatic disease in premenopausal or postmenopausal patients with hormone receptor–positive tumors

b. Response to hormonal therapy is dependent on the status of hormone receptors

c. Tamoxifen is the therapeutic agent of choice.

(1) Competitive antagonist of estrogen. Binds to estrogen receptors and prevents binding of estrogen.

(2) As effective as any other form of hormonal therapy, including oophorectomy

(3) If chemotherapy is used, tamoxifen therapy should start after completion of chemotherapy.

(4) Tamoxifen therapy should be continued for at least 2 years.

(5) The role of tamoxifen prophylactically in patients at high risk for breast cancer is currently under investigation.

25

DISEASES OF THE BREAST

HORMONE RECEPTOR STATUS

Receptor	Response Rate (%)
ER+, PgR+	78
ER+, PgR–	34
ER–, PgR+	45
ER–, PgR–	10

ER = estrogen receptor; PgR = progesterone receptor.

    d. Alternatives to tamoxifen
      (1) Progestation agents (progestins)
      (2) Luteinizing hormone–releasing analogs
      (3) Aminoglutethimide—Aromatase inhibitor; decreases circulating levels of estrogen by blocking the peripheral conversion of androstenedione to estrogen (medical adrenalectomy)
      (4) Antiprogestins—New class of drugs being evaluated in clinical trials
      (5) Oophorectomy—Only indication is in the treatment of metastatic breast cancer in premenopausal, hormone receptor–positive patients. Tamoxifen, however, has been shown to be equally effective and should be used first.

J. BREAST CANCER AND PREGNANCY

1. Incidence of breast cancer detected during pregnancy is 2 per 10,000 gestations, accounting for 2.8% of all breast cancers.
2. Diagnosis is more difficult and frequently delayed due to breast engorgement, tenderness, and increased nodularity.
3. Suspicious masses detected during pregnancy should undergo FNA or excisional biopsy.
4. If malignancy is identified, subsequent treatment decisions are influenced by specific trimester of pregnancy. The goal of treatment is the cure of breast cancer without injury to the fetus.
a. Studies have demonstrated that termination of pregnancy, in hopes of decreasing hormonal tumor stimulation, has no added benefit.
b. For cancer detected during first and second trimesters, MRM is the treatment of choice. However, immediate breast reconstruction should not be performed because a symmetrical result is impossible until the postpartum appearance of the contralateral breast is known.
c. Breast conservation therapy is complicated by fact that radiation therapy is contraindicated in pregnancy. For cancer detected during the third trimester, WLE and axillary node dissection may be safely performed, with radiation therapy delayed until after delivery.
d. For those requiring adjuvant chemotherapy, studies have shown no increased risk of fetal malformation for chemotherapy administered during the second and third trimesters. There is, however, an increased incidence of spontaneous abortion and congenital malformation associated with chemotherapy administered during the first trimester.

K. MALE BREAST CANCER

1. ≈1% the incidence of that in women
2. Increased risk may be associated with hyperestrogenic states—Klinefelter's syndrome, liver disease, and exogenous estrogen use (metastatic prostate cancer, transvestites). Low-dose radiation also implicated.
3. Usually diagnosed at a later age than in women—Mean age at diagnosis is 60-65 years.
4. Delay in diagnosis may result in more advanced stage at presentation and worse prognosis.
5. Infiltrating ductal carcinoma is most common histologic type of breast cancer in men. Lobular carcinoma occurs rarely.
6. Due to scant breast tissue in men, the pectoralis major muscle is more often involved.
7. Node-negative disease—Prognosis similar to that in women
   Node-positive disease has a significantly worse prognosis than in women.
8. Treatment—Depends on stage and local extent of tumor
a. If underlying pectoralis major muscle is involved, a radical mastectomy should be performed. Otherwise, MRM is the procedure of choice.
b. Postoperative radiation therapy may be considered due to local aggressiveness of these tumors; improves local control but does not affect survival
c. Adjuvant chemotherapy or hormonal therapy should be offered to node-positive or high-risk node-negative patients. Since >80% of male breast cancers are hormone receptor positive, tamoxifen may play an important role.

L. BREAST RECONSTRUCTION FOLLOWING MASTECTOMY

1. No evidence to suggest that breast reconstruction following mastectomy compromises efficacy of adjuvant chemotherapy, increases incidence of local recurrence, or delays diagnosis of recurrence on chest wall
2. Significantly improves patient's concept of body image
3. May be performed immediately or may be delayed until after completion of adjuvant chemotherapy or radiation therapy. Recent trend is toward immediate reconstruction.
4. Types of reconstructive procedures
a. Prosthetic breast implant—Filled with silicone or saline; inserted subpectorally
b. Myocutaneous flap reconstruction—More complicated procedure, but better long-term cosmetic results
   (1) Transverse rectus abdominis flap—Based on superior mesenteric artery and vein; entire contralateral rectus abdominis muscle is transposed with transverse ellipse of skin and SQ tissue from lower abdomen
   (2) Latissimus dorsi flap—Based on thoracodorsal artery and vein

25

DISEASES OF THE BREAST

    (3) Free rectus abdominis flap—Thoracodorsal or anterior serratus vessels are anastomosed to inferior epigastric vessels to maintain blood supply to the flap.

    (4) Greater omentum pedicle flap covered with a skin graft

    (5) Gluteus maximus free flap

c. Nipple-areolar reconstruction may be performed as a secondary procedure following prosthetic breast implant or myocutaneous flap reconstruction; typically delayed 6-12 weeks to allow reconstructed breast to attain its final shape and position

5. Complications of breast reconstruction

a. Infection

b. Tissue loss—Especially flap loss due to vascular compromise

c. Poor cosmetic result

d. Slippage of prosthetic implant or capsular contraction

Thyroid

Richard A. Falcone, Jr., MD

I. INTRODUCTION

A. GENERAL
1. Diseases of the thyroid gland are among the most common endocrine disorders seen by clinicians.
2. Thyroid disorders fall into three broad categories.
a. Hypofunction
b. Hyperfunction
c. Enlargements
    (1) Diffuse—Termed *goiter* regardless of functional status
    (2) Nodule

B. CLINICAL MANIFESTATIONS
1. Hyperthyroidism is suggested by weight loss, irritability, heat intolerance, thinning hair, palpitations, and tachycardia.
2. Hypothyroidism is suggested by weight gain, lethargy, coarse hair, cold intolerance, thick skin, slowed muscle reflexes, constipation, and slowed mentation.
3. Common clinical causes of hyperthyroidism and hypothyroidism

Hyperthyroidism	Hypothyroidism
Graves' disease	Autoimmune thyroiditis
Toxic solitary nodule	Thyroidectomy
Multinodular goiter	Iodine deficiency
	Dyshormonogenesis

II. ANATOMY

A. NORMAL WEIGHT
Normal weight is from 15-20 g.

B. BLOOD SUPPLY
1. Superior thyroid arteries—Branches off external carotid artery
2. Inferior thyroid arteries—Branches off thyrocervical trunk
3. Thyroidea ima—Directly off the aorta (not consistently present)

C. LARYNGEAL NERVES
1. Recurrent laryngeal—Variable positions. ≈70% run in the tracheoesophageal groove, 60% posterior to inferior thyroid artery. *It is important to always identify the nerve.*
2. Superior laryngeal nerve—Runs near the superior thyroid arteries

III. THYROID FUNCTION TESTS

The initial work-up of a patient suspected of hypothyroidism or hyperthyroidism should consist of serum thyroid-stimulating hormone (TSH), T_4 (thyroxine), and T_3 (triiodothyronine) radioiodine uptake (T_3RU). T_4 multiplied by T_3RU gives the free T_4 index (FT_4I), the level of circulating T_4 that has been corrected for changes in transport protein levels.

	Pituitary Failure	Hypothyroid	Hyperthyroid
FT_4I	Low	Low	High
TSH	Low	High	Low

IV. SURGICAL THYROID DISEASE

Surgeons are called on to manage three types of thyroid disease:
(1) enlargement causing compression; (2) certain types of hyperthyroidism; and (3) thyroid nodules.

A. COMPRESSION
1. Dyspnea, dysphagia, tracheal or esophageal deviation clinically or radiographically are indications for surgical debulking of the goiter.
2. Chest and neck radiographs along with thyroid function tests should be obtained.
3. Compression symptoms suggest substernal extension of the thyroid. CT scan of the neck and chest may be indicated.

B. HYPERTHYROIDISM
1. Surgical management is indicated for Graves' disease, toxic multinodular goiter, and toxic solitary nodule. In all three entities the medical control of thyrotoxicosis is crucial if thyroid storm is to be prevented.
a. Propylthiouracil (PTU)—300-600 ng/day 6-8 weeks preoperatively
b. Propranolol—40-480 mg/day 6-8 weeks preoperatively
c. SSKI or Lugol's solution—1 or 2 drops t.i.d. 1 week preoperatively
2. Graves' disease
a. Autoimmune disorder with pathogenic thyroid-stimulating antibodies
b. Diagnosis is by the identification of a diffusely enlarged gland with autonomous thyroid function.
c. Total thyroidectomy cures Graves' disease, with 100% postoperative hypothyroidism. Leaving a 6-8 g remnant cures 96% of patients, with postoperative hypothyroidism in 20-30%.
3. Toxic multinodular goiter (Plummer's disease)
a. Multiple nodules secreting thyroid hormone independent of TSH
b. Clinically more mild symptoms than Graves' disease, palpable nodules
c. Treatment is bilateral subtotal lobectomies
4. Toxic solitary nodule
a. Single autonomously functioning nodule
b. Palpable nodule with symptoms of hyperthyroidism
c. Surgical treatment is by lobectomy

5. Thyroid storm

Thyroid storm is life threatening and can be induced in hyperthyroid patient by any stress, especially surgery.

a. Symptoms—Hyperpyrexia, tachycardia, numbness, irritability, vomiting, diarrhea, and proximal muscle weakness. Cause of death is usually due to high-output cardiac failure.

b. Treatment—Prevention is the best treatment. During thyroid storm, treatment should be with mechanical cooling, oxygen, and volume resuscitation, 100 mg hydrocortisone IV piggyback to prevent adrenal insufficiency, propranolol 1-2 mg IV piggyback followed by 50-100 mg/min IV drip to control symptoms, IV sodium iodide (1-2.5 g), and q 2 h glucose management with D-50 for blood sugars <100. PTU therapy should begin during acute management.

C. NODULES

1. 4-8% of the U.S. population has palpable nodules.

2. The differential includes the following.

a. Adenoma

b. Cyst

c. Thyroiditis

d. Graves' disease

e. Teratoma

f. Metastasis to thyroid (breast, lung, kidney, and melanoma)

g. Thyroid carcinoma

3. Physical exam—Stand behind patients and have them swallow some water to help palpate thyroid masses. Thyroid masses move with swallowing because of the tracheal attachment. Note size, consistency, tenderness, and nodularity of the gland.

4. Thyroid function tests cannot be used to differentiate benign from malignant lesions.

5. Thyroid scanning with ^{123}I can indicate the functional activity of a nodule. Cold nodules have a 10-25% chance of malignancy. Hot nodules have a 1% chance of malignancy.

6. Ultrasound is helpful for detecting nonpalpable nodules and differentiating solid from cystic nodules.

7. Fine-needle aspiration is the single most useful test in evaluating thyroid nodules.

a. Insert 20-22 gauge needle.

b. Apply suction and fan needle.

c. Release suction, then remove needle.

d. Expel contents onto slide and fix.

e. Results

    (1) 7% nondiagnostic

    (2) Reliable for all cancers except follicular, because the cytology of follicular adenoma and follicular carcinoma are the same; determination of capsular or vascular invasion necessary to differentiate the two

26

THYROID

(3) Surgical excision is necessary for follicular neoplasms.
(4) Intermediate lesions have a 20-60% malignancy rate.
(5) Positive cytology is diagnostic except in follicular neoplasms.
(6) There is a 20% false-negative rate; thus, if malignancy is suspected clinically, negative cytology should never delay or deter surgical excision.

f. Cysts should be drained completely, which is curative in 75%.

V. THYROID CANCER

In thyroid cancer, 20-30% of nodules are malignant.

A. CLINICAL CHARACTERISTICS THAT SUGGEST MALIGNANCY
1. Male gender and age <15 and >60 years
2. History of head and neck radiation or thyroiditis
3. Family history of thyroid cancer
4. Rapidly enlarging nodule
5. Hard, single nodule and/or nodules fixed to surrounding structures
6. Hoarseness
7. Cervical lymphadenopathy

B. FREQUENCY AND TYPES
Thyroid cancer is the most common endocrine malignancy, occurring in 4/100,000 people (Table 26-1).

1. Papillary carcinoma—Slow growing, 60% multicentric, male-to-female ratio is 1:3, 80-90% of postradiation cancers of the thyroid, spread by lymphatics (50% have positive nodes at diagnosis). Presence of nodes does not affect prognosis. If tumor is >3 cm, male >40 years, female >50 years, distant metastasis or angioinvasion, then total thyroidectomy is indicated because of poor prognosis. AGES and MACIS scales may be used for prognosis.
2. Follicular carcinoma—More aggressive, unifocal, male-to-female ratio is 1:3, angioinvasive, metastasis to lung and bone
3. Mixed papillary-follicular carcinoma behaves and is treated like papillary carcinoma.
4. Hürthle cell tumor—Intermediate aggressiveness, unifocal, male-to-female ratio is 2:1, spread by lymphatics
   a. Thallium scan for metastatic localization
   b. Does not take up 131I, so surgery is only chance for cure
5. Lymphoma—Usually intermediate lymphomas, usually female, may have history of Hashimoto's thyroiditis; rapid enlargement, compressive symptoms common. Chemotherapy and radiation therapy sensitive.
6. Medullary thyroid cancer—Aggressive tumors, 90% sporadic, 10% in association with multiple endocrine neoplasia (MEN) type 2; amyloid stroma histologically, 95% produce calcitonin, 85% produce carcinoembryonic antigen. Sporadic form is unifocal, occurs around 45 years of age, and carries a worse prognosis. Familial form is multifocal, occurs around 35 years of age, and carries a better prognosis.

TABLE 26-1
ENDOCRINE MALIGNANCIES—SURGERY AND SURVIVAL

	Papillary	Follicular	Hürthle Cell	Lymphoma	Medullary	Anaplastic
Incidence (%)	70	10	5	5	7	3
Type of surgery	Lobectomy	Total thyroidectomy	Total thyroidectomy	For diagnosis and compressive symptoms	Total thyroidectomy	? Debulking thyroidectomy
10-Year survival (%)	85	40	60	40-50	30-40	<2

26

THYROID

C-cell hyperplasia is the precursor to medullary thyroid cancer in MEN 2.

a. Does not concentrate 131I.

b. Thallium, MIBG, DMSA are used to localize metastatic disease if calcitonin begins to rise.

c. All patients with medullary thyroid cancer should be screened for a pheochromocytoma (MEN 2), which should be resected first.

7. Anaplastic carcinoma—Very aggressive; 30% develop in a well-differentiated carcinoma; must be differentiated from lymphoma

a. Chemotherapy and radiation may slightly improve survival.

b. Mean survival is 2-4 months.

C. POSTOPERATIVE CARE

1. Position patient with elevated head of bed, provide cool misted oxygen.

2. Hypocalcemia—Calcium is checked postoperatively, then q 8 h × 24 hours, then q day. Patients may exhibit tingling and numbness around the lips and fingers and a positive Chvostek's sign.

3. Hypothyroidism

a. Levothyroxine (Synthroid) replacement 1 µg/lb to prevent hypothyroidism and suppress TSH (a growth factor for well-differentiated cancers, e.g., papillary, follicular, mixed and Hürthle cell)

b. Hold levothyroxine prior to postoperative iodine scan (performed 2-3 months postoperatively) so TSH will be elevated and residual or metastatic tissue will have maximal stimulation for iodine uptake.

c. Liothyronine (Cytomel), 75 µg/day, is given as thyroid replacement in the interim, and then discontinued 2 weeks before scan.

4. Have a tracheostomy tray available in case of airway compromise.

D. COMPLICATIONS

1. Vocal cord paralysis due to recurrent laryngeal nerve damage—1% if nerve is visualized, 4% if nerve is "avoided"

2. Hypoparathyroidism in total thyroidectomy—1-2% permanent, 10-20% temporary

3. Hypothyroidism—100% in total thyroidectomy, 20-30% if 6-8 g of tissue is left

4. Pneumothorax—Infrequent

5. Wound hematoma—If this occurs and the patient has respiratory distress, open the wound at the bedside.

RECOMMENDED READINGS

Gharib H: Fine-needle aspiration biopsy of thyroid nodules: Advantages, limitations, and effect. Mayo Clin Proc 69:44, 1994.

Hurley DL, Gharib H: Evaluation and management of multinodular goiter. Otolaryngol Clin North Am 29:527, 1996.

Mazzaferri EL: An overview of the management of papillary and follicular thyroid carcinoma. Thyroid 9:421, 1999.

Parathyroid

Richard A. Falcone, Jr., MD

I. PARATHYROID EMBRYOLOGY AND ANATOMY

A. EMBRYOLOGY
1. Inferior parathyroids originate from the third branchial pouch in conjunction with the thymus. They are therefore associated with or embedded in the thymus anywhere from the base of the skull to the anterior mediastinum.
2. Superior parathyroids arise from the fourth branchial pouch in conjunction with the thyroid. Enlarged glands tend to descend in the tracheoesophageal groove and can be found in the posterior mediastinum.

B. ANATOMY
1. Normal parathyroid usually weighs <50 mg and measures $3 \times 3 \times 3$ mm.
2. The superior parathyroid glands tend to be in a more posterior plane than the inferior parathyroids.

II. PRIMARY HYPERPARATHYROIDISM

A. GENERAL
1. One or more glands elaborate inappropriately increased amounts of parathyroid hormone (PTH) relative to the serum calcium level.
2. Occurs in 1:1000 population; recently diagnosed more frequently because of availability of routine serum calcium determinations

B. HISTOLOGIC PATTERNS
1. Single adenoma—90% of cases. A rim of normal parathyroid tissue around the adenoma distinguishes adenoma from hyperplasia.
2. Hyperplasia—10% of cases. No rim of normal tissue and lack of stromal fat. All four glands are involved. The hyperparathyroidism of multiple endocrine neoplasia syndromes is due to hyperplasia.
3. Parathyroid carcinoma—<1% of cases. Exceptionally high calcium level or palpable neck mass should raise suspicion. Excision with thyroid lobectomy indicated. Radical neck dissection for recurrent disease. Recur locally in 30%; distant metastasis to lung, liver, and bone in 30%.

C. CLINICAL PRESENTATION
1. 70% are asymptomatic, diagnosed incidentally by routine lab studies
2. Nephrolithiasis or nephrocalcinosis ("stones"). Present in 10-20% of patients, usually calcium phosphate. Calcium oxalate stones are less common.

27

3. "Bones"—Bone pain, arthralgias, and muscular aches
a. Present in 20% of symptomatic patients
b. Cortical resorption with medullary bone sparing secondary to increased turnover
c. Osteitis fibrosa cystica is the condition where resorption leads to "brown cysts" in the bone; it predisposes to fractures.
4. "Groans"—Peptic ulcer disease and pancreatitis; present in 20% of symptomatic patients
5. "Psychic overtones"—Fatigue, depression, anxiety, irritability, lack of concentration, and sleep disturbances
a. Present in 40% of symptomatic patients
b. No relationship of PTH or calcium levels to the severity of symptoms
c. Surgery improves all symptoms except anxiety.

D. PHYSICAL EXAM
1. Usually not helpful in diagnosis
2. If a mass is palpable, suspect thyroid pathology or parathyroid carcinoma.

E. DIAGNOSTIC WORK-UP
1. Hypercalcemia, hypophosphatemia, and hypercalciuria are the classic hallmarks of hyperparathyroidism.
2. The serum calcium may be intermittently normal with hyperparathyroidism, so three separate determinations should be made.
3. With the availability of PTH assay, the diagnosis is made when PTH levels are elevated relative to the serum ionized calcium level, which need not be markedly elevated and may fall into the upper limit of normal.
a. The N terminal of PTH confers the biologic effect—Half-life is several minutes
b. C terminal is inactive, but better for determining hyperparathyroidism—Half-life is 1-2 hours
c. Elevated PTH levels may occur with renal failure and do not necessarily imply hyperparathyroidism.
d. The humoral hypercalcemia of malignancy (hypercalcemia without bone metastasis) is mediated by PTH-like molecules that are not picked up on serum PTH assays, except with ovarian cancer, which may produce normal PTH.
4. Serum phosphorus level is low in primary hyperparathyroidism and high in secondary hyperparathyroidism.
5. Chloride is high secondary to renal HCO_3 wasting (direct effect of PTH).
a. Chloride-to-phosphorus ratio of >33 is diagnostic of primary hyperparathyroidism.
b. "Poor man's" PTH assay
6. Only 20% of hypercalcemia is caused by hyperparathyroidism.
7. Other causes of hypercalcemia must be ruled out (Table 27-1)

TABLE 27-1

CAUSES OF HYPERCALCEMIA

Cause	Specific Type
Malignancy (>50% of hypercalcemia)	Hematologic, lung, bone, breast, lymphoma, pancreas, ovary, prostate
Other endocrine disorders	Hyperthyroidism, adrenal insufficiency, pheochromocytoma
Vitamin D toxicity	—
Granulomatous disease	Sarcoidosis, histoplasmosis, leprosy, tuberculosis, coccidioidomycosis
Drugs	Thiazides, milk-alkali syndrome, lithium
Immobilization	—

F. RADIOGRAPHIC EXAM

Radiographic examination may show subperiosteal resorption in the classic distribution on the radial aspect of the second and third phalanges, distal phalangeal tufts, and distal clavicles.

1. Solitary bone cysts (brown tumors)
2. IV pyelogram may show urolithiasis or nephrocalcinosis.

G. MEDICAL TREATMENT OF HYPERCALCEMIC CRISIS

1. Symptoms include anorexia, nausea, vomiting, polyuria, polydipsia, abdominal pain, lethargy, bone pain, and muscular weakness.
2. If untreated, hypercalcemia may progress to dehydration, oliguria, acute tubular necrosis, and delirium within hours.
3. Rapid rehydration with normal saline to restore urine output is required.
4. Following rehydration, begin forced diuresis with furosemide drip (10-20 mg/h).
5. Steroids may be useful in a hypercalcemic crisis due to malignancy.
6. Etidronate disodium 7.5 mg/kg IV daily for 3 days followed by 5-20 mg/kg PO daily inhibits bone metabolism in hypercalcemia of malignancy. This should not be used in patients with renal failure.
7. Mithramycin (25 μg/kg over 4 hours IV piggyback) may be used as a last resort. If not used properly, this drug can lead to aplastic anemia.
8. Dialysis can be used to lower serum calcium emergently.
9. Surgery is treatment for the hypercalcemia of hyperparathyroidism, but only after hydration with adequate urine output is established.

H. SURGICAL INDICATIONS

1. Parathyroid carcinoma
2. Asymptomatic patients
a. Persistent calcium elevation of 1-1.6 mg/dL above normal
b. Calciuria >400 mg/24 h
c. Decreased bone density >2 SDs

d. Creatinine clearance decreased by 30% below normal without other causes
e. Age <50 years
3. Symptomatic patients
a. Urolithiasis or nephrocalcinosis
b. Peptic ulcer disease
c. Musculoskeletal symptoms
d. Pancreatitis

I. SURGICAL MANAGEMENT
1. With single adenoma, resection is curative.
2. For hyperplasia, $3^1/_2$-gland resection or 4-gland resection with $1/_2$ gland reimplanted in the forearm or sternocleidomastoid muscle is indicated.
3. For parathyroid carcinoma, wide excision including the involved structures is indicated.
4. Initial exploration is successful in 90-95% of cases without preoperative localization studies.
5. Ectopic locations
a. Thymic, substernal—20%
b. Posterior neck—5-10%
c. Intrathyroid—5%
d. Carotid sheath—1%
e. Anterior mediastinum—1-2%
6. If initial exploration fails, localization studies are indicated.
a. Ultrasound—80% accuracy for glands as small as 3 mm; does not detect mediastinal tumors
b. CT scan/MRI—Detects mediastinal tumors >2 cm
c. Thallium-technetium subtraction scan—80% accuracy
d. Arteriography—50% accuracy
e. Selective venous sampling for PTH—70% accuracy

J. POSTOPERATIVE CARE
1. Tracheostomy tray to bedside in case of hematoma causing airway compromise
2. Recurrent laryngeal nerve palsy 1-3%—only 10% of these are permanent
3. Hypocalcemia is common and occurs almost immediately.
a. Determine serum calcium in postanesthesia care unit, then q 8 h × 24 hours, then q AM.
b. Symptoms—Anxiety, hyperventilation, Chvostek's and Trousseau's signs, acral and circumoral paresthesias
c. Some advocate treating only symptomatic hypocalcemia.
d. Treat hypocalcemia with calcium carbonate 1 g PO q 6 h, or with IV calcium gluconate for severe hypocalcemia (<7.0).
e. Vitamin D supplementation may be necessary for refractory hypocalcemia.

III. SECONDARY HYPERPARATHYROIDISM

A. GENERAL
1. Hyperparathyroidism secondary to malfunction of another organ system
2. Usually occurs in patients with chronic renal failure, but may also be due to osteogenesis imperfecta, Paget's disease, or multiple myeloma
a. Pathophysiology in renal failure is increased phosphate because of poor renal excretion leading to decreased serum calcium, decreased gut absorption of calcium due to decreased renal hydroxylation of vitamin D_2, and decreased renal clearance of PTH breakdown products.
b. Clinically manifests as psychiatric disorders, headache, muscle weakness, weight loss, fatigue, renal osteodystrophy (bone resorption with pathologic fractures) and soft tissue calcifications (vessels, tendons, joint sheaths)

B. TREATMENT
1. Medical treatment is directed at the underlying disorder— Phosphate-binding antacids, oral calcium and vitamin D, increased calcium dialysate for chronic renal insufficiency patients
2. Surgery is indicated for uncontrolled symptoms—Either $3^1/_2$-gland parathyroidectomy or 4-gland parathyroidectomy with implantation of minced glands into sternocleidomastoid or forearm muscles marked by a surgical clip

IV. TERTIARY HYPERPARATHYROIDISM

A. GENERAL
1. Persistent hyperparathyroidism and hypercalcemia following successful renal transplant or resolution of underlying disorder
2. Occurs in up to 30% of patients who have pretransplant hyperparathyroidism
3. Pathophysiology is irreversible parathyroid gland hyperplasia with autonomous PTH production.

B. TREATMENT
Surgery is indicated for symptomatic patients or patients unresponsive to medical management 6 months after transplant—either $3^1/_2$-gland or 4-gland parathyroidectomy with implantation of minced glands into muscle.

RECOMMENDED READINGS

Cheung PSY, Borgstrom A, Thompson NW: Strategy in reoperative surgery for hyperparathyroidism. Arch Surg 124:676, 1989.
Udelsman R, Donovan PI, Sokoll LJ: One hundred consecutive minimally invasive parathyroid explorations. Ann Surg 232:331, 2000.

27

PARATHYROID

The Adrenal Gland

Philip K. Frykman, MD, PhD

I. EMBRYOLOGY

A. CORTEX
1. Derived from mesoderm of the urogenital ridge
2. During fetal development, the cortex has a thick inner "fetal zone" and a thin outer neocortex. During development, the inner zone produces steroids that are converted into estrogens by the placenta.
3. At midgestation, the adrenal is larger than the kidney.
4. The inner zone involutes shortly after birth and only the outer cortex persists.

28

B. MEDULLA (ECTODERM)
1. At the 20th week of gestation, cells from the neural crest invade the cortex to form the medulla.
2. Neuroblasts also arrive and form sympathetic ganglia.

II. ANATOMY

A. GENERAL
1. Inner medulla surrounded by outer cortex
2. Cortex is divided into three layers, with each producing different hormones.
a. Zona glomerulosa—Aldosterone
b. Zona fasciculata—Androgens, cortisol
c. Zona reticularis—Estrogens, androgens, cortisol

B. VASCULAR SUPPLY
1. Arterial supply—Inferior phrenic, renal, and aorta
2. Venous drainage is the inferior vena cava on the right and the renal vein on the left.

III. PHYSIOLOGY

A. HYPOTHALAMIC-PITUITARY-ADRENAL AXIS
1. Corticotropin-releasing hormone (CRH) is released from the anterior hypothalamus, which stimulates the anterior pituitary gland to secrete adrenocorticotropic hormone (ACTH).
2. ACTH stimulates the adrenal gland to secrete cortisol and mineralocorticoids.

B. ADRENAL CORTEX GLAND
1. The adrenal cortex gland makes three classes of hormones: glucocorticoids, mineralocorticoids, and androgens.

2. All cortical hormones are derived from cholesterol.
3. Hormones circulate in bound and unbound forms.
4. Free steroid hormones enter the cytosol and bind with receptors, and then the complex enters the nucleus to bind to DNA and activate messenger RNA synthesis.

C. CORTISOL
1. 75% bound to transcortin (increases with pregnancy or exogenous estrogens), 15% bound to albumin, 10% unbound (active form)
2. Circadian rhythm—highest in AM, lowest in PM
3. Metabolized by the liver (90-minute half-life)
4. Metabolites, 17-hydroxy/ketosteroids, cleared by kidneys
5. Effects of cortisol
  a. Increased gluconeogenesis, proteolysis, lipolysis
  b. Increased free fatty acids, triglycerides
  c. Increased glycogen deposition in the liver
  d. Decreased glucose uptake peripherally
  e. Anabolic in the liver, catabolic peripherally
  f. Immunosuppressant
  g. Anti-inflammatory (stabilizes lysosomal membranes)
  h. Decreased wound healing
  i. Increased bone reabsorption

D. ADRENAL SEX STEROIDS
1. Androgens from the adrenal guide fetal development of the external genitalia, vas deferens, prostate, and epididymis (Wolffian system).
2. Postnatally, androgens stimulate deepening of the voice, phallus growth, and development of skeletal muscle and body hair.
3. Estrogen from the adrenal in females stimulates breast and vaginal development.

E. MINERALOCORTICOID—ALDOSTERONE
1. From the zona glomerulosa
2. Degraded by the liver (15-minute half-life)
3. Secretion from the adrenal is stimulated by angiotensin II and K^+ increase.
4. Aldosterone acts on the distal renal tubule to increase Na^+ reabsorption with loss of K^+ and H^+ (sodium-potassium pump).

F. PHYSIOLOGY OF THE ADRENAL MEDULLA
1. Tyrosine is converted into L-dopa, then dopamine, then norepinephrine, then epinephrine.
  a. 80% of catecholamines are stored as epinephrine, 20% as norepinephrine
  b. Release is under sympathetic control. The medulla receives preganglionic sympathetic innervation from the splanchnic plexus.

c. Activity of catecholamines
    (1) Increase glycogenolysis
    (2) Increase gluconeogenesis
    (3) Increase glucagon secretion
    (4) Decrease glucose uptake
2. The medulla receives blood rich in glucocorticoids from the cortex, which influences catecholamine secretion.
3. Catecholamines act locally and systemically on α and β receptors
4. Catecholamines are cleared by the urine, by peripheral enzymatic degradation, and by uptake at nerve endings.
a. The monoamine oxidase system of the liver, kidney, intestine, and stomach clears norepinephrine.
b. Metabolites of catecholamines—Normetanephrine, metanephrine, vanillylmandelic acid (VMA), and methoxyhydroxyphenylglycol

IV. DISEASES OF THE ADRENAL CORTEX

A. CUSHING'S SYNDROME
1. Described in 1932 by Harvey Cushing
2. Hypercortisolism can result either from overproduction of cortisol autonomously from the adrenal or secondarily from ACTH overproduction from either the pituitary or an ectopic site.
3. Affects women nine times as often as men
4. Symptoms—Centripetal obesity, moon facies, buffalo hump, acne, purple striae, hirsutism, weakness, menstrual irregularity, increased blood pressure, glucose intolerance, pancreatitis, peptic ulcer disease
5. Etiologies of hypercortisolism
a. Pituitary—Hypercortisolism from a pituitary adenoma with increased secretion of ACTH is called *Cushing's disease*. This is the most common cause of hypercortisolism (60-70%).
b. Adrenocortical—Adrenal adenomas cause 10-20% of Cushing's syndrome. Of these cases, 10% are bilateral.
c. Ectopic ACTH production—10-15% of hypercortisolism originates from ectopic ACTH production. These patients do not appear cushingoid. They are cachectic from their underlying cancer. Etiologies are the following.
    (1) Lung (small cell), 50%
    (2) Pancreatic
    (3) Thymoma
    (4) Bronchial carcinoid tumors
d. Diagnosis is based on very high ACTH levels as well as increased cortisol and 17-ketosteroid levels.
e. Adrenocortical carcinoma—Rare cause of Cushing's syndrome. Aggressive tumor with poor prognosis. Most are secretory (60%), and many are palpable at presentation (50%).

28

THE ADRENAL GLAND

6. Diagnosis

a. Cortisol levels—Serum increased in 80%

b. The best screening test is measurement of 24-hour urinary free cortisol level.

c. Low-dose dexamethasone suppression test—Dexamethasone is a stronger suppressant of ACTH secretion than cortisol is. A 2-mg dose given the night before suppresses morning urinary cortisol level in normal individuals but not those with hypercortisolism.

d. Tests to localize the cause

(1) ACTH—Elevated in pituitary disease, very elevated when from an ectopic site, and low in adrenal disease

(2) High-dose dexamethasone suppression—8 mg given over 24 hours. Suppresses urinary levels of free cortisol to <50% of baseline levels in patients with pituitary adenomas only. Urinary free cortisol levels are not suppressed in patients with ectopic ACTH production or adrenal adenoma. ≈95% accurate.

(3) Metyrapone stimulation test—Inhibits the enzymatic production of cortisol, causing increase in ACTH and urinary excretion of cortisol precursors in normal individuals. In hypercortisolism from a pituitary adenoma, ACTH as well as cortisol precursors increases. In hypercortisolism from primary adrenal source, no change in precursors is noted.

(4) CRH—Administration of CRH to normal patients should cause a slight increase in cortisol levels. With Cushing's disease, cortisol levels are markedly increased. With ectopic ACTH secretion or adrenal adenomas, there is no change in cortisol levels.

7. Treatment

a. Pituitary—Trans-sphenoidal hypophysectomy for tumors <1 cm allows pituitary function to be preserved in many cases. Transfrontal resection for tumors extending outside the sella turcica. Radiation is used if the tumor is unresectable. Bilateral adrenalectomy is used in the past for unresectable disease. Pharmacologic therapy occasionally is used preoperatively or early postoperatively to control cortisol levels.

b. Adrenal—Adrenalectomy is curative for adrenal adenomas. Posterior approach is associated with decreased morbidity. If cancer is suspected, an anterior approach is indicated. Must guard against possible stress-induced adrenal insufficiency with perioperatively dosed hydrocortisone IV. Contralateral adrenal function may take weeks to recover. For bilateral adrenal hyperplasia, bilateral adrenalectomy is indicated.

8. Cushing's syndrome in children

a. Most common cause is a neoplasia, the majority being malignant

b. Affects females more than males (3:1).

c. Cushing's disease and ectopic ACTH production are rare in children.

9. Nelson's syndrome—Complication found in 10% of patients after bilateral adrenalectomy. ACTH and melanocyte-stimulating hormone (MSH) levels are increased, causing an increase in skin pigmentation.

B. CONN'S SYNDROME (LOW-RENIN HYPERALDOSTERONISM)

1. Surgical cause of hypertension, though hypertension is not as severe as seen in renovascular hypertension
2. Diagnosis
   a. Suggested by diastolic hypertension, hypokalemia, metabolic alkalosis (40% of hypertensive patients with hypokalemia have Conn's syndrome). Confounding factor in the diagnosis is diuretic use for the treatment of hypertension.
   b. Serum renin and aldosterone levels (to distinguish from renovascular hypertension)
   c. 24-Hour urine collection for aldosterone while off potassium-sparing diuretics (spironolactone) >24 hours
   d. Sometimes a high-sodium diet or an IV infusion of Na^+ is used to further elevate the aldosterone level to make the diagnosis (95% sensitivity).
3. Differential diagnosis of decreased renin, increased aldosterone
   a. Adrenocortical adenoma
   b. Bilateral adrenal hyperplasia
   c. Adrenal carcinoma
   d. Aldosterone-secreting ovarian tumor
4. 80% are single adrenal adenomas, whereas 15% are bilateral adrenal hyperplasia. These must be distinguished because only 20% of patients with hyperplasia are cured surgically. CT/MRI can distinguish bilateral/unilateral disease. ^{131}I-iodocholesterol uptake scans can be performed in cases of equivocal localization.
5. Confirmatory test is a captopril challenge.
   a. Essential hypertension—Captopril decreases the plasma levels of aldosterone and increases renin.
   b. Conn's syndrome—Administration of captopril does not change levels of aldosterone and renin.
   c. Postcaptopril aldosterone level >15 ng/dL *and* aldosterone-to-renin ratio >50 is diagnostic.
6. Management
   a. Nonoperative therapy—Spironolactone opposes the action of aldosterone; can cause gynecomastia and hyperkalemia; treatment of choice for bilateral adrenal hyperplasia
   b. For adenomas, unilateral adrenalectomy with a posterior approach is curative in 90% of patients.

C. ADRENOGENITAL SYNDROMES

1. Definition—Syndrome of salt wasting and ambiguous genitalia arising from enzymatic deficiencies of cortisol synthesis
   a. Low cortisol level allows ACTH levels to rise, stimulating the adrenal gland to produce more cortisol precursors
   b. Androgens cause virilization (increased phallus size, muscle mass, body hair) in males, usually presenting at puberty. Males can present in infancy with salt wasting and hypertension.

c. Females present at birth with ambiguous genitalia (fused labia, enlarged clitoris) but normal internal reproductive organs.

d. When children present later, they often have an early period of rapid growth followed by premature closure of growth plates (short stature).

2. 21-Hydroxylase deficiency

a. Most common enzymatic deficiency in these patients (94%)

b. Common in Inuits

c. Presentation—Virilizing in females, precocious sexual development in males. A complete lack of the enzyme presents with salt wasting (40%).

d. Diagnosed by low cortisol levels and increased 17-hydroxyprogesterone

e. Treatment—Aldosterone and cortisol replacement

3. 11-Hydroxylase deficiency

a. 5% of individuals with adrenogenital syndrome

b. Present with hyperpigmentation, virilization, hypertension, and low cortisol

D. ADRENAL NEOPLASMS ASSOCIATED WITH INCREASED SEX STEROIDS

1. Virilizing tumors

a. Females more often affected than males (2:1)

b. Usually present after the first year of life as clitoral enlargement, increased pubic hair in girls, enlarged phallus, hirsutism in males

c. Tumors secrete androgen precursors.

d. These slow-growing tumors must be excised, because they are not suppressed by dexamethasone.

2. Feminizing adrenal tumors

a. Rare tumors that present with bilateral gynecomastia, rapid growth, and increased bone age in young males (20-40 years)

b. Diagnosed by increased 17-ketosteroids, estrogens

c. Women present with precocious puberty and an abdominal mass.

d. Half are benign.

E. ADRENOCORTICAL INSUFFICIENCY (ADDISON'S DISEASE)

1. Bilateral adrenocortical destruction

a. Chronic steroid use with suppression of the adrenal gland is the most common etiology.

b. Most common noniatrogenic etiology—Idiopathic; presumed to be autoimmune mediated (associated with hyperthyroidism, diabetes mellitus)

c. Females more often affected than males (2:1)

d. Tuberculosis found in 20% of patients

e. Metastatic carcinomas (lung) can also cause Addison's disease

2. Clinical presentation

a. Fatigue, weight loss, anorexia, nausea/emesis, abdominal pain, diarrhea, hyperpigmentation

b. Decreased Na^+, increased K^+, azotemia, hypoglycemia, increased calcium

3. Diagnosis

a. Can present in addisonian crisis with fever, abdominal pain, hypotension, vomiting, lethargy

b. Can occur after stopping steroids, stress, infection, hemorrhage, Waterhouse-Friderichsen syndrome

c. Cortisol levels low

4. Treated acutely with 100 mg hydrocortisone, normal saline, then chronic steroid replacement

F. ADRENOCORTICAL CARCINOMA

1. Rare tumor with very poor prognosis

2. Affects males and females equally, usually in 40s

3. Most (75%) are functional

4. Presentation—Abdominal pain, mass, anemia, fever, virilization, feminization

5. Diagnosis

a. Assess if functional—Urine cortisol, serum ACTH, low-dose dexamethasone test

b. Most are >5 cm, seen on CT scan

c. T2-weighted MRI images can distinguish carcinoma from adenomas.

d. Chest radiograph, CT scan of the liver to rule out metastatic disease

e. Malignant vs. benign—Histologically can be difficult to determine. Characterization based on radiographic findings: if >6 cm, metastatic, and locally invasive, then likely malignant.

6. Treatment

a. 60% are metastatic at diagnosis.

b. En bloc resection (often includes nephrectomy)

c. Nonsurgical

(1) Most patients benefit from debulking.

(2) Mitotane improves symptoms but has many side effects and often requires steroid replacement.

(3) Radiation and chemotherapy have no proven roles.

7. Results—25%, 5-year survival; 40% if localized disease

V. PHEOCHROMOCYTOMA

A. GENERAL

1. Clinically presents with hypertension, headaches, palpitations

2. Equally affects males, females, aged 20-50 years

3. Hypertension (50-70%) usually sustained. Episodes can be elicited by physical exertion and emotional stress and can last 15-30 minutes.

4. Episodes also associated with consumption of foods rich in tyramine, e.g., beer, wine, and cheese.

5. Nonfunctioning tumors are rare.

6. 10-20% of pheochromocytomas are the following.

a. Malignant

b. Extra-adrenal in location
c. Multiple
d. Associated with other conditions—Multiple endocrine neoplasia (MEN) type 2, neurofibromatosis 1
e. In children

7. Associated conditions

a. MEN 2a—Medullary carcinoma of the thyroid, parathyroid hyperplasia, pheochromocytoma. Autosomal dominant, with all affected individuals developing medullary thyroid carcinoma (MTC). 50% develop parathyroid hyperplasia or pheochromocytomas.
b. MEN 2b—MTC, pheochromocytomas, mucosal neuromas, ganglioneuromatosis; rare syndromes, autosomal dominant or sporadic
c. Neurocutaneous disorders—5-10% of patients with pheochromocytomas have neurofibromatosis; also associated with tuberous sclerosis, Sturge-Weber syndrome, and von Hippel-Lindau syndrome

8. Pheochromocytoma in pregnancy

a. Associated with a 50% fetal mortality
b. If condition unknown, 60% maternal mortality; if known, 18% mortality
c. Can cause hypertensive crisis up to 48 hours postpartum
d. Can be excised if diagnosed before third trimester or α blockade can be initiated and the child carried to term
e. Child should be delivered by cesarean section and the tumor excised immediately

9. Pheochromocytoma in childhood

a. Males most commonly affected
b. 10% of pheochromocytomas in individuals <20 years of age
c. 40% bilateral, and more often extra-adrenal
d. Presents with sweating, hypertension, polyuria, polydipsia

10. Malignant pheochromocytomas

a. 10-40% are malignant
b. Females affected more than males (3:1)
c. Hypertension, symptoms more consistent if malignant
d. Associated with extra-adrenal pheochromocytomas
e. Associated with increased dopamine levels
f. Malignancy determined by demonstration of metastases or local invasion since difficult to determine histologically
g. Cytoreduction either by debulking or preferably by resection

11. Extra-adrenal pheochromocytomas

a. 90% of pheochromocytomas are found in the adrenal, 98% are within the abdomen
b. Other locations—Bladder, organ of Zuckerkandl (anterior aorta, near inferior mesenteric artery), carotid body, or sympathetic ganglia
c. Organ of Zuckerkandl most common site; difficult to excise from anterior border of aorta; suspect if only norepinephrine is elevated.

B. CLINICAL PRESENTATION

1. Hypertension (usually sustained, but can be episodic), headache, sweating, palpitations, chest pain, anxiety, fever, abdominal pain
2. Suspect in cases of refractory hypertension, hypertension in children or pregnancy

C. DIAGNOSIS

1. The best screen study is a 24-hour urine collection for catecholamines, metanephrines, and VMA levels. A 24-hour VMA level is 97% sensitive and 91% specific for pheochromocytoma.
2. Catecholamines can also be elevated in essential hypertension.
3. Stimulation tests
   a. Glucagon—Used if blood pressure is normal. When used for this indication, it has few side effects. A threefold increase of catecholamines is diagnostic.
   b. Clonidine suppression test—Central α agonist that decreases catecholamine release. In patients with pheochromocytomas, catecholamine levels are unchanged.
4. Localization
   a. CT scan readily detects tumors >1 cm with 87-100% sensitivity.
   b. MRI—Especially with T2-weighted images, can better distinguish anatomic extension; also can distinguish medullary and cortical neoplasms, as well as malignancy from benign processes (adenoma)
   c. MIBG scan—MIBG (metaiodobenzylguanidine) is a norepinephrine analog that accumulates in chromaffin cells and shows rapid uptake in pheochromocytomas. In multi-institutional studies, the sensitivity is 77-87% and specificity is 96-100%. This is an excellent study for diagnosing extra-adrenal pheochromocytoma.

D. SURGICAL TREATMENT

1. Preoperative preparation
   a. α Blockade (phenoxybenzamine, phentolamine, metyrosine) should be started 2 weeks before surgery to control hypertension and restore the blood volume.
   b. β Blockade—May begin only after α blockade; β blockade alone can worsen congestive heart failure and hypertension by blocking epinephrine-induced vasodilation; only used if patient is hypertensive
   c. Selective α_1 antagonists terazosin and doxazosin in combination with nifedipine and nicardipine have been as effective at blood pressure control as phenoxybenzamine.
   d. With α blockade, will reduce hypertension intraoperative with manipulation of the pheochromocytoma
   e. Without α blockade, increased risk of postoperative hypotension
2. Anesthesia management
   a. Reverse Trendelenburg can increase venous capacitance.

b. Nipride or phentolamine (short-acting α blocker) for intraoperative blood pressure control. Norepinephrine may be necessary postoperatively for hypotension.

c. Lidocaine is often necessary to control catecholamine-induced arrhythmias.

d. Arterial line, central venous pressure, Foley catheter for monitoring

e. Halothane is associated with less cardiac stimulation.

f. Sedate preoperatively.

3. Technical aspects

a. Anterior approach used because of risk of multiple primary tumors, bilateral disease, malignancy, and ectopic location

b. Laparoscopic approach can be used in experienced hands.

c. Remove with capsule intact to decrease risk of recurrence.

d. Manipulate as little as possible.

e. Identify and ligate veins early to prevent hypertensive episodes.

E. PROGNOSIS

1. Normal life expectancy

2. 10-30% recur

F. PARAGANGLIOMA

1. Nonfunctional medullary neoplasm

2. Presents as an abdominal mass

3. First, rule out functional mass, then excise

4. 50% have recurrence or metastatic disease

5. 75% 5-year survival

VI. METASTATIC DISEASE TO THE ADRENAL

A. GENERAL

1. Most frequent site of metastatic disease (by weight)

2. Most common—Breast, lung, kidney, pancreas

3. Can cause Addison's disease, though masked by other symptoms of end-stage cancer

4. 40% bilateral

5. Best diagnosed by CT; can be resected in certain circumstances

VII. ADRENAL IMAGING

A. NONINVASIVE TECHNIQUES

1. Ultrasonography—Must be 2-3 cm to visualize

2. CT scan—Effective in imaging masses ≥ 1 cm

3. MRI—Allows imaging without radiation or IV contrast exposure, T2-weighted images with similar sensitivity to CT

4. Radionuclide imaging—MIBG (^{131}I-metaiodobenzylguanidine) scintigraphy can effectively demonstrate intra-abdominal and

extra-abdominal pheochromocytomas; can also be used therapeutically in cases of unresectable tumors

VIII. INCIDENTAL ADRENAL MASSES

A. GENERAL
1. Frequency—0.6% of abdominal CTs
2. With history of carcinoma, must rule out metastatic disease
3. Most incidental masses are benign cortical adenomas.
4. Check functional status by history, physical exam, serum potassium, 24-hour urine collection for free cortisol, VMA, metanephrines, catecholamines

B. DIAGNOSIS AND TREATMENT
1. Fine-needle aspiration may be indicated in cases of suspected metastatic disease, once a pheochromocytoma has been ruled out biochemically.
2. MRI, with T2-weighted images, can give additional information.
3. If mass >5 cm, check functional status, then excise.
4. If mass <3.5 cm and nonfunctional, follow with CTs at 6 months.
5. If functional tumor, then treatment is excision
6. 3.5-5.0 cm—Debatable

28

THE ADRENAL GLAND

RECOMMENDED READINGS

Brunt LM, Halverson JD: The endocrine system. In O'Leary JP (ed):
    The Physiologic Basis of Surgery, 2nd ed. Baltimore, Williams & Wilkins,
    1996, pp 331-340.
Gagner M, Pomp A, Heniford BT, et al: Laparoscopic adrenalectomy:
    Lessons learned from 100 consecutive cases. Ann Surg 226:238, 1997.
Perry RR, Nieman LK, Cutler GB Jr, et al: Primary adrenal causes of
    Cushing's syndrome: Diagnosis and surgical management. Ann Surg
    210:59, 1989.
Ross NS, Aron DC: Evaluation of the patient with an incidentally
    discovered adrenal mass. N Engl J Med 323:1401, 1990.

Neuroendocrine Tumors

Amod A. Sarnaik, MD

I. APUD (amine *p*recursor *u*ptake and *d*ecarboxylation) CELL

A. DEFINITION
1. A group of cells (presumed endodermal origin) that share similar histologic and functional features
2. Most notably, they are capable of producing >40 distinct, hormonally active polypeptides.

B. CHARACTERISTICS
1. Found in the GI system, thyroid, parathyroid, adrenal medulla, carotid body, lung, and neural cells
2. Neoplastic transformation, termed *apudomas*, can result in autonomous overproduction of hormonally active polypeptides that result in symptoms.
3. All tumors may potentially be multihormonal, with predominant symptoms related to the most biochemically potent product.

II. CARCINOID TUMORS (Table 29-1)

A. GENERAL
1. Most common GI apudoma and most common tumor of small bowel
2. All potentially malignant tumors typically arising from enterochromaffin (Kulchitsky) cells found in the crypts of Lieberkühn

B. ORIGIN
1. Can originate from foregut (including bronchial tree, pancreas, gallbladder), midgut (jejunum, ileum, appendix, proximal colon), or hindgut (distal colon, rectum)
2. Bronchial and metastatic small bowel carcinoids most likely to cause carcinoid syndrome
3. Appendix—Most common site (41%), followed by small bowel (20%), rectum (16%) (overall 85-90% in the GI tract); lungs (10%); larynx, thymus, kidney, ovary, prostate, skin (5%)
4. Except for appendiceal and rectal carcinoid, lesions tend to be multifocal.
5. Survival depends on mitotic rate and the presence or absence of metastases.

C. HORMONE PRODUCTION
1. Serotonin predominates; may also produce kallikrein, substance P, many others
2. Hindgut tumors produce hormones that do not typically cause symptoms (e.g., human chorionic gonadotropin [HCG]).

TABLE 29-1

CHARACTERISTICS OF NEUROENDOCRINE TUMORS

Tumor	Site	Predominant Hormone(s)	Symptoms
Carcinoid	Appendix, ileum Other GI sites, bronchial tree Multifocal	Bradykinin, serotonin	Flushing, diarrhea, cramping, right-sided heart failure
Gastrinoma	Pancreas, duodenum Ectopic	Gastrin	Severe peptic ulcer disease, diarrhea, abdominal pain
Insulinoma	Pancreas (β cell)	Insulin	Symptoms of hypoglycemia often misdiagnosed as neurologic or psychiatric problem
Glucagonoma	Pancreas (α cell) (50% in tail)	Glucagon	Migratory necrolytic erythema, anemia, mild diabetes, cachexia, thrombosis
VIPoma	Pancreas (D cell), (80% body/tail) 10-20% extrapancreatic	Vasoactive intestinal polypeptide	WDHA (watery diarrhea, hypokalemia, achlorhydria) syndrome
Somatostatinoma	Pancreas (D cell)	Somatostatin	Mild diabetes, steatorrhea, indigestion, often asymptomatic and found incidentally

3. Hormones may be inactivated by the liver prior to entering systemic circulation.

D. SYMPTOMS

1. 40-60% of patients are asymptomatic and are diagnosed incidentally. Symptoms, when present, are dependent on site of involvement.
2. Midgut—Abdominal pain/mechanical bowel obstruction due to tumor or secondary desmoplastic reaction
3. Foregut—Hematemesis/hemoptysis, anemia, recurrent respiratory infection
4. Hindgut—Hematochezia, distal bowel obstruction
5. Metastatic—Carcinoid syndrome that requires elaboration of active hormone by tumor *outside* the portal venous drainage
6. Most common symptoms of carcinoid syndrome and probable cause
   a. Flushing (94%)—Kallikrein (bradykinin)
   b. Diarrhea (78%)—Serotonin
   c. Cramping (51%)—Serotonin
   d. Fibrotic right-sided valvular heart lesions (50%)—Serotonin (pathogenesis remains unknown)
   e. Pellagra (5%)—Depletion of niacin stores due to overproduction of serotonin
7. Other symptoms can include telangiectases, bronchoconstriction, and facial edema.

E. DIAGNOSIS

1. Most are found at autopsy or during surgery for intestinal obstruction or appendectomy; preoperative search unusual, but angiography, endoscopy, barium studies, and CT scan all can be useful; bronchial lesions diagnosed by chest radiograph and/or bronchoscopy
2. 5-Hydroxyindoleacetic acid (HIAA) levels >10 mg in 24-hour urine is diagnostic of hormonally active extraportal tumor; 80% sensitive and 99% specific if the patient is not on phenothiazines (results in false negative); test also requires that patient not eat serotonin-containing foods (e.g., pineapple, chocolate, bananas, walnuts, avocados)
3. Bronchial carcinoids may cause elevated 5-hydroxytryptophan (HTP) levels with normal 5-HIAA values.
4. Octreotide scintigraphy—Identifies hormonally active primary tumors and metastases

F. SURGICAL TREATMENT

Surgical resection is the most likely chance for cure. *Always* consider lesions to be malignant.

1. Appendiceal carcinoid <1.5 cm—Simple appendectomy
2. Appendiceal carcinoid >1.5 cm, located at base of cecum, serosal with invasion, or local nodal disease—Right hemicolectomy

29

NEUROENDOCRINE TUMORS

3. Treatment of small bowel carcinoids—Wide resection including mesenteric nodes. There is a high incidence of other primary tumors.

4. Rectal carcinoids—Locally excised unless >2 cm, locally invasive, or associated with nodal disease, in which case abdominoperineal resection is recommended, or low anterior resection if possible.

5. Often multifocal, thus careful exploration is necessary; all gross disease should be resected to reduce hormone production.

6. Gastric/duodenal carcinoids <2 cm—Local/endoscopic excision; >2 cm—partial or total gastrectomy with regional node excision

7. Hepatic metastases may be resected to provide palliation of symptoms.

8. Bronchial carcinoids are resected as indicated based on location.

9. If preoperative diagnosis is made (e.g., carcinoid syndrome), the patient should be prepared for surgery with hydration, serotonin antagonists, and possibly β- and/or α-adrenergic blockers to avoid extreme response to tumor manipulation (see Chap. 28 section VI).

G. MEDICAL TREATMENT

1. Antihormonal measures—Octreotide is the sole agent demonstrated to alleviate carcinoid syndrome. By blocking serotonin receptors, symptoms from diarrhea and flushing are ameliorated. May be given preoperatively to reduce risk of intraoperative carcinoid crisis.

2. Some reports of long-term remission with hepatic artery embolization for liver metastases

3. Chemotherapy (5-fluorouracil [5-FU], streptozocin, doxorubicin, interferon α)—Confers variable results in small studies; most patients respond poorly.

H. PROGNOSIS (5-YEAR SURVIVAL)

1. Overall—65-80%
2. Localized disease—up to 95%
3. Regional nodal disease—≈65%
4. Distant metastases—20%
5. Appendix highest survival (99%); lungs and bronchi next (96% local disease, 87% all stages)

III. GASTRINOMA (ZOLLINGER-ELLISON SYNDROME) (see Table 29-1)

A. GENERAL

1. 85% are located in the gastrinoma triangle (Fig. 29-1); 15-20% duodenal or ectopic (splenic hilum, gastric wall, mesentery, liver)

2. >50% are malignant, and due to delay in diagnosis, >50% of those are metastatic at time of presentation.

3. Common sites of metastasis include lymph nodes, liver, spleen, peritoneum, and mediastinum. Very slow-growing tumors; prolonged

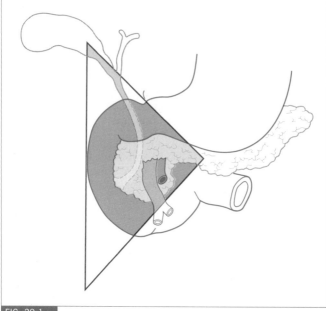

FIG. 29-1

The gastrinoma triangle.

survival if ulcers are controlled. Of patients with peptic ulcer disease, 0.1-1% have a gastrinoma.
4. Duodenal tumors are usually solitary, and 75% are benign; benign tumors elsewhere tend to be multifocal, with the head of the pancreas most common.

B. CLINICAL PRESENTATION
Gastrinoma is severe peptic ulcer disease with atypical location of multiple ulcers, often resistant to medical therapy. Associated complications (bleeding, perforation, outlet obstruction) are common.
1. Diarrhea—May be the only symptom in up to 40% of patients. Diarrhea results from acid secretion, inactivated enzymes, and gastrin-stimulated increased motility.
2. Epigastric pain—Present in >90% of patients; may become malnourished/dehydrated
3. Reflux—90% have ulceration, with the proximal duodenum most commonly involved.
4. Associated with parathyroid and pituitary tumors (multiple endocrine neoplasia [MEN] type 1) in 25% of patients

C. DIAGNOSIS

Diagnosis is determined by an elevated fasting gastrin level (>500 pg/mL) in a patient with *increased* gastric acid. Differential diagnosis includes gastrinoma, retained antrum, gastric outlet obstruction, renal failure, and short bowel syndrome. If gastric acidity is *decreased*, elevated gastrin is secondary to chronic gastritis, gastric carcinoma, pernicious anemia, vagotomy, H_2 blockers, or omeprazole (Prilosec).

1. If gastrin level >normal (20-150 pg/mL) but <500 pg/mL, need provocative test (off H_2 blockers at least 24-48 hours)
2. Secretin stimulation (positive in >90% of cases; peak usually at 2-5 minutes)—Test of choice
   - Measure serum gastrin, *then*
   - Administer secretin 2 U/kg IV bolus, *then*
   - Administer serum gastrin at 2, 5, 10, 20, 30 minutes after infusion
   Positive test if gastrin increased 100-200 pg/mL above baseline
3. Calcium stimulation (may cause arrhythmias, need to monitor)—80% sensitive, 50% specific
   - Monitor patient
   - Ca^{2+} gluconate 5 mg/kg/h infusion × 3 hours
   - Serum gastrin every 30 minutes
   Positive test is 300-400 pg/mL rise above baseline
4. Acid output measurement
   a. Basal acid output (BAO) >15 mEq/h or >100 mmol HCl/12 h suggests gastrinoma.
   b. Maximal acid output (MAO) with pentagastrin stimulation shows minimal increase over BAO with gastrinoma. BAO/MAO ratio is usually >0.6 with gastrinoma. Parietal cells are already maximally stimulated endogenously.
   c. Acid outputs less accurate than secretin stimulation test
5. Gastrin levels >5000 pg/mL, or presence of β-HCG in serum suggests metastatic disease.
6. Always check serum Ca^{2+} to screen for MEN 1.

D. LOCALIZATION

It is often not possible to identify a gastrinoma preoperatively owing to small size of tumors (<3 cm). Duodenal tumors can sometimes be identified endoscopically. Endoscopic ultrasound may be used to visualize the gastrinoma triangle.

1. Transhepatic portal venous sampling/mapping—Up to 80% success reported but is operator dependent
2. CT scan—20-80% success; various series, most on lower end of range. Angiography, ultrasound <25% successful.
3. Intraoperative ultrasound is successful and when combined with thorough palpation of the pancreas can locate most gastrinomas.
4. Octreotide scintigraphy is 90% sensitive, 100% specific, and less invasive than angiography.

E. TREATMENT

1. High-dose H_2 blockade often controls secretory diarrhea and peptic ulcer disease symptoms, but breakthrough acid secretion can occur with time; some patients never respond.
2. Omeprazole (H^+,K^+ adenosine triphosphatase inhibitor) provides better control of acid secretion at doses up to 60 mg b.i.d.
3. All patients with Zollinger-Ellison syndrome should be explored to attempt curative resection (20% of patients are cured with complete resection).
4. Some authors report good symptomatic results with tumor debulking combined with parietal cell vagotomy and H_2 blockade when the tumor is unresectable.
5. Classic surgical approach in the past was total gastrectomy. This is rarely necessary due to improvement in medical management of acid secretion and earlier diagnosis.

IV. INSULINOMA (see Table 29-1)

A. GENERAL

1. Functional β-cell tumor of pancreatic islet; second most common endocrine tumor of pancreas
2. 10% malignant, 10% multiple, 4-10% associated with MEN 1; multiple lesions associated with MEN 1 >50% of the time
3. Tumors are small (60-70% <1.5 cm), equally distributed through pancreas; up to 90% solitary and benign; usually are resectable
4. Insulin is produced as proinsulin that is cleaved into C-peptide and insulin.

B. CLINICAL

1. Symptoms of hypoglycemia (primarily neurologic) with reactive epinephrine release. Usually brought on by fasting or exercise; often occurs in AM; patients are often obese owing to learned habit of frequent ingestion of sweets to alleviate the symptoms.
2. Hypoglycemic symptoms of diplopia, blurred vision, confused behavior, amnesia, weakness, focal or generalized seizures, paralysis, and coma. Accompanying adrenergic symptoms are sweating, hunger, tremor, palpitations.
3. With repeated attacks, permanent neurologic damage can occur; often initially confused with neuropsychiatric problems; mean of 33 months from onset of symptoms to diagnosis
4. Nesidioblastosis—Diffuse microadenomata of the pancreas seen in neonates causing neonatal hypoglycemia

C. DIAGNOSIS

1. Whipple's triad strongly suggests diagnosis
a. Symptoms of hypoglycemia with fasting

29

NEUROENDOCRINE TUMORS

b. Blood glucose <50 mg/dL at time of symptoms

c. Symptoms relieved by glucose

2. 72-hour fast-test of choice—Measure insulin and glucose levels every 6 hours. Sensitivity is 95% with most developing symptoms of hypoglycemia in <12 hours. Fasting insulin/glucose (I/G) ratio >0.30 or serum insulin level >6 μU/mL is diagnostic.

3. Must rule out factitious hyperinsulinemic hypoglycemia; to exclude a factitious disorder, measure insulin antibodies, urinary sulfonylureas, proinsulin/C-peptide (both *low* with self-administered human insulin).

4. C-peptide suppression test—Used in euglycemic patients and is rarely necessary. Requires administration of *both* insulin and glucose (to maintain euglycemia). Test is positive if C-peptide does not decrease.

5. Provocative tests (tolbutamide, calcium gluconate infusion) are less reliable than 72-hour fast; provocative tests risk severe side effects; not recommended by most authors

6. Malignancy is suggested by very high proinsulin level and/or presence of HCG in serum.

D. LOCALIZATION

Localization is difficult due to small size of the tumors.

1. Endoscopic ultrasound—85% sensitive, 95% specific to evaluate pancreatic disease

2. Angiography with subtraction techniques can be up to 90% successful; shows localized, dense tumor blush on capillary phase; false-positive results can occur (accessory spleens, inflamed lymph nodes); test invasive

3. CT scan/conventional ultrasound in general are <50% successful in localizing these small tumors, but if positive, they save the patient from angiography.

4. Percutaneous transhepatic portal vein sampling (PTPVS)—Has variable but encouraging results when other methods fail; however, PTPVS is invasive, tedious, and expensive and requires a skilled angiographer

5. Intraoperative ultrasound is extremely accurate (and should be available) when combined with intraoperative bimanual pancreatic palpation.

E. TREATMENT

Surgical resection is the goal, with up to 90% cure rate.

1. Preoperative maintenance of glucose levels with frequent meals and/or glucose infusion; frequent intraoperative glucose measurements

2. Mobilize and palpate entire gland, even if single tumor localized preoperatively (Kocher maneuver and mobilization of pancreatic tail and spleen)

3. Enucleate small tumors near surface; pancreatic resection for others, including Whipple's procedure if necessary for tumor located in head;

frozen section to confirm pathology. Enucleation in tail or deep within the head may damage the pancreatic duct.

4. If tumor is not found, intraoperative ultrasound should be performed.

a. Biopsy or resection of pancreatic tail—If frozen section reveals nesidioblastosis (microadenomatosis), 75-80% resection is said to provide best palliation of symptoms with the least morbidity; may require subsequent medical therapy

b. Do not blindly resect the head of the pancreas.

5. Complications of operative resection include postoperative diabetes, abscess, pseudocyst, and postoperative fistula.

6. Metastatic disease should be treated by debulking tumor mass (cytoreduction).

7. Medical treatment—For patients who cannot tolerate general anesthesia, for control of symptoms preoperatively, or to treat metastatic disease

a. Diazoxide—Inhibits insulin release, decreases peripheral glucose utilization; multiple side effects may preclude use (edema, hirsutism, nausea, bone marrow depression, hyperuricemia); diuretic may control edema; must stop 7 days prior to general anesthesia secondary to hypotension at induction

b. Streptozotocin with 5-FU to treat malignant insulinoma; 50-66% achieve partial remission, 17-33% with complete remission; up to 95% experience nausea and vomiting, sometimes severe; renal tubular, hepatic toxicity also possible

c. Octreotide—Used to treat infants with nesidioblastosis

V. GLUCAGONOMA (see Table 29-1)

A. GENERAL

Glucagonoma is a rare α-cell pancreatic islet tumor (<100 reported cases).

B. CLINICAL

Patients with glucagonoma present with cachexia, deep venous thrombosis/pulmonary embolus, hypoaminoacidemia, and mild and easily controlled diabetes mellitus.

C. DIAGNOSIS

1. Skin lesions are best clue—Migratory annular erythematous eruptions, superficial necrosis ("migratory necrolytic erythema") involves pretibial, perioral, and intertriginous areas

2. Confirm with elevated plasma glucagon (>500 pg/mL).
   Note: Levels may also be elevated with renal failure, liver failure, and severe stress.

3. Provocative test—Arginine infusion, which elevates plasma glucagon in patient with glucagonoma, is rarely needed.

29

NEUROENDOCRINE TUMORS

D. LOCALIZATION

Arteriography, CT scan, and selective venous sampling all can localize tumor. MRI appears best for liver metastases, and ultrasound is occasionally useful.

1. Most are bulky (>3 cm) and vascular, therefore easier to find.
2. 50% in tail, 50% malignant, 50% metastatic at time of exploration (to nodes, liver, adrenal, spine)

E. TREATMENT

Treatment is by surgical excision if possible; ≈30% are completely resectable.

1. Debulking unresectable primaries and metastases has resulted in prolonged survival.
2. Chemotherapy for recurrent or unresectable tumors can ameliorate symptoms; DTIC (dacarbazine), or 5-FU/streptozotocin have both been used.
3. Hepatic artery embolization has been used for liver metastases.
4. Somatostatin analog (octreotide) has been effective in treating symptoms.
5. Rash is treated with zinc, high-protein diet, and control of the diabetes. Preoperative total parenteral nutrition is often necessary to improve nutritional status.

VI. VIPoma (see Table 29-1)

VIPoma is also known as Verner-Morrison syndrome, pancreatic cholera syndrome, or WDHA (*w*atery *d*iarrhea, *h*ypokalemia, *a*chlorhydria) syndrome.

A. GENERAL

1. Rare syndrome due to production of vasoactive intestinal polypeptide (VIP), which is normally a neurotransmitter, from a pancreatic islet cell tumor (70%), extrapancreatic tumor (10-20%; includes duodenal, ganglioneuroblastoma, adrenal medulla, pulmonary sites), or possibly islet cell hyperplasia (10-20%)
2. About 50-60% are malignant and most are metastatic at the time of diagnosis. Extrapancreatic tumors are *rarely* malignant.

B. CLINICAL

WDHA—2-10 L/day of *w*atery *d*iarrhea, resulting in dehydration, *h*ypokalemia, acidosis; associated with *a*chlorhydria (hypochlorhydria more common) due to suppressive action of VIP on gastric acid secretion

1. Up to 20% of patients exhibit spontaneous flushing similar to carcinoid syndrome.

2. Hyperglycemia/hypercalcemia occur in 50-75% of VIPoma patients for unclear reasons.
3. Occasionally associated with MEN 1

C. DIAGNOSIS

Diagnosis is made by documenting the presence of WDHA syndrome (with associated electrolyte abnormalities) with low gastric acid secretion and elevated fasting VIP levels.
1. VIP is invariably elevated, but assay is difficult and requires a reliable laboratory.
2. Pancreatic polypeptide (PP) may also be elevated with pancreatic VIPomas.

D. LOCALIZATION

Use CT and/or ultrasound first; 80% is body or tail. If unsuccessful, use angiography; transhepatic venous sampling may prove helpful in difficult cases.

E. TREATMENT

1. Vigorous preoperative fluid resuscitation/electrolyte replacement, then surgical resection, which is usually curative
2. If no tumor is found, some authors believe that subtotal pancreatectomy is indicated if tumor markers (VIP, PP) are consistently elevated preoperatively.
3. For unresectable/metastatic disease, debulk; some recommend hepatic artery embolization.
a. Steroids may provide symptomatic relief in 50%, but relapse is common.
b. >90% remission rate with streptozotocin, many lasting for years; DTIC and 5-FU have also been used successfully.
4. Preoperative octreotide reduces VIP levels and reduces diarrhea 80% in of cases.

VII. SOMATOSTATINOMA (see Table 29-1)

A. GENERAL

1. Very rare tumor of pancreatic islet; duodenal tumors also reported
2. Termed *inhibitory syndrome*; classic triad of gallstones, diabetes, and steatorrhea is relatively nonspecific, and duodenal tumors are usually asymptomatic. Thus, most tumors are discovered late in the course with metastases already present.
3. In general, these are malignant, solitary, and virulent.

B. SYMPTOMS

Symptoms are due to inhibition of exocrine and endocrine pancreas, gallbladder contraction, and gastric emptying (resulting in bloating, indigestion, nausea, and vomiting).

29

NEUROENDOCRINE TUMORS

C. DIAGNOSIS

Somatostatinoma is usually discovered *incidentally* at cholecystectomy; plasma somatostatin can be measured and is markedly elevated. Duodenal tumors are associated with von Recklinghausen's disease.

D. LOCALIZATION

Most somatostatinomas are discovered incidentally, but CT and angiography are useful.

E. TREATMENT

Resection should be attempted, if possible; however, most patients' tumors are unresectable at presentation, in which case debulking is recommended.
1. Duodenal somatostatinomas should be treated like carcinomas.
2. Tumor is rare; no information on chemotherapy is available.

F. PROGNOSIS

Prognosis in cases described is poor, with most patients surviving several months; early diagnosis and resection might be curative.

VIII. MULTIPLE ENDOCRINE NEOPLASIA SYNDROMES

All are autosomal dominant.

MEN 1	MEN 2a	MEN 2b
Pituitary adenoma	Medullary thyroid carcinoma	Medullary thyroid carcinoma
Parathyroid hyperplasia	Pheochromocytoma	Pheochromocytoma
Pancreatic islet cell tumor	Parathyroid hyperplasia	Multiple mucosal neuromas

A. MEN 1

MEN 1 is also referred to as Wermer's syndrome or the "3 Ps" (pituitary, parathyroid, pancreas).
1. 15% of all neuroendocrine tumors are secondary to MEN 1. The syndrome is due to germline mutation in tumor suppressor gene, *menin*, found on the long arm of chromosome 11. Tumors demonstrate loss of heterozygosity.
2. Peak incidence in 20s for women, 30s for men; most commonly present with peptic ulcer disease symptoms/complications; next most common is hypoglycemia (insulinoma); less common are headaches, visual field deficits, amenorrhea (pituitary adenoma)
3. Pituitary—60-70% have adenoma, usually chromophobe with hypofunction; occasionally have functional tumor; prolactinomas most common
4. Parathyroid—Most consistent lesion; >90% with generalized hyperplasia and hypercalcemia; may have renal stones, peptic ulcer disease

5. Pancreas—80% with pancreatic lesion; most commonly gastrinoma, followed by insulinoma; *any* islet cell tumor is possible, including simple islet cell hyperplasia; tumors usually multifocal, often malignant, but slow growing

6. Diagnosis

a. Screen all patients with pancreatic tumor for hyperparathyroidism (Ca^{2+}, parathyroid hormone).

b. Screen all family members of patients with gastrinoma or any other MEN 1–associated lesions (pituitary, parathyroid).

c. Pancreatic polypeptide may be good marker; seems to be elevated in nearly *all* cases

7. Treatment

a. Hyperparathyroidism—Treat first, with four-gland parathyroidectomy with autotransplantation or with subtotal parathyroidectomy; if peptic ulcer disease is present and persists with normal Ca^{2+}, do work-up for gastrinoma.

b. Because gastrinomas and other pancreatic lesions in MEN 1 are often multiple and/or malignant, surgery may not be curative.

c. Pituitary lesions—Addressed surgically as indicated

B. MEN 2a (SIPPLE'S SYNDROME) AND 2b

1. Both MEN 2a and 2b are autosomal dominant, but sporadic cases have been reported.

2. Caused by mutation in the proto-oncogene *c-Ret*, a transmembrane receptor tyrosine kinase. MEN 2a is caused by a mutation in the ligand-binding domain, and MEN 2b is caused by a mutation in the kinase domain; both mutations result in constitutive kinase activity.

a. Patients with MEN 2a classically develop medullary thyroid carcinoma, bilateral pheochromocytoma, and parathyroid hyperplasia.

b. Patients with MEN 2b classically develop medullary thyroid carcinoma, multiple neuromas of the buccal mucosa, marfanoid habitus, GI ganglioneuromas, and megacolon. MEN 2b is not associated with hyperparathyroidism.

3. Medullary thyroid carcinoma, preceded by thyroid C-cell hyperplasia, is present in 100% of patients with MEN 2. Tumors are multifocal and bilateral, unlike sporadic cases; they are much more aggressive tumors in MEN 2b, making early total thyroidectomy critical for long-term survival.

4. Pheochromocytoma—Present in 40-50%; 80% bilateral, almost always benign; peak incidence in teens, 20s

5. Parathyroid hyperplasia is present in approximately 60% of patients with MEN 2a.

6. Diagnosis—Elevated plasma calcitonin level

a. Measurement of plasma calcitonin after pentagastrin stimulation (0.5 μg/kg IV, measure calcitonin at 1-3 minutes and 30 minutes) detects

29

NEUROENDOCRINE TUMORS

medullary thyroid carcinoma in normal patients who will have microscopic disease when thyroid is removed.

b. Symptoms of pheochromocytoma (see Chap. 28 section VI for work-up)

c. Blood Ca^{2+}, parathyroid hormone levels for hyperparathyroidism

7. Treatment

a. Look for and treat pheochromocytoma first—Abdominal, bilateral exploration due to frequency of bilateral lesions

b. Total thyroidectomy, with resection of nodes between the jugular veins from thyroid cartilage to sternal notch; neck dissection for more extensive lymphatic involvement; follow pentagastrin stimulation test to check for adequacy of resection, recurrence

c. Subtotal parathyroidectomy for MEN 2a patients with hyperparathyroidism, or total parathyroidectomy with reimplantation of partial gland in sternocleidomastoid muscle or in forearm

8. Prognosis

a. Related to the extent of thyroid tumor

b. Extremely variable, even in same family. Overall, 10-year survival of patients with medullary thyroid carcinoma is 50%.

Note: *Medullary thyroid carcinoma is responsible for most of the mortality associated with MEN 2.*

The Esophagus

Wilson M. Clements, MD

I. ANATOMY

A. GENERAL DESCRIPTION

1. A muscular tube ≈25 cm long that begins 15 cm from incisors, at the cricopharyngeus muscle, and ends at the gastroesophageal (GE) junction. It is narrowed at the level of the cricopharyngeal muscle (narrowest point), the aortic arch, the left main stem bronchus, and the diaphragmatic hiatus.
2. The esophagus enters the abdomen via the esophageal hiatus at the T11 level and is accompanied by the vagal trunks. The distal 2-4 cm is intra-abdominal (Fig. 30-1).

30

B. BLOOD SUPPLY AND NERVES

1. Arterial supply is segmental from superior and inferior thyroid, aortic and esophageal branches, inferior phrenic, and left gastric arteries
2. Venous drainage is to the hypopharyngeal, azygos, hemiazygos, intercostal, and gastric veins. All are a potential source of varices if portal hypertension is present.
3. Nerve innervation is from both parasympathetic and sympathetic systems. Right and left vagal trunks lie posterior and anterior, respectively, on the distal esophagus.

C. HISTOLOGY

1. The mucosa is lined by squamous epithelium, changing to columnar epithelium at or near the GE junction.
2. The submucosa contains glands, arteries, Meissner's neural plexus, lymphatics, and veins.
3. The muscularis is composed of two layers, an outer longitudinal and an inner circular layer. Nerves and blood vessels run between the layers. The upper one third is composed of striated muscle, and the lower two thirds is smooth muscle.
4. The lack of a serosal layer potentially contributes to an increase in anastomotic leaks and early mediastinal invasion by cancer.

II. PHYSIOLOGY

The esophagus functions to transport swallowed material, in a coordinated fashion, from the pharynx to the stomach with voluntary and involuntary actions.

A. PERISTALSIS

1. Primary peristalsis—Initiated by relaxing the upper esophageal sphincter (UES) that propels swallowed material from pharynx to stomach in a progressive and sequential manner

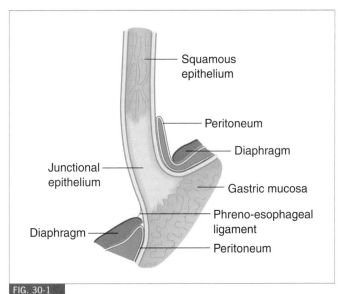

FIG. 30-1
Anatomy of the esophagus.

2. Secondary peristalsis—Involuntary waves, initiated in the smooth muscle layer, clear locally distended segments of the esophagus
3. Tertiary peristalsis—Repetitive, nonprogressive, and uncoordinated smooth muscle contractions

B. SPHINCTERS
1. UES is ≈3 cm long with resting pressure of 20-60 mm Hg.
2. Lower esophageal sphincter (LES)
a. Not an anatomically defined sphincter in humans; more appropriately referred to as a zone of high pressure that serves to reduce gastric regurgitation and reflux. It is located in distal 3-5 cm of esophagus and defined by "pull-back" manometric studies. Its normal resting pressure is 10-20 mm Hg.
b. Varies with respiration; increases with inspiration and drug and/or hormone levels
   (1) Pressure increased by gastrin, caffeine, α-adrenergic drugs, bethanechol, and metoclopramide
   (2) Pressure decreased by secretin, cholecystokinin, glucagon, progesterone, alcohol, nitroglycerin, nicotine, anticholinergics, and β-adrenergic drugs

c. Abdominal pressure transmitted to distal esophagus important for competence. The intra-abdominal position of the lower segment of the esophagus is maintained by the phrenoesophageal ligament.

III. MOTILITY DISORDERS

A. DEFINITION
Motility disorders are conditions that interfere with swallowing and are not caused by intraluminal obstruction or external compression.

B. HISTORY
1. A careful, detailed history should be obtained.
2. Dysphagia with liquids more than solids suggests motility disorder.
3. Dysphagia progressive from solids to liquids suggests mechanical obstruction.
4. Odynophagia suggests spasm or esophagitis. Increased pain with cold liquids is suggestive of spasm.
5. Difficulty with swallowing or nasopharyngeal reflux suggests a neurologic or muscular disorder.
6. Symptoms of reflux
7. Duration of symptoms
8. Hematemesis, weight loss, and alcohol/tobacco use should be questioned.
9. Gurgling with swallowing or regurgitation of undigested food suggests a Zenker's diverticulum.

C. UES DYSFUNCTION—CRICOPHARYNGEAL ACHALASIA
1. Caused by abnormalities in central and peripheral nervous systems; metabolic, inflammatory myopathy; GE reflux; and others
2. Patients complain of a "lump" in the throat, excessive expectoration of saliva, weight loss, and intermittent hoarseness
3. Diagnosis by barium swallow and manometric studies; however, these may be normal
4. Treatment depends on the cause—Antireflux procedure, bougienage, or cervical esophagotomy

D. ESOPHAGEAL BODY DISORDERS
1. Achalasia—Failure of relaxation
a. Abnormal peristalsis secondary to absence or destruction of Auerbach's (myenteric) plexus and failure of LES to relax; affects body and distal esophagus
b. Etiology unknown, multiple associations
c. Patients complain of dysphagia, regurgitation, weight loss, retrosternal chest pain, and recurrent pulmonary infections
d. Barium swallow demonstrates "bird's beak" narrowing of distal esophagus with proximal dilation

30

THE ESOPHAGUS

e. Manometric studies show incomplete LES relaxation and lack of progressive peristalsis. Aperistalsis is observed in the esophageal body. An elevated LES pressure (<6 mm Hg) is common.

f. 1-10% of patients develop squamous cell carcinoma after 15-25 years of disease.

g. Treatment is palliative.

   (1) Nonsurgical treatment includes sublingual nitroglycerin, calcium channel blockers, botulinum toxin injection, and repeated dilation. 65% improve with pneumatic or hydrostatic dilation.

   (2) Surgical treatment is a longitudinal (Heller) esophagotomy. 85% of patients improve; there is a 3% rate of reflux following this procedure. The Heller procedure may be done laparoscopically or thorascopically, and some surgeons include a Toupet antireflux procedure.

   (3) End-stage patients with megaesophagus may require an esophagectomy.

2. Diffuse esophageal spasm

a. Repetitive, simultaneous, high-amplitude contractions

b. Pain greater than dysphagia; symptoms increased by emotional stress

c. Diagnosis by motility studies. Barium swallow may show "coiled spring" or "corkscrewing."

d. Medical treatment includes small, soft meals and calcium channel blockers.

e. Surgical treatment is extended esophagomyotomy.

3. Nutcracker esophagus

a. Defined as a manometric abnormality with hypertensive contractions with mean pressures in the distal esophagus >180 mm Hg

b. A normal peristaltic sequence occurs in the body of the esophagus.

c. Complaints include chest pain and dysphagia.

d. Medical therapy is indicated for these patients.

e. Most common esophageal motility disorder

4. Hypertensive LES

a. Defined as an elevated LES pressure ≥45 mm Hg with normal LES relaxation

b. Main complaints are chest pain and dysphagia.

c. Medical therapy and dilation are the first line of therapy.

d. Myotomy may be indicated in those failing medical therapy and dilation.

5. Scleroderma

a. Fibrous replacement of esophageal smooth muscle and atrophy

b. LES loses tone and normal response to swallowing; results in GE reflux

c. Medical/surgical treatment directed at antireflux measures to decrease esophagitis

d. Operative therapy usually avoided in these patients

IV. DIVERTICULA

A. DEFINITION
Diverticula are epithelial-lined mucosal pouches that protrude from the esophageal lumen.

B. PHARYNGOESOPHAGEAL (ZENKER'S DIVERTICULUM)
1. Located between oblique fibers of the thyropharyngeus muscle and the horizontal fibers of the cricopharyngeus
2. Most common esophageal diverticula (pseudodiverticulum) that contains only mucosa and submucosa
3. Pulsion-type diverticula created by increased intraluminal pressure
4. Patients are usually 30-50 years of age and complain of cervical dysphagia, effortless regurgitation of undigested food, choking, gurgling in throat, and recurrent aspiration
5. Diagnosis is made with a barium swallow
6. Treatment includes diverticulectomy with myotomy of the cricopharyngeus muscle
7. Low mortality and recurrence rates—2% and 4%, respectively

C. PERIBRONCHIAL
1. Located near tracheal bifurcation
2. Traction diverticulum resulting from inflammatory reaction, typically mediastinal granulomatous disease of adjacent lymph nodes that adhere to the esophagus and pull on wall during healing
3. Rarely symptomatic, tend to be very small, and are discovered incidentally

D. EPIPHRENIC
1. Located in distal 10 cm of esophagus
2. Pulsion-type, arising from distal obstruction or motor dysfunction
3. Patients complain of regurgitation, dysphagia, and retrosternal chest pain.
4. Treatment—Usually none. If the diverticulum is large, the appropriate treatment is a long extramucosal thoracic myotomy and diverticulectomy.

V. HIATAL HERNIA AND GASTROESOPHAGEAL REFLUX

A. ANATOMY
1. Normally, the distal 2-3 cm of esophagus is intra-abdominal.
2. Endoabdominal fascia (continuous with transversalis fascia) inserts into the esophageal wall at the esophageal hiatus.
3. No discrete LES in humans

B. PATHOPHYSIOLOGY
1. Decreased LES tone
2. Delayed gastric emptying

30

THE ESOPHAGUS

3. Increased intra-abdominal pressure due to obesity, tight garments, or large meal
4. Motor failure of esophagus with loss of peristalsis
5. Iatrogenic injury to LES

C. ACID-PROTECTING MECHANISMS
1. Distal esophagus prevents reflux through influence of intra-abdominal pressure.
2. Peristalsis rapidly clears gastric acid.
3. Bicarbonate-rich saliva (1000-1500 mL/day)

D. REFLUX ESOPHAGITIS
1. Gastric acid and pepsin are corrosive to the esophageal mucosa.
2. Complications
a. Pain and spasm
b. Stricture
c. Hemorrhage
d. Shortening of esophagus
e. Ulceration
f. Barrett's esophagus
   (1) Definition—Squamous to columnar metaplasia of the distal esophagus
   (2) Associated with an increased risk of developing adenocarcinoma (10-15%) over 10 years
   (3) Correction of reflux does not prevent malignant transformation, and it requires serial endoscopic surveillance and possible biopsy. Esophageal resection is indicated for severe dysplasia.
g. Dysmotility
h. Schatzki's ring—A constrictive band at the squamocolumnar junction composed of mucosa and submucosa, not esophageal muscle
i. Aspiration pneumonia
3. Symptoms
a. Heartburn, retrosternal pyrosis
b. Regurgitation of sour or bitter liquids, aggravated by postural changes
c. Nocturnal aspiration with recurrent pneumonia, lung abscesses, or bronchiectasis
d. Dysphagia secondary to obstruction or motility disorder
4. Diagnosis
a. Upper GI series
   (1) Spontaneous reflux in 40% of patients with true GE reflux
   (2) Able to document stricture or ulcer
b. Esophagoscopy combined with mucosal brushings and biopsy is essential to diagnosis for reflux esophagitis.
c. Esophageal pH probe
   (1) Accurate for determining magnitude and duration of reflux
   (2) 24-hour test most precise and quantitative method

        (3) Acid reflux test—HCl is placed into the stomach; esophageal pH proximal to LES is monitored as intragastric pressure is increased; a pH <4 is a positive test

d. Bernstein test (infrequently used in modern practice)
   (1) Reproduction of pain during instillation of acid into midesophagus. Acid is alternated with saline.
   (2) Normal individual is able to clear acid.

e. Manometry
   (1) Does not test reflux; however, reflux more common with low LES pressure (<6 mm Hg)
   (2) Useful in identifying underlying motility disorder (present in up to 25% of patients)

5. Treatment

a. Medical
   (1) Dietary
      (a) Avoid substances that decrease LES tone, i.e., cigarette smoking, chocolate, alcohol, and fatty foods
      (b) Do not eat 2 hours prior to sleeping.
      (c) Avoid excessive eating; eat small meals.
   (2) Avoid anticholinergics, tranquilizers, and muscle relaxants.
   (3) Reduce weight, if obese.
   (4) Elevate head of bed 6 inches on blocks.
   (5) Increase LES pressure
      (a) Metoclopramide 10 mg q 8 h.
      (b) Bethanechol 10-50 t.i.d. or q.i.d.
   (6) Decrease gastric acid.
      (a) Antacids
      (b) H_2 blockers
      (c) Proton-pump inhibitors

b. Surgical—Antireflux procedures
   (1) Goals
      (a) Restore segment of intra-abdominal esophagus.
      (b) Maintain distal esophagus as small-diameter tube.
      (c) Narrow the hiatus.
      (d) Avoid increasing the resistance of the relaxed sphincter to level that exceeds peristaltic force of esophagus.
   (2) Indications
      (a) Failure of medical therapy
      (b) Esophagitis with frank ulceration or stricture
      (c) Complications of reflux esophagitis
      (d) Severe symptoms or progressive disease
   (3) Procedures
      (a) Nissen fundoplication—A 360-degree fundoplication. Currently, the accepted first-line procedure is the laparoscopic procedure. Provides symptomatic relief for most patients. The Nissen may also be performed as an open abdominal or thoracic operation.

    (b) Partial fundoplications such as the Belsey Mark IV or the Toupet are indicated if esophageal motility is poor. The Belsey is a transthoracic open procedure done with the additional indication of a foreshortened esophagus, whereas the Toupet is a laparoscopic operation. Both feature a 270-degree fundoplication designed to limit reflux but allow transit of esophageal contents.

    (c) Other older, rarely indicated, antireflux operations

        (i) Hill gastropexy—Features a 180-degree wrap with the phrenoesophageal ligament anchored to the median arcuate ligament of the diaphragm

        (ii) Collis gastroplasty—Used in patients with an extremely foreshortened esophagus. The esophagus is lengthened with a gastric tube, allowing a tension-free fundoplication around the new esophagus.

    (d) In the morbidly obese patient (body mass index >35) with other comorbid conditions, performing a laparoscopic or open Roux-en-Y gastric bypass is the surgical treatment for reflux disease.

  (4) Complications

    (a) Perforation of the esophagus—Most dreaded complication. Prompt intraoperative recognition is crucial for repair and prevention of potential mediastinitis.

    (b) Excessively tight wrap–dysphagia—This decreases with increasing experience and can be prevented with intraoperative manometry.

    (c) Excessively loose or short wrap–reflux

    (d) "Slipped-Nissen" occurs when wrap slides down, the GE junction retracts into the chest, and the stomach is partitioned. This is usually due to a foreshortened esophagus unrecognized at the first operation.

    (e) "Gas bloat syndrome" is described as difficult eructation due to swallowed air in the stomach of a patient with a restored LES.

    (f) Incidence of splenectomy is very low at 1-2%.

E. HIATAL HERNIA

1. Type I (sliding or axial) (Fig. 30-2)

a. GE junction migrates above diaphragm; phrenoesophageal membrane intact; no true peritoneal sac

b. Most common hiatal hernia—90%

c. Significant only if reflux symptoms

d. Etiology

  (1) Chronically increased intra-abdominal pressure, including obesity

  (2) Weakness of supporting structures at esophageal hiatus

2. Type II (paraesophageal)

a. Herniated gastric fundus with GE junction in normal position

b. Peritoneal sac

c. Reflux rare

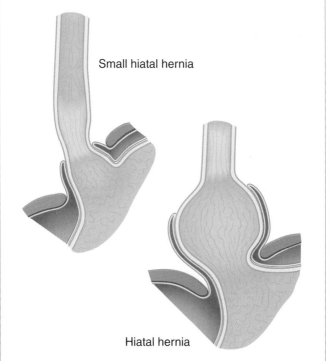

Small hiatal hernia

Hiatal hernia

FIG. 30-2
Type I hiatal hernia.

d. Uncommon type of hernia
e. Can result in gastric volvulus or strangulation
f. All type II hernias should be repaired
3. **Type III—A combination of types I and II**

VI. BENIGN TUMORS OF THE ESOPHAGUS

The incidence of benign tumors of the esophagus is rare (<1% of esophageal tumors).

A. LEIOMYOMA

1. Most common benign tumor of esophagus—75%
2. Less common in esophagus than stomach or small bowel
3. Usually located in distal two thirds of esophagus
4. Lesions <5 cm are usually asymptomatic.

5. Multiple in 3-10% of patients
6. 97% are intramural (within the circular muscle layer); histologically appear as interlacing smooth muscle bundles
7. Symptoms
a. Progressive intermittent dysphagia
b. Vague retrosternal ache
c. Heartburn
d. Odynophagia
e. Regurgitation
8. Diagnosis by chest radiograph, barium swallow, and endoscopy (avoid biopsy if suspected). Endoscopic ultrasound is the gold standard for diagnosis.
a. Five discrete layers exist on ultrasound.
b. Alternating layers of hyperechoic and hypoechoic concentric rings
c. The ultrasonographic layers from intraluminal to periesophageal—Superficial mucosa, deep mucosa, submucosa, muscularis propria, and periesophageal tissue
d. Esophageal leiomyoma are found in the fourth layer, the muscularis propria.
e. Ultrasound also allows for fine-needle aspiration of nodes in the periesophageal tissue.
9. Treatment
a. Excision of leiomyoma via thoracotomy, mortality <2%
b. Tumors not amenable to enucleation (10%) may require esophageal resection (mortality 10%)

B. OTHER BENIGN TUMORS
1. Esophageal cysts—20%
2. Polyps
3. Lipomas
4. Hemangiomas

VII. ESOPHAGEAL CARCINOMA

A. INCIDENCE
1. Male-to-female ratio—3:1
2. Black-to-white ratio—4:1
3. Peak incidence—50-70 years of age

B. RISK FACTORS
1. Alcohol and tobacco use
2. Diet
a. Nitrosamines
b. Betel nuts
c. Chronic ingestion of hot foods and beverages
3. Lower socioeconomic level

4. Caustic ingestion (1-5% incidence)
5. Achalasia (2-8% incidence of squamous cell carcinoma)
6. Plummer-Vinson syndrome—Esophageal webs, anemia, brittle nails, glossitis
7. Vitamin and mineral deficiencies
8. Barrett's esophagus—10% incidence of adenocarcinoma
9. GE reflux disease (GERD)—Additional risk factor for esophageal adenocarcinoma
10. High-risk patients for adenocarcinoma are young white men with GERD.

C. PATHOLOGY
1. 70% are squamous cell carcinomas
a. Cervical—8%
b. Upper or middle half of esophagus—55%
c. Distal esophagus—37%
2. Adenocarcinomas arise from gastric cardia or Barrett's esophagus, mostly in the distal third.
3. Incidence increasing in the United States
4. Three growth patterns
a. Fungating—60%
b. Ulcerative—25%
c. Infiltrative—15%
5. Tumors spread circumferentially and longitudinally via lymphatics, vascular invasion, and direct extension.
6. 75% of patients present with lymph node metastasis at the time of diagnosis. Common distant metastatic sites are liver, lung, and bone.

D. TNM CLASSIFICATION
1. Primary tumor (T)
   T0: No evidence of a primary tumor
   Tis: High-grade dysplasia/carcinoma in situ
   T1: Tumor invading lamina propria (T1a), the muscularis mucosae (T1a), or submucosa (T1b) but does not breach the submucosa
   T2: Tumor invades muscularis propria
   T3: Tumor invades the adventitia
   T4: Invasion of adjacent structures
   TX: Tumor cannot be assessed
2. Regional lymph nodes (N)
   N0: No lymph node involvement
   N1: Regional node involvement
   NX: Regional node status cannot be assessed
3. Distant metastases (M)
   MX: Presence of distant metastasis cannot be assessed
   M0: None
   M1a: Nonregional lymph node metastases
   M1b: Other distant metastases

30

THE ESOPHAGUS

E. STAGING

Stage O: Tis NO MO
Stage I: T1 NO MO
Stage IIA: T2 NO MO, T3 NO MO
Stage IIB: T1 N1 MO, T2 N1 MO
Stage III: T3 N1 MO, T4 any N MO
Stage IVa: any T or N M1a
Stage IVb: any T, any N, M1b

F. CLINICAL PRESENTATION

1. Insidious onset, beginning as indigestion or retrosternal discomfort. Dysphagia, progressing from solids to liquids, is present in >80% of patients. Dysphagia occurs when the lumen narrows to <13 mm. Pain is a late symptom indicating extraesophageal involvement.
2. Weight loss
3. Odynophagia
4. Regurgitation
5. Anemia
6. Hematemesis
7. Vocal cord paralysis, left more than right
8. Aspiration pneumonia
9. Tracheoesophageal or bronchoesophageal fistula

G. DIAGNOSIS

1. Barium swallow has 92% accuracy in demonstrating mucosal irregularity and annular constrictions but less accurately identifies abnormal peristalsis.
2. Fiberoptic endoscopy with biopsy or brushing is confirmatory in 95% of cases.
3. Bronchoscopy with biopsy to rule out involvement of the bronchus in upper-two-third tumors and a synchronous lung primary.
4. Nasopharyngoscopy and direct laryngoscopy to rule out synchronous head and neck lesions and vocal cord involvement
5. CT scan of chest with extension to liver and adrenals to assess tumor spread
6. Endoscopic ultrasound allows assessment of depth of invasion (T) and assessment of regional lymph nodes

H. THERAPY

1. Principles
a. Most patients have advanced disease at presentation and are surgically incurable.
b. 50% of tumors are resectable at presentation. Preoperative chemotherapy increases operability rates.
c. Treatment must be modified by the patient's cancer stage.

d. Operative therapy is done ideally for a cure but can offer excellent long-term palliation.

2. Surgical

a. Curative in early lesions (high-grade dysplasia and T1a) and as part of a multimodal therapy in advanced cases. Resection should not be performed in patients with distant metastases or contraindications to operative therapy.

b. Esophagectomy techniques

    (1) Ivor-Lewis

        (a) Involves esophagectomy, gastric mobilization, and GE anastomosis in the chest or neck

        (b) Midline abdominal incision and right thoracotomy are performed.

        (c) Predominantly for T1b N0 M0 and T2 N0 M0 tumors

    (2) Trans-hiatal

        (a) Via neck and abdominal incisions

        (b) Blunt esophagectomy, gastric mobilization, and GE anastomosis in neck

        (c) Useful for high-grade dysplasia and T1a lesions

    (3) Esophageal reconstruction can also be completed with colon or jejunal interposition or as free graft

    (4) Overall mortality rate is 5% and morbidity rate is 25%.

    (5) Survival not improved with radical en bloc resections

3. Radiation

a. Dosages to the mediastinum range from 4000 to 6000 cGy.

b. Primary treatment for poor-risk patients and palliation for unresectable lesions with obstructive symptoms

c. May have some utility in postoperative therapy for residual mediastinal disease; however, there is no proven survival benefit

d. 5-year survival for patients treated with radiation alone only slightly worse than surgery alone

4. Chemotherapy

a. Current regimen—5-Fluorouracil, cisplatin, and paclitaxel (Taxol)

b. Increased disease-free and long-term survival when given preoperatively and postoperatively to responding tumors

c. May decrease tumor mass preoperatively

5. Multimodal

a. Preoperative chemotherapy, esophagectomy, and postoperative chemotherapy for responding tumors and radiation to residual mediastinal disease is the current treatment of choice.

b. 70% survival at 12 months in nonrandomized trials

6. Palliation

a. Resection or bypass is best long-term palliation

b. Laser fulguration for relief of obstruction

c. Repeated dilation and pulsion placement of endoprosthesis is reserved for poor-risk, terminal patient. There is a 14% mortality and 25% morbidity rate.

30

THE ESOPHAGUS

7. Prognosis
a. Mortality at 1 year—80%
b. Overall 5-year survival—<10%
c. Radiation therapy—6-10% survival
d. Surgery—2-24%, average 10% 5-year survival
e. Multimodal therapy 5-year survival rates pending

VIII. ESOPHAGEAL RUPTURE AND PERFORATION

A. ETIOLOGY
1. Iatrogenic—Most common
a. Endoscopic injury more common with rigid vs. flexible scope and occurs most commonly at pharyngoesophageal junction. Direct injury frequently results from foreign body removal.
b. Dilation (balloon or bougienage)
c. Biopsy
d. Intubation (esophageal or endotracheal)
e. Operative—Devascularization or perforation with pulmonary resection, vagotomy, or antireflux procedure
f. Placement of nasoenteric tubes
2. Noniatrogenic
a. Barogenic trauma
 (1) Postemetic (Boerhaave's syndrome)—Transmural tear following forceful or repeated vomiting. Usually associated with gluttony, bulimia, or alcoholic binge. Esophageal and gastric contents forced into chest under pressure.
 (2) Blunt chest or abdominal trauma
 (3) Other—Labor, convulsions, defecation
b. Penetrating neck, chest, or abdominal trauma
c. Foreign body
d. Postoperative—Anastomotic disruption
e. Corrosive injury
f. Erosion by adjacent inflammation
g. Carcinoma

B. CLINICAL PRESENTATION
1. Can be dramatic and catastrophic with tachycardia, hypotension, and respiratory compromise
2. Others include dyspnea, neck or chest pain, fever, subcutaneous emphysema, and pneumothorax

C. DIAGNOSIS
1. Chest radiograph may reveal pneumothorax, pneumomediastinum, pleural effusion, or subdiaphragmatic air.
2. Contrast swallow—Controversy whether water-soluble or barium swallow is best. Most would perform water-soluble study first

because its effects on mediastinum are less than barium if
perforation is present. However, this material is worse if aspirated.
Barium study can be obtained if initial study is negative and suspicion
remains high.

D. TREATMENT

1. Early recognition and treatment are essential to survival.
   The differential diagnosis also must include myocardial infarction,
   perforated viscus, dissecting aortic aneurysms, and pulmonary
   embolus.
2. Basics
   a. Drainage
   b. NPO
   c. Fluid resuscitation
   d. Broad-spectrum antibiotics
   e. Nutritional support in recovery period; parenteral route is preferred
   f. If perforation occurs in the presence of other pathology, the underlying
      disease must be treated at the time of surgery or the repair will
      break down.
3. Nonoperative management of esophageal perforation
   a. Controversial; applicable only in patients with the following.
      (1) Hemodynamic stability
      (2) Small perforation
      (3) Cervical perforation
      (4) A contained leak
      (5) No evidence of sepsis
      (6) Wide drainage back into esophagus on esophagram
   b. Nasogastric suction, antibiotics, and close observation
4. Operative management depends on the location and extent of the
   perforation.
   a. Cervical
      (1) Limited extravasation and extrathoracic perforation may initially be
          managed nonoperatively.
      (2) Patient with crepitus or increased extravasation—Operative
          drainage, antibiotics, closure of rupture if possible and potentially a
          cervical esophagostomy
   b. Thoracic
      (1) Mortality—10-15% in patients treated within 24 hours of injury
          and increases to >50% if diagnosis delayed >24 hours
      (2) Early—Suture closure, wide drainage, and antibiotics. Bolstering
          repair with patch is of controversial benefit.
      (3) Late—Operative drainage and antibiotics. Suture closure is unlikely
          to succeed. Some advocate esophagectomy, oversewing the cardia,
          and creating a cervical esophagostomy.
5. Complications of esophageal perforation include sepsis, abscess,
   fistula, empyema, mediastinitis, and death.

30

THE ESOPHAGUS

IX. CAUSTIC INJURY

A. BACKGROUND
1. Usually results from ingestion of alkalis, acids, bleach, or detergents
2. Patients usually <5 years old or adolescent or adult attempting suicide
3. Alkalis cause liquefactive necrosis that results in greater depth of injury.

B. CLINICAL PRESENTATION
1. Oral and oropharyngeal burns (pseudomembranes)
2. Signs and symptoms of laryngotracheal edema (hoarseness, stridor, aphonia, and dyspnea)
3. Signs and symptoms of esophageal or gastric perforation
4. In the absence of perforation, acute manifestations resolve in a few days. Clinical improvement may continue for several weeks.
5. Stricture can occur as a late complication.

C. DIAGNOSIS
1. Upper endoscopy to establish severity of the injury
2. Contrast exam of esophagus can demonstrate injury as well as suspected perforation.

D. TREATMENT
1. Initial therapy
a. Induction of emesis should be avoided, as should attempts to dilute the caustic agent (damage is nearly instantaneous, and intake of large volumes of fluid may only cause distention and emesis).
b. NPO
c. IV hydration
d. Broad-spectrum antibiotics after diagnosis confirmed
e. Efficacy of corticosteroids in attempt to limit stricture is debatable.
2. Operative intervention
a. Patients with evidence of esophageal or gastric perforation require immediate operation.
   (1) Best explored through abdominal incision, but patient is prepped from mandible to pubis to allow for possibility of cervical incision
   (2) Restoration of alimentary continuity should await resolution of the acute insult.
b. Stricture formation tends to be the rule.
   (1) Dilation is traditional therapy.
   (2) Stricture that cannot be dilated or remains refractory to dilation after 1 year requires esophageal substitution
      (a) Stomach is preferred substitute but often is unusable secondary to scarring from original injury
      (b) Esophagus should be excised.

Gastric Tumors

Andrew W. Knott, MD

I. ADENOCARCINOMA OF THE STOMACH

A. EPIDEMIOLOGY
1. 90-95% of all gastric tumors
2. Eighth most common cause of cancer mortality in United States
3. Declining incidence (10 per 100,000 in United States)
4. Male-to-female ratio—2:1
5. 70% of patients >50 years old (peak, 7th decade)
6. Incidence highest in Japan (80 times higher than United States)

B. RISK FACTORS
1. Environment
a. Diet—Smoked foods, nitrosamine compounds, polycyclic hydrocarbons, and low consumption of fruits and vegetables
b. Occupational—Heavy metals, rubber, asbestos
c. Cigarette smoking, alcohol consumption
d. Low socioeconomic status
2. Genetic
a. Associated with blood type A—Relative risk 1.2
b. Hereditary nonpolyposis colon cancer syndrome—Lynch's syndrome II
c. *P53* mutation
d. Germline mutation of e-cadherin
e. Black race
f. Family history gastric cancer (first-degree relatives have two or three times the risk)

C. PRECURSOR CONDITIONS
1. Partial gastrectomy for benign disease
a. Most cases occur following Billroth II—5% risk
b. Usually >15 years after primary surgery—Relative risk 1.5-3
c. Chronic exposure to biliary, pancreatic, and intestinal secretions with resultant gastritis
2. Gastric polyps
a. Inflammatory—75-90% incidence
b. Adenomatous polyps—10-20% incidence associated with gastric cancer
   (1) <2 cm—2-4% risk of adenocarcinoma
   (2) >2 cm—20-40% risk of adenocarcinoma. Malignancy more common in villous adenomas.
   (3) Adenomatous polyps associated with increased risk of adenocarcinoma elsewhere in the stomach
c. Foveolar hyperplasia
3. Chronic atrophic gastritis
a. Hypertrophic gastritis (Ménétrier's disease)

      (1) Inflammatory disease of gastric epithelium
      (2) Up to 10% risk of malignant change
  b. Pernicious anemia
      (1) Association with achlorhydria and atrophic gastritis
      (2) Increased risk of gastric cancer—2-10%, controversial
4. Peptic ulcer disease—<1% risk of malignant change
5. *Helicobacter pylori*
  a. Gram-negative microaerophilic bacterium, possible promoter agent of gastric carcinoma
  b. Patients with *H. pylori* infection have three to six times increased risk of gastric cancer; also increased infection rate in patients with cancer
  c. Increased incidence *H. pylori* infection in China, where rate of gastric cancer is high

D. PATHOLOGY
1. Histology types
  a. Intestinal (most common overall; most common type in Japan)—Associated with Erb B-2 and Erb B-3 receptor stimulation
  b. Diffuse or signet-ring cell—Most common in United States
2. Location of primary tumor
  a. Pyloric canal or antrum—30%
  b. Body—20%
  c. Cardia—37%
  d. Entire stomach—12%
3. Borrmann's classification
      Type I (3%): Nonulcerated, polyploid, growing intraluminal
      Type II (18%): Ulcerated, circumscribed with sharp margins
      Type III (16%): Ulcerated, margin *not* sharply circumscribed
      Type IV (63%): Diffuse, infiltrating, may be ulcerated; may involve entire stomach (linitis plastica)
4. Routes of developing metastatic disease
  a. Direct extension to adjacent organs
  b. Lymphatic
      (1) Regional nodes—Greater/lesser curve, celiac axis
      (2) Supraclavicular (Virchow's node)
      (3) Umbilical (Sister Mary Joseph's node)
  c. Hematogenous via portal or systemic circulation—Ascites, jaundice, liver mass, pelvic mass
  d. Peritoneal seeding to omentum, parietal peritoneum, ovaries (Krukenberg's tumor), or cul-de-sac (Blumer's shelf)

E. CLINICAL FEATURES
The following characteristics are rarely present with early gastric carcinoma.
1. Weight loss—62%
2. Pain and dyspepsia—52%
3. Anemia—40-50%

4. Palpable abdominal mass—30-50%
5. Nausea and emesis—34%
6. Dysphagia—26%
7. Hematemesis is rare; melena—20%
8. Early satiety—18%
9. Ascites, pleural effusion, or lymphadenopathy from metastasis

F. DIAGNOSIS
1. Radiology
a. Barium upper GI series with air contrast—90% accurate
   (1) Evaluate for ulcer, mass, or infiltrating lesions
   (2) Sensitivity is poor if previous gastric surgery; 10-20% false-negative rate for early-stage disease
b. Abdominal CT
   (1) Delineates extent (invasion into surrounding structures) of primary tumor and presence of metastatic disease
   (2) Accuracy 80% for regional node metastases >1 cm, especially liver metastases
2. Endoscopy
a. 90-95% accurate in diagnosing advanced cancers
b. Multiple biopsies (four to six), brush and lavage cytology improve accuracy
c. <3% gastric ulcers evaluated by endoscopy/biopsy are malignant
3. Endoscopic ultrasound (EUS)
a. More accurate than CT for depth, regional nodes, and invasion of adjacent structures
   (1) Accuracy of EUS for determining T stage—80-92%
   (2) Accuracy in detecting N stage—65-87%
b. Used together with CT; ultrasound unable to identify distant metastases
c. Performed only in patients being evaluated for neoadjuvant trials
4. Laparoscopy and laparoscopic ultrasound with peritoneal washings
a. Laparoscopy may be used to determine M stage.
   (1) Suspicious lymph nodes should be biopsied.
   (2) Peritoneal spread can be directly visualized. Laparoscopic ultrasound can be used to detect small hepatic metastases.
b. Using combined diagnostic modalities allows more accurate preoperative staging and may prevent unnecessary laparotomy.

G. TNM CLASSIFICATION
1. Primary tumor (T)
   T1: Tumor limited to mucosa or submucosa
   T2: Tumor extends to subserosa
   T3: Tumor penetrates serosa
   T4: Tumor invades adjacent structures
2. Regional lymph nodes (N)
   N0: No metastases to regional lymph nodes

N1: Tumor spreading to 1-6 lymph nodes
N2: Tumor spreading to 7-15 lymph nodes
N3: Tumor spreading to >15 lymph nodes

3. Distant metastases (M)

MO: No known distant metastasis
M1: Distant metastasis present

4. Surgical results (R)

RO: No residual tumor
R1: Microscopic residual tumor
R2: Macroscopic residual tumor

H. TREATMENT

1. Lymphadenectomy (Fig. 31-1)

a. Value of extended procedure is controversial.
b. Benefit in patients with local or regional disease
c. D1—Resection of stomach, omentum, and perigastric lymph nodes
d. D2—R1 resection with en bloc resection of superior leaf of transverse mesocolon, pancreatic capsule, celiac artery lymph nodes, infraduodenal, and supraduodenal areas
e. D3—R2 resection with aortic and paraesophageal lymph node resection; also includes the spleen and pancreatic tail

2. Surgical resection

a. Indicated for both curative intent and palliation
b. Curative resection

(1) Cardia, fundus—Total gastrectomy including regional lymphadenectomy; reconstruction by Roux-en-Y esophagojejunostomy. In lesions confined to the cardia, proximal subtotal gastrectomy with lymphadenectomy is an alternative. Esophagogastrectomy is usually performed for tumors of the gastroesophageal junction.

(2) Body—Carcinomas can involve all regional nodal areas draining stomach. Options include radical subtotal or total gastrectomy. Total gastrectomy is associated with improved survival in patients with early gastric cancer.

(3) Antrum and pylorus—Subtotal gastrectomy with regional lymphadenectomy; optimal reconstruction by antecolic gastrojejunostomy. Need at least 1-cm margin in first part of duodenum and 5- to 7-cm margin in proximal stomach. Obtain frozen-section evaluation of margins prior to anastomosis.

(4) Splenectomy increases morbidity and has no survival benefit.

c. Palliative surgery

(1) 65% have advanced disease such that curative resection is not possible; performed to relieve obstruction, bleeding, or pain

(2) Subtotal gastrectomy better than gastroenterostomy bypass; good control of symptoms in 50%

(3) Endoscopic laser ablation or intubation

3. Minimally invasive resection

a. Early gastric cancer—Defined as tumors confined to mucosa and submucosa. Resection based on macroscopic appearance and depth of invasion by endoscopy and endoscopic ultrasound. Resection without need for lymphadenectomy if tumor invasion is limited to superficial submucosa, <3 cm, and minimally elevated or flat.

(1) Interventional flexible endoscope—Preferred method if tumor does not involve submucosa. Tumor injected with epinephrine, excised to level of submucosa, and laser ablated.

(2) Combined endoscopic/laparoscopic approach—Best method for posterior wall tumors involving only mucosa.

(3) Transgastrostomal endoscopic approach—Another alternative for posterior wall tumors without need for stomach insufflation. More suitable for full-thickness tumors. Resection performed through small midline incision and limited anterior gastrotomy. A short operating proctoscope is placed through the gastrotomy and resection is performed with endoscopic instruments.

(4) Laparoscopic wedge resection—Small, superficial lesions without deep submucosal invasion located on anterior wall of stomach near lesser curvature. Tumors may be resected without lymphadenectomy.

(5) Laparoscopic gastrectomy—Reserved for lesions >3 cm with deep submucosal invasion. Total gastrectomy for middle- and upper-third tumors. Distal gastrectomy is sufficient for tumors of the antrum. All gastrectomies should include omentectomy. Follow-up period at this time is too limited to compare to open resection.

b. Advanced gastric cancer—Invasion through submucosa

(1) Laparoscopic gastrectomy and extensive lymph node resection controversial because of risk of tumor spillage and less than adequate node dissection

(2) Laparoscopic gastrectomy for stages I and II tumors may be of benefit to elderly patients with coexisting medical morbidity.

4. Adjuvant therapy

a. SWOG 9008—5-fluorouracil (5-FU) plus radiation improves survival vs. observation alone

b. Advanced disease—5-FU plus epirubicin leads to significantly longer survival vs. 5-FU, doxorubicin (Adriamycin), and methotrexate.

5. Intraperitoneal chemotherapy

a. Continuous hyperthermic peritoneal perfusion with mitomycin C with or without other agents (5-FU or cisplatin)

b. Studies from Japanese literature have shown decreased peritoneal recurrence for all stages and survival advantage in stage III patients.

6. Neoadjuvant therapy

a. Unresectable and locally advanced disease

(1) Preoperative and postoperative 5-FU and cisplatin

(2) Overall curative resection significantly higher (79% vs. 61%)

(3) Down-stages advanced tumors to allow resection

31

GASTRIC TUMORS

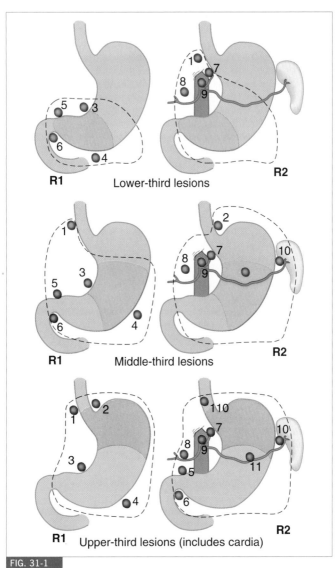

R1

Lower-third lesions

R2

R1

Middle-third lesions

R2

R1 Upper-third lesions (includes cardia)

R2

FIG. 31-1

Legend on opposite page.

b. Potentially resectable disease
  (1) Preoperative 5-FU, cisplatin, doxorubicin, and methotrexate
      followed by intraperitoneal 5-FU has shown improved response
      rates, resection rates, and median survival for resectable disease
      in phase II clinical trials.

I. PROGNOSIS (5-YEAR SURVIVAL, WESTERN SERIES)
1. Overall 5-year survival—10-21%
2. Survival of patients undergoing resection with curative intent—20-25%
3. Survival of patients with early gastric cancer (T1)—90%
4. Survival of patients with cancer of the cardia—<10%
5. Survival of patients with linitis plastica—<5%

31

II. GASTRIC LYMPHOMA

GASTRIC TUMORS

A. GENERAL
1. 5% of primary gastric malignancies; two thirds of GI lymphomas
2. 2% of all non-Hodgkin's lymphoma; most common extranodal lymphoma

B. CLINICAL PRESENTATION
1. Indistinguishable from presentation of gastric adenocarcinoma
2. Up to 42% present as emergencies (bleeding, perforation, obstruction).

C. HISTOLOGY
1. Predominant histology—Histiocytic

D. DIAGNOSIS
1. Endoscopy with biopsy and brush cytology—80% accuracy
2. Staging—Chest radiograph, chest and abdominal CT scan,
   bone marrow biopsy, pedal lymphangiography, and biopsy of enlarged
   peripheral node

FIG. 31-1—cont'd

Structures involved in lymphadenectomy. See text for explanation of illustrations.
*(Adapted from Smith JW, Shiu MH, Kelsey L, Brennan MF: Morbidity of radical
lymphadenectomy in the curative resection of gastric carcinoma. Arch Surg
126:1469, 1991.)*

1. Right cardiac	7. Left gastric artery
2. Left cardiac	8. Hepatic artery
3. Lesser curvature	9. Celiac
4. Greater curvature and short gastric	10. Splenic hilar
5. Suprapyloric (optional)	11. Splenic artery
6. Infrapyloric (optional)	110. Paraesophageal (cardia lesions)

E. TREATMENT
1. Radiation therapy achieves nearly the same remission rate as resection and with less morbidity.
2. Resection reserved for bulky lesions that produce gastric outlet obstruction followed by postoperative radiation therapy. Some centers use chemotherapy (doxorubicin and cyclophosphamide [Cytoxan]) and reserve surgery for incomplete responses or recurrent disease.

F. PROGNOSIS
1. Prognosis is better than adenocarcinoma.
2. 5-year survival—80% for stages I and II tumors

III. GASTROINTESTINAL STROMAL TUMORS (GIST)

A. CHARACTERISTICS
1. <1% of all GI malignancies
2. Previously described as leiomyoma, leiomyoblastoma, and epithelioid leiomyosarcoma
3. 94% of GISTs express *CD117* (c-*kit*)
4. Stem cell is the interstitial cell of Cajal (ICC) that variably expresses (94%) *CD117* and histologic features of smooth muscle and neural tissue.
5. Mutation of the *CD117* proto-oncogene results in ligand-independent activation of the Kit receptor tyrosine kinase and unopposed cell cycle stimulation.

B. GASTRIC GIST
1. Most common site of GIST—52%
2. 1-3% of primary gastric malignancies
3. Presentation—Usually presents as a bulky mass with central area of necrosis. Tumor develops submucosally.
4. Diagnosis—Similar work-up as other GI tumors
a. Upper GI—Smooth-lined filling defect with sharp borders
b. Endoscopic ultrasound—Hypoechoic mass contiguous with muscularis propria. Tumors >4 cm, irregular extraluminal border, echogenic foci, and cystic foci associated with malignancy
c. Endoscopy—Endophytic lesion seen on gastric wall. Overlying mucosa is usually intact; ulceration and/or bleeding not uncommon. If mucosa is intact, biopsy is not indicated.
5. Pathology
a. Heterogenous histology ranging from well-differentiated tumors (myoid, neural, or ganglionic features) to incomplete or mixed differentiation
b. Malignancy associated with tumors >10 cm, invasion of adjacent organs/structures, ≥5 mitoses/30 high-power field (HPF), missense mutation of c-*kit* gene that codes for *CD117*

6. Treatment
a. Total excision, if possible
b. Hematogenous spread common; liver frequently involved
c. No literature to support the use of chemotherapy or radiation. There are ongoing preliminary trials using imatinib (Gleevac, a platelet-derived growth factor receptor inhibitor that also inhibits c-*kit*), which may be effective as a neoadjuvant and adjuvant therapy.

7. Prognosis
a. Low grade—<9 mitoses/10 HPF associated with 100% 5- and 10-year survival
b. High grade—>10 mitoses/10 HPF associated with 25% and 13% 5- and 10-year survival, respectively
c. Overall 5-year survival—30-50%

IV. BENIGN TUMORS OF THE STOMACH

A. GENERAL
1. Overall incidence—7%
2. Most common in the antrum and body

B. CLASSIFICATION
1. Hyperplastic polyp—40%
2. Leiomyoma—40%
3. Gastric adenoma—10%
4. Heterotopic pancreas—7%

C. PRESENTATION
Presentation depends on tumor size and location and its histologic nature.

D. DIAGNOSIS
Diagnosis is by endoscopy with biopsy and brush cytology.

E. TREATMENT
Therapy depends on tumor size and type.
1. Remove symptomatic polyps endoscopically.
2. Open surgical excision is indicated for lesions >2 cm, incomplete endoscopic excision, or if malignant neoplasm is identified.

RECOMMENDED READINGS

Davila RE, Faigel DO: GI stromal tumors. Gastrointest Endosc 58:80-83, 2003.

Sipponen P, Marshall BJ: Gastritis and gastric cancer: Western countries. Gastroenterol Clin North Am 29:579-592, 2000.

Stein HJ, Sendler A, Fink U, Siewert JR: Multidisciplinary approach to esophageal and gastric cancer. Surg Clin North Am 80:659-682, 2000.

31

GASTRIC TUMORS

Peptic Ulcer Disease

Andrew W. Knott, MD

I. DUODENAL ULCER

A. PATHOGENESIS

1. Higher rates of basal and stimulated acid secretion (noted in 40% of patients with duodenal ulcers)
2. Increased number of parietal cells and enhanced gastrin sensitivity
3. Disturbances in gastric motility (accelerated gastric emptying)
4. *Helicobacter pylori*—Gram-negative organism associated with peptic ulcer disease
a. Although 70-90% of patients with duodenal ulcer and 50-70% of patients with gastric ulcer have concomitant *H. pylori* infection, not all patients with *H. pylori* have peptic ulcer disease.
b. Pathogenesis is unclear, but infection may disrupt protective mucosal layers and predispose to peptic ulcer disease.
c. Diagnosis is established with antral biopsy and *Campylobacter*-like organism (CLO) test, or serology.
d. Treatment (see section I. E) accelerates healing and decreases rate of ulcer recurrence.

B. PATHOLOGY

1. Usually located 1-2 cm distal to the pylorus, commonly on the posterior wall, but can occur anteriorly and in the pyloric channel
2. Duodenal ulcers are rarely malignant.
3. Multiple ulcers or those that occur in the second and third portions of the duodenum should raise suspicions of gastrinoma (Zollinger-Ellison syndrome [see Chap. 29]).

C. CLINICAL PRESENTATION

1. Duodenal ulcers are most common in the younger population (25-35 years old), with a male predominance.
2. Increased familial incidence
3. Risk factors—Alcohol, tobacco, aspirin, coffee, and steroids
4. Pain typically presents as a burning sensation when the stomach is empty (i.e., several hours after eating) and is relieved by ingestion of food or antacids that act to buffer acid secretion.
5. Epigastric tenderness may be present on physical exam.

D. DIAGNOSTIC STUDIES

1. Endoscopy is 95% accurate for diagnosis and may detect other lesions of the esophagus, stomach, and duodenum.
2. Upper GI series is 75-80% accurate and may reveal a duodenal lesion.

32

E. MEDICAL MANAGEMENT

Medical management should include discontinuation of risk factors and ulcerogenic medications when possible. Therapy is aimed at reducing acid output, increasing mucosal protection, and eliminating infectious agents.

1. Acid-reducing medications

a. Antacids should be given 1 hour before and 3 hours after each meal. Those containing magnesium can produce diarrhea, whereas those with aluminum can produce constipation. Antacids are associated with healing rates of 80% at 4 weeks.

b. H_2 receptor antagonists (cimetidine, ranitidine, famotidine) have ulcer healing rates that exceed 80% at 4 weeks; ≈5-10% of duodenal ulcers are refractory to H_2 receptor therapy, with recurrence rates up to 30% with long-term maintenance therapy.

c. Omeprazole (Prilosec)—Blocks the proton pump and reduces acid secretion by 99%. Promotes faster ulcer healing than other medications now available. Useful in ulcers refractory to H_2 blockers.

d. Pantoprazole (Protonix I.V.)—IV proton-pump inhibitor indicated for short-term treatment of gastroesophageal reflux disease in patients unable to tolerate oral intake

2. Cytoprotective agents

a. Sucralfate (Carafate)—Basic aluminum sucrose sulfate that dissociates in an acidic medium

  (1) The negatively charged polymerized molecule adheres to proteinaceous deposits found in the ulcer base. Binding lasts ≈6 hours with little systemic absorption.

  (2) Sucralfate requires an acidic medium and should be taken on an empty stomach. The standard dose is 1 g/h before each meal and at bedtime. Concomitant antacid use should be avoided.

  (3) Healing action may result from the physical barrier that prevents acid and pepsin from acting further on the ulcer. Healing rates (95% at 12 weeks) are similar to those of H_2 blockers.

  (4) Most common side effect is constipation (7.5%).

b. Misoprostol (Cytotec)—Prostaglandin E_2 analog that is the only treatment with demonstrated effectiveness in prophylaxis of nonsteroidal anti-inflammatory drug-induced ulcer disease

3. Treatment of infectious agents

a. Treatment of *H. pylori* infection has been shown to increase the rate of ulcer healing and decrease the rate of recurrence.

b. At present, first-line treatment of *H. pylori* infection includes 10-day course with each of the following: lansoprazole (Prevacid) 30 mg b.i.d., amoxicillin 1 g b.i.d., and clarithromycin (Biaxin) 500 mg b.i.d.

c. Alternative treatments include combinations of bismuth, metronidazole, and tetracycline for 2 weeks, but there are often side effects of nausea, vomiting, or diarrhea.

4. Following diagnosis, a course of medical therapy (most often H_2 antagonist and/or antacids) should be tried. After 6-8 weeks,

repeat diagnostic tests are indicated to document healing. Ulcers that do not heal after 8-12 weeks of medical management may require surgical intervention.

F. INDICATIONS FOR OPERATION
Only 10-20% of patients with peptic ulcer disease require surgical intervention.
1. Bleeding—Most cases stop spontaneously. Typically seen with posterior ulcers that erode into the gastroduodenal artery. Surgery is indicated for acute bleeds that require transfusion of ≥6 units of blood.
2. Perforation
a. Typically seen in anterior wall duodenal ulcers
b. Indication for surgery in up to 30% of patients
c. Classic presentation is sudden onset of severe generalized abdominal pain associated with a rigid abdomen
d. Free air under the diaphragm on upright chest radiograph is seen in 75% of cases.
3. Gastric outlet obstruction
a. Usually seen with prepyloric or duodenal ulcers; results from edema during acute phase or scarring of the duodenal bulb
b. History of emesis of undigested food shortly after eating; usually long history of peptic ulcer disease
c. Characteristic electrolyte abnormalities (hypokalemia, hypochloremia, and metabolic alkalosis)
d. Saline load test for diagnosis. Empty stomach with nasogastric tube and instill 750 mL of normal saline. Place patient in sitting position for 30 minutes, then aspirate. Test is positive if aspirate >400 mL.
4. Intractable pain despite maximal medical therapy
5. Failure of medical management

G. SURGICAL TREATMENT
1. Resections
a. Subtotal gastrectomy—Operative mortality 2-4%, recurrence rate 4%. Rarely performed today due to increased incidence of postgastrectomy syndromes.
b. Vagotomy and antrectomy—Mortality 1-3%; has the lowest recurrence (<2% at 5 years) but a high incidence of postoperative diarrhea and dumping (10-20%)
c. The most common reconstructions used after gastric resection procedures
    (1) Billroth I—Gastroduodenostomy (Fig. 32-1)
    (2) Billroth II—Gastrojejunostomy with closure of the duodenal stump (Fig. 32-2)
    (3) Roux-en-Y gastrojejunostomy (Fig. 32-3)
2. Vagotomy and drainage (pyloroplasty or gastrojejunostomy)— A mortality rate of 1% with recurrence rate of 5-10%. This procedure

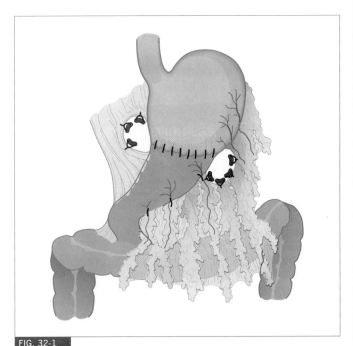

FIG. 32-1

Billroth I reconstruction.

is useful in cases of active bleeding but should be performed in conjunction with oversewing of the bleeding ulcer.

3. Selective vagotomy—The entire stomach is denervated with preservation of the celiac and hepatic branches of the vagal nerves. A drainage procedure is often required as gastric emptying is delayed.

4. Highly selective vagotomy/parietal cell vagotomy

a. Only the parietal cell mass is denervated.

b. As the motor function of the antrum and pylorus remains intact, no drainage procedure is needed; very low incidence of postgastrectomy syndromes

c. Results are highly dependent on operator experience. Mortality rate is 0.1-0.3%, with long-term recurrence rate of 15%.

d. Contraindicated for prepyloric or pyloric channel ulcers—Higher recurrence rate due to inadequate isolation of all parietal cell innervations

5. Omental (Graham) patch for perforated ulcer may be an adequate procedure in patients without prior history of chronic ulcer disease, since 30% have no further manifestation of their disease.

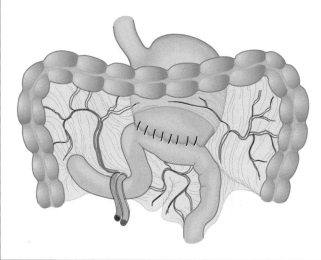

FIG. 32-2
Retrocolic Billroth II reconstruction.

H. POSTOPERATIVE COMPLICATIONS
1. Recurrent ulcers
a. More common with duodenal ulcers
b. Usually occur at the anastomotic site (intestinal side) within the first 2 years after surgery ("marginal ulcer")
c. Most commonly caused by incomplete vagotomy
d. Can be treated with medical management but should be re-explored if these measures fail
2. Early postprandial dumping—Most common postgastrectomy complication
a. Rapid emptying of hyperosmolar chyme causes intravascular fluid shifts, resulting in gastrointestinal and vasomotor symptoms.
b. Symptoms of abdominal pain and fullness, vomiting, diarrhea, flushing, palpitations, and dizziness occur within 30 minutes of a meal.
c. Symptoms are relieved with supine position and prevented by frequent, small, high-protein and low-carbohydrate meals.
d. If surgical intervention is required, an antiperistaltic jejunal loop between the gastric remnant and the small intestine or a Roux-en-Y loop may be successful.
3. Late postprandial dumping/reactive hypoglycemia.
a. Large amounts of carbohydrates stimulate insulin release that produces hypoglycemia several hours after eating.

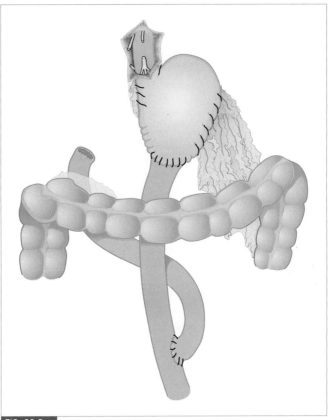

FIG. 32-3
Roux-en-Y gastrojejunostomy.

b. Symptoms include tachycardia, dizziness, and diaphoresis 1.5-2 hours after a meal.
c. Treatment consists of low-carbohydrate meals with the ingestion of carbohydrates once symptoms begin.
d. Surgical intervention consists of an antiperistaltic jejunal loop to delay gastric emptying.
4. **Afferent loop syndrome**
a. Postprandial distention, nausea, and right upper quadrant pain relieved by bilious emesis
b. Acute form may be related to postoperative edema at the gastrojejunostomy, obstructing the afferent loop. Hyperamylasemia is

common secondary to reflux of the duodenal contents into the pancreatic duct.

c. Chronic form is caused by intermittent obstruction of a long afferent limb and results in bilious emesis without the presence of food.

d. Operative correction of chronic form involves conversion to a Roux-en-Y gastrojejunostomy.

5. Postvagotomy diarrhea is typically episodic and may occur in up to 30% of patients. First-line therapy includes constipating agents or cholestyramine to bind bile acids. Operative intervention using a reversed jejunal segment is rarely necessary.

6. Bile reflux gastritis presents as epigastric pain often associated with nausea and vomiting. Treatment is initiated with H_2 blockers or sucralfate. Surgical options include conversion to a Roux-en-Y or Tanner-19 gastrojejunostomy.

II. GIANT DUODENAL ULCERS

A. PATHOGENESIS
1. Defined as a duodenal ulcer >2cm that is usually full thickness and occupies most of the duodenal bulb
2. Although typical duodenal ulcers have a high association with *H. pylori* infection (70-90%), ≈40% of patients with giant duodenal ulcer are *H. pylori* positive.

B. CLINICAL PRESENTATION
1. Most common in men 55 to 60 years old with long-standing history of ulcer symptoms
2. Symptoms are similar to typical duodenal ulcer disease. However, most patients present with pain and GI hemorrhage.
3. Obstructive symptoms more common with giant duodenal ulcer because of chronic inflammation, scarring, and edema.

C. DIAGNOSTIC STUDIES
1. Upper GI series—Findings are subtle radiographically. Lack of normal peristalsis, loss of mucosal pattern, air-fluid levels within the ulcer crater, and constant size and appearance of the ulcer during the study are suggestive of giant duodenal ulcers.
2. Endoscopy—Now the gold standard for diagnosis. Findings include a widened, edematous pyloric sphincter with immobile pylorus. The ulcer itself usually has necrotic slough with a visible vessel at the base.

D. MANAGEMENT
1. Medical management
a. 70% can be treated successfully with omeprazole 40 mg/day.
b. Treat *H. pylori* infection if positive

2. Surgical management

a. Indications for operation are the same as for duodenal ulcer.

b. In a recent series from the University of Cincinnati, stigmata of bleeding and negative *H. pylori* status were associated with a higher incidence of requiring surgical intervention (63%).

III. GASTRIC ULCERS

A. PATHOGENESIS

1. Type I—Most common and present as a solitary ulcer on the lesser curve

a. Caused by the reflux of duodenal contents through an incompetent pylorus, resulting in atrophic gastritis

b. Ulceration occurs at the junction of acid-secreting and nonacid-secreting mucosa.

c. Most clearly related to defects in mucosal resistance. Nearly one third of gastric ulcers are related to aspirin or nonsteroidal drugs.

2. Type II—Associated with concomitant duodenal ulcer

3. Type III—Prepyloric ulcers (located within 2 cm of the pylorus) are similar in etiology to duodenal ulcers.

B. PRESENTATION AND DIAGNOSIS

1. Gastric ulcers are less common than duodenal ulcers and occur in older patients.

2. Pain is the most common complaint, but there is less correlation with meals. The pain may actually be exacerbated by food. Completely asymptomatic lesions are also common.

3. 5-10% of gastric ulcers are malignant, with those >2 cm in size having a higher rate of malignancy.

4. Endoscopy and radiographic studies are used to confirm the diagnosis. Endoscopy is preferred, because biopsies can be taken at the time of diagnosis to distinguish benign from malignant ulcers. All gastric ulcers should be biopsied to rule out malignancy.

C. MEDICAL TREATMENT

1. Medical treatment is similar to that of duodenal ulcers except that antacids are less effective.

2. Failure to heal suggests malignancy.

3. Complications of gastric ulcer are more frequent than duodenal ulcer; relapse rates are as high as 60% within 2 years.

D. INDICATIONS FOR SURGERY

1. Failure to heal after 3 months of conservative therapy

2. Dysplasia or carcinoma

3. Recurrence

4. Poor medical compliance

5. Complications—Bleeding (>6 units acutely or recurrent), perforation

E. SURGICAL INTERVENTION

1. Type I ulcers are treated with distal gastrectomy (antrectomy) to include the ulcer without concomitant vagal section. Cure rate is about 95%.
2. Type II and type III ulcers should be treated as duodenal ulcers.
3. Proximal ulcer may be treated with local excision and closure; consider antrectomy or drainage if gastric stasis is a contributing factor.

IV. STRESS GASTRITIS

A. PATHOLOGY

1. Occurs in the setting of severe and prolonged physiologic stress, e.g., critically ill patients with severe trauma, burns, acute respiratory distress syndrome, renal failure, and sepsis.
2. Multiple superficial punctate lesions arise acutely in the proximal stomach. In 20% of patients these can progress and coalesce to form multiple hemorrhagic ulcerations (acute hemorrhagic gastritis).
3. Etiology appears to be a defect in mucosal membrane protection, because stress gastritis is not associated with acid hypersecretion.
4. Patients should receive stress ulcer prophylaxis if one primary or two secondary risk factors are present.

a. Primary (one or more)
   (1) Coagulopathy (one or more of the following: platelets <50,000, INR >1.5, partial thromboplastin time >2 times normal value)
   (2) Mechanical ventilation >48 hours
   (3) History of previous upper GI bleed or pelvic ulcer disease
   (4) Solid organ transplantation
   (5) Thermal injury >35% total body surface area

b. Secondary (two or more)
   (1) Severe head injury (Glasgow Coma Scale score <10 with or without spinal cord injury)
   (2) Shock and hypotension
   (3) Sepsis
   (4) Organ failure (renal or hepatic)
   (5) Major trauma and/or surgery
   (6) Acute or chronic steroid use

B. DIAGNOSIS

Diagnosis is established with endoscopy.

C. TREATMENT

1. The most effective form of treatment is prevention. Maintain intraluminal pH >4.5 with H_2 blockers or antacids. Sucralfate is also an effective prophylactic agent.
2. In severe hemorrhage endoscopy with coagulation, intra-arterial vasopressin or embolization can be used (see Chap. 20).

3. Surgical procedures used only if nonoperative management fails; associated with high rebleeding rates (25-50%) and mortality (30-40%)
a. Oversewing of bleeding points and a vagotomy and drainage
b. Vagotomy and drainage for bleeding from the distal stomach is preferred to prevent rebleeding.
c. Hemorrhage not controlled by a. or b. may require near-total gastrectomy.

V. ZOLLINGER-ELLISON SYNDROME

See Chapter 29.

Inflammatory Bowel Disease

KuoJen Tsao, MD

I. INFLAMMATORY BOWEL DISEASE (IBD)

The term *inflammatory bowel disease* refers to the following two diseases, which are distinctly different but difficult to differentiate clinically (Table 33-1).

A. ULCERATIVE COLITIS (UC)
UC is a diffuse inflammatory disease limited to the *mucosa* of the colon and rectum. Operative therapy is almost always curative.

B. CROHN'S DISEASE (CD)
CD is a chronic, relapsing, *transmural*, usually segmental, and often granulomatous inflammatory disorder that can involve any portion of the GI tract. Surgical intervention is reserved for the treatment of complications or intractable disease.

33

II. ULCERATIVE COLITIS

A. ETIOLOGY
Unknown, multifactorial, multiple theories:
1. Infectious—Viral, bacterial, mycobacterial
2. Immunologic—Possible defect in regulation of mucosal immunity with poorly regulated inflammatory response to exogenous antigens
3. Autoimmune
4. Genetic—Increase in whites, females, and Jews (two to four times higher risk); familial disposition; association with certain HLA phenotypes
5. Environmental—Increased in urban dwellers

B. PATHOPHYSIOLOGY
UC results from an increased production of mucosal immunoglobulins in response to initiating antigens, recruitment of inflammatory cells, and altered mucosal function and permeability.

C. EPIDEMIOLOGY
1. Age of onset—Bimodal, 15-30 and 50-70 years of age
2. Females > males (1.3:1)
3. Family history in 10-20% of cases
4. Incidence—5-12/100,000
5. Prevalence—400,000
6. Smoking—Suggested to be protective

D. CLINICAL MANIFESTATIONS AND DIAGNOSIS
1. Signs and symptoms

TABLE 33-1

COMPARISON OF THE TWO TYPES OF INFLAMMATORY BOWEL DISEASE

Characteristic	Ulcerative Colitis	Crohn's Disease
Epidemiology	Bimodal: 15-30/50-70 years of age	20-40 years of age
	Females > males	Females = males
Clinical presentation	Bloody diarrhea	Nonbloody diarrhea
	Rectal bleeding	Colicky abdominal pain
	Tenesmus	Anorectal lesions
	Weight loss	Weight loss
	Abdominal pain	Intermittent periods of active disease
Gross pathology	Continuous disease	Skip lesions
	Friable mucosa	Longitudinal fissures
	Pseudopolyps	Focal strictures
	Stovepipe narrowing	Bowel wall thickening
	Granular irregularity	"Cobblestoning"
Microscopic pathology	Mucosal	Transmural
	Loss of goblet cells	Granulomas
	Crypt abscesses	Mesenteric adenopathy
	Plasma cell infiltrate	—
GI distribution	Continuous from anus	30% small bowel only
	<5% rectal sparing	55% small bowel and colon
	No skip lesions	15% colon only
	10% terminal ileitis	30% rectal involvement
	—	20% skip lesions
	—	50% perianal disease
Complications	Toxic megacolon	Abscesses
	Perforations	Fistulas
	Sclerosing cholangitis	Intestinal obstruction
	Extraintestinal less common	Extraintestinal more common
	Malnutrition	—
	Colon cancer	—
Surgical intervention	Used for cure	Reserved for complications, not curative
Mortality	2-3% elective surgery	3-6% elective surgery
	8-25% emergent surgery	—

a. Ranked by frequency
　(1) Most common—Diarrhea, rectal bleeding, tenesmus
　(2) Less common—Abdominal pain, weight loss, fever, malnutrition
　(3) Rare—Vomiting, perianal disease, abdominal mass
b. Onset may be insidious, or acute and fulminant (15%)
c. Extraintestinal manifestations (see section II. E. 1)
2. Disease distribution
a. Confined to colon and rectum, no skip lesions

b. Almost always involves the rectum (95%)

c. "Backwash" ileitis (10%), resolves after colonic resection

3. Laboratory findings

a. Anemia, leukocytosis, elevated erythrocyte sedimentation rate

b. Negative stool cultures for ova and parasites

c. Severe disease—Hypoalbuminemia, dehydration, electrolytes/vitamin depletion, steatorrhea

4. Serological markers—Perinuclear antineutrophil cytoplasmic antibody (pANCA)

a. Expressed in 60-80% of patients

b. Only 20-30% of patients with CD

c. <5% in normal patients

5. Radiographic findings

a. Plain abdominal films—Follow colonic size during acute phase to exclude toxic megacolon; free air for perforation

b. Barium enema—Mucosal irregularity, "collar-button" ulcers, and pseudopolyps; chronic disease characterized by loss of haustrations and by colonic shortening and narrowing; ileum typically spared; strictures are late manifestations and should imply malignancy

6. Endoscopy

a. Essential for diagnosis and extent of disease

b. 90% accurate with biopsy to diagnose IBD

c. 10% failure rate in differentiating IBD during fulminant colitis

d. Uniform disease pattern

e. Findings

    (1) Early—Edema, confluent erythema, rectal involvement

    (2) Moderate—Granularity, contact bleeding

    (3) Late—Discrete ulcers, pus

f. Biopsy findings—Mucosal depletion of goblet cells, inflammatory polyps in healing stage, crypt abscess

g. Colonoscopy—Valuable for specific investigations (stricture, malignancy) and cancer surveillance

E. COMPLICATIONS

1. Extraintestinal manifestations (1/3 of cases)

a. Skin—Erythema nodosum, pyoderma gangrenosum, erythema multiforme, aphthous ulcers, stomatas

b. Eyes—Conjunctivitis, iritis (uveitis), episcleritis

c. Joints—Arthritis, sacroiliitis, ankylosing spondylitis (associated with HLA-B27 antigen in conjunction with IBD)

d. Hepatobiliary—Fatty liver, pericholangitis, hepatitis, bile duct carcinoma, sclerosing cholangitis

2. Anorectal disease—Hemorrhoids, anal fissures, rectal strictures

3. Toxic colitis with or without megacolon—10% of patients

a. Leading cause of death in University of Cincinnati Medical Center; 40% of cases are fatal

33

INFLAMMATORY BOWEL DISEASE

b. May be initial presentation of UC in 30% of cases

c. Highest risk for perforation with initial attack of toxic megacolon

d. Pathology—Inflammation extends into muscle layers of bowel wall; perforation causing localized abscess or generalized peritonitis

e. Etiology—Many theories including paralysis of smooth muscle by inflammatory infiltration, destruction of myenteric plexus between circular and longitudinal muscles, destruction of Auerbach's plexus with preservation of Meissner's plexus, increase production of nitric oxide, leading to smooth muscle relaxation.

f. Clinical findings—Fever, abrupt onset of bloody diarrhea, abdominal pain, nausea, vomiting, abdominal distention, systemic toxicity

g. Radiographic findings—Transverse colon 8-10 cm in diameter on plain abdominal films for megacolon

h. Mortality with perforation 40%; only 2-8% for surgery before perforation

i. Treatment

    (1) IV fluids and electrolyte resuscitation

    (2) NPO, nasogastric tube decompression

    (3) Broad-spectrum parenteral antibiotics

    (4) Consider total parenteral nutrition (TPN)

    (5) Medical treatment includes high-dose steroids (hydrocortisone 100 mg q 6 h, methylprednisolone 16-20 mg q 8 h, or prednisone 20 mg q 8 h) and/or immunosuppression (cyclosporine, 6-mercaptopurine).

    (6) Surgery indicated if conservative therapy fails after 2-5 days. Subtotal colectomy, Brooke ileostomy, and Hartmann closure of rectum is standard procedure in the setting of acute disease; reserve proctectomy and ileoanal anastomosis for when patient is stable

    (7) Emergent surgery indicated in free perforation, peritonitis, or massive hemorrhage

4. **Massive hemorrhage—Can occur in toxic colitis. Treatment is subtotal colectomy, Brooke ileostomy, and Hartmann closure of rectum; allows for future sphincter-sparing operation.**

5. **Carcinoma of colon/rectum**

a. Begins to appear after 5-10 years of active disease. More common in patients with initial colitis prior to age 25 years.

b. Five times normal risk, related to severity of disease

c. Incidence

    (1) 10 years—2-5%

    (2) 20 years—20%

    (3) 1-2% per year if disease present >10 years

d. Predictors—Dysplasia (if severe, then 10% chance of invasive carcinoma at distant site), extent of colitis, persistent disease

e. Surveillance with colonoscopy

    (1) After 7 years for patients with pancolitis

    (2) After 10 years for patients with left-sided disease

    (3) Then, q 1-2 years

      (4) Must include random segmental biopsies as well as biopsies of suspicious lesions

f. Strictures—Must rule out neoplasm

g. Short-term prognosis is worse than with idiopathic colon cancer; long-term (5-year) survival is equivalent.

6. Malnutrition—With acute, severe episodes; growth retardation in children

F. MEDICAL MANAGEMENT

1. Aminosalicylates—Sulfasalazine, mesalamine, olsalazine, balsalazide

a. Sulfasalazine—Metabolized by bacteria to 5-aminosalicylic acid (5-ASA), the active component; and sulfapyridine, which is responsible for major side effects

      (1) Conjugated to prevent small bowel absorption

      (2) Good for sustaining remission and mild/moderate disease

      (3) Enemas may be used for distal colitis and proctitis.

b. Proposed mechanisms

      (1) Inhibit prostaglandins and leukotriene production

      (2) Inhibit bacterial peptide-induced neutrophil chemotaxis

      (3) Scavenge reactive oxygen metabolites

c. Side effects—Dose-related toxicity

      (1) Oligospermia

      (2) Inhibits folate absorption

      (3) Hemolytic anemia

      (4) Nausea, vomiting, headache, abdominal discomfort

      (5) Allergic hypersensitivity—10-15%

d. Mesalamine

      (1) Fewer side effects than sulfasalazine at comparable doses

      (2) Various formulations allow different distribution of delivery.

         (a) Rowasa, Canasa—Rectal

         (b) Asacol, Salofak—pH dependent, distal ileum and colon

         (c) Pentasa—Time release, jejunum to colon

2. Corticosteroids

a. Used to control acute inflammatory activity. Does not prevent relapse. No proven maintenance benefit.

b. IV steroids—For severe or fulminant disease

      (1) Hydrocortisone 100-300 mg/day

      (2) Prednisolone 20-80 mg/day

      (3) ACTH 20-40 units/day as continuous infusion

c. Oral steroids—Prednisone 20-60 mg/day, for less severe or improving disease

d. Enemas or topical for distal colitis or proctitis

3. Immunosuppressives

a. Azathioprine (6-mercaptopurine, active metabolite)

      (1) Used for refractory disease or disease in remission. Allows gradual tapering of corticosteroids. May be required up to 6 months.

      (2) Possible increased risk of lymphoma

33

INFLAMMATORY BOWEL DISEASE

       (3) Side effects—Bone marrow suppression, hepatotoxicity, pancreatitis

       (4) Unknown mechanism of action. Suspected to suppress T-cell activity, thus prolonging therapeutic response.

b. Cyclosporine

       (1) Used in severe, acute toxic colitis otherwise needing urgent proctocolectomy refractory to high-dose corticosteroids

       (2) Presumed to block lymphocyte activation

       (3) Short-term, can be controlled; up to 50% eventually need proctocolectomy within a year.

G. SURGICAL MANAGEMENT

1. Indications

a. Severe, acute attack unresponsive to intense medical therapy

b. Colonic complications—Perforation, toxic megacolon, massive hemorrhage, obstruction

c. Chronic, debilitating disease

d. Carcinoma or high risk for carcinoma

e. Growth failure in children

f. Severe extraintestinal complications (see section II. E. 1)

2. Surgical procedures (total proctocolectomy is curative)

a. Total abdominal colectomy, mucosal proctectomy, ileal reservoir, and ileoanal anastomosis

       (1) Curative procedure

       (2) Sphincter-sparing procedure preserves continence

       (3) Failure rate—10%

       (4) 4-8 bowel movements per day

       (5) Minimal bladder and sexual dysfunction

       (6) Disadvantages include pouch fistulas, frequent soiling, nighttime incontinence, pouchitis, anal excoriation and risk of intestinal obstruction.

       (7) Contraindications include CD, diarrhea, and distal rectal cancer.

       (8) Pouch created from 30 cm of terminal ileum with anastomosis to anus

         (a) J pouch—Simple

         (b) S pouch—Larger capacity with less tension to anus

b. Total proctocolectomy with standard (Brooke) ileostomy

       (1) Until recently was the gold standard operation; now replaced by sphincter-sparing operations to preserve continence

       (2) One-step operation

       (3) Curative procedure, no contraindications

       (4) Disadvantages include incontinence and ileostomy, and 10-15% of male patients develop impotence.

       (5) Complications include stoma revisions, perineal wound infections, small bowel obstructions, bladder dysfunction, and sexual dysfunction.

       (6) Must empty ostomy bag four to eight times per day

       (7) 1-3% elective operative mortality

c. Total proctocolectomy with continent (Kock) ileostomy
  (1) Avoid need for conventional ileostomy/appliances
  (2) Major problem—Stability of continent nipple valve within ileal reservoir (40-50% require reoperation)
  (3) Use is now limited to patients who strongly desire continence-restoring procedure following total proctocolectomy.
d. Total abdominal colectomy with ileostomy, rectal preservation
  (1) Reserved for emergency procedures (hemorrhage, toxic megacolon) to decrease operative morbidity and mortality (3-10%)
  (2) Mucosal proctectomy and ileoanal anastomosis can be subsequently performed to control proctitis, reduce cancer risk, and preserve continence.

H. PROGNOSIS
1. Mortality
a. 5% death rate over 10 years (pancolitis)
b. Elective surgery—2%
c. Emergent surgery—8-15%
2. Left-sided colitis and pancolitis
a. Acute intermittent—60%; most relapses within first year
b. Chronic, unremitting—20%
c. Fulminant—10%
d. Up to 50% require colectomy in first 10 years
3. Ulcerative proctitis
a. ≈20% develop left-sided colitis
b. Only 2-15% reported to progress to pancolitis

III. CROHN'S DISEASE

A. ETIOLOGY
The etiology of CD is unknown, although many theories exist.
1. Infectious
a. Typical *Mycobacteria (Mycobacteria paratuberculosis, Mycobacteria avium)*
b. Measles virus
c. *Yersinia enterocolitica*
2. Genetic
a. *NOD2*—Chromosome 16
b. 15-20% of patients have a positive family history of IBD
3. Environmental—Temperate climates
4. Smoking—Two to four times increased risk, increased relapse

B. EPIDEMIOLOGY
1. Bimodal—Peak incidence between 20-30 years of age, late peak ages 50-60 years.
2. Equal sex distribution

33

INFLAMMATORY BOWEL DISEASE

3. Incidence—3-6/100,000
4. Prevalence—400,000
5. Highest incidence—North America and northern Europe

C. CLINICAL MANIFESTATIONS AND DIAGNOSIS

1. Diagnosis takes longer than UC due to nonspecific, indolent symptoms. Mean time from onset to diagnosis is 35 months.
2. Chronic granulomatous disease with intermittent periods of exacerbation and remission
3. Early superficial aphthous ulcers progress to transmural inflammation
a. Linear ulcers produce transverse clefts and sinuses ("cobblestoning")
b. Submucosal/muscularis inflammation causes bowel lumen narrowing
4. Signs and symptoms
a. Diarrhea—90% of cases, usually nonbloody
b. Recurrent abdominal pain—Mild colicky pain, often initiated by meals, relieved by defecation
c. Abdominal distention, flatulence
d. Fever, malaise
e. Anorectal lesions—Chronic recurrent or nonhealing anal fissures, ulcers, complex anal fistulas, perirectal abscesses (may precede bowel involvement)
f. Malnutrition—Protein-losing enteropathy, steatorrhea, mineral and vitamin deficiencies, growth retardation
g. Acute onset—Acute appendicitis-like presentation due to acute inflammation of the distal ileum; only 15% of these patients with isolated terminal ileitis develop chronic CD
h. Extraintestinal manifestations in 30% (see section II. E. 1)
5. Disease distribution
a. May involve any segment of entire GI tract (from mouth to anus)
b. Distal ileum is most frequently involved
c. Skip regions—12-35%
d. Small bowel only—30%
e. Distal ileum and colon—55%
f. Colon only—15%
6. Laboratory findings
a. Anemia—Iron or vitamin B_{12}/folate deficiency
b. Hypoalbuminemia or steatorrhea
c. Tests of bowel function (D-xylose absorption, bile acid breath test) are abnormal with extensive disease.
7. Serologic markers—Anti-*Saccharomyces cerevisiae* antibody (ASCA)
a. 60% of patients with CD
b. 5% of patients with UC
c. <5% in normal population
8. Radiographic findings
a. Upper GI with small bowel follow-through or enteroclysis—If small bowel disease is suspected

      (1) Narrowed terminal ileum (Kantor's [string] sign)
      (2) Fistulas
      (3) Nodules, sinuses, clefts, linear ulcers
  b. Barium enema—Thickened bowel wall, longitudinal ulcers, transverse fissures, cobblestone formation, and rectal sparing. Terminal ileum, demonstrated by reflux from barium enema, may contain strictures (string sign).
  c. Abdominal CT—Intra-abdominal abscesses

9. **Endoscopy**
  a. Normal rectum in 40-50% of patients with colonic disease. Random biopsies are required because grossly normal-appearing rectum may reveal histologic disease.
  b. Characteristic lesions
      (1) Aphthous ulcers
      (2) Mucosal ulcerations
      (3) Anal fissures
      (4) Cobblestoning
  c. Segmental lesions

10. **Intraoperative findings**
  a. Creeping of mesenteric fat toward antimesenteric border
  b. Serosal and mesenteric inflammation
  c. Bowel wall thickening, strictures
  d. Shortening of bowel and mesentery
  e. Mesenteric lymphadenopathy
  f. Inflammatory masses, abscesses, adherent bowel loops

D. COMPLICATIONS
  1. Intestinal obstruction
  2. Abscess formation
  3. Fistula—Internal and external
  4. Anorectal lesions—Abscess, fistula, fissures
  5. Free perforation and hemorrhage—Rare
  6. Carcinoma—Less common than UC
  7. Toxic megacolon—Occurs in 5% of colonic involvement, responds to medical therapy better than UC
  8. Extraintestinal (see section II. E. 1)
  a. More common with colonic involvement
  b. Urinary—Cystitis, calculi (oxalate), ureteral obstruction

E. MEDICAL MANAGEMENT
For additional discussion on medical management, also see section II. F.
  1. Aminosalicylates—Oral agent (mesalamine) used for mild to moderate disease
  2. Corticosteroids—Used in acute exacerbations, may be useful in combination with sulfasalazine to maintain short-term remission.

33

INFLAMMATORY BOWEL DISEASE

Budesonide is a U.S. Food and Drug Administration–approved agent for distal ileitis and right-sided colonic disease; 90% first-pass metabolism results in fewer systemic effects.

3. Immunosuppressants

a. Azathioprine, 6-mercaptopurine, cyclosporine—Useful during remission to decrease steroid requirements, usually added after 7-10 days of high-dose IV steroids. May be required for 2-3 months.

b. Methotrexate—Used in steroid-dependent active disease and to maintain remission

4. Metronidazole—May help anal complications; requires long-term use

5. Supportive measures

a. NPO, IV fluids, nasogastric decompression

b. TPN—Fistulas and malnutrition

c. Low-residue/high-protein diet for mild disease

F. SURGICAL MANAGEMENT

Surgical intervention is eventually necessary in 70-75% of cases over the lifetime of the disease. It is reserved for treating complications only.

1. Indications for surgery

a. Small bowel obstruction—Indication in 50% of surgical cases

b. Fistula

c. Abscess

d. Hemorrhage

e. Perianal disease—Unresponsive to medical therapy

f. Disease intractable to medical management

g. Failure to thrive—Chronic malnutrition, growth retardation

h. Toxic megacolon

2. Surgical procedures—Not curative

a. Conservative resection of diseased or symptomatic bowel segment, primary end-to-end anastomosis

   (1) Only resect grossly diseased bowel with small "normal-appearing" margins; unnecessary to get histologically free margins for anastomosis

   (2) Distal ileum and cecal resection with ileocolostomy is a common procedure.

   (3) 60% recurrence in long-term follow-up

b. Stricturoplasty—Relieves obstruction in chronically scarred bowel without resection; especially useful for multiple symptomatic strictures

c. Exclusion bypass—Higher incidence of recurrence and carcinoma; may be indicated in the following

   (1) Bypass unresectable inflammatory mass

   (2) Gastroduodenal CD

   (3) Multiple, extensive skip lesions

d. Continent (Kock) ileostomy and mucosal proctectomy procedures are contraindicated.

G. PROGNOSIS
In chronic disease, cure is not possible by either medical or surgical therapy.

1. Medical therapy—Does not avoid surgery

2. Recurrence rates 10 years after initial operation

a. Ileocolic disease—50%

b. Small bowel disease—50%

c. Colonic disease—40-50%

3. Reoperation rates at 5 years

a. Primary resection—20%

b. Bypass—50%

4. 80-85% of patients who require surgery lead normal lives.

5. Mortality rate—15% at 30 years

33

RECOMMENDED READINGS

Berg DF, Bahadursingh AM, Kaminski DL, Longo WE: Acute surgical emergencies in inflammatory bowel disease. Am J Surg 184:45-51, 2002.

Pikarsky A, Zmora O, Wexner SD: Immunosuppressants and operation in ulcerative colitis. J Am Coll Surg 195:251-260, 2002.

Podolsky DK: Inflammatory bowel disease. N Engl J Med 347:417-429, 2002.

INFLAMMATORY BOWEL DISEASE

Appendicitis

Russell J. Juno, MD

I. EPIDEMIOLOGY

A. GENERAL
1. Appendicitis is the most common cause of acute abdomen requiring surgery, with ≈300,000 cases/year in the United States and affecting 7% of the population.
2. Peak incidence is in adolescents and young adults, with a slight male predominance.
3. The incidence of perforation is 12%.
4. Overall incidence of normal appendices after appendectomy is 10-15%.

34

B. MORBIDITY AND MORTALITY
1. Overall mortality is 0.1% for nonperforated cases and 5% for perforated cases.
2. Infants and elderly have a much higher morbidity and mortality—≈85% for infants and 65-75% for elderly adults owing to an increase in the perforation rate

II. PATHOPHYSIOLOGY

A. GENERAL
1. Obstruction of the appendiceal lumen is thought to be the initiating event in two thirds of cases, most commonly secondary to a fecalith in adults and lymphoid hyperplasia in children.
2. With continued mucosal secretion, luminal pressure rises and eventually exceeds capillary venous and lymphatic pressures, causing venous infarction in watershed areas (middle and proximal antimesenteric regions).
3. Bacterial overgrowth occurs in the inspissated mucus.
4. Polymicrobial infection with anaerobes > aerobes 3:1
5. *Escherichia coli*, *Bacteroides fragilis*, *Pseudomonas* spp present in 80%, 70%, and 40%, respectively.

B. COMPLICATIONS
1. Worsening edema, high luminal pressure, and bacterial proliferation lead to occlusion of arterial blood flow and gangrenous appendicitis
2. Transmural necrosis and bacterial penetration into the appendiceal wall is associated with perforation, which may be either walled off by omentum or spread throughout the abdomen, inducing diffuse peritonitis
3. Overall incidence is 12% for perforation.

III. PRESENTATION

A. HISTORY
  1. Patient may give history of indigestion lasting hours to 1 day prior to a painful attack.
  2. Pain usually begins as vague midabdominal discomfort, due to appendiceal distention and referred pain along lesser splanchnics.
  3. Anorexia and nausea occur almost uniformly *after* the pain. Almost all adults have anorexia, whereas children with appendicitis may remain hungry.
  4. Pain localizes to the right lower quadrant (RLQ) as the parietal peritoneum in that area becomes irritated.
  a. If the appendix lies in the pelvis or retrocecal area, the location of the pain (and tenderness) will change accordingly with peritoneal irritation.
  b. If perforation occurs, diffuse peritonitis ensues with pain throughout the abdomen.
  5. Patients may have constipation, diarrhea, or no change in bowel habits.
  a. A history of late onset of loose stools may indicate pelvic peritonitis after perforation.

B. PHYSICAL EXAMINATION
  1. Fever may be present, but the temperature is rarely higher than 38°C (101°F), unless perforation and/or abscess formation has occurred.
  2. When appendix lies anteriorly, tenderness is present at McBurney's point (one third the distance between the anterior superior iliac spine and the umbilicus).
  3. Abdominal wall muscular rigidity may be present.
  4. With peritoneal irritation, guarding, rebound, and indirect rebound tenderness may occur.
  5. Rovsing's sign is pain in RLQ with palpation of the left lower quadrant.
  6. Cutaneous hyperesthesia may be present in distribution of T10-T12 in the RLQ and is tested by rolling the skin between the thumb and forefinger, which normally does not cause pain.
  7. Rectal exam elicits suprapubic pain if the inflamed appendix tip lies in the pelvis.
  8. The psoas sign is pain occurring with extension of the right thigh and indicates an irritative focus overlying that muscle.
  9. The obturator sign is pain with passive internal rotation of the flexed right thigh and indicates inflammation overlying that muscle.
  10. Males may have pain in the right, left, or both testicles, because both are innervated by T10.

C. LAB AND RADIOLOGIC FINDINGS
  1. The diagnosis of appendicitis is largely a clinical one; however, some objective data may be useful.

2. White blood cell (WBC) elevation from 10,000 to 18,000/mm^3 is expected, with a left shift on differential.
a. WBC count is normal in approximately 10% of patients.
b. Patients who are HIV positive have the same symptoms, but usually the WBC count is normal.
3. Urinalysis may be normal or reveal few red blood cells (RBCs) or WBCs only, especially in retrocecal or pelvic appendix.
4. Abdominal radiographs are usually nonspecific but may show a fecalith in the RLQ, loss of the right psoas shadow (fat pad) paucity of RLQ gas, and/or a few dilated loops of bowel.
5. Barium enema, though not specific, may rule out appendicitis if normal filling of the appendix occurs.
a. Mass effect on the cecum or terminal ileum is seen with appendicitis.
b. 10% false-negative rate
6. CT scan has been shown to be superior to ultrasound in diagnosing acute appendicitis in both pediatric and adult populations.
a. Both are helpful when pain is associated with an RLQ mass to rule out phlegmon vs. abscess.
b. CT scan should also be used to aid diagnosis in patients with atypical presentation.

IV. DIFFERENTIAL DIAGNOSIS

A. **GASTROENTERITIS**

B. **DIVERTICULITIS (ADULTS)**

C. **ACUTE MESENTERIC ADENITIS (CHILDREN)**

D. **MECKEL'S DIVERTICULITIS**

E. **INTUSSUSCEPTION (INFANTS AND CHILDREN)**

F. **REGIONAL ENTERITIS**

G. **PERFORATED PEPTIC ULCER**

H. **PERFORATING CARCINOMA OF CECUM OR SIGMOID COLON**

I. **URINARY TRACT INFECTION**

J. **URETERAL STONE**

K. **GYNECOLOGIC DISEASE (E.G., PELVIC INFLAMMATORY DISEASE, ECTOPIC PREGNANCY, OVARIAN CYST)**

34

APPENDICITIS

L. MALE UROLOGIC DISEASE (E.G., TESTICULAR TORSION, EPIDIDYMITIS)

M. EPIPLOIC APPENDAGITIS

N. SPONTANEOUS BACTERIAL PERITONITIS

O. HENOCH-SCHÖNLEIN PURPURA

P. YERSINIOSIS

V. COMPLICATIONS

A. PERFORATION
1. Occurs more in patients >50 and <10 years of age
2. Associated with more diffuse pain *after* localized tenderness
   a. Initially pain may be relieved, followed by peritonitis
3. Uncommon for perforation to occur within 24 hours of onset of abdominal pain

B. PERITONITIS
1. Occurs after perforation
2. Localized peritonitis refers to peritonitis that is microscopic and contained by surrounding viscera or omentum, whereas generalized peritonitis refers to gross spillage into the peritoneal cavity
3. Associated with high fever and may lead to sepsis

C. ABSCESS
1. Associated with an RLQ mass on physical exam
2. CT scan should be performed along with percutaneous drainage.
3. The patient is then treated with antibiotics and an interval appendectomy is performed.
4. If present at the time of operation, the appendix should be removed and drains placed.
5. Appendicitis recurs in 10% of patients treated with antibiotics and drainage alone.

VI. TREATMENT

A. GENERAL
1. The treatment of appendicitis is surgical and requires removal of the inflamed appendix, except in cases of appendiceal perforation, in which treatment can vary (drainage and antibiotic treatment).
2. Appendectomy can be performed either open and laparoscopically.
3. Perioperative antibiotics have been shown to be beneficial in lowering the infectious complications, and many authors recommend 3-5 days of antibiotics in patients with confirmed appendicitis.

B. TECHNIQUE

1. With the open technique, use a McBurney (or Rockey-Davis) incision over McBurney's point with a muscle-splitting technique (Fig. 34-1).
2. If there is reasonable doubt about the diagnosis, some surgeons prefer a paramedian or midline incision.
3. After resection of the appendix, the ligated stump is usually inverted.
4. In the case of a perforated appendix with phlegmon formation (or significant cecal inflammation), an "interval" (or delayed) appendectomy is usually performed. Drains are brought out to drain discrete collections only, and the fascia is closed while the skin and subcutaneous tissue are left open.
5. Patients with a walled-off abscess may be managed by ultrasound- or CT-guided percutaneous drainage, followed by interval appendectomy 6-8 weeks later.
6. If no appendiceal inflammation is present, a careful search for other causes of the symptom should be undertaken.

34

APPENDICITIS

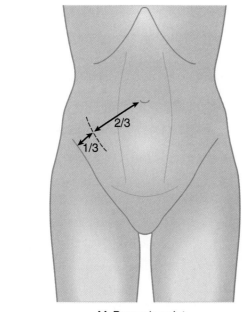

McBurney's point

FIG. 34-1

Diagram of method used to locate McBurney's point.

a. Examination of pelvic organs
b. Gallbladder and gastroduodenal area are inspected
c. Gram stain of any peritoneal exudate
d. Inspection of the mesentery for lymph nodes
e. Thorough examination of the small bowel to rule out regional enteritis and Meckel's diverticulum
f. Palpation of the colon and kidneys

C. LAPAROSCOPY
Laparoscopic appendectomy has no major differences in results when compared to open appendectomy.
1. Some advantages
a. Evaluation of the abdomen/pelvis when the diagnosis is in question
   (1) Women in childbearing years—Can visualize pelvis, fallopian tubes, and ovaries
   (2) Elderly—Can evaluate for perforated cecal cancer or diverticulitis
b. Postoperative stay is less, with some patients being discharged the day of surgery
c. Time of return to normal activity is shorter.
d. The procedure is technically easier in obese patients.
e. In the case of a perforated appendix, there is better visualization of the peritoneum, allowing more adequate drainage.
f. Lower incidence of wound infections
2. Procedure—Multiple variations exist. In general, the technique at the University of Cincinnati Medical Center is as follows.
a. Performed under general anesthesia with bladder and stomach decompression
b. The appendix is grasped with a forceps to expose its base through the right upper quadrant cannula.
c. Using either a vascular stapler or clips to ligate vessels, the mesoappendix is taken down.
d. The appendix can either be amputated with a linear stapler or excised after an endoloop is placed at its base.
e. The appendix is placed in a bag and removed through the 10-12 mm cannula, with care taken not to contact the subcutaneous tissue with the inflamed appendix.

VII. SPECIAL CIRCUMSTANCES

A. ELDERLY
1. Account for >50% of the deaths from appendicitis
2. Higher mortality is due to delay of definitive treatment, uncontrolled infection, and a high incidence of coexistent disease.
3. Constellation of symptoms is usually much more subtle.
a. Abdominal pain may be minimized.

b. Fever and leukocyte count are less reliable signs.
4. Perforation rates reach 75%.
5. Morbidity and mortality are much higher due to the delay in accurate diagnosis.

B. INFANTS
1. Similarly high rates of rupture and secondary complications as in the elderly, due to delayed or atypical presentation
2. Accurate diagnosis is made more difficult by the fact that infants are unable to give a history, the index of suspicion is usually lower, and progression of disease is usually faster.
3. The ability of the infant to wall off perforated appendicitis is inefficient and results in rapid, diffuse peritonitis and distant abscesses.

C. PREGNANCY
1. Although appendicitis is the most common extrauterine surgical emergency in pregnant patients, it occurs with the same frequency in pregnant women as it does in nonpregnant women.
2. It does occur more frequently in the first two trimesters than in the third.
3. Diagnosis is obscured by the lateral and superior displacement of the appendix by the gravid uterus with an accompanying change in the point of maximum tenderness.
a. The appendix is in its "normal" position until 12 weeks, when it is displaced upward and laterally.
b. It reaches the umbilicus by 20 weeks and the iliac crest at 24 weeks.
4. Diagnosis also made more difficult by the fact that abdominal pain, nausea, vomiting, and an elevated WBC count are normal findings during pregnancy.
a. However, an elevated neutrophil count is not a normal finding.
b. Ultrasound may be helpful, especially in the first trimester.
5. Laparoscopy is as safe as laparotomy in the first and second trimesters.
6. Although maternal mortality is very low, early operative intervention is essential as perforation and peritonitis result in fetal mortality rates as high as 35%.
7. Risk of premature delivery is highest during the first week after surgery and then returns to baseline.

VIII. APPENDICEAL TUMORS
Tumors are found in almost 5% of removed appendices.

A. CARCINOID
1. Carcinoid tumors are most commonly located in the appendix and are usually benign.
2. Appendectomy is the treatment unless there is nodal involvement, the tumor is >2 cm, or the mesoappendix or base of cecum is involved.
3. Right hemicolectomy is then the treatment of choice.

34

APPENDICITIS

B. ADENOCARCINOMA
1. Adenocarcinoma of the colon can arise in the appendix.
2. Most of these case present as acute appendicitis.
3. A right hemicolectomy should be performed.

C. PSEUDOMYXOMA
1. Pseudomyxoma arises in the appendix in half of patients with pseudomyxoma peritonei.
2. Appendiceal mucocele or fluid-filled cyst can be seen on imaging and may be associated with gelatinous ascites.
3. Both ovaries should be examined in females for secondary disease.
4. In a patient with a preoperative diagnosis of appendicitis, surgical debulking of all gross disease is the treatment, along with adjuvant chemotherapy after tissue diagnosis of pseudomyxoma.
5. Patients with undiagnosed disease should undergo a right hemicolectomy without penetration of the tumor. Once the diagnosis is confirmed, further cancer work-up and treatment are then performed.

RECOMMENDED READINGS

Maxwell JG, Robinson CL, Maxwell TG, et al: Deriving the indications for laparoscopic appendectomy from a comparison of the outcomes of laparoscopic and open appendectomy. Am J Surg 182:687-692, 2001.

Piskun G, Kozik D, Rajpal S, et al: Comparison of laparoscopic, open, and converted appendectomy for perforated appendicitis. Surg Endosc 15:660-662, 2001.

Rice HE, Brown RL, Gollin G, et al: Results of a pilot trial comparing prolonged intravenous antibiotics with sequential intravenous/oral antibiotics for children with perforated appendicitis. Arch Surg 136:1391-1395, 2001.

Wilson EB, Cole JC, Nipper ML, et al: Computed tomography and ultrasonography in the diagnosis of appendicitis: When are they indicated? Arch Surg 136:670-675, 2001.

Colorectal Cancer

Bruce W. Robb, MD

I. INCIDENCE

A. ANNUAL
1. Colorectal cancer accounts for 14% of all cases of cancer, excluding skin malignancies. There are ≈150,000 new cases of colorectal cancer annually.
2. Colorectal cancer accounts for 14% (≈57,000) of all yearly cancer deaths (second only to lung cancer).

B. OTHER
1. Colorectal cancer is second in incidence only to breast cancer in females and third in incidence in males behind prostate cancer and lung cancer.
2. The peak incidence is in the 7th decade of life.

II. ETIOLOGY

A. ENVIRONMENTAL FACTORS
1. Western countries have a higher incidence of colorectal cancer than countries in Asia and Africa. Immigrants from Asia and Africa have higher incidence of colorectal cancer than their countrymen, suggesting an environmental etiology such as the low-fiber, high-fat diet common in the West.
2. Routine use of nonsteroidal anti-inflammatory drugs may be associated with a lower incidence of polyp and cancer formation.

B. GENETIC PREDISPOSITION
1. Genetic syndromes account for <5% of colorectal cancers.
2. Well-described polyposis syndromes include the following.
a. Familial polyposis—Adenomatous polyposis of the colon with a 100% risk of malignancy; may also occur in the proximal GI tract; autosomal dominant inheritance
b. Gardner's syndrome—Polyposis associated with exostoses, soft tissue tumors, and osteomas; also has a 100% incidence of malignant degeneration
c. Turcot's syndrome—Polyposis of the colon associated with CNS tumors; autosomal recessive inheritance
d. Cronkhite-Canada syndrome—GI polyposis with alopecia, nail dystrophy, hyperpigmentation; minimal malignant potential; no inheritance pattern
e. Peutz-Jeghers syndrome—Hamartomatous polyps of the entire GI tract with mucocutaneous deposition of melanin in lips, oral cavity, and digits; slightly increased potential; autosomal dominant inheritance

35

C. INFLAMMATORY BOWEL DISEASE

1. Ulcerative colitis and, to a lesser extent, Crohn's disease are associated with increased rates of colon cancer.
2. After 10 years, the risk of cancer in ulcerative colitis is 1-2% per year.

D. ADENOMATOUS POLYPS

Adenomatous polyps are probably premalignant lesions. They are thought to represent transformation of normal mucosa to cancer, although most polyps do not progress to carcinoma. Increasing size and increased number of polyps are associated with an increased risk of developing cancer.

1. Tubular adenomas—65% of adenomas; 15% have carcinoma in situ or frank invasive cancer
2. Tubulovillous adenomas—25% of adenomas; 19% have carcinoma in situ or invasive cancer
3. Villous adenomas—10% of adenomas; 25% have carcinoma in situ or invasive cancer

E. SUMMARY OF MAJOR RISK FACTORS

1. Hereditary polyposis syndromes
2. Adenomatous polyps
3. Previous colorectal cancer
4. Inflammatory bowel disease
5. Family history of colorectal cancer
6. Age >50 years

III. DIAGNOSIS

A. SIGNS AND SYMPTOMS

Colorectal cancer may present with different symptoms and manifestations related to the region of the bowel from which it arises.

1. Right-sided lesions are typically bulky, fungating, ulcerative lesions that project into the lumen.
   a. Anemia—Microcytic; chronic, intermittent occult blood loss in the stool
   b. Systemic complaints—Anorexia, fatigue, weight loss, or dull persistent abdominal pain; abdominal mass with more advanced tumors
   c. Obstruction is rare secondary to the liquefied consistency of the stool and the large diameter of the bowel.
   d. Triad—Anemia, weakness, right lower quadrant mass
2. Left-sided lesions—Annular, "napkin ring" lesions that often obstruct the bowel
   a. Change in bowel habits—Obstipation, alternating constipation and diarrhea, small-caliber "pencil" stools
   b. Obstructive symptoms are more prominent due to growth pattern of tumor, small caliber of bowel, and solid stool
3. Rectal cancer—Blood streaking in stools, tenesmus. This finding must *not* be attributed to hemorrhoids without further investigation.

Obstruction is uncommon but is a poor prognostic sign when present.
4. Abdominal pain is the most common presenting symptom for lesions in all locations.

B. SIGNS OF LOCAL EXTENSION OR METASTASIS
1. Abnormal liver function tests, jaundice, or hepatomegaly
2. Fistula formation
3. Mass fixed to sacrum on rectal exam

C. DIAGNOSTIC STUDIES
1. Rectal exam—All patients undergo rectal exams. Up to 10% of lesions are palpable on rectal exam.
2. Stool guaiac—Up to 50% of positive tests are due to colorectal cancer. It should be repeated yearly on at least three separate occasions in patients >40 years old.
3. Barium enema or flexible sigmoidoscopy for routine screening every 3-5 years in patients >50 years of age. Flexible sigmoidoscopy should detect almost 50% of colorectal cancers.
4. Colonoscopy every 10 years for routine screening (may be both diagnostic and therapeutic)
5. Work-up for metastatic disease in biopsy-proven cases
a. Must evaluate the entire colon; 6% incidence of synchronous lesions
b. Chest radiograph (some surgeons advocate chest CT)
c. Liver function tests
d. Abdominal CT for intra-abdominal metastasis and extracolonic spread
e. Carcinoembryonic antigen (CEA) preoperatively
f. IV pyelogram—Optional in patients with low-lying lesions or urinary symptoms

IV. PATHOLOGY

A. GENERAL
The majority are located in the distal colon; however, there is an increasing incidence of right-sided lesions.

B. GROSS DESCRIPTION
1. Polypoid—Bulky polypoid lesions are more common in the right colon.
2. Scirrhous—Annular ("apple core") lesions. More common in the left colon
3. Ulcerated
4. Nodular

C. ROUTES OF SPREAD
1. Intramural—Along bowel wall
2. Direct extension into surrounding tissues—E.g., ovary, small bowel
3. Intraluminal

35

COLORECTAL CANCER

4. Peritoneal
5. Lymphatic
6. Hematogenous

D. HISTOLOGIC STAGING
Dukes' classifications are used for histologic staging. There have been several modifications to the original classification.
1. **Astler-Coller modification (1959) is most commonly used.**
   Stage A: Limited to mucosa (above lymphatic channels)
   Stage B1: Into the muscularis propria
   Stage B2: Through the muscularis propria
   Stage C1: Into the muscularis propria, with positive nodes
   Stage D (not part of the original classification): Metastases or unresectable
2. **American Joint Committee for the Cancer Staging and End Results (TNM)**
a. Primary tumor (T)
   Tx: Primary tumor cannot be assessed
   T0: No evidence of primary tumor
   Tis: Intraepithelial, carcinoma in situ
   T1: Tumor invades the submucosa
   T2: Tumor invades the muscularis propria
   T3: Tumor invades into the subserosa or nonperitonealized pericolic structures
   T4: Tumor directly invades other organs or perforates
b. Regional lymph nodes (N)
   Nx: Regional lymph nodes cannot be assessed
   N0: No regional lymph node metastasis
   N1: Metastasis in 1-3 pericolic lymph nodes
   N2: Metastasis in 4 or more pericolic lymph nodes
   N3: Other distant lymph node metastasis
c. Distant metastasis (M)
   Mx: Presence of metastases cannot be assessed
   M0: No distant metastases
   M1: Distant metastases
3. **Prognosis is related to the stage of disease, not size of the tumor.**
a. Five-year survival using the Astler-Coller modification

Stage A, >90%	TNM stage I
Stage B1, 70-85%	TNM stage II
Stage B2, 55-65%	TNM stage II
Stage C1, 45-55%	TNM stage III
Stage C2, 20-30%	TNM stage III
Stage D, <5%	TNM stage IV

Patients with isolated hepatic metastases that undergo resection for cure have a 5-year survival rate of 15-25%.

b. Rectal cancer has a higher local recurrence rate and smaller 5-year survival than colonic tumors.
c. Only 70% of colorectal cancer patients can undergo resection for cure at presentation.
   (1) 10% of primary lesions are unresectable.
   (2) 20% of patients have distant metastases at presentation.
d. 45% of patients are cured by primary resection.
e. Of the 25% of patients who develop a recurrence, 20% will be cured by further resection.
f. Overall 5-year disease-free survival is ≈50% for colon cancer and ≈40% for rectal cancer resected for cure.

V. TREATMENT

A. GENERAL
1. An adequate cancer operation requires resection of tumor-containing bowel with 3- to 5-cm margins and resection of the mesentery at the origin of the arterial supply, including the primary lymphatic drainage of the tumor.
2. Recent studies suggest that 90% of tumors can be adequately handled by 2-cm margins.
3. This is especially important for lesions of the lower third of the rectum, which may be managed with a low anterior resection and primary anastomosis.

B. PREOPERATIVE PREPARATION
1. Mechanical bowel preparation and preoperative oral antibiotics have been shown to reduce wound and intra-abdominal infections.
2. Perioperative systemic antibiotics may decrease the incidence of infectious complications.
3. CEA level must be obtained prior to operation.

C. CHOICE OF OPERATION (Fig. 35-1)
1. Lesions of the cecum and ascending colon are treated by resection of the distal ileum to the mid-transverse colon, including the ileocolic, right colic, and middle colic vessels with accompanying mesentery.
2. Tumors in the left transverse colon and splenic flexure require resection of the transverse and proximal descending colon. The middle and left colic arteries are removed.
3. Tumors in the descending and sigmoid colon require removal from the splenic flexure to the rectosigmoid. The left colic and sigmoidal arteries are removed.
4. Tumors in the upper third of the rectum are treated by an anterior resection.
5. Lesions between 5 and 10 cm from the anal verge are treated by a low anterior resection or an abdominal-sacral resection (Kraske, York-Mason).

35

COLORECTAL CANCER

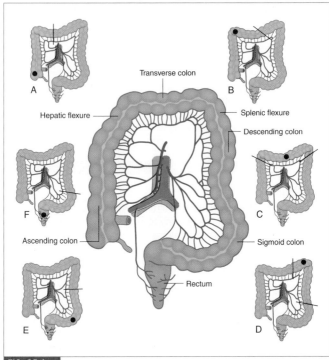

Anatomic resection commonly employed for cancer at different sites within the large bowel. *A*, Right hemicolectomy. *B*, Extended right hemicolectomy. *C*, Transverse colectomy. *D*, Left hemicolectomy. *E*, Sigmoid colectomy. *F*, Abdominal perineal resection. Black circles signify the location of the cancer.

6. Lesions in the lower third of the rectum (0-5 cm) usually require an abdominoperineal resection (Miles procedure) with a permanent end-sigmoid colostomy; may be amendable to a low anterior resection with anastomosis using a stapler (EEA). At least 4 cm of rectal stump is necessary for fecal continence.
7. Preoperative multimodality therapy using both chemotherapy and radiation may aid in down-staging locally advanced rectal carcinoma so that otherwise unresectable lesions may be resected.
8. Selected patients with rectal cancer have equal survival following either wide local excision via a transanal approach or a more aggressive resection such as an abdominoperineal resection. Criteria for local excision are the following.
a. Mobile tumor in the lower third of the rectum
b. Size <3 cm

c. Stage A or B1 by endorectal ultrasound
d. Well or moderately differentiated histology
e. No detectable pararectal lymph node involvement clinically or by endorectal ultrasound.

9. Bilateral oophorectomy may be reasonable at the time of initial resection, because about 6% of female patients will have microscopic involvement of the ovaries.

10. Direct adherence of the tumor to adjacent structures may result from inflammation rather than from tumor extension. A cure in the presence of local invasion may still be possible with resection of the involved structures, or if local invasion is more extensive, by total pelvic exenteration.

D. ADJUVANT THERAPY

1. For patients with Dukes' C colon adenocarcinoma, postoperative therapy with 5-fluorouracil (5-FU) and levamisole or leucovorin has been shown to be effective in improving both disease-free and overall survival. Radiation therapy has not been shown to be an effective adjuvant treatment for colon adenocarcinoma.

2. For patients with Dukes' B2 or C rectal carcinoma, postoperative combined modality therapy with radiation and chemotherapy improves both disease-free and overall survival and also improves local tumor control and should be considered standard therapy after either abdominoperineal or low anterior resection. Some recent data suggest chemotherapy alone may be just as beneficial, however. The use of preoperative radiation is controversial but may be helpful, especially with large, bulky tumors.

VI. POSTOPERATIVE FOLLOW-UP

A. GENERAL

Approximately 80% of recurrences occur within 2 years of resection, most often in the form of hepatic metastases or local recurrence.

B. DIAGNOSIS AND TREATMENT

1. Detection and treatment of recurrent disease remain problematic.
2. Careful history, physical exam, liver function tests, CEA screening, and stool guaiacs detect >90% of recurrent disease.
3. Follow-up protocol
a. Routine physical exam, stool guaiac, CBC, liver function tests— q 3 months for 2 years, then q 6 months for 2 years, then annually.
b. CEA—q 3 months for 2 years, then q 6 months for 2 years, then annually.
c. Colonoscopy—Baseline at 3-6 months, then annually for 4 years, then q 2-3 years. Barium enema should be performed if complete visualization is not achieved by colonoscopy.

35

COLORECTAL CANCER

4. CEA helpful only if initially elevated and returns to normal postresection

5. An increase in CEA (>5 ng/mL) requires prompt investigation, including abdominal CT scans, chest radiograph, and colonoscopy or barium enema. If no abnormalities are found, some advocate a second-look laparotomy. Whether this results in increased 5-year survival is controversial. However, recurrences detected by frequent CEA screening alone are more frequently respectable than recurrences detected by the appearance of symptoms.

6. Other screening tests—Tissue peptide antigen and CA 19-9 are not as sensitive or specific as CEA.

C. TREATMENT OF RECURRENT DISEASE

1. Local recurrence

a. Should attempt a cure by resection in selected patients or to palliate symptoms whenever possible

b. Resectability can be determined only by re-exploration. Debulking procedures (tumor resections with gross disease left behind) are rarely indicated.

c. Recurrence following low anterior resection usually requires an abdominoperineal resection.

d. Pelvic recurrences following abdominoperineal resection are usually unresectable, but occasionally pelvic exenteration is possible.

2. Distant metastases

a. Involve the liver, lung, bone, brain (in order of frequency)

b. ≈35-50% of all colorectal carcinoma patients develop hepatic metastases during the course of their disease.

c. 10-20% of patients with hepatic metastases may benefit from resection, with 5-year survival of 25% in some studies. Relative contraindications to resection are the following.

(1) Positive hepatic nodes

(2) Extrahepatic metastases

(3) >4 hepatic metastases

d. When synchronous hepatic metastasis is found during operation for primary colorectal malignancy, the hepatic lesion may be removed simultaneously or at second operation 2-3 months later.

e. No difference in survival has been demonstrated for lobectomy vs. wedge resection (when possible).

f. For unresectable hepatic metastases, an implantable pump for intra-arterial (hepatic artery) infusion of 5-FU or floxuridine (FUDR) has shown tumor response rates of 40-60%; however, toxicity remains a significant problem.

g. Pulmonary metastases most often present as disseminated disease. For metastatic nodules, up to 38% 5-year survival has been demonstrated with surgical resection (usually wedge). Patients with solitary nodules and nodules <3 cm in size may have better survival.

h. For unresectable systemic disease, chemotherapy (5-FU and leucovorin) is used, but results continue to be disappointing.

Diverticular Disease of the Colon

Lawrence E. Stern, MD

I. DIVERTICULOSIS

A. DEFINITION
Diverticulosis is a saccular outpouching of mucosa through the colonic musculature.

1. Acquired diverticula
a. Most common type of diverticulum
b. Contain only the mucosal and submucosal layers (false or pseudodiverticula)
c. These diverticula occur at weak points in the bowel wall where the vasa recta penetrate the circular muscle layer, primarily on the mesenteric side of the two antimesenteric tenia and adjacent to the two borders of the mesenteric tenia.
d. Do not occur below the peritoneal reflection
e. Diverticula may occur throughout the GI tract but are most common in the large bowel, with 95% of patients having diverticula in the sigmoid colon.

2. Congenital diverticula
a. Contain all layers of the bowel wall (true diverticula)
b. Rare and usually single
c. Predominantly located in the right colon, in or near the cecum

B. INCIDENCE
1. Male = female
2. Age—<5% at 40 years of age; 65% in those >85 years old
3. Region—Higher in Western nations

C. PATHOPHYSIOLOGY
1. 80% are asymptomatic.
2. Symptoms (secondary to hypermotility, not to the diverticula themselves)—Pain, diarrhea, constipation
3. 65% of cases are limited to the sigmoid colon.
4. The etiology is presumed to result from elevated intraluminal pressure.
a. Increased elastin is laid down in a contracted form, causing bunching of the circular muscle and shortening of the tenia.
b. Laplace's law states that the pressure within a tube varies directly with wall tension and inversely with the radius of the lumen; therefore, the thickened wall results in a greater intraluminal pressure.
c. The sigmoid colon, the narrowest region of the colon, has the highest incidence of diverticular disease.

36

5. Dietary fiber content has been inversely related to the incidence of diverticular disease. Regions of the world with low fiber intake have higher rates of diverticulosis. Animal studies have provided some support for this theory.

D. COMPLICATIONS
1. Inflammation of a diverticulum is referred to as *diverticulitis* and may lead to infection, perforation, bleeding, fistulization, and obstruction.
2. 10-25% of patients with diverticulosis develop diverticulitis or hemorrhage, and 30% of these require operative intervention.
a. Diverticulitis (see section II).
b. Hemorrhage (see Chap. 20)
    (1) The close anatomic relationship between the diverticulum and the penetrating artery provides the opportunity for bleeding.
    (2) 70% of lower GI bleeding is caused by diverticulosis.
        (a) 70% of bleeds secondary to diverticulosis stop spontaneously.
        (b) 75% of those that stop spontaneously do not recur.
    (3) Differential diagnosis
        (a) Angiodysplasia
        (b) Upper GI bleeding (rapid)
        (c) Hemorrhoids
        (d) Carcinoma/polyps
        (e) Colitis (ischemic, inflammatory)

E. TREATMENT
1. Prevention—High-fiber diet decreases incidence of symptomatic disease. The most protective fiber is from fruits and vegetables, rather than cereal fibers. Intake of total fat and red meat increases the risk of symptomatic disease.
2. Surgery may be required for complications (see section II. E).

II. DIVERTICULITIS

A. EPIDEMIOLOGY AND PATHOPHYSIOLOGY
1. Age—Occurs in 20% of patients >40 years of age with diverticulosis
2. Inspissated stool lodges in the diverticulum, producing increased intraluminal pressure with impairment of venous return. Venous hypertension with impaired capillary filling results in ischemia and mucosal injury with subsequent inflammation.
3. Ischemia usually leads to a "microperforation," a contained perforation into the mesentery or pericolic fat, causing focal inflammation and localized peritonitis.
4. 10-15% of patients with diverticulitis have free perforation, producing generalized peritonitis. This is more common in immunosuppressed, debilitated, and steroid-dependent patients.

B. PRESENTATION

1. Symptoms

a. Classic triad of left lower quadrant pain, fever, and leukocytosis

    (1) Pain—Most common symptom, usually in left lower quadrant, but may be anywhere in lower abdomen due to the redundancy of the sigmoid colon (or right sided diverticulitis). The pain is typically dull and achy but may be crampy and associated with tenesmus.

    (2) Fever, malaise, anorexia, nausea with/without emesis

b. Change in bowel habits—Diarrhea, constipation, alternating diarrhea and constipation, change in stool caliber, obstipation, tenesmus

c. Urinary symptoms—Frequency, nocturia, and/or dysuria due to pericystic inflammation; pneumaturia (presenting symptoms in 3-5%) and/or polymicrobial urinary tract infection in noncatheterized patients are seen with colovesical fistulas.

2. Signs

a. Tenderness and guarding

b. Distention due to ileus or mechanical bowel obstruction

c. Palpable tender mass, especially on pelvic or rectal exam

d. Hypoactive or absent bowel sounds with peritonitis

e. Hyperactive, high-pitched bowel sounds with obstruction

f. Guaiac-positive stools

3. Laboratory exam

a. Mild to moderate leukocytosis, often with a shift to immature forms

b. Urinalysis—Leukocytes may be present as a result of inflammation around the ureters and bladder.

4. Differential diagnosis

a. Acute appendicitis

b. Crohn's disease

c. Carcinoma

d. Colitis—Pseudomembranous, infectious, and ischemic

e. Gynecologic—Ruptured ovarian cysts, ovarian torsion, ectopic pregnancy, and pelvic inflammatory disease

C. DIAGNOSTIC TESTS

Initial diagnosis is made on clinical assessment—diagnostic studies are performed for confirmation of clinical suspicion. Ten to 20% of patients diagnosed with diverticulitis on clinical grounds subsequently are found to have carcinoma of the colon; therefore, it is necessary to rule out carcinoma following resolution of the acute attack.

1. CT scan—Study of choice

a. Therapeutic advantage of percutaneous abscess drainage

b. Superior to contrast enemas for defining pericolic inflammation and evaluating complications of diverticulitis

c. 90-95% sensitivity, 72% specificity, and false-negative rate of 7-21%

2. Contrast enema

a. Barium enema deferred until peritoneal signs subside (usually 2-4 weeks) due to risk of perforation and resulting barium peritonitis

b. Water-soluble contrast enema has 94% sensitivity and accuracy of 77%

3. Ultrasonography—Low cost, reasonable sensitivity (84-93%), but highly operator dependent

4. Flexible sigmoidoscopy (with minimal insufflation) can be used to rule out a perforated colon cancer.

5. Colonoscopy—Mandatory once acute process has resolved (6-8 weeks) in the case of bleeding or the possibility of cancer based on radiographic studies

D. TREATMENT

1. Nonoperative management

a. Outpatient

(1) Oral antibiotics—Appropriate for mild tenderness and low-grade fever. Coverage should last 7-10 days and should include anaerobes and gram-negative rods.

(a) Amoxicillin plus clavulanic acid.

(b) Sulfamethoxazole-trimethoprim and metronidazole

(c) Quinolone and metronidazole

(2) Low-residue diet once symptoms improve

(3) Admission criteria include high fever, increasing abdominal pain, inability to tolerate enteral nutrition, and/or failure to improve on oral antibiotics.

b. Inpatient

(1) NPO, IV hydration, and nasogastric suction (if ileus or small bowel obstruction is present)

(2) Parenteral antibiotics—Gram-negative and anaerobic coverage. Continue for 7-10 days, or until afebrile with normal white blood cell (WBC) count and nontender exam

(3) Pain control with meperidine

(4) Serial abdominal exams to detect worsening or complicated disease

(5) Oral antibiotics—Continue for 1-2 weeks after discontinuation of parenteral antibiotics for severe attacks.

(6) Diet—Clear liquids once symptoms have improved. Low-residue diet for 2-4 weeks after an acute attack. Patients are then placed on a high-fiber diet including psyllium. This may decrease the rate of further symptoms but probably does not decrease the incidence of complications.

2. Surgical management

a. 50-70% of all patients admitted to the hospital resolve their diverticulitis with conservative therapy. Only 25% return with a subsequent attack (half within 1 year, 90% within 5 years).

b. Of the patients who do not respond during initial hospitalization

(1) 60% do not resolve (or recur) after discontinuation of antibiotics.

Diverticular Disease of the Colon

431

(2) 30% have free perforation, requiring immediate surgery.
(3) 9% have urinary fistulas.
(4) 1% have a solitary right-sided diverticulum.
c. Indications for operation
  (1) Repeated attacks (two or more)
    (a) In patients >50 years of age, response rate to conservative therapy is 70% after the second attack and only 6% after the third attack.
    (b) The rate of complications is <20% with the first occurrence but increases to 60% with subsequent attacks.
  (2) Complications—Abscess, obstruction, fistula, stricture
  (3) Failure to improve with conservative management after 3-4 days
  (4) First episode in patients <40 years of age (controversial)
  (5) Inability to exclude carcinoma
  (6) Right-sided diverticulitis (see section III)
d. Operative procedures
  (1) Single-stage—Resect all diverticulum-bearing colon with a primary anastomosis, usually an elective operation on prepared bowel.
    (a) Open technique—Proximal margin should be soft pliable bowel; 2% incidence of ureteral injuries
    (b) Laparoscopic technique—Decreased pain and shorter hospitalization; improved cosmesis with potential acceptance of colectomy in younger patients
  (2) Two-stage—The safe creation of an anastomosis is not possible in the presence of edematous bowel or gross contamination because of the high incidence of resultant leaks.
    (a) First stage—Primary resection of diseased colon with end colostomy and Hartmann pouch or mucous fistula. Diversion without resection is associated with a higher mortality rate (12% vs. 29%).
    (b) Alternative first stage—Primary resection and anastomosis with a proximal diverting colostomy
    (c) Second stage—Reanastomosis after 2-6 months
  (3) Three-stage—Rarely used
    (a) Employed for severe peritonitis with localized abscess cavity, on an unstable patient, or for a prohibitively difficult resection
    (b) Disadvantage—Leaves diseased colon holding column of stool in place
    (c) First stage—Drainage of abscess and proximal diverting colostomy
    (d) Second stage—Resection of involved colon with anastomosis
    (e) Third stage—Closure of diverting colostomy

36

DIVERTICULAR DISEASE OF THE COLON

E. COMPLICATIONS
1. Abscess
a. CT-guided drainage

(1) Effective drainage of an abscess can allow the performance of an elective procedure when the acute process has subsided, with lower morbidity and mortality than an emergent one, and can avoid the need for a colostomy.

(2) A one-stage operation is possible in 50-90% of patients after effective percutaneous drainage.

b. Hartmann's operation is usually indicated during a celiotomy in the setting of an undrained abscess.

2. Fistula

Fistula occurs in 2-4% of patients with diverticular disease and in 20% of patients undergoing surgery for diverticular disease.

a. Colovesical fistula.

(1) Accounts for 65% of fistulas secondary to diverticulitis

(2) Cancer is the second most common cause of colovesical fistulas (after diverticulitis) and must be ruled out.

(3) 3:1 male-to-female preponderance owing to absence of interposed uterus and adnexa

(4) Ascending infections (i.e., pyelonephritis) are rare, except in the face of distal obstruction.

(5) Presentation—Typically fecaluria, pneumaturia, or recurrent urinary tract infections. Major abdominal symptomatology is the exception, not the rule.

(6) Diagnosis

(a) CT with intraluminal contrast is the most sensitive test. Air will be seen in the bladder in 90% of patients.

(b) Barium enema is <50% sensitive.

(c) Cystoscopy—Usually only induration and edema are seen.

(7) Treatment

(a) 50% close spontaneously.

(b) If the fistula was caused by colon cancer, the resection must include a disc of bladder; otherwise, the colon may be dissected free, leaving the bladder intact.

(c) Methylene blue distention of the rectum or bladder may help delineate a hard-to-find fistula tract.

b. Colovaginal fistula

(1) Almost all patients have had a hysterectomy.

(2) Barium enema is <50% sensitive.

(3) Speculum exam—Fistula is visible in 85%.

c. Coloenteric fistula—Usual treatment in single-stage en bloc resection and primary anastomosis of both colon and small bowel

3. Perforation

a. Associated with generalized peritonitis

b. Sepsis must be controlled.

c. Primary resection should be performed whenever possible (lower mortality rate compared to simple diversion).

III. RIGHT COLON (ISOLATED) DIVERTICULOSIS

A. GENERAL
1. May be a congenital (true) or acquired (false) diverticulum
2. High incidence in Asia (35-84% of cases)

B. LOCATION
1. Cecum—Usually congenital with ≈1-2% incidence. Most patients are asymptomatic. The most common complication is inflammation.
2. Ascending colon—Most are acquired; most common complication is bleeding

C. PRESENTATION
1. Usually occurs in younger (30-40 year-old) age group
2. Often mimics appendicitis
3. Symptoms may be prolonged and persistent

D. DIAGNOSIS
1. CT scan—For atypical presentation of appendicitis, particularly in older patients
2. Barium enema or flexible colonoscopy if no perforation
3. Must rule out malignancy
4. The diagnosis usually is not made preoperatively.

E. THERAPY
1. Isolated ileo-right colectomy is often required.
2. Conservative treatment with antibiotic therapy or more limited diverticulectomy may be effective in mild cases.

RECOMMENDED READINGS

Stollman NH, Raskin JB: Diverticular disease of the colon. J Clin Gastroenterol 29:241-252, 1999.

Wolff BG, Devine RM: Surgical management of diverticulitis. Am Surg 66:153-156, 2000.

Young-Fadok TM, Roberts PL, Spencer MP, Wolff BG: Colonic diverticular disease. Curr Probl Surg 37:459-514, 2000.

36

DIVERTICULAR DISEASE OF THE COLON

Colitis and Enteric Infections

Amod A. Sarnaik, MD

I. MICROBIOLOGY

A. GENERAL
1. The colon is sterile at birth.

B. FLORA
1. Normal fecal flora comprises ≈400 bacterial species, which vary by site
   a. Stomach—*Helicobacter pylori*
   b. Small intestine—*Streptococcus* spp, *Staphylococcus* spp, *Lactobacillus* spp, *Bacteroides fragilis*
   c. Large intestine—*B. fragilis*, *Streptococcus* spp, *Escherichia coli*, *Clostridium* spp
2. 99% of bacteria are anaerobic (*B. fragilis* is most prevalent at 10^{10}/g).
3. 1% aerobic—Coliforms (*E. coli*—10^7/g; *Klebsiella* spp, *Proteus* spp, *Enterobacter* spp) and enterococcus

II. HOST DEFENSE

A. PERISTALSIS
1. Peristalsis limits bacterial stasis and subsequent overgrowth.
2. Pharmacologic inhibition of motility with opioids or diphenoxylate (Lomotil) results in increased bacterial counts, increased relative number of anaerobic bacteria, and increased frequency of bacterial translocation.

B. GASTRIC ACID
1. Gastric acid reduces normal flora bacterial counts and reduces the incidence of colonization with pathogenic organisms.
2. ICU patients treated with an H_2 receptor antagonist have been shown to have increased incidence of gram-negative pneumonia vs. ICU patients treated with sucralfate.

C. ILEOCECAL VALVE
1. The ileocecal valve provides an anatomic barrier that prevents retrograde migration of colonic flora into terminal ileum.
2. Damage or operative resection of the ileocecal valve causes increased bacterial counts in the distal ileum as well as malabsorption of vitamin B_{12} and bile acids.

D. NORMAL FLORA
1. Normal flora limits the growth of pathogenic strains of bacteria.

37

2. The mechanism is thought to be due to consumption of nutrients, inhibition of adherence, and elaboration of metabolic waste products that inhibit growth of pathogenic bacteria.

III. DIARRHEA

A. DEFINITION
1. Increased number of stools and increased fluid loss (controversial)

B. NORMAL STOOL
1. <200 g/day
2. Diarrhea—>250 g/day or more than three liquid stools per day

C. MECHANISMS
1. Increased motility, presence of osmotically active substances, inflammatory exudate, increased secretion by mucosa

D. BACTERIAL TOXINS
1. Cause increased mucosal secretion
2. Cytotoxic (e.g., cholera, enterotoxigenic *E. coli*)—Do not damage mucosal epithelium; increase mucosal secretion by increasing cyclic adenosine monophosphate via activation of adenylate cyclase
3. Cytotoxic (e.g., *Shigella*, enterohemorrhagic *E. coli*)—Cause direct damage to epithelium

E. DIAGNOSIS
1. Stool smear
a. White blood cells (WBCs)—Likely an exudative process, e.g., inflammatory bowel disease (IBD) or infectious enteritis
b. Red blood cells, no WBCs—Ischemia, cancer, amebic colitis, pseudomembranous colitis
2. High stool fat content—Malabsorption due to IBD, short gut, pancreatic insufficiency, infection, or interruption of enterohepatic bile circulation
3. Osmolarity—Mucosa is permeable to water; therefore, stool and serum osmolarity should be approximately equal. If stool osmolarity is > serum osmolarity by ≥50 mOsm, then an osmotically active cation is likely present.

IV. PSEUDOMEMBRANOUS COLITIS

A. PATHOGENESIS
1. Almost always due to *Clostridium difficile*, a gram-positive obligate anaerobe, that readily forms spores that are highly resistant to antiseptic agents
a. 3-5% of the population is a carrier. Asymptomatic carriage is common in infants.

b. Can be found in 15-20% of asymptomatic patients treated with antibiotics

c. Most common cause of nosocomial diarrhea in United States

2. Nosocomial transmission

a. Opportunity for epidemic outbreaks, particularly on surgical wards and ICUs

b. *Hand washing* is the primary means of controlling spread of the disease.

3. Antibiotic use causes alterations in the normal flora of the colon, allowing for overgrowth of *C. difficile*. Almost all antibiotics have been implicated (although clindamycin, ampicillin, and the cephalosporins are most common).

4. Damage to the mucosal integrity is caused by two exotoxins produced by the bacteria. The precise mechanism of action is unknown but is thought to involve disruption of intestinal epithelial cytoskeleton leading to cell death, and induction of inflammatory cytokines leading to pseudomembrane formation.

a. Toxin A (enteropathic)—More cytotoxic than toxin B in vivo

b. Toxin B (cytopathic)—More cytotoxic than toxin A in vitro but requires toxin A for effect in vivo

5. Pseudomembranes—Dead mucosal cells and WBCs, along with mucus and fibrin, that give a characteristic histologic appearance

6. Usually most severe in the sigmoid and rectum, but 10% of cases are located solely on the right side; involvement proximal to ileocecal valve is rare

B. SIGNS AND SYMPTOMS

1. Severity may vary from mild to severe, with complications including perforation and toxic megacolon

2. Copious watery diarrhea (rarely grossly bloody), crampy pain, fever, and leukocytosis

3. Typically occurs 5-10 days after starting the offending antibiotic, but up to 20% of cases are seen as long as 6 weeks after discontinuation

C. DIAGNOSIS

1. WBCs are present in <50% of patients' stools. Therefore, a positive test rules out benign etiologies, but a negative one is not necessarily helpful.

2. Detection of *C. difficile* toxin A or B in stool by enzyme-linked immunosorbent assay is ≈85% sensitive and ≈95% specific. Up to 20% of cases may require multiple stool samples to detect toxin. Stool culture is used less frequently.

3. Colonoscopy is reserved for use in severe cases due to risk of perforation.

D. TREATMENT

1. Stop the offending antibiotic if possible, and replace fluid and electrolyte losses.

2. In toxic, elderly, and immunocompromised patients, start therapy empirically while waiting for toxin titers to return.
3. Do not use an antiperistaltic agent.
4. Vancomycin—100% of cases are sensitive. The drug is poorly absorbed from the GI tract. 125 mg PO q 6 h has been shown to be equivalent to 500 q 6. Parenteral vancomycin is not efficacious.
5. Metronidazole—≈90% of cases are sensitive. It is the drug of choice because it is significantly cheaper than vancomycin and reduces incidence of vancomycin-resistant bacteria. Its use is contraindicated in infants and pregnant patients. Dosage is 500-750 mg PO t.i.d. or 250 mg q.i.d. Oral formation is favored over parenteral.
6. There is a 20% recurrence rate, despite drug choice. Occurs 1-5 weeks following treatment. Recurrence is more common in patients with renal failure and patients being treated concurrently with antibiotics for additional infection. Recurrent infection may be eliminated by tapering metronidazole or vancomycin over 4-6 weeks.
7. Cholestyramine—Binds to toxin. Less efficacious than vancomycin or metronidazole. Mainly used in the setting of relapsing disease or treatment failure. Also binds to and inhibits the action of vancomycin.
8. *Lactobacillus* and *Saccharomyces boulardii/cerevisiae*—Used to reconstitute the beneficial effect of normal flora. Fecal enemas have also reportedly been used for the same goal but are not approved for use in the United States.

V. ULCERATIVE COLITIS
See Chapter 33.

VI. CROHN'S COLITIS
See Chapter 33.

VII. ISCHEMIC COLITIS
See Chapter 52.

VIII. NEUTROPENIC COLITIS

A. GENERAL
1. Occurs with acute myelogenous leukemia (25%), aplastic anemia, and chemotherapy
2. Primarily affects the cecum and ascending colon

B. PATHOGENESIS
1. Unknown, though hypothesized to be secondary to necrosis of intramural leukemic cells that then cause mucosal ulceration

C. SIGNS AND SYMPTOMS
1. Diarrhea, abdominal pain, fever, distention, right lower quadrant tenderness

D. TREATMENT
1. Hydration, nasogastric decompression, antibiotics, and administration of a granulocyte stimulant
2. Operative intervention is reserved for complications (perforation, hemorrhage, obstruction) or unresponsive sepsis.

IX. ENTERIC INFECTIONS

A. AMEBIC COLITIS *(Entamoeba histolytica)*
1. Typically a tropical disease, although 5% of U.S. citizens are carriers
2. The most common complication is hepatic abscess formation.
3. Fecal-oral transmission
4. Trophozoite—Invasive, motile form causes ulcerations in the colon, primarily the cecum
5. Cyst—Infective form
6. Most infected people are carriers.
7. Symptoms/signs—Mild dysentery to severe colitis
8. Diagnosis—Trophozoites show microscopically in the stool in 90% of cases. Differentiation from ulcerative colitis is critical, because steroids can cause colonic perforation and lead to dissemination.
9. Ameboma—An inflammatory mass in the wall of the colon that can cause obstruction and may mimic a colon cancer diagnostically
10. Treatment—Metronidazole kills the invasive trophozoite. Iodoquinol kills the organisms within the lumen of the bowel. Operative therapy is indicated for an ameboma that is unresponsive to antibiotics.

B. GIARDIA *(Giardia lamblia)*
1. A protozoan infection obtained from drinking contaminated water. Most frequent parasitic pathogen in the United States.
2. Primarily involves the duodenum and jejunum
3. Symptoms/signs—Cramps, anorexia, steatorrhea
4. Diagnosis—50% detection in the stool; duodenal biopsy is most sensitive
5. Treatment—Metronidazole. Infection is prevented by water filtration.

C. CYTOMEGALOVIRUS COLITIS
1. 90% of AIDS patients are infected (in various organs) with cytomegalovirus (CMV).
2. 10% of AIDS patients get CMV colitis.
3. The most frequent cause for emergent exploration of the abdomen in AIDS patients
4. Symptoms/signs—Diarrhea, hematochezia, fever
5. Diagnosis—CMV inclusions are demonstrated on biopsy.
6. Treatment—Ganciclovir
7. Survival—50% at 6 months

37

COLITIS AND ENTERIC INFECTIONS

D. CHAGAS' DISEASE *(Trypanosoma cruzi)*
1. A protozoan endemic to South America
2. Destroys the myenteric plexus of Auerbach, primarily in the rectum, creating a functional obstruction that can cause megacolon proximal to lesion
3. Treatment—Resection

E. BACTERIA
1. *E. coli*—"Traveler's diarrhea"
a. Present in all stool
b. Most treated with trimethoprim-sulfamethoxazole (TMP-SMZ), but resistance is emerging.
c. Five pathogenic strains—Enterotoxigenic, pathogenic, hemorrhagic, invasive, and adherent
d. 0157:H7 strain—Most common cause of hemorrhagic colitis in the United States. Associated with hemolytic-uremic syndrome characterized by triad of microangiopathic hemolytic anemia, thrombocytopenia, and renal failure
2. *Shigella*—Noted for adherence to and penetration of mucosa. Treat with TMP-SMZ or tetracycline. Plasmid-mediated resistance is common.
3. *Salmonella*—Typhoid fever
a. Penetration of mucosa → lymphatic invasion → access to blood stream → reticuloendothelial system → recurrent bacteremia
b. Hyperplasia of Peyer patches can cause ulceration and/or perforation.
c. Treatment—Ampicillin or TMP-SMZ; however, resistant strains are emerging.
4. *Campylobacter*—No. 1 cause of bacterial diarrhea in United States
5. *Yersinia*—Suspect at negative appendectomy with findings of mesenteric adenitis and inflammation of the terminal ileum

F. ACTINOMYCOSIS *(Actinomyces israelii)*
1. Gram-positive anaerobic bacteria
2. Normal oral flora
3. Typically a head and neck infection—20% primarily involve the chest; 20% the abdomen. Abdominal involvement most commonly occurs as a cecal infection following an appendectomy.
4. Causes chronic inflammation and sinus formation
5. Treatment—Drainage and antibiotics (tetracycline or penicillin)

G. FOOD POISONING
1. Results from bacterial toxins produced in the food prior to ingestion. Inadequate cooking heat to kill the bacteria allows for multiplication and toxin elaboration while food is cooling, prior to eating.
2. Causes
a. *Clostridium perfringens*—12-hour, self-limited illness involving severe crampy pain without vomiting

b. *Staphylococcus aureus* (coagulase positive)—24-48 hours primarily of vomiting, but also involving cramping and diarrhea

c. *Bacillus cereus*—Both diarrheal and vomiting forms

X. INFECTIONS OF THE ANORECTUM

See Chapter 38.

Anorectal Disorders

Harry T. Papaconstantinou, MD

I. ANATOMY

A. RECTUM
1. The rectum is 12-15 cm in length and extends from the sacral promontory to the levator ani muscles.
2. The three teniae coli spread out at the rectosigmoid junction and fuse into a continuous smooth muscle layer with obliteration of the haustral markings.
3. Three horizontal rectal mucosal folds are visible internally as the *valves of Houston.*
4. The proximal third of the rectum is covered by peritoneum anteriorly and laterally. The anterior peritoneal reflection extends deep into the pelvis to ≈7 cm above the anal verge and lies behind the bladder in males and behind the uterus (pouch of Douglas) in females.

B. ANAL CANAL
1. Anatomic anal canal is 3 cm in length and extends from the dentate line to the anal verge.
2. Surgical canal—Extends from the top of the anorectal ring to the anal verge
3. The rectum is lined by colonic columnar epithelium. The transitional zone is lined with cuboidal epithelium that lines the anal canal from the columns of Morgagni to the dentate line. Anal glands located in the intersphincteric plane drain into the anal crypts that are pockets formed between each column. Below the dentate line the anal canal is lined by squamous epithelium.
4. Internal sphincter (involuntary)—Thickened continuation of the circular smooth muscle of the rectum under control of the autonomic nervous system
5. External sphincter (voluntary)—Downward extension of the puborectalis, which is striated muscle with somatic innervation (branch of the internal pudendal nerve S2-S4)

C. LEVATOR ANI MUSCLE
Composed of *iliococcygeus* and *pubococcygeus*, the levator ani muscle constitutes the pelvic floor and is innervated by the fourth sacral nerve.

D. BLOOD SUPPLY AND LYMPHATIC DRAINAGE
1. Arterial supply—Segmental but with rich anastomoses
a. Superior hemorrhoidal—Last branch of the inferior mesentery artery (IMA)
b. Middle hemorrhoidal—Branch of the internal iliac artery
c. Inferior hemorrhoidal—Branch of the internal pudendal artery

38

2. Venous drainage—Parallels the arterial supply

a. Superior hemorrhoidal—Drains the rectum and upper part of anal canal into the portal system

b. Middle hemorrhoidal—Drains rectum and upper anal canal into internal iliac vein (systemic circulation)

c. Inferior hemorrhoidal vein—Drains rectum and lower anal canal into the systemic venous return

d. The superior, middle, and inferior hemorrhoidal veins converge to form the inferior hemorrhoidal plexus in the submucosa of the columns of Morgagni.

3. Lymphatic drainage follows the paths of the arteries.

a. Superior and middle rectum—Drains into the IMA nodes

b. Lower rectum and upper anal canal—Drains into the superior rectal lymphatic (leading to the IMA) and to the internal iliac nodes

c. Anal canal distal to the dentate line—Has dual drainage to the inguinal nodes and the internal iliac nodes

II. HEMORRHOIDS

A. TYPES

1. Internal hemorrhoids—Cushions of dilated submucosal veins of the superior rectal plexus that lie proximal to the dentate line and are covered by transitional or columnar epithelium. Typically found in three locations

a. Left lateral—3 o'clock

b. Right posterolateral—7 o'clock

c. Right anterolateral—11 o'clock

d. Classification

First degree: Painless bleeding usually associated with defecation
Second degree: Protrude during defecation but spontaneously reduce
Third degree: Protrude during defecation and must be manually reduced
Fourth degree: Permanently prolapsed

2. External hemorrhoids—Dilated veins arising from the inferior hemorrhoidal plexus below the dentate line that are covered with squamous epithelium; generally asymptotic, unless thrombosed

B. SIGNS AND SYMPTOMS

1. Pain, pruritus, rectal bleeding (usually bright red with spotting of the toilet paper) with or without iron deficiency anemia, perianal moistness, or drainage

2. Symptoms are most commonly due to prolapsing internal hemorrhoids. Mucoid discharge and soiled undergarments occur when columnar mucosa is prolapsed beyond the anal verge, resulting in irritation and inflammation of the perianal skin.

3. Severe pain is not typically associated with internal hemorrhoids but is commonly seen with thrombosed external hemorrhoids.

C. TREATMENT

Although internal hemorrhoids are the most common cause of rectal bleeding, it is important to exclude other sources. Depending on the age of the patient, proctosigmoidoscopy or colonoscopy may be required to exclude more proximal sites of bleeding.

1. Initial treatment is nonoperative, except with symptomatic thrombosed hemorrhoids. Regulation of diet and bowel movement and avoidance of prolonged straining during defecation are used for mild symptoms. Sitz baths provide symptomatic relief and improve hygiene. Increasing dietary fiber, stool softeners, and bulk agents (psyllium) minimizes constipation and straining. Hydrocortisone acetate (Anusol-HC) suppositories and Tucks pads help resolve inflammation.
2. Nonoperative treatment—Usually used for first- and second-degree internal hemorrhoids
a. Rubber band ligation—Used in the treatment of internal hemorrhoids, rubber bands must be placed above the dentate line where somatic pain innervation is absent. Usually only one to two hemorrhoids are ligated per week. Further ligations can be performed every 4 weeks until symptoms have resolved.
b. Sclerotherapy—Submucosal injection of hemorrhoid with sclerosing agent, which obliterates the hemorrhoid by fibrosis
c. Other therapies—Include cryotherapy, bipolar diathermy, infrared coagulation, and direct current therapy
3. Hemorrhoidectomy indicated for prolapse, incarceration, pain, or persistent bleeding.
a. Dissection should be carried out in no more than three quadrants of the anal canal to avoid stricture formation (Whitehead's deformity).
b. The hemorrhoidal vein is ligated and then dissected free. The mucosa is closed for homeostasis but is left open distally for drainage.
c. Injection of long-acting local anesthetic is helpful.
d. Rectal packs may aid homeostasis but can be quite uncomfortable.
e. Sitz baths are started the next day as well as stool softeners or bulk laxatives.
f. Alternatively, circumferential stapled hemorrhoidectomy technique is emerging as a safe and effective alternative to traditional hemorrhoidal excision.
4. Thrombosed external hemorrhoids—These can be extremely painful and should be excised if seen within 48 hours. Beyond this time, conservative therapy with analgesics and sitz baths is appropriate.

III. ANAL FISSURE

Anal fissure is considered one of the most frequent causes of severe anal pain.

38

ANORECTAL DISORDERS

A. GENERAL
1. Represents an acute or chronic tear in the anal squamous epithelium usually in the posterior midline. The fissure extends from the dentate line to the anal verge. Lateral or multiple fissures should raise suspicion of trauma, inflammatory bowel disease, lymphoma, neoplasm, or infection and require further investigation such as proctosigmoidoscopy.
2. Equal frequency among males and females and most common in young adults
3. Typically associated with spasm of the internal sphincter

B. SIGNS AND SYMPTOMS
1. Sharp tearing or burning pain is associated with defecation. Blood may streak the toilet paper.
2. Physical exam may reveal a sentinel tag or hypertrophied papilla. Internal sphincter muscle fibers may be seen at the base of the fissure.

C. TREATMENT
1. Nonoperative therapy is used in anal fissures with mild or moderate symptoms.
a. Stool softeners and bulk laxatives relieve straining.
b. Sitz baths offer symptomatic relief and improve hygiene.
c. Anesthetic suppositories and nitroglycerine 0.2% cream may be helpful.
d. Botulinum toxin 20 units administered as two injections on each side of the anterior midline of the internal anal sphincter.
2. **Operative therapy indicated for failure of conservative management. The goal of surgery is to break the cycle of internal anal sphincter spasm and pain.**
a. Anal dilation—Disrupts the internal sphincter in an unpredictable way. May lead to incontinence.
b. Lateral-internal sphincterotomy—Predictable and effective. The lateral-internal sphincter is divided to relieve the spasm and pain. Most fissures heal with continued conservative care.

IV. ANORECTAL ABSCESS

Anorectal abscesses originate from an infection arising from the anal glands that communicate with the anal crypts. The acute phase of the infection causes an anorectal abscess, whereas the chronic stage is referred to as a *fistula*. An anorectal abscess typically forms in the intersphincter space. Subsequent spread can occur along various paths (Fig. 38-1). The exact etiology of anorectal abscess is not known. Factors implicated in the development of abscess include constipation, diarrhea, trauma, Crohn's disease, tuberculosis, actinomycosis, anorectal malignancy, leukemia, and lymphoma. The disease is more common in diabetic and immunocompromised patients than in the general public, and the incidence is much higher in men (3:1). Typically polymicrobial (*Escherichia coli, Proteus* spp, *Streptococcus* spp, and *Bacteroides* spp).

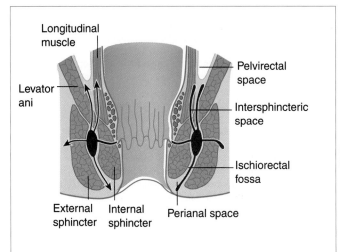

FIG. 38-1

Pathways of infection in perianal spaces.

A. CLASSIFICATION

1. Perianal abscess—Superficial abscess that lies beneath the skin of the anal canal but does not traverse the external sphincters.
2. Ischiorectal abscess—Occupy the ischiorectal fossa below the levators and lateral to the sphincters. The abscess can cross the midline to form bilateral abscess called a *horseshoe abscess*.
3. Intersphincteric abscess—Located between the external and internal sphincter muscle. Most common in the posterior quadrant. Typically without evidence of perianal swelling or induration.
4. Supralevator abscess—Occurring above the levators. More difficult to diagnose and drain. Can mimic an intra-abdominal condition.

B. SIGNS AND SYMPTOMS

1. Usually presents with extreme perianal pain
2. A mass is commonly felt on rectal exam. Cellulitis and fluctuance are often seen.
3. Systemic symptoms of fever, chills, and leukocytosis warrant urgent surgical decompression.
4. Vague pain and a high, ill-defined mass may be evidence for a supralevator abscess.

C. TREATMENT

1. Surgical drainage is always indicated, and drainage alone is usually sufficient therapy.

2. Most small, superficial perianal abscesses can be drained in the emergency department. Packing is left in overnight and removed with the institution of sitz baths or showers. Alternatively, long-term indwelling mushroom-tip catheters may be used.
3. Broad-spectrum antibiotics are indicated for diabetic or immunocompromised patients or patients with valvular heart disease or prosthetic implants.
4. Ischiorectal abscesses and all abscesses in diabetics or immunocompromised patients should be drained in the OR. Necrotizing fasciitis and Fournier's gangrene are feared complications if left undrained.
5. Supralevator abscesses may require CT-guided drainage or proximal fecal diversion in complex cases.
6. If not previously performed, a proctosigmoidoscopy should always be performed to rule out other proximal causes.

V. FISTULA IN ANO

A. GENERAL
1. An abnormal communication between the anal canal (internal opening) at about the level of the dentate line and the perianal skin (external opening)
2. Typically represents the incomplete healing of a drained anorectal abscess and is commonly secondary to a pyogenic process and, less frequently, a granulomatous disease
3. Those fistulas arising above the dentate line are typically secondary to diverticulitis neoplasm or trauma.

B. CLASSIFICATION
1. Intersphincteric fistula (70%)—Located in the intersphincteric space with external opening typically on the perianal skin near the anal verge
2. Trans-sphincteric fistula (23%)—Starts in the intersphincteric space, traverses the external sphincter into the ischiorectal fossa, with external opening lateral to the perianal skin. Horseshoe fistula falls into this category.
3. Suprasphincteric fistula (5%)—Starts in the intersphincteric space, passes above the puborectalis muscle and tracks laterally between the levator and the puborectalis muscle
4. Extrasphincteric fistula (2%)—Complicated fistula. Passes from the perianal skin through the ischiorectal fossa and levator ani muscles and subsequently through the rectal wall

C. GOODSALL'S RULE (Fig. 38-2)
1. Relates the position of the internal opening of a fistula to the external opening

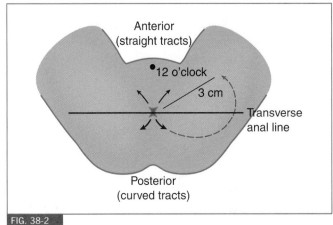

FIG. 38-2
Goodsall's rule.

2. Fistulas with external openings anterior to a transverse line through the anal opening have a fistula tract that extends directly to the anal canal anteriorly.
3. Those fistulas with an external opening posterior or >3 cm from the verge have a tract that curves and have their internal opening in the posterior midline. Fistulas defying this rule should raise the suspicion of inflammatory bowel disease. Anterior midline is the 12 o'clock position by convention.

D. SIGNS AND SYMPTOMS
1. Chief complaint is typically intermittent or constant drainage. A history of recurrent perianal abscess may be found.
2. The external opening is represented by a red cluster of granulation tissue. A cordlike tract may be palpated on rectal exam.

E. TREATMENT
1. Delineation of the fistula tract is most important but is possible in only two thirds of cases. This must be performed as an exam under appropriate anesthesia.
2. The entire tract must be unroofed for drainage. The wound heals secondarily. Actual excision of the tract (fistulectomy) is rarely necessary.
3. Fistulas traversing both internal and external sphincters require placement of a seton to prevent incontinence (Fig. 38-3). A heavy suture or vascular loop is passed through the tract to improve drainage and stimulate fibrosis of the tract. The seton may be sequentially

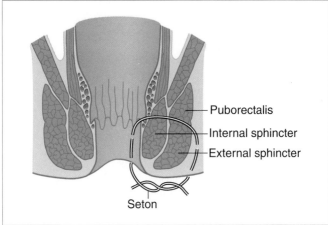

FIG. 38-3

Use of a seton in a high fistula.

tightened, and after significant fibrosis the tract is ultimately opened
with a greatly reduced risk of incontinence.
4. Horseshoe fistulas involve infection of the deep postanal space with
extension into the ischiorectal spaces on both sides. These can be
treated by opening the postanal space and placing appropriate
counterincisions laterally for drainage.

VI. PILONIDAL DISEASE

A. GENERAL
1. A common skin lesion of the sacrococcygeal area
2. Most frequently seen in young men after puberty and rarely after
40 years of age
3. The prevalence in adolescent males suggests a hormonal relationship.
However, it is believed to be a result of obstruction of the hair follicles in
this area, which then leads to formation of cysts, sinuses, or abscesses.
4. Sinuses or cysts are typically seen in the midline.
5. Most patients present with pain and swelling resulting from infection.

B. TREATMENT
1. Acute abscess—Incision and drainage with curettage of the cavity.
Impacted hair is removed. The wound is packed open. Up to 40% of
patients develop chronic draining pilonidal sinuses, which will require
further treatment.
2. Chronic pilonidal sinus—Many treatment options are available, and
their use depends on the severity of disease.

a. Lay open technique—Open sinus with incomplete excision and curettage; recurrence rate 15%; prolonged wound healing is 6 weeks

b. Excision and marsupialization—Recurrence rate 5-15%; accelerated healing

c. Simple pilonidal cystectomy with primary closure—Recurrence rate 15%; primary healing within 2 weeks

VII. ANAL AND PERIANAL INFECTIONS

A. CONDYLOMATA ACUMINATA

1. General—Condylomata acuminata (venereal warts) are caused by human papillomavirus and may occur on perianal skin, anorectal mucosa, or genital region. The incubation period is 1-6 months. Presenting symptoms include a lump in the perianal region, pruritus ani, bleeding, or pain. Examination reveals coliform-like masses that are typically pink or white and tend to grow in rows. There is a high incidence of dysplasia and an increased risk for cancer.

2. Treatment—Combination of local ablation and improved hygiene with concomitant treatment of sexual contacts. Genital lesions should be treated concurrently.

a. Podophyllin resin—25% solution in mineral oil or tincture of benzoin for small, scattered lesions

b. Fulguration under anesthesia for extensive involvement

c. Surgical excision of large masses may be necessary.

d. Giant condyloma (Buschke-Lowenstein tumor) may appear histologically benign but is locally invasive and malignant. May require wide local excision or abdominoperineal resection.

B. ANORECTAL HERPES

1. Usually presents with severe pain.

2. Characteristic herpetic lesions are seen on exam and are confirmed by Giemsa (Tzanck prep) stain, viral culture, and biopsy.

3. Treatment—No cure exists for herpes; however, antiviral agents such as acyclovir shorten the clinical course and the frequency of recurrence. Acutely, treatment includes oral acyclovir 200-400 mg five times daily for 10 days, whereas maintenance suppressive dosing of 400 mg b.i.d. for 1 year is recommended.

C. GONOCOCCAL PROCTITIS

1. Symptoms of gonococcal proctitis include pain and discharge.

2. Anoscopy reveals mucosal erythema and purulence of the anal crypts. *Gonococcus* is confirmed by Gram stain and culture.

3. Treatment—Owing to the rise in prevalence of penicillinase-producing *Neisseria gonorrhoeae*, ceftriaxone 250 mg IM (single dose) followed by doxycycline 100 mg PO b.i.d. for 7 days is recommended.

VIII. PRURITUS ANI

Perianal itching occurs in up to 1-5% of the population. Men are affected more commonly than women by a ratio of 4:1, and it is most common in the 5th and 6th decades of life. Pruritus ani begins insidiously, but the area of involvement spreads as intensity of itching increases and the patient starts scratching and irritating the skin, creating a vicious cycle.

A. GENERAL

1. There is a long list of causes, but in general any condition that leads to moisture, drainage, or soiling increases its prevalence. Therefore, it is important to obtain a careful history to aid in identifying the etiology. History should include, but not be limited to, dietary and bowel habits, hygiene practice, menopausal state, systemic diseases, prior anorectal surgeries, and previous radiation.
2. A careful examination of the perianal skin and anorectum is required. Biopsy and specimens for cultures are obtained when necessary.
3. Hygiene is the mainstay of treatment even when surgically correctable problems such as hemorrhoids exist. Improved hygiene may solve pruritus and improve other symptoms, obviating surgery.

B. CAUSES

1. Hemorrhoids, fissures, fistula
2. Other causes include fungi, pinworms, other infectious agents
3. Underlying disease—Diabetes, jaundice, Crohn's disease
4. Topical or dietary sensitivities
5. Neoplasm—Carcinoma, melanoma, Paget's disease of bone, Bowen's disease
6. >50% ultimately are classified as idiopathic.

C. TREATMENT

1. Goal is to keep perianal skin clean and dry by using appropriate hygiene
2. If symptoms continue in the compliant patient despite aggressive therapy, a second opinion from a dermatologist should be considered.

IX. ANAL NEOPLASM

Malignancies of the anal canal are relatively uncommon and represent only 2-3% of all anorectal carcinomas. The position of the tumor in the anal canal relative to the dentate line is important with regard to the biologic behavior of the tumor. This is based on the lymphatic drainage in these two areas. Most tumors spread by direct extension and lymphatic drainage. Hematologic spread is less common. Anal tumors are classified into two groups based on location: (1) anal canal tumors and (2) anal margin tumors.

A. TUMORS OF THE ANAL CANAL

1. Epidermoid carcinoma (1-2% of all colorectal carcinomas) are referred to as squamous, basaloid, cloacogenic, or transitional carcinomas. Although each has different histologic features, they exhibit similar biologic behavior and are thus grouped together.

a. Typically seen in patients 50-70 years of age

b. Seen more frequently in women

c. Two cell types—Squamous cell (keratinizing) and transitional cell (nonkeratinizing)

d. Rectal pain, bleeding, or mass are common presenting symptoms.

e. 40-50% have pelvic lymph node involvement at diagnosis, whereas 15-36% have inguinal nodal involvement and 10% have distant metastasis.

f. Excellent prognosis when discovered prior to nodal involvement and invasion to adjacent structures. 80% of tumors are cured by chemotherapy/radiation therapy alone.

g. Chemotherapy with mitomycin C and 5-fluorouracil combined with radiation is the treatment of choice. This may be followed by surgical resection. Abdominoperineal resection is indicated for residual disease or recurrence.

2. Malignant melanoma—0.5-1% of malignant anal tumors

a. Anal canal is the third most common site after skin and eyes.

b. Typically occurs adjacent to the dentate line

c. Rectal bleeding is the most frequent complaint.

d. Most are not highly pigmented, and diagnosis is difficult.

e. Tumor is aggressive and often widely metastatic. Abdominoperineal resection is indicated in selected patients.

f. Tumors often radioresistant and unresponsive to chemotherapy.

g. 5-year survival is <15%.

B. TUMORS OF THE ANAL MARGIN

1. These tumors are similar to skin tumors elsewhere and are treated likewise.

2. Include squamous cell and basal cell carcinomas, Bowen's disease, and Paget's disease of bone.

X. RECTAL PROLAPSE

A. CLASSIFICATION (Fig. 38-4)

Type I (false prolapsed or mucosal prolapsed): Redundant prolapsed rectal mucosa with radial folds in orientation

Type II (incomplete prolapsed): Rectal intussusception without a sliding hernia

Type III (true prolapsed or complete prolapsed): Protrusion of the entire rectal wall through the anal orifice with herniation of the pelvic peritoneum or cul-de-sac; circular mucosal folds are seen; most common type

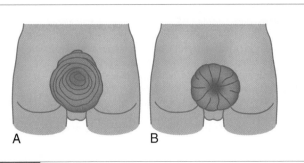

FIG. 38-4
Depiction of a true rectal prolapse *(A)* and a type I mucosal prolapse *(B)*.

B. CLINICAL FEATURES

1. 85% of patients are female with maximal incidence in the 5th and subsequent decades. Also seen in children <5 years old.
2. Many patients have had prior gynecologic surgery.
3. In men, the incidence is more evenly distributed throughout the age range.
4. High incidence of associated chronic neurologic or psychiatric disorders (5-50%)
5. Possible pathogenesis include either sliding-type hernia, where the rectum herniates through a defect in the pelvic fascia, or intussusception of the rectum.
6. Presenting complaints may be related to the prolapse itself or to the disturbance of anal continence that frequently coexists and includes the following.
a. Extrusion of a mass with defecation, exertion, coughing, sneezing, and so forth
b. Difficulty in bowel regulation—Tenesmus, constipation, fecal incontinence
c. Permanently extruded rectum with excoriation, ulceration, and constant soiling
d. Associated urinary incontinence or uterine prolapsed
7. Physical findings
a. Demonstrated prolapse during Valsalva's maneuver
b. Compromised sphincter tone
c. Excoriation or circumferential inflammation of mid-rectum on proctosigmoidoscopy

C. EVALUATION

1. Reduce the prolapsed segment, if possible, and perform sigmoidoscopy to determine the condition of the bowel and the presence of any associated lesion or carcinoma.

2. Assess sphincter tone and the degree of fecal continence by exam defecography and manometry. Many patients with rectal prolapse have poor sphincter tone.
3. Barium enema or colonoscopy
4. IV pyelogram—The ureters may be pulled with the rectum into the sliding hernia.
5. Radiographs of the lumbar spine and pelvis—Look for neurologic disease.
6. Cinedefecography—Useful in the evaluation of occult prolapse (type II)
7. Anal manometry and pudendal terminal motor nerve latencies may be indicated to assess sphincter function prior to operation. Identification of a nonrelaxing puborectalis may be useful in planning additional therapy such as biofeedback.
8. Transit time studies document functionally delayed transit (colonic inertia) as a cause of chronic constipation and straining and assess the need for colon resection.

D. TREATMENT OPTIONS
1. False prolapse
a. Common in very young children. Conservative therapy is often successful. Gently replace the prolapsed rectum after each defecation or straining. Excision of redundant mucosa is rarely necessary.
b. In adults, hemorrhoidectomy with excision of redundant mucosa is effective. Circumferential stapled hemorrhoidectomy may be used with similar results.
2. True prolapse—Typically a progressive disorder that is not responsive to nonsurgical therapy. Many procedures have been described that indicate the difficulty and chronicity of the problem. Basic features of the repairs include correction of the following anatomic characteristics.
a. Abnormally deep or wide cul-de-sac
b. Weak pelvic floor with diastasis of the levators
c. Patulous anal sphincter
d. Redundant rectosigmoid
e. Lack of fixation of the rectum to the sacral hollow with abnormal mobility and loss of the normal horizontal position of the lower rectum
f. Associated incontinence is not treated initially because it may resolve after treatment of the prolapse.

E. ABDOMINAL APPROACHES
1. Abdominal proctopexy with sigmoid resection. The lateral rectal stalks are used to anchor the rectum to the presacral fascia and periosteum. This is a treatment option in young, healthy patients and can be performed laparoscopically.
2. Rectal sling (Ripstein procedure)—The rectum is fixed to the sacrum using a sling of synthetic mesh. This must be loose enough to prevent obstruction. Foreign material makes concomitant sigmoid resection more hazardous and provides an increased risk of pelvic sepsis.

3. Ivalon sponge—Popular in Europe. The rectum is mobilized posteriorly and attached to the sacrum with a polyvinyl alcohol sponge.

F. PERINEAL APPROACH
The perineal approach is useful in debilitated patients who would not tolerate an abdominal incision.

1. Perineal rectosigmoidectomy (Altemeier procedure)—Involves resection of the redundant prolapsing bowel with primary anastomosis, high ligation of the hernia sac, and approximation of the levator ani muscles. This is well tolerated even in high-risk patients and may be performed under regional anesthesia.
2. Thiersch procedure—Of historical note only and is rarely (if ever) done. This technique was used in those too ill to tolerate even a perineal resection. The sphincters are encircled with a wire or band of synthetic material.

G. TRANS-SACRAL APPROACH
The trans-sacral approach is resection of the coccyx and lower sacrum with subsequent resection of the redundant prolapsing bowel with primary anastomosis. This technique has not gained popularity.

XI. ANOSCOPY

A. GENERAL
1. Examination of the lower rectum and anal canal
2. Patient preparation is not necessary; however, an enema may improve the exam depending on the clinical situation.

B. TECHNIQUE
1. Position the patient in right or left lateral decubitus position with hips and knees flexed. Alternatively, an examining table providing prone jackknife positioning is ideal.
2. Inspection—Note the presence of fissures, hemorrhoids, skin tags, blood, or pus.
3. Palpation—Digital exam must be done prior to anoscopy.
a. Note masses, induration, spasm, tenderness, or discharge.
b. Palpate normal structures, including prostate.
c. Inspect examining finger for blood, pus, stool, or mucus. Stool should be analyzed for occult blood.
4. Anoscopy
a. Lubricate generously and insert obturator.
b. Introduce anoscope into anus and point in direction of umbilicus. Once the upper end of the anal canal is reached, direct the anoscope posteriorly toward sacral hollow.
c. Note the character of mucosa, presence of lesions, masses, or foreign body.

d. Slowly withdraw scope, observing the mucosa as the scope passes.

XII. RIGID SIGMOIDOSCOPY

A. GENERAL
Rigid sigmoidoscopy reaches to 25-30 cm.

B. PATIENT PREPARATION
1. Gentle lavage such as magnesium citrate the evening before procedure
2. Clear liquids after midnight
3. The patient is given an enema in the morning or prior to the procedure.

C. TECHNIQUE
1. Position the patient in the lateral decubitus position or in elbow-to-chest position over a sigmoidoscopy table. Alternatively, an examining table providing prone jackknife positioning is ideal.
2. Inspect the perianal area and perform a digital exam, as in anoscopy.
3. Insert the scope into the anus directed toward the umbilicus.
4. As soon as the rectum is entered, remove the obturator and close the window. The scope should be advanced further only under direct visualization of the lumen. Insufflation is used as needed.
5. Slowly advance the scope though the lumen of the bowel. Movements are initially posterior into the sacral hollow, then anterior and left into the sigmoid colon.
6. Once the scope is fully inserted, it is slowly withdrawn in a circular fashion to carefully examine sigmoid and rectal mucosa.
7. Biopsy should be performed last so that blood does not obscure the rest of the exam.
8. Before the scope is removed, insufflated air should be evacuated for the patient's comfort.

RECOMMENDED READINGS

Brisinda G, Maria G, Bentivoglio AR, et al: A comparison of injections of botulinum toxin and topical nitroglycerine ointment for the treatment of chronic anal fissure. N Engl J Med 341:65-69, 1999.

Disorders of the Anorectum. Gastroenterol Clin North Am 30(1):entire issue, 2001.

Anorectal Surgery. Surg Clin North Am 74(6):entire issue, 1994.

ANORECTAL DISORDERS

Gynecologic Oncology

Russell J. Juno, MD

I. CERVICAL CANCER

The incidence of *invasive cancer* has steadily declined due to the Papanicolaou (Pap) smear, but the frequency of diagnosis of *carcinoma in situ* has increased. Therefore, cervical cancer is preventable disease. The lifetime risk of developing a cervical malignancy is <1%. It is second only to breast cancer as the leading cause of cancer death in women. Significant risk factors are young age at first intercourse, multiple sexual partners, high parity, low socioeconomic status, and cigarette smoking. These are all linked to sexual behavior and human papillomavirus (HPV) infection. Preinvasive intraepithelial carcinoma occurs primarily in women 20-30 years of age, whereas invasive carcinoma usually presents between 40 and 60 years of age. Cervical malignancy is predominantly squamous cell carcinoma (85-90%) or adenocarcinoma (10-15%). Other types include adenosquamous carcinoma, small cell variants, and cervical lymphoma. Adenocarcinoma appears to be more aggressive and appears at a more advanced stage, owing to its common location within the endocervix.

A. CLINICAL PRESENTATION

1. Presents (in decreasing frequency) with vaginal bleeding, abnormal Pap smear, lower abdominal pain, or vaginal discharge
2. Advanced lesions present with pain (pelvic, lower back, and/or lower extremity), dysuria, hematuria, and weight loss. The lesions may be exophytic, ulcerative, or endophytic.

B. DIAGNOSTIC WORK-UP

1. Yearly routine Pap smears recommended beginning at age 18 years or at initiation of sexual activity.
2. Low-grade squamous intraepithelial lesions and atypical glandular cells of undetermined significance—Repeat Pap smear every 4-6 months for 2 years. If a repeat is abnormal, then follow with colposcopy and biopsy. After three consecutive normal smears, resume annual screening. May also elect to go directly to colposcopy and endocervical curettage (ECC).
3. High-grade squamous intraepithelial cells require colposcopy and biopsy. Some advocate loop excision if the entire high-grade lesion is seen on colposcopy.
4. Cone biopsy if the following
   a. ECC shows intraepithelial or microinvasive carcinoma.
   b. Cytologic abnormality (Pap) is not consistent with tissue diagnosis.
   c. The entire transformation zone is not visible.
   d. Microinvasive carcinoma is diagnosed by direct biopsy.
   e. Premalignant or malignant glandular epithelium is detected.

5. Staging provides the basis for therapeutic decisions and prognosis and requires tissue and histologic diagnosis, a thorough history and physical exam (including bimanual pelvic and rectal exams), and radiologic and laboratory studies as appropriate.

C. STAGING

Cervical cancer is still staged *clinically*.

Stage 0: Carcinoma in situ, squamous intraepithelial lesions (SIL), or cervical intraepithelial neoplasia (CIN)

Stage I: Confined to the cervix; (IA) preclinical, with microscopic invasion <3 mm (IA1), or with invasion 3-5 mm in depth from the base of the epithelium (IA2), and a maximum of 7 mm horizontal spread. All tumors larger than IA2 are IB. Tumors <4 cm in size are IB1 and those >4 cm are IB2. *Overall 5-year survival is 65-90%.*

Stage II: Extends beyond cervix, including upper two thirds of vagina, but not to the pelvic wall (IIA); no obvious parametrial involvement (IIA) or with parametrial involvement (IIB). *Overall 5-year survival is 45-80%, 30-40% if adenocarcinoma.*

Stage III: Either extends to pelvic wall or invades the lower third of the vagina (III). IIIA extends to the lower vagina, while IIIB either extends to the wall and/or is associated with hydronephrosis or a nonfunctioning kidney. *The 5-year survival is as high as 61%, 20-30% if adenocarcinoma.*

Stage IV: Extension beyond the true pelvis or has clinically involved the mucosa of the bladder or rectum; spread to adjacent organs (IVA), or spread to distant organs (IVB). *The overall 5-year survival is <15%.* Other prognostic factors include age, tumor volume, histologic grade, lymphatic and vascular invasion, performance status, *HER2/neu* and c-*myc* oncogene overexpression, and tumor aneuploidy.

D. MANAGEMENT

Stage 0: Excision or ablation via cold-knife conization, laser cone, loop electrosurgical excision, cryotherapy, laser or electrocoagulable ablation. Some oral topical retinoids and 5-fluorouracil (5-FU) are under investigation.

Stage IA: Conservative surgery (conization, simple hysterectomy) for lesions with <3 mm stromal invasion, no invasion of blood or lymphatic channels, no areas of confluence, and negative margins. Conization is especially helpful in patients who wish to preserve fertility. Other lesions should be treated like stage IB lesions, and poor surgical candidates can be treated with intracavitary radiation.

Stage IB: 15% of patients have metastases to pelvic lymph nodes, and therefore options include radical hysterectomy and pelvic lymphadenectomy, or external pelvic combined with intracavitary irradiation

Stage IIA: Most recommend combination radiation therapy, although radical hysterectomy with lymphadenectomy may be appropriate for small-volume lesions

Stages IIB, III, IVA: Primarily with external and intracavitary irradiation, combined with radiosensitizing agents (hydroxyurea, 5-FU, cisplatin). External-field irradiation for para-aortic lymph nodes has shown to be of some benefit in long-term survival. Stage IVA, barring evidence of distant or unresectable disease, can occasionally be cured with pelvic exenteration.

Stage IVB: Treated with chemotherapy (primarily cisplatin), radiation given for palliation.

E. RECURRENCE

1. ≈35% have recurrent or persistent disease that generally develops within 2-3 years.
2. The pelvis is the most common site of recurrence, followed by the uterus and distant organs (lungs and bone).
3. Signs and symptoms include unexplained weight loss, lower extremity edema, pelvic and lower extremity pain, serosanguineous vaginal discharge, progressive ureteral obstruction, and lymphadenopathy.
4. *For locally recurrent cervical cancer,* after previous irradiation, treatment includes pelvic exenteration or, rarely, hysterectomy. If previously treated with surgery, irradiation therapy is appropriate. 25-50% of exenterations result in cure.
5. *For metastatic cervical cancer,* systemic chemotherapy (cisplatin) is the treatment of choice.
6. Overall prognosis is poor, with a 10-15% 1-year survival for all patients with recurrent disease.

F. SURVEILLANCE

1. Physical and pelvic exam, and Pap smear q 3 months for the first year, q 4 months for the second year, q 6 months for years 3-5, and annually thereafter.
2. Radiologic and laboratory studies include annual chest radiograph (may not be necessary in stages I-IIA), IV pyelogram annually, or at any time for patients with hydronephrosis (also may not be necessary for stages I-IIA), and CBC, BUN, creatinine q 6 months to yearly.

II. ENDOMETRIAL CANCER

Endometrial cancer is the most common gynecologic malignancy in the United States and the fourth most common malignancy in women. Mean age of onset is 63 years, but ≈25% of cases occur in premenopausal women. The lifetime risk of development is 1 in 38. Chronic, unopposed exposure to estrogen is the principal predisposing factor; other risk factors include early menarche, late menopause, obesity, chronic anovulation, nulliparity, estrogen-secreting tumors, complex atypical hyperplasia, and ingestion of unopposed estrogen (progestins can nullify this risk). Other associations include pelvic radiation, hypertension, diabetes mellitus, and a history of breast or ovarian malignancy. The use of oral contraceptives is *negatively* correlated with the incidence of endometrial cancer. Histologically, about 75% are adenocarcinomas, followed by adenosquamous (15-20%), papillary serous, and clear cell. Other types include mucinous carcinoma, squamous, undifferentiated, and mixed type.

A. CLINICAL PRESENTATION AND DIAGNOSIS

1. Presenting signs and symptoms include any bleeding or abnormal vaginal discharge in postmenopausal women or abnormal menstruation or intermenstrual bleeding in perimenstrual and premenopausal women.
2. Diagnostic work-up in suspected patients includes a careful inspection of the vulva, anus, vagina, and cervix; a Pap smear; transvaginal ultrasonography; and endometrial biopsy, curettage, or aspiration.
3. Once confirmed, pretherapy work-up includes physical exam for adenopathy (supraclavicular and inguinal), ascites, and liver size. A chest radiograph to look for lung metastases should be performed. Further evaluation should be tailored to the patient's specific symptoms or findings.

B. STAGING AND GRADING

1. Staging

Staging for endometrial cancer is surgical. Once cancer is biopsy proven, a total abdominal hysterectomy and bilateral salpingo-oophorectomy, peritoneal cytology, and pelvic and periaortic node dissection are done.

Stage I: Confined to the body of the uterus with tumor limited to the endometrium (IA), or invasion to less than (IB) or more than (IC) half of the myometrium. *The overall 5-year survival is 75-100%.*

Stage II: Involves the uterine body and cervix with endocervical glandular involvement only (IIA) or cervical stromal invasion (IIB). *The 5-year survival is ≈60%.*

Stage III: Extends outside the uterus, but confined to the true pelvis or involves para-aortic nodes; IIIA invades uterine serosa and/or adnexa and/or has positive peritoneal cytology, IIIB has vaginal metastasis, and IIIC involves pelvic and/or para-aortic lymph nodes. *The 5-year survival is 30-50%.*

Stage IV: Involves adjacent bladder and/or bowel mucosa (IVA) or distant metastases (IVB). *The 5-year survival is 10-20%.*

2. Histopathologic grading

Grade 1: ≤5% of a nonsquamous or nonmorular solid growth pattern
Grade 2: 6-50% of a nonsquamous or nonmorular solid growth pattern
Grade 3: >50% of a nonsquamous or nonmorular solid growth pattern

Note: *Although staging and grade usually correlate, the clinical stage is more influential in the prognosis.*

C. MANAGEMENT

1. Low-risk disease is grade 1 or 2 tumors confined to the endometrial cavity (IA)—Require no further therapy
2. Intermediate-risk disease is grade 1 or 2 tumors with middle third invasion and no extrauterine spread (IB-C, II)—Postoperative radiation (whole-pelvis or intracavitary) is questionable.
3. High-risk disease is extrauterine disease or grade 3 tumors with any invasion—Benefits from adjuvant therapy. If positive aortic nodes are found, whole-pelvis radiation is given.
4. Intra-abdominal metastatic disease—May benefit from debulking surgery and adjuvant whole-abdomen radiation therapy, chemotherapy (doxorubicin, cisplatin, or multiagent), or progestin therapy combined with radiation
5. Distant metastatic disease—Usually treated with single agent or combination chemotherapy

D. RECURRENT DISEASE

Recurrent endometrial cancer is managed with radiation therapy for patients originally treated with radiation alone or with chemotherapy or progestin therapy for patients having received radiation.

Postoperative follow-up should be q 3 months for the first year, then q 3-4 months for the next, q 6 months for the third year, and then annually. Pap smears should be done annually and CA-125 levels checked in patients who had initial elevations and extrauterine disease.

E. TAMOXIFEN

Used in breast cancer treatment as an antiestrogen, tamoxifen has weak estrogen effects on the uterine lining. Its use, especially after 5 years, has been associated with an increased incidence of endometrial cancer. However, the benefit of therapy for breast cancer far outweighs the potential increase. Some advocate annual screening with vaginal ultrasonography or hysteroscopy. All breast cancer patients, and postmenopausal women, should undergo annual gynecologic evaluation and endometrial samplings for abnormal vaginal bleeding or discharge.

III. OVARIAN CANCER

Ovarian cancer accounts for ≈25% of all gynecologic malignancies but for ≈50% of gynecologic cancer-related deaths because of the usual advanced stage at presentation. Risk of developing ovarian cancer is 1 in 70 women in her lifetime and increases with age until 70 years. Other risk factors include positive family history, low parity, decreased fertility, and delayed childbearing. In contrast, high parity, oral contraceptive use, tubal ligation, and hysterectomy have been shown to decrease the risk of epithelial ovarian cancer. Most (85-90%) are epithelial in origin, with the other types (germ cell and sex cord-stromal tumors) rarer.

39

GYNECOLOGIC ONCOLOGY

A. SCREENING

1. Unfortunately, no effective screening program exists; therefore, most patients present clinically with advanced-stage carcinoma, with only 30% of the cases confined to the ovaries.
2. Careful pelvic examination remains the only effective screening method to date.
3. Transvaginal ultrasonography offers some promise; however, tumor markers such as CA-125 are not sensitive or specific enough to be helpful as a *screening tool*, especially in early-stage disease.

B. CLINICAL PRESENTATION AND DIAGNOSIS

1. Most presenting symptoms are those associated with increasing tumor mass, spread of tumor along the surfaces of other organs, and disseminated disease. These include abdominal discomfort, upper abdominal fullness, early satiety, constipation, dysuria, polyuria, vaginal bleeding, and constitutional symptoms.
2. Physical findings include pelvic tenderness and ascites associated with a pelvic mass. An adnexal mass that is bilateral, irregular, solid, or fixed is suggestive of malignancy, although not diagnostic.
3. All masses, both solid and cystic, found in premenarchal girls and postmenopausal women should be considered abnormal and potentially malignant.
4. Work-up includes a thorough history and physical exam, including pelvic and rectal examination and Pap smear; pelvic ultrasound (as discussed above), CT or MRI to detect extraovarian disease and lymphadenopathy; chest radiograph to rule out metastatic disease or pleural effusion; and blood tests including CA-125 (elevated in 80-85%). Other tumor markers such as CA-19-9 (mucinous epithelial ovarian carcinomas), α-fetoprotein and human chorionic gonadotropin (germ cell tumors), lactate dehydrogenase (dysgerminoma), and carcinoembryonic antigen (epithelial ovarian carcinoma) may also be useful.
5. Postmenopausal women with completely cystic lesions without septations and normal serum markers may be treated conservatively. They must be followed up in 3 months for signs of change.
6. All solid masses found in premenarchal girls are considered neoplastic, and surgery is indicated.
7. For women of reproductive age, a unilateral cystic lesion <8 cm can be followed up in 4-6 weeks. For solid, bilateral or >8-cm, cystic lesions, surgery is indicated.

C. STAGING

Ovarian cancer is surgically staged by laparotomy, noting any ascites and performing cytologic washes on entering the abdomen. The abdominal cavity should then be explored systematically and biopsies taken as indicated.

Stage I: Growth limited to one ovary (IA) or both ovaries (IB) with no tumor on external surface, capsule intact and no malignant ascites; or involving the surface of one or both ovaries, capsule ruptured or with peritoneal washings containing malignant cells (IC). *The 5-year survival is 60-90%.*

Stage II: Growth involving one or both ovaries with extension and/or metastases to the uterus and/or tubes (IIA), extension to other pelvic tissues (IIB), or pelvic extension with malignant ascites or washings (IIC). *The 5-year survival is 40-70%.*

Stage III: Tumor involving one or both ovaries grossly limited to the true pelvis with negative nodes but with microscopic seeding of abdominal peritoneal surfaces (IIIA); macroscopic implants of abdominal peritoneal surfaces, none >2 cm in diameter and negative lymph nodes (IIIB) or abdominal implants >2 cm in diameter and/or positive retroperitoneal or inguinal lymph nodes (IIIC). *The overall 5-year survival is 4-15%.*

Stage IV: Involves one or both ovaries with distant metastasis, positive pleural effusion cytology, or parenchymal liver metastasis. *The 5-year survival is 0-5%.*

D. MANAGEMENT

1. Surgical management is aimed at confirming the diagnosis, staging early disease, and resecting as much of the tumor as possible in advanced disease.

a. If a malignant tumor is identified, thoroughly inspect the abdomen and pelvis, remove the primary tumor, submit free fluid for cytology, or send peritoneal washings.

(1) If fertility is not desired, the patient should undergo total abdominal hysterectomy and bilateral salpingo-oophorectomy, biopsy of the peritoneum or suspicious areas and the right hemidiaphragm, removal of the infracolic omentum or other diseased portion, and sampling of the pelvic and periaortic nodes. If there is no extraovarian spread, care should be taken not to rupture the capsule when removing the adnexa, because this may seed the peritoneal cavity and increase the stage of the cancer.

(2) If fertility is desired, the contralateral adnexa and uterus can be preserved in women with stage IA disease. Laparoscopy must be performed by an experienced operator, because it increases the risk of rupturing the primary tumor.

b. Cytoreductive surgery and debulking procedures in which residual disease is minimized, ideally to <2 cm of residual disease, have been shown to improve long-term survival in stage II and III cancers and may provide palliation in stage IV, and therefore should be performed.

2. Adjunctive therapy

a. Stage I lesions that are poorly differentiated or associated with dense adhesions to adjacent structures or stage IC disease warrant

further therapy. Multiagent chemotherapy including cisplatin has been shown to be as effective as intraperitoneal chromium phosphate ^{32}P.
b. Stage II lesions can be managed with intraperitoneal ^{32}P, total abdominal irradiation, or systemic chemotherapy followed in 1 year by a second-look surgery with similar survival statistics.
c. Stage III lesions are treated with removal of as much tumor as possible, followed by combination chemotherapy (cisplatin and cyclophosphamide [Cytoxan]).
d. Stage IV lesions are treated similar to stage III lesions; however, the overall results are disappointing.

E. RECURRENT DISEASE
1. Platinum-based chemotherapeutic agents, if not used in the past or used >6 months prior to recurrence, are the standard regimen. No survival advantage over supportive therapy alone has been shown.
2. Second-line agents, including paclitaxel (Taxol) (≈30% response rate), are used for patients not meeting this criterion.
3. Cytoreductive surgery is used only in those who have had a long disease-free survival and if the recurrent disease is amenable to surgery.

F. SPECIAL CONSIDERATIONS
1. Borderline epithelial tumors account for ≈15% of epithelial tumors, are of low malignant potential, and usually occur in premenopausal women. Stage I tumors can even be treated with unilateral salpingo-oophorectomy if preservation of fertility is desired, whereas more advanced tumors are treated similar to the usual epithelial ovarian cancers.
2. Germ cell tumors account for 2-3% of ovarian cancers and usually occur in younger women. Most are unilateral, and unilateral salpingo-oophorectomy can be performed for stage IA lesions if the contralateral ovary appears normal (biopsies are often taken). Chemotherapeutic agents such as BEP (bleomycin, etoposide, Platinol) are often used, even for IA lesions.
3. Sex cord–stromal tumors account for ≈2% of ovarian cancers and include granulosa cell and Sertoli–Leydig cell tumors. Most are unilateral and can be managed similar to the germ cell tumors.

G. OVARIAN CANCER HEREDITARY SYNDROMES
1. Breast and ovarian cancer syndrome—Both cancers occur at higher rates in individuals with the *BRCA1* and *BRCA2* genes than in the general public.
2. Site-specific ovarian cancer syndrome—Probably a form of breast and ovarian cancer syndrome that is found too early for breast cancer to be seen. Linked to the *BRCA1* gene.
3. Ovarian cancers associated with higher rates of colorectal and endometrial cancers. Hereditary nonpolyposis colorectal cancer is seen with 10-15% of all hereditary ovarian cancers.

IV. VULVAR CANCER

Vulvar cancer accounts for only 5% of gynecologic malignancies, with 80% of them being of squamous cell origin. Risk factors include advanced age, low socioeconomic status, smoking, hypertension, obesity, diabetes, previous neoplasm of the cervix or vagina, and immunosuppression. HPV infection has been associated with vulvar cancer, but the relationship is not as clear as in cervical cancer. Syphilis, lymphogranuloma venereum and granuloma inguinale have also been cited as antecedent infections. Clinical signs and symptoms include a mass or a lump on the vulva and vulvar itching and/or irritation. Bleeding, discharge, and dysuria are less common. On physical examination, the lesion is usually raised and may appear fleshy or ulcerated. Diagnosis is based on biopsy, and evaluation should include a thorough pelvic and rectal examination with colposcopy because vulvar cancer is associated with other malignancies of the lower genital tract. Fine-needle aspirates of suspected groin lymph nodes may aid in diagnosing advanced disease. Vulvar cancer spreads by (1) direct extension to adjacent structures; (2) lymphatic embolization to regional lymph nodes; and (3) hematogenous spread to distant organs including the liver, lungs, and bone.

A. STAGING

Stage 0: Carcinoma in situ; intraepithelial carcinoma

Stage I: Confined to the vulva and/or perineum; ≤2 cm in greatest diameter (<1 cm IA and >1 cm <2 cm IB); no nodal metastasis. *The 5-year survival is ≈90%.*

Stage II: Confined to the vulva and/or perineum; >2 cm in greatest diameter; no nodal metastases. *The 5-year survival is 75-80%.*

Stage III: Tumor of any size with (1) adjacent spread to the distal urethra and/or the vagina, or the anus, and/or (2) unilateral regional lymph node metastasis. *The overall 5-year survival is ≈50%.*

Stage IV: Tumor invades proximal urethra, bladder, rectum, bone and/or bilateral regional node metastasis (IVA), or involves distant metastasis, including pelvic lymph nodes (IVB). *The overall 5-year survival is 20-70%, depending on extent of metastasis.*

B. MANAGEMENT

1. Radical vulvectomy with bilateral inguinal lymphadenectomies through separate incisions and occasional bilateral pelvic lymphadenectomy is the preferred treatment for most vulvar cancers but is associated with a high morbidity rate.

2. Preoperative radiation and neoadjuvant combined-modality therapy can be used in patients with locally advanced disease to reduce the need for exenteration. Postoperative radiation is often used to decrease the incidence of inguinal node recurrence in patients with ≥2 positive inguinal lymph nodes.

3. Cancers that are not poorly differentiated and <2 cm in diameter and no more than 1 mm thick can often be treated with deep and wide

excision (1 cm) alone, without lymph node dissection. Locally advanced lesions can be treated with external-beam radiation with radiosensitizing agents followed by excision.

C. FOLLOW-UP
A pelvic exam and Pap smear should be done q 3 months for 2 years, q 6 months for 5 years, and then yearly.

D. OTHER VULVAR CARCINOMAS
1. Melanoma is the second most common vulvar malignancy and presents as a raised, nodular pigmented lesion. Most patients are >50 years of age. Diagnosis is confirmed by biopsy, and the primary lesion should be excised with at least a 2-cm margin. Tumors with invasion of more than 0.75 mm should be removed en bloc with removal of the regional nodes. Prognosis is related to the thickness, with overall 5-year survival about 30-35%.
2. Bartholin's gland carcinoma accounts for 5% of vulvar cancers but is often misdiagnosed. Any persistent mass in the region of the gland, especially in patients >50 years of age, should be biopsied. Radical vulvectomy with bilateral inguinal node dissection is the traditional treatment, but less radical surgery such as hemivulvectomy or radical local excision may be as effective. Postoperative radiation may reduce the incidence of local recurrence.
3. Paget's disease of the vulva predominantly affects postmenopausal white women and presents with pruritus and local soreness and an erythematous, scaly appearing lesion. Second primary lesions occur in ≈30% and usually involve the GU or GI tract or the breasts. Treatment requires wide local excision. If an underlying adenocarcinoma or underlying stromal invasion is present, a more radical local excision or radical vulvectomy is needed combined with a regional lymphadenectomy.
4. Verrucous carcinoma is rare and requires an adequate biopsy to distinguish it from a benign condyloma or a squamous cell carcinoma. These tumors are slow growing, are locally destructive, and usually occur in postmenopausal women. Treatment should be by radical local excision.

V. VAGINAL CANCER
Vaginal cancer is defined as tumor confined to the vagina with no involvement of the cervix or vulva. It accounts for only 1-2% of all gynecologic malignancies. Most malignancies in the vagina are metastatic. The mean age at occurrence is 60-65 years; 80-90% are squamous and are usually located in the upper posterior wall of the vagina. Clear cell adenocarcinoma is a rare vaginal carcinoma, seen more commonly in diethylstilbestrol-exposed women. Patients usually present with abnormal vaginal bleeding or discharge, whereas pelvic pain and dysuria are late

symptoms. Physical examination requires careful inspection and palpation of the vagina, and colposcopy and/or biopsies are performed as appropriate. After diagnosis, work-up should include a chest radiograph and exam under anesthesia with cystoscopy and proctoscopy. A CT scan may also help with staging.

A. STAGING

Stage 0: Carcinoma in situ. *The 5-year survival is 95%.*
Stage I: Confined to the vaginal wall. *The 5-year survival is 80%.*
Stage II: Involves subvaginal tissue, but not into parametrium.
   The 5-year survival is 50%.
Stage III: Extending to the pelvic sidewall. *The 5-year survival is 35%.*
Stage IV: Extending beyond true pelvis to bladder or rectum or
   metastasis outside true pelvis. *The 5-year survival is 10%.*

B. MANAGEMENT

1. Carcinoma in situ is usually managed by surgical excision, laser ablation, topical 5-FU, or high-dose brachytherapy. Frequent follow-up with Pap smears is needed.
2. For stage I lesions that do not involve the upper vaginal fornices, radiation therapy (usually intracavitary) is the standard form of treatment.
3. Stage I lesions involving the upper fornices can be treated with a radical hysterectomy, pelvic lymphadenopathy, and partial vaginectomy.
4. Stage IIA lesions are usually treated with external radiation ± intracavitary radiation. More advanced tumors are also treated with external-beam and intracavitary radiation.
5. Recurrent disease is usually treated with surgery, from wide local excision to pelvic exenteration.
6. Chemotherapy has also been tried with varying degrees of success.
7. Clear cell adenocarcinoma usually requires radical hysterectomy, pelvic lymphadenectomy, and removal of most of the vagina with reconstruction.
8. Advanced lesions are treated with radiation, similar to squamous cell neoplasms.

VI. CANCER OF THE FALLOPIAN TUBE

Cancer of the fallopian tube is the rarest of gynecologic malignancies, accounting for only 0.3-1% (metastatic disease to the fallopian tube is 10 times more common than primary tumors) and affects primarily older women.

A. CLINICAL PRESENTATION AND DIAGNOSIS

1. Although the combination of abnormal vaginal bleeding, discharge, lower abdominal pain, and an adnexal mass in a postmenopausal woman is considered pathognomonic, these signs and symptoms are not common.

2. Usually, the diagnosis is made on surgical exploration, and most are adenocarcinoma. There are no official staging criteria for fallopian tube carcinoma, but the prognosis is related to the spread of the disease to adjacent organs, the peritoneum, and regional and para-aortic lymph nodes.

B. MANAGEMENT
1. Treatment includes a total abdominal hysterectomy, bilateral salpingo-oophorectomy, peritoneal cytology, and lymph node dissection. Postoperative intraperitoneal ^{32}P or whole-abdominal radiation is indicated for positive peritoneal cytology, and abdominoperineal radiation including to the para-aortic lymph nodes is used when spread involves adjacent organs. Combination chemotherapy is also often used for intraperitoneal spread or recurrent disease.
2. Overall 5-year survival is ≈40%.

Jaundice

Burnett S. Kelly, Jr., MD

Jaundice is a readily visible sign of various diseases. By definition, jaundice is the icteric manifestation of abnormal bilirubin metabolism. A thorough patient history, physical examination, and the appropriate laboratory and diagnostic studies can assist in identifying surgically treatable jaundice.

I. GENERAL CONSIDERATIONS

A. NORMAL BILIRUBIN METABOLISM

1. Bilirubin is derived from hemoglobin (70-90%) and nonhemoglobin (10-30%) sources via microsomal heme oxygenase.

a. Hemoglobin of senescent erythrocytes
b. Myoglobin and other hemoproteins
c. Hepatic hemoproteins (cytochrome P-450)
d. Ineffective erythropoiesis

2. Indirect—Bilirubin noncovalently bound to albumin; water insoluble (unconjugated)

3. Direct—Bilirubin conjugated by glucuronic acid; water soluble (conjugated)

a. Bilirubin—Albumin transported across the hepatic sinusoid into the hepatocyte.
b. Within the hepatocyte, bilirubin is bound to glutathione-S-transferase.
c. Conjugation occurs within the endoplasmic reticulum of the hepatocyte.
   (1) Diglucuronide—Normal
   (2) Monoglucuronide—Present in hepatocyte injury; may react as "direct"
d. Conjugated bilirubin secreted into canalicular system

B. ENTEROHEPATIC CIRCULATION

Conjugated bilirubin is excreted by the liver into the bile ductile system and then the duodenum. Bilirubin is reduced to urobilinogen by small intestine bacteria. In the terminal ileum, 10-20% is absorbed and re-excreted by the liver and kidneys. 80% of bile acids are neosynthesized daily.

C. CLINICAL JAUNDICE

Jaundice is evident when total bilirubin >2 mg/dL. Consuming large quantities of carotenes or lycopenes, or drugs such as rifampin or quinacrine, can give the false appearance of jaundice.

II. HISTORY AND PHYSICAL EXAM

A. HISTORY

1. Abdominal pain, fever, nausea, and vomiting
2. Dark urine, light stools
3. Itching

4. Diarrhea, malabsorption
5. Alcohol, IV drug abuse

B. PHYSICAL EXAM
1. Clinical jaundice—Skin, sclera, oral mucosa under tongue
2. Abdominal tenderness
3. Abdominal masses
a. Hepatomegaly, splenomegaly
b. Palpable gallbladder
4. Stigmata of chronic liver disease
a. Spider angiomata, palmar erythema, caput medusae
b. Ascites, muscle wasting (malar or hypothenar wasting most notably)
c. Asterixis, encephalopathy
d. Testicular atrophy
e. Malnutrition

III. LABORATORY TESTS

Lab studies are conducted to differentiate hepatic from posthepatic causes of jaundice. Blood tests in combination with a physical exam and history can have >95% positive predictive value.

A. BILIRUBIN
In jaundice of hemolysis and hepatocellular disease, indirect bilirubin makes up 90-95% of the total bilirubin. In obstructive jaundice, direct bilirubin makes up >50% of total bilirubin.

	Normal (mg/dL)	Hemolysis	Hepatocellular Disease	Bile Duct Obstruction
Serum bilirubin				
Indirect	0.2-1.3	Increased	Increased	Normal
Direct	0-0.3	Normal	Increased	Increased
Urine				
Urobilinogen	2-4	Increased	Increased	Absent
Bilirubin	Negative	Negative	Positive	Positive
Fecal				
Urobilinogen	40-280	Increased	Decreased	Absent

B. CBC
1. Microcytic anemia with an increased reticulocyte count suggests hemolysis. Peripheral smear reveals sickle cells, spherocytes, and target cells.
2. Increased white blood cell (WBC) count is consistent with infectious etiology but is nonspecific.

C. TRANSAMINASES
Transaminases are increased with hepatocellular injury (viral, alcoholic, or drug-induced hepatitis).

1. Serum glutamic-pyruvic transaminase (SGPT) or alanine aminotransferase (ALT)—More specific for liver than SGOT
2. Serum glutamic-oxaloacetic transaminase (SGOT) or aspartate aminotransferase (AST)—Found in liver, heart, skeletal muscle, kidney, pancreas

D. ALKALINE PHOSPHATASE
There is increased production of alkaline phosphatase by proliferating terminal biliary ductules in response to intrahepatic or extrahepatic obstruction.
1. Sources—Liver, bone, placenta, kidney, WBCs, intestine
2. Increased level may also be due to hepatic infiltrative diseases (tuberculosis, sarcoid, lymphoma), space-occupying lesions (abscess, neoplasm), bone disease, and pregnancy.

E. 5'-NUCLEOTIDASE
5'-Nucleotidase shows comparable sensitivity to alkaline phosphatase but with increased specificity. Sources are liver (bile canaliculi and sinusoidal membranes), intestine, heart, brain, blood vessels, and endocrine pancreas (also increase during third trimester of pregnancy).

F. GAMMA GLUTAMYL TRANSFERASE (GGT)
The sensitivity and specificity of GGT is greater than alkaline phosphatase.

G. PROTHROMBIN TIME (PT)
1. Dependent on hepatic synthesis of factors V, VII, and X, prothrombin and fibrinogen, and intestinal absorption of vitamin K
2. Helpful in assessment of hepatic synthetic function and reserve
3. If PT >3 seconds above control, treat with vitamin K 10 mg SQ or IV
a. Corrects within 48 hours if due to cholestasis or deficiency
b. Remains prolonged if due to hepatocellular insufficiency

H. ALBUMIN
1. Reflection of hepatic synthetic function and nutritional status
2. Half-life of approximately 15-20 days. Not as valuable in detecting acute liver injury. Short-turnover proteins (lactate dehydrogenase, transferrin, prealbumin, and retinol-binding protein) are more indicative of current synthetic status.

I. UROBILINOGEN
The total absence of urobilinogen from urine and feces indicates complete biliary obstruction.

J. HEPATITIS SEROLOGY (Table 40-1)
1. Hepatitis A
a. IgM—Acute and transient
b. IgG—Appears during recovery and persists

TABLE 40-1		
SEROLOGIC FEATURES OF VIRAL HEPATITIS		
Form of Infection	Serologic Markers	Interpretation
Hepatitis A	IgM anti-HAV	Acute disease
	IgG anti-HAV	Remote infection and immunity
Hepatitis B	HBsAg	Acute or chronic disease
	HBeAg	Active replication
	IgM anti-HBc (high titer)	Acute disease
	IgG anti-HBc	
	IgG anti-HBc positive	Past infection and immunity
	IgG anti-HBc negative	Immune response from vaccination
Hepatitis C	Anti-HCV	Acute, chronic, or resolved disease
Hepatitis D	HBsAg and anti-HDV	Acute disease
	IgM anti-HBc positive	Co-infection
	IgG anti-HBc negative	Super-infection
Hepatitis E	None	

HAV = hepatitis A virus; HBsAg = hepatitis B surface antigen; HBeAg = hepatitis Be antigen; HBc = hepatitis B core; HCV = hepatitis C virus; HDV = hepatitis D virus; Ig = immunoglobulin.

2. Hepatitis B (Fig. 40-1)

a. HBsAg—Surface antigen; first marker to appear; absent by 3 months

b. HBcAg—Core antigen

c. HBeAg—Internal component of the nucleocapsid gene of hepatitis B virus (HBV). Indicates ongoing viral replication. HBV is most infectious when this is detected in the serum

d. HBsAb—Surface antibody; presence suggests "recovery" and immunity from HBV infection

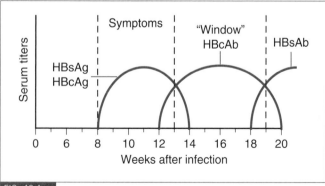

FIG. 40-1

Serology of hepatitis B virus. HBsAg = hepatitis B surface antigen; HBcAg = hepatitis B core antigen; HBsAb = hepatitis B surface antibody; HBcAb = hepatitis B core antibody.

e. HBcAb—Core antibody; present during "window" period when HBsAg and HBsAb are too low to measure

f. Important risk factor for hepatocellular carcinoma

g. HBV DNA replication correlates with active viral replication

3. Hepatitis C

a. Responsible for >90% of post-transfusion hepatitis

b. Chronic hepatitis develops in 50% of patients.

c. Anti-hepatitis virus C is not detectable in 10-20% of chronic hepatitis C patients.

4. Hepatitis D

a. Can develop in patients with HBsAg in serum

b. IV drug abusers and hemophiliacs at particular risk

5. Hepatitis E

a. "Enterically transmitted non-A, non-B hepatitis"

b. Transmitted by contaminated water

c. Does not lead to chronic infection

IV. DIAGNOSTIC STUDIES

Imaging studies are designed to delineate the etiology, presence, and level of posthepatic jaundice.

A. ABDOMINAL FLAT PLATE

1. Gallstones—15% are radiopaque

2. Gas in biliary tree—Seen in gallstone ileus and surgical anastomoses with intestinal tract, cholangitis with gas-producing organism

3. Emphysematous cholecystitis—Gas in gallbladder wall, extremely rare, is usually seen in diabetics

B. ULTRASONOGRAPHY

1. Accuracy >90% for cholelithiasis

2. Can identify dilated intrahepatic and extrahepatic ducts, common duct stones, hepatic and pancreatic masses

3. Accuracy affected by obesity, ascites, bowel gas, skill of technician and radiologist

C. NUCLEAR BILIARY SCAN (HIDA AND OTHERS)

1. Unreliable test if serum bilirubin >20 mg/dL (hepatic secretion of agent decreases as serum bilirubin >5 mg/dL)

2. Visualization of bile ducts but not gallbladder suggests cystic duct obstruction; 95% sensitive for acute cholecystitis

3. Visualization of the duodenum rules out *complete* common duct obstruction.

D. LIVER SCAN

Liver scan reveals liver and spleen size, masses (>2 cm), and parenchymal disease better than HIDA scan.

40

JAUNDICE

E. COMPUTED TOMOGRAPHY
CT scan is most effective in identifying liver and pancreatic masses and the level of extrahepatic biliary obstruction.

F. PERCUTANEOUS TRANSHEPATIC CHOLANGIOGRAPHY (PTC)
1. Identifies cause, site, extent of obstruction prior to surgery
2. Provides therapeutic drainage as well as diagnostic imaging of the obstruction and biliary anatomy
3. Obtainable in 95% of patients with dilated ducts secondary to extrahepatic biliary obstruction
4. Contraindications
a. Coagulopathy—Prolonged PT, partial thromboplastin time; platelets <40,000/mm^3
b. Ascites—Unable to tamponade liver puncture
c. Perihepatic or intrahepatic sepsis
d. Disease of right lower lung or pleura
5. Complications (4%)—Bile peritonitis, bilothorax, pneumothorax, sepsis, hemobilia, bleeding

G. ENDOSCOPIC RETROGRADE CHOLANGIOPANCREATOGRAPHY (ERCP)
1. Visualization of upper GI tract, ampullary region, biliary and pancreatic ducts
2. Allows collection of cytology and biopsy specimens
3. Complications—Traumatic pancreatitis (1-2%), pancreatic or biliary sepsis. Preprocedure coverage with broad-spectrum antibiotic is recommended.

H. PERCUTANEOUS LIVER BIOPSY
1. Histologic evaluation of liver parenchyma
2. Determines hepatic causes of jaundice
3. Contraindications—See section IV. F. 4

I. MAGNETIC RESONANCE CHOLANGIOPANCREATOGRAPHY (MRCP) AND ENDOSCOPIC ULTRASOUND (EUS)
1. Newer modalities
2. MRCP allows midresolution imaging of the biliary system with accompanying imaging of the liver. Indicated for patients with immediate contraindication to ERCP or PTC.
3. EUS is an invasive procedure that is most beneficial in facilitating a biopsy or duct brushings
a. Complications—Esophagus, gastric, or duodenal perforation, and bleeding
b. Lower false-negative (sampling error) rate than duct brushing

J. CHOLANGIOSCOPY
1. New modality, not widely practiced
2. Fiberoptic scope inserted through side-viewing endoscope
3. Facilitates tissue sampling and stone removal

K. BILIARY OPTICAL COHERENCE TOMOGRAPHY
Biliary optical coherence tomography is largely experimental at this time

V. DIFFERENTIAL DIAGNOSIS OF JAUNDICE

A. PREHEPATIC JAUNDICE
1. Hemolysis
a. Increased indirect bilirubin; unconjugated bilirubin is bound with albumin and cannot be excreted in urine
b. Production of bile pigments can raise total bilirubin by only 3 mg/dL (total bilirubin >5 mg/dL indicates associated liver disease or biliary obstruction).
2. Gilbert's disease—Defect in hepatocyte uptake of indirect (unconjugated) bilirubin and a deficiency in bilirubin conjugation. Good prognosis with this disease.
3. Crigler-Najjar (types 1 and 2)—Decreased conjugation secondary to profound deficiency in uridine diphosphate (UDP)–glucuronyl transferase activity
a. Type 1 is an autosomal recessive disease associated with absence of UDP–glucuronyl transferase and early childhood death. The cause of death is most frequently kernicteric brain injury. The disease is unresponsive to phenobarbital. Treatment is with orthotopic liver transplant.
b. Type 2 is an autosomal recessive disease characterized by decreased UDP–glucuronyl transferase activity. This disease is responsive to phenobarbital administration.

B. HEPATIC JAUNDICE
1. Viral hepatitis
a. Insidious onset of symptoms—Anorexia, malaise, fever, nausea, arthralgias, myalgias, headache, photophobia, pharyngitis, cough, coryza, and low-grade fever. Usually precede abdominal pain.
b. Tender enlarged liver
c. Serologic markers (see section III. J)—Cytomegalovirus titers
2. Alcoholic hepatitis—Long history of alcohol abuse
3. Drug-induced hepatitis—Acetaminophen, halothane, erythromycin, isoniazid, chlorpromazine, valproic acid, phenytoin, oral contraceptives, 17,α-alkyl, substituted anabolic steroids, chlorpropamide, and methimazole
4. Cirrhosis (see Chap. 41)

5. Dubin-Johnson syndrome—Impaired hepatic excretion of conjugated bilirubin
6. Cholestatic jaundice of pregnancy (see Chap. 19)
7. Rotor's syndrome—Autosomal recessive condition marked by cholestasis and increased urine coproporphyrin level

C. POSTHEPATIC/OBSTRUCTIVE JAUNDICE
1. General considerations
a. Increased total bilirubin, bilirubin present in urine (dark-colored, "Coca-Cola" urine), clay-colored stool
b. When total bilirubin is >3 mg/dL, both direct and indirect fractions are increased.
c. Abdominal pain usually precedes symptoms of systemic disease.
d. Painless jaundice with palpable gallbladder suggests cancer distal to the cystic duct (Courvoisier's law).
e. Charcot's triad—Fever, right upper quadrant (RUQ) pain, jaundice; suggests extrahepatic obstruction with ascending cholangitis; a surgical emergency
f. Reynolds' pentad—Charcot's triad, shock, mental obtundation
2. Choledocholithiasis (see Chap. 42)
3. Cholangitis (see Chap. 42)
4. Sclerosing cholangitis
a. Nonbacterial inflammatory narrowing of bile ducts—Predominantly affects men ages 20-50 years; etiology unknown
b. Presents with fatigue, weight loss, anorexia, insidious development of jaundice and pruritus, intermittent RUQ pain
c. Estimated that 50% of patients with sclerosing cholangitis have or will develop ulcerative colitis
d. ERCP and biopsy used for diagnosis—Rule out malignancy
e. Treatment
    (1) Medical—Corticosteroids, long-term antibiotics to prevent cholangitis, immunosuppression, bile-acid binding agents, penicillamine
    (2) Surgical—T tube, transhepatic stent, other decompressive procedure
f. May progress to secondary biliary cirrhosis with ascites, varices, and hepatic failure requiring transplantation
5. Benign biliary stricture
a. 95% caused by surgical trauma; 5% caused by abdominal trauma, chronic pancreatitis or impacted stone
b. Presents with intermittent cholangitis, jaundice
c. Diagnosis with PTC or ERCP—Stricture usually within 2 cm of bifurcation
d. Treatment
    (1) Antibiotics for cholangitis
    (2) Surgical repair requires tension-free anastomosis and mucosal apposition—Choledochoduodenostomy, choledochojejunostomy or end-to-end bile duct anastomosis

e. Complications (if untreated)
   (1) Infection—Cholangitis, abscess, sepsis
   (2) Liver/biliary disease—Cirrhosis, portal hypertension
6. Cholangiocarcinoma (Altemeier-Klatskin tumor)
a. Diagnosis usually made in 7th decade—Commonly metastatic at presentation
b. Associated conditions—Ulcerative colitis (incidence unaffected by colectomy), *Clonorchis sinensis* infection (oriental liver fluke), chronic typhoid carrier state, choledochal cyst, sclerosing cholangitis
c. Presentation includes insidious onset of jaundice, pruritus, anorexia, pain, and possible cholangitis.
d. Diagnosis—PTC or ERCP with abdominal CT scan
e. Bismuth (modified) classification of intrabiliary cancer extent
   Type 1: 2 cm below hepatic duct bifurcation
   Type 2: At level of bifurcation
   Type 3a: Through the common duct with extension up the right hepatic duct system
   Type 3b: Through the common duct with extension up the left hepatic duct system
   Type 4: Through the common duct with extension up the bilateral hepatic ducts
f. Therapy
   (1) Curative resection (rarely possible)—Wide resection and reconstruction of biliary tree
   (2) Palliative resection—Cholecystojejunostomy, choledochojejunostomy, U tube or percutaneous drainage catheters
   (3) Both postoperative and palliative radiation may prolong life.
g. Prognosis—5-year survival is 10-15%.
7. Carcinoma of the head of pancreas—See Chapter 44
8. Carcinoma of the ampulla of Vater.
a. 10% of obstructing tumors of common duct; either ampullary or duodenal carcinoma
b. Presentation—Early jaundice, occult blood in stool
c. Diagnosis with CT and biopsy during ERCP
d. Spread locally with slow rate of metastasis
e. Therapy—Pancreaticoduodenectomy
   (1) 5-10% operative mortality
   (2) Prognosis—5-year survival is 39%.
9. Choledochal cyst—Congenital cyst of the extrahepatic biliary tree
a. Classic triad consists of RUQ mass, jaundice, and pain.
b. Four times more common in females
c. One third diagnosed before age 10 years
d. Natural history—If left untreated, may progress to complete biliary obstruction, cholangitis, secondary biliary cirrhosis, spontaneous rupture (frequently occurs during pregnancy), or carcinoma
e. Five subtypes—All treated surgically

40

JAUNDICE

Type I: Cystic dilation of entire common hepatic and common bile duct. Excision of cyst with Roux-en-Y hepaticojejunostomy is the procedure of choice.

Type II: Diverticulum of common bile duct. Excise diverticulum.

Type III: Cystic dilation of the distal common bile duct (choledochocele). Marsupialize the diverticulum with a long sphincteroplasty or divide the common bile duct with Roux-en-Y choledochojejunostomy.

Type IV: Extrahepatic and intrahepatic biliary cystic dilation (Caroli's disease)

Type V: Fusiform extrahepatic and intrahepatic dilatation. Both types IV and V are treated by Roux-en-Y hepaticojejunostomy with transhepatic stent placement.

RECOMMENDED READINGS

Blumgart LH, Fong Y (eds): Surgery of the Liver and Biliary Tract, 3rd ed. London, WB Saunders, 2002, pp 218-221.

Frank BB: Clinical evaluation of jaundice: A guideline of the Patient Care Committee of the American Gastroenterological Association. JAMA 262:30-31, 1989.

Schiff ER, Sorrell MF, Maddrey WC (eds): Schiff's Diseases of the Liver, 8th ed. Philadelphia, Lippincott-Raven, 1999, p 119.

Cirrhosis

Burnett S. Kelly, Jr., MD

Cirrhosis is defined by the formation of scar tissue and is the end result of parenchymal liver damage and failed hepatocyte regeneration. With scar formation there is a change in liver architecture such that resistance to blood flow, especially portal blood flow, increases. The result is portal hypertension and the formation of spontaneous compensatory portosystemic shunts and hepatocellular failure.

I. ETIOLOGY

A. ETHANOL ABUSE
Ethanol abuse is responsible for up to 70% of cases of cirrhosis in the United States.

B. VIRAL HEPATITIS (B and C)

C. HEREDITY
Hemolytic anemia and α_1-antitrypsin deficiency are inherited disorders.

D. BILIARY OBSTRUCTION

E. PRIMARY BILIARY CIRRHOSIS

F. AUTOIMMUNE HEPATITIS

G. OCCUPATIONAL EXPOSURE
Exposure to chemicals, e.g., carbon tetrachloride, beryllium, and vinyl chloride, can cause cirrhosis.

H. SCHISTOSOMIASIS

I. NUTRITIONAL
Cirrhosis can result from long-term total parenteral nutrition (TPN).

J. CONGESTIVE HEART FAILURE (CHRONIC)

II. DIAGNOSIS

A. HISTORY
1. Cirrhosis is a chronic disease process.
2. Patients are often aware of their diagnosis and have a history consistent with the etiologic factor.

B. PHYSICAL EXAM

1. Examine for the stigmata of hepatocellular failure and portal hypertension—Jaundice, dark urine, muscle wasting, ascites, peripheral edema, purpura, encephalopathy, splenomegaly, spider angiomata, caput medusae, asterixis, gynecomastia, testicular atrophy, "venous hum" over the right upper quadrant, palmar erythema, loss of body hair, and Dupuytren's contractures.

2. Liver may be enlarged due to vascular congestion or shrunken due to chronic disease. Patients should also be evaluated for hemorrhoids (less specific finding).

C. LIVER FUNCTION TESTS

1. Bilirubin

a. Direct hyperbilirubinemia—Due to excess conjugated bilirubin owing to overproduction or underexcretion

b. Indirect hyperbilirubinemia—An inability to conjugate and clear bilirubin (excess unconjugated bilirubin)

c. Clinical jaundice is apparent when total bilirubin is >2 mg/dL.

d. Conjugated bilirubin is water soluble and excreted by the kidney.

2. Serum enzymes

a. Alkaline phosphatase

    (1) Produced in bone, placenta, and liver

    (2) Excreted in bile

    (3) Elevated alkaline phosphatase can signal obstruction of bile ducts (in the absence of bone disease and pregnancy)

b. Transaminases

    (1) Aspartate aminotransferase (AST; serum glutamic-oxaloacetic transaminase [SGOT])

    (2) Alanine aminotransferase (ALT; serum glutamic-pyruvic transaminase [SGPT])

    (3) ALT > AST in viral hepatitis

    (4) AST > ALT in alcoholic hepatitis

    (5) Transaminase may be normal in long-standing disease, despite acute exacerbation.

3. Serum proteins (measure synthetic function)

a. Albumin—Low when hepatic function is impaired

b. Coagulation factors

    (1) Prothrombin time (PT) reflects adequate fibrinogen, prothrombin, and coagulation factor (V, VII, IX, X) production.

    (2) PT is prolonged when fat absorption, and subsequent vitamin K absorption, are impaired (i.e., biliary obstruction, malnutrition, and hepatocellular insufficiency).

D. RADIOLOGIC PROCEDURES

1. Scintillation scans—Reflect hepatic functional capacity; "cold spot" seen when hepatocyte function is decreased or absent

2. CT scan—Assesses liver size, ascites, and presence of varices
3. Ultrasonography
4. Angiography—Can directly measure hepatic artery pressures as well as define portal vein flow during the venous phase (see section IV). CT angiography can be useful in determining portal and systemic vessel patency as well as hepatobiliary pathology.

E. PERCUTANEOUS LIVER BIOPSY
1. Allows histologic diagnosis
2. Contraindications—Coagulopathy, thrombocytopenia, cholangitis, tense ascites
3. Complications—Bile leak or peritonitis, pneumothorax, bleeding, pain

F. PARACENTESIS
1. Relieves dyspnea and anorexia due to increased intra-abdominal pressure
2. Cytologic exam of ascitic fluid—Can distinguish cause (cancer vs. cirrhosis) and diagnose spontaneous bacterial peritonitis
3. Complications—Infection, bleeding, perforation of viscus

III. CIRRHOSIS AND LIVER FUNCTION

To appreciate the impact of cirrhosis, it is important to understand that the liver is the "metabolic clearinghouse" and regulates almost every aspect of metabolism. Although cirrhosis implies nothing about the state of hepatic function, a cirrhotic liver is metabolically dysfunctional.

A. CARBOHYDRATE METABOLISM
1. Glycogenesis $\leftrightarrow$ glycogenolysis
2. Glycolysis $\leftrightarrow$ gluconeogenesis
3. Derangements result in hyperglycemia (early cirrhosis) and hypoglycemia (sine qua non of profound advanced failure).

B. PROTEIN METABOLISM
1. Amino acids and bacterially produced ammonia from the gut are metabolized to urea by the liver. (Hyperammonemia may be present during encephalopathy, but 10% of encephalopathic patients have a normal serum ammonia level.)
2. Proteins synthesized in the liver include blood clotting factors, albumin, transferrin, and immunologic proteins. Decreased production results in ascites, edema, and coagulopathy.

C. FATTY ACID METABOLISM
1. Fatty infiltration of the liver may be seen when fatty acids cannot be metabolized.
2. Serum cholesterol levels may be lowered in liver disease states.

41

CIRRHOSIS

D. HORMONE METABOLISM

1. Both activation and inactivation of various hormones (estrogen, testosterone, thyroxine, corticosteroids, aldosterone) are carried out in the liver
2. Altered hormonal metabolism may result in gynecomastia, testicular atrophy, loss of axillary and pubic hair, palmar erythema, and increased total body water.

E. DRUG METABOLISM

1. Uptake, detoxification, and excretion of drugs occur in the healthy liver.
2. Dosage requirements in cirrhotic patients may be different for drugs including antibiotics, anti-inflammatory agents, antiarrhythmics, and anticonvulsants.

IV. PATHOPHYSIOLOGY

Alterations in liver function and the development of portosystemic shunts result in the pathophysiologic disease processes that characterize a patient with cirrhosis.

A. PORTAL HYPERTENSION

1. Defined as portal venous pressure >12-15 mm Hg by direct measurement, or a wedged hepatic vein pressure (WHVP) >4 mm Hg above inferior vena cava (IVC) pressure; usually becomes clinically significant when WHVP >12 mm Hg above IVC pressure.
2. Portal hypertension is commonly classified by the level of venous obstruction.
   a. Prehepatic (or presinusoidal)—Portal vein thrombosis, tumor encasement, primary biliary cirrhosis, and schistosomiasis
   b. Intrahepatic (sinusoidal)—Alcoholic and postnecrotic viral cirrhosis
   c. Post-hepatic (or post-sinusoidal)—Hepatic vein occlusion (Budd-Chiari syndrome), vena caval web (most prominent in Japanese)
   d. In the absence of obstruction, portal hypertension can occur with increased portal flow, i.e., splenic arteriovenous (AV) fistula or hepatic artery–portal vein AV fistula
3. Portal vein pressure is decompressed through portosystemic collateral veins (Fig. 41-1)
   a. Esophageal (esophageal venous plexus, coronary vein)
   b. Gastric (coronary vein)
   c. Abdominal wall (umbilical vein)
   d. Hemorrhoidal (inferior mesenteric vein, veins of Retzius)
   e. Diaphragm (diaphragmatic veins of Sappey)
4. Diagnosis
   a. Portal venography—Obtained by venous phase imaging during mesenteric arteriography
      (1) Defines size and location of dilated veins and provides qualitative estimate of hepatic portal perfusion

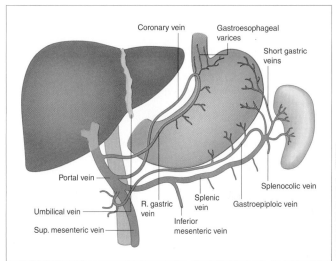

FIG. 41-1

Portal venous anatomy.

      (2) Hepatopedal flow (away from liver) vs. hepatofugal flow
         (toward liver)
  b. Hepatic vein wedge injection
      (1) Visualize portal vein if hepatopedal flow present
      (2) Used to determine adequacy of portal perfusion
  c. Measurement of portal pressure
      (1) Direct—Measured during operation or venography
      (2) Indirect—WHVP; compare to IVC pressure (see section IV. A. 1)

B. ASCITES
1. Local causes
a. Portal hypertension—Increased hydrostatic pressure
b. Lymphatic outflow obstruction—Ascitic fluid can be seen weeping from
   surface of liver at surgery
2. Systemic causes
a. Hypoalbuminemia—Results in low intravascular oncotic pressure, with
   water loss into the extravascular space
b. Secondary hyperaldosteronism
     (1) Due to increased secretion and/or decreased inactivation of
        aldosterone by the impaired liver
     (2) Results in increased total body water and sodium, due to
        augmented sodium resorption in the distal tubule

c. Increased antidiuretic hormone secretion
   (1) Due to relative hypovolemia, as detected by the carotid body and the CNS
   (2) Results in decreased free water clearance

C. CARDIOVASCULAR CHANGES
1. High cardiac output and low systemic vascular resistance (SVR) may cause cardiac failure.
2. Low SVR is not completely understood, but several contributing factors are hypothesized.
a. Peripheral shunting (splanchnic, muscle, skin)
b. Putative vasodilatory agents include prostaglandins, γ-aminobutyric acid, vasoactive intestinal polypeptide, substance P, insulin, glucagon, and bile acids.
c. Decreased estrogen metabolism
d. Accumulation of "false" or "weak" neurochemical transmitters (phenylethylamine, tyramine, octopamine), displacing sympathetic adrenergic transmitters (norepinephrine)

D. RENAL DYSFUNCTION
Hepatorenal syndrome may result (Table 41-1), including oliguria with elevated BUN and creatinine levels.
1. Type 1—Resolved by relief of ascites and improved volume status/renal perfusion
2. Type 2—Resolved by improved hepatic function and increased SVR
3. Urine sodium < 10 mEq/L

E. ENCEPHALOPATHY
1. Characterized by altered consciousness, asterixis ("liver flap"), rigidity, hyperreflexia, electroencephalographic changes
2. May be seen in acute or chronic hepatic dysfunction
3. Etiology—Shunting of portal blood, containing toxins and nutrients metabolized by healthy hepatocytes, around the liver. Factors implicated include ammonia, mercaptans, aromatic amino acids, and others.
4. Precipitating factors
a. GI hemorrhage.
b. Portosystemic shunting procedure
c. Infection, especially spontaneous bacterial peritonitis
d. Excessive dietary protein
e. Constipation
f. Narcotics and sedatives

V. CHILD'S CLASSIFICATION
Patients with cirrhosis are at increased risk during any kind of surgery. When elective surgery is being considered, prophylactic treatment for the

TABLE 41-1

CLASSIFICATION OF HEPATORENAL SYNDROME

Characteristic	Type 1	Type 2
Blood pressure	Normal or low	Increased
Cardiac index	Normal or decreased	Increased
Peripheral resistance	Normal or increased	Decreased
Intravascular volume	Low	Normal
Urinary sodium	<10 mEq/L	<10 mEq/L
Pathophysiology	Effective hypovolemia Portoreflex	Maldistribution of blood flow
Associated findings	Intractable ascites	Hepatic encephalopathy
	Pressure gradient between IVC and right atrium	Acute hepatic insult
	High hepatic vein wedge pressure	
Therapy	Volume infusion	α-Adrenergic agents and
	Ascites reinfusion (rare)	levodopa—neither of
	Peritoneal-atrial shunt	these results in survival
	Side-to-side portal decompression	unless hepatic function improves

IVC = inferior vena cava.

41

CIRRHOSIS

complications of cirrhosis should be considered (see section VI. A). Child's classification (Table 41-2) originally was designed as a prognostic guide for patients receiving portal decompressive surgery. It has been modified to extrapolate surgical risk in cirrhotic patients receiving other surgical procedures. With proper preoperative intervention (i.e., nutritional support, bowel preparation with antibiotics), liver function can be improved (as indicated by improved Child's class) and the risk of surgery reduced.

The cumulative score determines the Child's classification.

Child's A = 5-7 points (2% mortality)
Child's B = 8-10 points (10% mortality)
Child's C ≥ 11 points (>50% mortality)

TABLE 41-2

CHILD-TURCOTTE-PUGH MODIFIED CLASSIFICATION

	1 Point	2 Points	3 Points
Ascites	None	Controlled	Uncontrolled
Bilirubin (mg/dL)	<2.0	2.0-2.5	>3.0
Encephalopathy	None	Minimal	Refractory
Prothrombin time (seconds)	1-4	4-6	>6
Albumin (g/dL)	>3.5	3.0-3.5	<3.0

VI. TREATING CIRRHOSIS COMPLICATIONS

A. PROPHYLAXIS
1. Ensure fluid and electrolyte management.
a. Sodium and water restriction
b. Cautious diuresis—Overdiuresing can result in intravascular dehydration and prerenal acute renal failure.
2. Maintain nutritional status.
a. Patients are hypermetabolic and require as much as 1.1 g protein/kg/day to maintain nitrogen balance.
b. Hepatamine is a specifically defined TPN solution that is high in branched-chain amino acids and low in aromatic amino acids that can be used in patients with liver dysfunction. Low-sodium enteral diet is still the preferred primary source of nutrition.
3. Prevent GI bleeding, which increases intraluminal protein load.
a. H_2 blockers
b. Neutralize gastric pH.
4. Reduce intestinal flora to decrease bacterial production of ammonia.
a. Oral neomycin (500 mg PO q 6 h) to decrease intraluminal bacterial counts
b. Lactulose (15-30 mL PO b.i.d.) is metabolized to organic acids in the colon; NH_3 (easily absorbed and delivered to the liver via the portal circulation) is readily converted to NH_4^+, which is poorly absorbed, due to the change in colonic pH.

B. GASTROINTESTINAL BLEEDING
1. Diagnosis
a. Endoscopy (esophagogastroduodenoscopy)
b. In cirrhotic patients, 50-90% of upper GI bleeds are due to variceal hemorrhage.
c. Remaining percentage due to Mallory-Weiss tears, portal hypertensive gastropathy, peptic ulceration, gastric or esophageal neoplasm
2. Natural history
a. 15-30% of cirrhotic patients have varices; <50% bleed from them.
b. 20-50% mortality from first variceal hemorrhage; of those who live, >70% rebleed within 1 year
c. Bleeding is rare unless WHVP exceeds IVC pressure by 12 mm Hg
3. Treatment
a. Nasogastric tube, saline lavage, Foley catheter
b. Volume resuscitation
    (1) Blood and blood products
    (2) Maintain hematocrit >27-30%
c. Correct coagulopathy
    (1) Fresh frozen plasma, cryoprecipitate, platelets as appropriate
    (2) Vitamin K, 10 mg IV (does not work immediately)

d. IV vasopressin—Controls bleeding in 75% of patients
  (1) Initial bolus of 20 units over 20 minutes
  (2) Continuous drip at 0.2-0.8 units/min
  (3) After bleeding stops, wean off by 0.1-unit increments over 48 hours; watch closely, because rebleeding is common.
  (4) Vasopressin is a potent splanchnic vasoconstrictor that should be combined with nitroglycerin 50 μg/min IV to protect against cardiac ischemia
e. Esophageal balloon tamponade (Sengstaken-Blakemore, Minnesota tubes)
  (1) Initial success rate is high, but rebleeding occurs in 40-70%.
  (2) Gastric erosion, gastric and esophageal perforation, and aspiration pneumonia are complications.
  (3) Consider prophylactic endotracheal intubation to prevent aspiration.
f. Endoscopic banding/sclerotherapy
  (1) Acute control of bleeding accomplished in up to 90% of patients, with 20-30% mortality.
  (2) With adequate visualization of bleeding site, banding of varices is technically easier and is associated with a higher success (lower rebleeding) rate than sclerotherapy.
  (3) Endoscopic banding/sclerotherapy is technically challenging in the presence of the following.
    (a) Bleeding that occurs at the gastroesophageal junction
    (b) Multiple (circumferential) varices
    (c) Excessive bleeding that obscures visualization
  (4) Sclerosing agents, including ethanolamine oleate, sodium morrhuate, and sodium tetradecyl sulfate—Administered into the varix directly, around the varix, or both, with similar results
g. Portal decompression
  (1) *Nonselective* shunt, e.g., portacaval—Eliminates portal venous flow; most effective at controlling bleeding, but followed by a high rate of encephalopathy and hepatic failure
  (2) *Selective* shunt, e.g., distal splenorenal—Preserves portal venous flow to the liver
  (3) Operative mortality may reach 40-50% in Child's class C patients.

4. Therapeutic options in prevention of recurrent variceal hemorrhage.
a. Pharmacologic therapy—β blockers, nitrates, and calcium channel blockers have been studied; most have not been demonstrated to be beneficial especially over the long term.
b. Endoscopic sclerotherapy
  (1) Decreases the frequency of recurrent variceal hemorrhage (48-58%) when compared to conventional medical management. 5-year survival not significantly different than in those patients who undergo portosystemic shunt procedures.
  (2) Injection sclerotherapy should be performed until all varices are eradicated. Despite complete eradication, varices have been shown

41

CIRRHOSIS

to recur at a mean interval of 1-2 years. Rebleeding rate is ≈15% per year after obliteration of varices is achieved.

    (3) Patients with gastric varices, or whose varices are difficult to eradicate or have recurrent bleeding during therapy, should have early consideration for portosystemic shunt.

c. Nonselective (total) portosystemic shunts (Fig. 41-2)

    (1) Portacaval shunt—End-to-side (Eck fistula) and side-to-side portacaval shunts are the gold standard by which other shunts are evaluated.

        (a) Prospective, randomized trials have failed to show any survival benefit compared to conventional medical therapy. When data from these trials are combined, however, some survival benefit is probable.

        (b) Highly effective in preventing recurrent variceal hemorrhage (>90%). Hepatic encephalopathy occurs in about 15-30% of cases, whereas hepatic failure is a major cause of postshunt mortality (13-18%).

        (c) The failure to show significant survival benefit has significantly decreased use of total portosystemic shunts. At present, the most common indications include the use of an end-to-side shunt in acute variceal hemorrhage and a side-to-side shunt in the treatment of refractory ascites.

    (2) Interposition H-graft shunts—Mesocaval, portacaval, and mesorenal

        (a) Grafts >10 mm diameter are generally considered total shunts.

        (b) Increased frequency of late thrombosis compared to conventional portacaval shunts

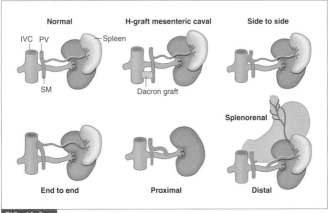

FIG. 41-2

Normal portacaval circulation (*upper, left*) and types of portosystemic shunts. IVC = inferior vena cava; SM = superior mesenteric; PV = portal vein.

(c) Useful in patients who are transplant candidates
(3) Central splenorenal shunt (Linton shunt)
    (a) Includes splenectomy with anastomosis of portal side of splenic vein to the left renal vein
    (b) Physiologically and hemodynamically similar to a side-to-side portacaval shunt
    (c) Results similar to those with portacaval shunts, but probably has a higher thrombosis rate
(4) Transjugular intrahepatic portosystemic shunt (TIPS)—Radiologically guided, percutaneously placed shunt. Obviates the need for surgery, useful in high-risk or pretransplant patients. Long-term data not yet available.

d. Selective portosystemic shunts
  (1) Distal splenorenal (Warren-Zeppa) shunt
    (a) Most commonly employed selective shunt used in United States. Splenic vein is divided and splenic side is anastomosed end-to-side to left renal vein. Spleen remains in situ and the coronary vein is ligated.
    (b) Varices are decompressed via the short gastric veins. Decompresses the varices while maintaining portal perfusion in ≈90% of patients.
    (c) Operative mortality (7-10%) and long-term survival are similar to nonselective shunts in patients with alcoholic cirrhosis. Survival seems to be improved in patients with nonalcoholic cirrhosis.
    (d) Possibly lower incidence of late hepatic failure and encephalopathy compared to nonselective shunts (in 3 of 6 studies)
    (e) Long-term survival (60% 5-year survival) following distal splenorenal shunt is similar to that of endoscopic sclerotherapy. Rate of rebleeding is higher in sclerotherapy, whereas shunting may lead to progression of liver dysfunction.
    (f) Splenic vein must be >7 mm in diameter, and ascites must be absent or medically controlled.
  (2) Small-bore (8-10 mm) portacaval H-grafts—May be effective in controlling rebleeding with less postshunt encephalopathy.
  (3) Left gastric-vena caval shunt—Not used much in United States
e. Esophageal transection (including stripping of coronary veins [Sugiura procedure])—Has met with limited success in the United States when compared with Japan
f. Orthotopic liver transplantation
  (1) Treats both portal hypertension and underlying liver disease
  (2) Limited availability of donor organs prevents routine use
  (3) 70% 5-year survival in major centers for predominantly nonalcoholic cirrhotic patients
  (4) Avoid portacaval shunt in patients awaiting transplant—Use sclerotherapy, TIPS, or selective shunting where possible.

g. Splenopneumopexy—Anastomosis of spleen to lung through the diaphragm to decompress varices through pulmonary circulation

C. SURGICAL TREATMENT OF ASCITES
1. Peritoneovenous shunt is the surgical treatment of choice for ascites.
2. Allows drainage of intraperitoneal fluid directly into the superior vena cava
3. LeVeen shunt has a one-way valve that opens when intra-abdominal pressure exceeds 3 cm H_2O.
4. Denver shunt incorporates an SQ pump that prevents clogging by active pumping.
5. Complications—Sepsis, congestive heart failure, disseminated intravascular coagulation (DIC), hypokalemia, shunt malfunction, air embolism, and superior vena cava thrombosis
6. Monitor for DIC postoperatively with serial fibrinogen levels, fibrin degradation products, and platelet counts. Shunt must be ligated if DIC cannot be controlled with coagulation factors

RECOMMENDED READINGS

Kamath PS, Wiesner RH, Malinchoc M, et al: A model to predict survival in patients with end-stage liver disease. Hepatology 33:464-470, 2001.

Maddery WC, Feldman M (eds): Atlas of the Liver, 2nd ed. Philadelphia, Current Medicine, 2000.

Zimmerman H, Reichen J: Assessment of liver function in the surgical patient. *In* Blumgart LH, Fong Y (eds): Surgery of the Liver and Biliary Tract, 3rd ed. London, WB Saunders, 2002, p 35.

Gallbladder and Biliary Tree

Eric Hungness, MD

I. CHOLELITHIASIS AND CHRONIC CALCULOUS CHOLECYSTITIS

A. INCIDENCE
1. Gallstones are found in 8% of male and 17% of female adults.
2. Predisposing conditions include obesity, multiparity, diabetes mellitus, cirrhosis, pancreatitis, chronic hemolytic states, malabsorption, inflammatory bowel disease, and certain racial/genetic factors (blacks, Pima Indians)

B. ETIOLOGY
The most important factor is composition of bile, which has three major constituents.
1. Bile salts (primary: cholic and chenodeoxycholic acids; secondary: deoxycholic and lithocholic acids)
2. Phospholipids—90% lecithin
3. Cholesterol—Although insoluble, both lecithin and cholesterol are incorporated along with bile salts into more soluble mixed micelles.
a. Conditions that affect the relative concentrations of these components give rise to lithogenic bile.
b. Bile containing excess cholesterol relative to bile salts and lecithin is predisposed to gallstone formation.

C. TYPES OF GALLSTONES
1. Mixed—75%
a. Most common, usually multiple
b. Cholesterol usually predominates—≈70% of content
c. 15-20% may ultimately calcify and therefore become radiopaque.
2. Pure cholesterol—l0%
a. Often solitary with large (>2.5 cm), round configuration
b. Usually not calcified
3. Pigment—15%
a. Composed of unconjugated bilirubin, calcium, and variable amounts of organic material
b. 50% are radiopaque
c. Black pigment stones are associated with cirrhosis and chronic hemolytic states. Bile is usually sterile, and choledocholithiasis is unusual.
d. Brown pigment stones are found more frequently in the biliary tree than in the gallbladder. Associated with states that predispose to bile stasis (i.e., biliary strictures).

D. NATURAL HISTORY
1. 80% of gallstones are asymptomatic. Each year, ≈2% of patients with asymptomatic stones develop symptoms, most commonly (75%) biliary colic.

42

2. Incidence of development of symptoms in patients with asymptomatic stones is ≈15-30% over 15 years.
3. Elective cholecystectomy is recommended for patients with cholelithiasis who develop symptoms.

E. BILIARY COLIC

Biliary colic is pain arising from a gallbladder without established infection. It is often difficult to differentiate between colic and intermittent chronic cholecystitis.

1. **Etiology**—Thought to be due to transient gallstone obstruction of the cystic duct resulting in gallbladder distention
2. **History**—Generally presents with moderate intermittent right upper quadrant (RUQ) and epigastric pain
a. Pain may radiate to back or below right scapula
b. Pain usually begins abruptly and subsides gradually, lasting from minutes to hours.
c. Pain of biliary colic is usually steady, not undulating like that of renal colic.
3. **Physical exam**
a. No associated fever
b. May have some mild epigastric or RUQ tenderness, or palpable gallbladder
4. **Differential diagnosis**—Pancreatitis, peptic ulcer disease, hiatal hernia with reflux, gastritis, hepatic flexure carcinoma, hepatobiliary carcinoma, cardiopulmonary disease
5. **Complications**
a. Prolonged cystic duct obstruction may allow bacterial growth and progress to acute cholecystitis.
b. Stones may pass into the common bile duct (CBD) with consequent obstruction or pancreatitis.

F. DIAGNOSIS

1. **Lab findings**
a. None are diagnostic.
b. Liver function tests (LFTs), amylase, and white blood cell (WBC) count should be obtained.
c. Elevation of alkaline phosphatase is common in biliary disease but is nonspecific.
2. **Plain films**
a. 30% of gallstones are radiopaque and may be detected
b. Can exclude other diagnoses
3. **Oral cholecystogram (Graham-Cole test)**—Evaluates presence of gallstones as well as gallbladder function. Rarely used today because of use of ultrasound. Unreliable in the presence of jaundice (bilirubin >3.0 mg/dL) or hepatic dysfunction; variable GI absorption of contrast medium.
4. **Ultrasound**

a. Has become the diagnostic procedure of choice. Identifies stones and determines wall thickness, presence of masses, ductal dilation, and fluid collections. Pancreatic head may also be examined

b. Technical difficulties include obese patients, large amount of bowel gas, and skill required for technician and interpretation.

c. Sensitivity 95%, with overall specificity ≈90%

5. **Radionuclide scan (HIDA)**

a. Diagnosis is acute cholecystitis (up to 95% accuracy) if gallbladder does not visualize within 4 hours of injection and the radioisotope is excreted in the CBD.

b. Reliable with a bilirubin up to 20 mg/dL

c. Cholecystokinin-HIDA

G. TREATMENT
Cholecystectomy should be performed in most patients with symptoms and demonstrable stones if symptoms cannot be attributed to other disease states.

H. MANAGEMENT OF ASYMPTOMATIC STONES
1. **Truly asymptomatic patients do not require cholecystectomy unless it can be performed safely during laparotomy for another condition ("incidental cholecystectomy"). Postoperative cholecystitis has been reported in up to 20% of patients with cholelithiasis undergoing a second major abdominal procedure.**

2. **Prophylactic cholecystectomy should be considered in asymptomatic patients in the following situations.**

a. Patients with sickle cell disease, on chronic total parenteral nutrition, or undergoing immunosuppression for solid organ transplants

b. The patient with a calcified "porcelain" gallbladder (15-20% associated with carcinoma)

c. Any patient with a history of biliary pancreatitis

II. ACUTE CALCULOUS CHOLECYSTITIS

A. GENERAL CONSIDERATIONS
95% of cases of acute cholecystitis are associated with obstruction of the cystic duct by a gallstone. Approximately 30% of patients with biliary colic develop acute cholecystitis within 2 years.

B. SYMPTOMS
Symptoms of acute calculous cholecystitis are constant, severe RUQ or epigastric pain that may radiate to the infrascapular region. Anorexia, nausea, and vomiting are common.

C. PHYSICAL EXAM
1. **RUQ tenderness on palpation and signs of focal peritoneal irritation may be present.**

2. Murphy's sign—Examiner palpates the RUQ and asks the patient to inhale deeply. The diaphragm descends and pushes the inflamed gallbladder against the examiner's fingertips, causing enough pain that patients arrest their inspiration.
3. Low-grade fever
4. Palpable gallbladder—Uncommon

D. LAB FINDINGS
1. Moderate leukocytosis—10,000-20,000/mm^3
2. Frequent mild elevation of bilirubin—Elevation >4 mg/dL is unusual in simple cholecystitis and suggests the presence of choledocholithiasis.
3. Frequent elevation of alkaline phosphatase; transaminases and amylase may be elevated.

E. DIFFERENTIAL DIAGNOSIS
The differential diagnosis of acute calculous cholecystitis includes acute peptic ulcer disease with or without perforation, pancreatitis, acute appendicitis, cecal volvulus, right lower lobe pneumonia, myocardial infarction, passive hepatic congestion, acute gonorrheal perihepatitis (Fitz-Hugh–Curtis syndrome), and viral or alcoholic hepatitis.

F. COMPLICATIONS
1. Hydrops—Cystic duct obstruction leads to a tense gallbladder filled with mucus ("lime bile"). May lead to gallbladder wall necrosis if pressure exceeds capillary blood pressure.
2. Gangrene and perforation—May be localized, leading to abscess that is confined by the omentum; or free perforation may occur, leading to generalized peritonitis and sepsis. Emergency laparotomy indicated.
3. Empyema of the gallbladder (suppurative cholecystitis)—Condition in which the gallbladder contains frank pus. The patient is often toxic, and urgent surgery is indicated.
4. Cholecystenteric fistula
a. Results from repeated attacks of cholecystitis
b. Duodenum, colon, and stomach involved, in decreasing order
c. Air is present in the biliary tree in 40% of cases (visible on plain films of the abdomen).
d. May not cause symptoms unless the gallbladder is partially obstructed by stones or scarring
e. Symptomatic cholecystenteric fistulas should be treated with cholecystectomy and fistula closure
5. Gallstone ileus—Gallstones causing the cholecystenteric fistula pass into the enteric lumen and cause intermittent bouts of small bowel obstruction ("tumbling ileus").
a. Symptoms of acute cholecystitis immediately preceding onset of bowel obstruction are uncommon (25-30%).

b. Stones <2-3 cm usually pass spontaneously and do not cause bowel obstruction.

c. Terminal ileum is the most common site of obstruction.

d. Overall, responsible for 1-2% of bowel obstructions.

e. Mortality l0-15%—Reflects elderly patients, in whom this is more common

f. Small bowel enterotomy proximal to the point of obstruction is usually required to remove the stone.

g. Immediate cholecystectomy is not warranted because <4% of patients have further symptoms.

G. MANAGEMENT OF ACUTE CHOLECYSTITIS

1. Preferred treatment is cholecystectomy (open procedure or laparoscopic) within 3 days of the onset of symptoms. Multiple prospective, randomized trials indicate that most patients benefit from early cholecystectomy (open or laparoscopic). In some high-risk patients (chronic steroid use, diabetes mellitus), immediate operative treatment is recommended. Conservative management with IV fluids and antibiotics (first- or second-generation cephalosporin) may be justified in some high-risk patients to convert an emergency procedure into an elective procedure. Lack of noticeable improvement within 1 to 2 days of initiation of conservative treatment suggests possible complicated acute cholecystitis, necessitating more urgent operative intervention. In extremely high-risk patients, cholecystostomy and drainage may be indicated to decompress the gallbladder, saving formal cholecystectomy until the patient is more stable. This can be done percutaneously with radiologic guidance.

2. The risk of gangrene and perforation is relatively low during the first 3 days after the onset of symptoms. After this period, the incidence increases to ≈10%.

3. Microbiology and antibiotics

a. *Escherichia coli, Klebsiella* spp*, Enterococcus* spp*,* and *Enterobacter* spp account for >80% of infections.

b. First- or second-generation cephalosporins are first choice of antibiotic coverage, although they do not cover *Enterococcus* sp*.*

c. Broader-spectrum antibiotics are used depending on the severity of the infection and the patient's response to treatment. Ampicillin, aminoglycoside, and metronidazole (or clindamycin) may be indicated in overtly septic patients.

H. ACUTE ACALCULOUS CHOLECYSTITIS

5% of cholecystitis occurs in the absence of cholelithiasis; 50-80% present in an advanced state (gangrene, perforation, abscess). This condition is associated with a 40% mortality rate.

1. Acalculous cholecystitis is primarily seen as a complication of prolonged fasting after an unrelated operation or trauma

42

GALLBLADDER AND BILIARY TREE

(e.g., acute burns, multiple organ failure, multiple fractures). Etiologies are believed to include the following.

a. Ischemia of the gallbladder during episodes of relative hypoperfusion.

b. Dehydration leads to formation of extremely viscous bile, which may obstruct or irritate the gallbladder.

c. Bacteremia may result in seeding of the stagnant bile.

d. Sepsis with resultant mucosal hypoperfusion may promote gallbladder wall invasion of organisms.

e. Bile stasis results from a lack of cholecystokinin-stimulated gallbladder contraction.

f. May be associated with large amounts of parenterally administered narcotics with resultant spasm of the sphincter of Oddi.

2. Acalculous cholecystitis may also be due to cystic duct obstruction by another process, e.g., tumor or nodal enlargement.

3. Diagnosis may be difficult and often delayed, because patients often are in the ICU setting with multiple medical problems; requires high degree of suspicion

4. Diagnosis is obtained by HIDA scan or ultrasound; treatment is emergent cholecystectomy.

I. LAPAROSCOPIC CHOLECYSTECTOMY

1. Indications—Similar to open procedure

2. Contraindications

a. Absolute

    (1) Coagulopathy

    (2) Suspicion of carcinoma

b. Relative

    (1) Diffuse peritonitis

    (2) Cholangitis

    (3) Cirrhosis or portal hypertension

    (4) Chronic obstructive pulmonary disease

    (5) Pregnancy

3. Advantages

a. Decreased postoperative pain

b. Smaller incision

c. Improved cosmesis

d. Quicker return to work

e. Quicker return of bowel function

f. Shorter hospital stay

4. Disadvantages

a. Lack of depth perception

b. Difficult to control hemorrhage

c. Potential CO_2 complications

d. Inability to palpate CBD

e. Slight increase in bile duct injuries

5. Pneumoperitoneum—Open (Hasson trocar) vs. closed (Veres needle)

6. Conversion to open procedure—up to 20% of cases

a. Unclear anatomy

b. Suspected injury to major vessel, viscus, or duct

c. Inability to remove CBD stone by minimally invasive techniques, including endoscopic retrograde cholangiopancreatography (ERCP)

7. Complications

a. Pneumoperitoneum—Mildly elevated Pco_2, decreased venous return, gas embolism, vagal reaction

b. Trocar insertion—Bleeding, injury to bowel

c. Cholecystectomy—Bile duct injury, wound infection

8. Bile duct injuries

a. Incidence

  (1) Open—0.2%

  (2) Laparoscopic—0.4-1.3%

b. Pathogenesis

  (1) Misidentification

  (2) Technical—Excessive traction, electrocautery

c. Types—Leaks and strictures

d. Clinical presentation

  (1) Leaks (usually earlier)—Pain, fever, occasionally sepsis, mildly elevated alkaline phosphatase and bilirubin

  (2) Strictures (usually later)—Jaundice, pain, elevated LFTs, pruritus

e. Diagnosis—CT scan good initial study, with percutaneous transhepatic cholangiography (PTC), ERCP, or magnetic resonance cholangiopancreatography to further characterize injury

f. Treatment—Roux-en-Y hepaticojejunostomy usually preferred

g. Complications—Hepatic fibrosis, atrophy, or portal hypertension

III. CHOLEDOCHOLITHIASIS

A. GENERAL CONSIDERATIONS

1. ≈8-16% of patients with cholelithiasis will be found to have stones in the CBD.

2. Most CBD stones arise from the gallbladder and pass into the CBD (secondary stones).

3. Stones forming de novo within the CBD are referred to as primary CBD stones; almost always associated with partial duct obstruction

4. Complications include biliary colic, cholangitis, pancreatitis, late benign biliary stricture, and biliary cirrhosis.

B. DIAGNOSIS

1. Elevations of serum bilirubin, alkaline phosphatase, and 5'-nucleotidase are characteristic; amylase is elevated with concomitant biliary pancreatitis. WBC elevated if cholangitis present, normal otherwise

2. Ultrasound is not useful in detecting CBD stones but is highly sensitive in detecting associated intrahepatic and extrahepatic ductal dilation

3. ERCP is procedure of choice after ultrasound
a. For CBD >9 mm, abnormal LFTs, or history of pancreatitis or jaundice
b. Can define biliary anatomy as well as upper GI anatomy
c. Can be therapeutic as well as diagnostic (e.g., sphincterotomy or placement of stents as necessary)
4. Intraoperative cystic duct cholangiography or intracorporeal laparoscopic ultrasonography should be performed in all patients at risk for choledocholithiasis or with uncertain anatomy.

C. TREATMENT
Surgical treatment of stones within the biliary tree requires evacuation of all stones and debris and establishment of free flow of bile into the GI tract. The procedure may be performed preoperatively via ERCP, intraoperatively via open, laparoscopic, or endoscopic (ERCP) techniques, or postoperatively via ERCP or T tube.
1. Absolute indications for CBD exploration
a. Palpable stones in the CBD—90% reliable
b. Jaundice with acute suppurative cholangitis
c. Proven presence of CBD stones on cholangiogram
2. Relative indications for CBD exploration
a. Dilated CBD >15 mm—35% reliable
b. Bilirubin >8 mg/dL
3. Choledochoenteric bypass (choledochoduodenostomy or choledochojejunostomy) may be performed in the presence of >five CBD stones, marked CBD dilation, impacted stones that cannot be removed safely, history of previous choledocholithotomy, and primary CBD stones.
4. Preoperative ERCP with endoscopic sphincterotomy
a. For patients with "high likelihood" of having a CBD stone (increased LFTs, bilirubin or alkaline phosphatase, jaundice, or dilated biliary tree)
b. Cholecystectomy should take place within 48 hours to minimize chance for new stone migration into CBD
c. Complications (6-10%)—Hemorrhage, pancreatitis, perforation, cholangitis
5. Intraoperative CBD exploration
a. Initial attempt—Transcystic approach
b. If fails, choledochotomy is required (T tube or antegrade stent necessary)
c. On-table ERCP with endoscopic sphincterotomy has been described, but this is institution and operator dependent
6. Postoperative T-tube extraction
a. 4-6 weeks required for mature tract to form
b. 80-95% successful
c. Management of T tube
   (1) T-tube cholangiogram on postoperative days 5-7
   (2) If no evidence of leakage or retained CBD stones, may clamp tube
   (3) Remove tube in 2-3 weeks on outpatient basis

7. Postoperative ERCP with endoscopic sphincterotomy
a. T tube not required (need not wait 4-6 weeks)
b. Recommended for elderly patients at high risk for complications with CBD exploration

D. RETAINED COMMON DUCT STONES
Retained common duct stones are found in up to 5% of patients undergoing CBD exploration.
1. Options for the patient with a T tube in place
a. Remove stones percutaneously with a basket passed through a mature T-tube tract (4 weeks) using fluoroscopic control (>90% success rate)
b. Endoscopic sphincterotomy for unstable patients, malfunctioning T tubes, or unsuccessful percutaneous extraction
c. Chemical dissolution or mechanical lithotripsy rarely indicated or successful
2. Patients without a T tube
a. Endoscopic sphincterotomy and "basket" removal of stones transduodenally
b. Reoperation
c. Percutaneous transhepatic approach
d. Extracorporeal shockwave lithotripsy

IV. CHOLANGITIS

A. GENERAL CONSIDERATIONS
1. A life-threatening disease that requires prompt recognition and treatment
2. Caused by obstruction of the biliary tract and biliary stasis, leading to bacterial overgrowth, suppuration, and subsequent biliary sepsis under pressure

B. ETIOLOGY
1. Choledocholithiasis—60%
2. Benign postoperative strictures
3. Pancreatic or biliary neoplasms
4. Miscellaneous—Invasive procedures, biliary-enteric anastomoses, foreign bodies, parasitic infections

C. CLINICAL FINDINGS
1. Charcot's triad—RUQ pain, jaundice, fever and chills. The classic Charcot's triad is seen in only 50-70% of cases.
2. Reynold's pentad may be seen—Charcot's triad, shock, and mental obtundation

D. DIAGNOSIS
1. Leukocytosis, hyperbilirubinemia, elevated LFTs

2. Initial study should be RUQ ultrasound; presence of ductal dilation and gallstones is suggestive. Thickening of bile duct walls, liver abscess, or gas in the biliary tree are strong supportive evidence.

E. MANAGEMENT

The immediate goal is to decompress the biliary tree. The method by which this is accomplished depends on the particular clinical situation.

1. Initially, provide supportive care with hydration, electrolyte correction, and broad-spectrum antibiotics (successful in up to 85% of patients).
2. The toxic patient is prepared for immediate surgical decompression by CBD exploration.
3. Patients with a protracted course usually have more complicated obstruction and may require percutaneous cholangiography or ERCP. PTC may be therapeutic in the acute situation by decompressing the biliary tree.
4. ERCP may be effective in decompressing the biliary tree by papillotomy or by the endoscopic placement of biliary stents or nasobiliary tube.

V. GALLBLADDER CARCINOMA

A. GENERAL CONSIDERATIONS

1. Associated with gallstones in >90% of cases
2. Increased incidence in patients with diffuse gallbladder wall calcification ("porcelain gallbladder"), cholecystenteric fistula, and adenoma
3. Male:female ratio—1:2
4. Adenocarcinoma most common cell type—82%

B. PRESENTATION

1. Most commonly found incidentally at the time of elective cholecystectomy. A loss of clear dissection planes in the gallbladder bed or near the hilum is common.
2. Symptoms include RUQ pain, jaundice, and symptoms secondary to metastases.

C. TREATMENT

1. In situ lesions require cholecystectomy only.
2. For advanced lesions, cholecystectomy with wedge resection of adjacent liver and regional lymphadenectomy; radical hepatic resections do not influence survival.
3. Relieve ductal obstruction if present.
4. Adjuvant chemotherapy or radiation therapy is largely ineffective.

D. PROGNOSIS

The prognosis of gallbladder carcinoma is poor, with 95% mortality at 5 years.

Liver Tumors

Eric Hungness, MD

I. DIFFERENTIAL DIAGNOSIS

A. BENIGN
1. Neoplastic
a. Cavernous hemangioma
b. Focal nodular hyperplasia
c. Adenoma
d. Hamartomas—Normal tissue arranged in a disorderly fashion
2. Non-neoplastic
a. Simple cysts
b. Polycystic liver disease—Other organ involvement
c. Choledochal cyst—Types IV and V
d. Echinococcal cyst

B. MALIGNANT
1. Primary
a. Hepatocellular carcinoma (HCC)—≈90% of primary malignant lesions
b. Cholangiocarcinoma—≈7% of primary malignant lesions
c. Hepatoblastoma
d. Sarcoma—Angiosarcoma, leiomyosarcoma, others
e. Epithelioid hemangioendothelioma
2. Metastatic

II. BENIGN LIVER TUMORS

A. CAVERNOUS HEMANGIOMA
1. The most frequent benign liver tumor
2. Most are small and do not cause symptoms; however, larger lesions can produce significant pain.
3. Rarely, may cause congestive heart failure secondary to a large arteriovenous shunt
4. Inappropriate use of percutaneous biopsy may lead to massive hemorrhage and therefore is contraindicated if hemangioma is suspected.
5. Accurate preoperative diagnosis can usually be made by a delayed-phase CT angiogram that demonstrates pooling of dye in the lesion.
6. T2-weighted MRI or ^{99m}Tc-labeled red blood cell scan
7. In general, it is not necessary to resect asymptomatic lesions.

B. FOCAL NODULAR HYPERPLASIA
1. Usually found in young women, but no oral contraceptive relationship
2. Etiology thought to be due to local ischemia and tissue regeneration
3. Rarely produces symptoms; rupture is exceedingly rare

4. On CT scan, a central stellate scar may be apparent, although often difficult to distinguish from adenomas
5. Usually <5 cm in diameter
6. Resection not necessary if diagnosis is secure

C. ADENOMA
1. Occurs primarily in young women in association with the use of oral contraceptives
2. Usually solitary, often present with abdominal pain and palpable mass
3. Should be resected, because approximately one third present with either rupture or bleeding
4. Malignant potential
5. Percutaneous biopsy is contraindicated secondary to bleeding potential.

III. MALIGNANT TUMORS OF THE LIVER

A. HEPATOCELLULAR CARCINOMA
1. Epidemiology
a. Relatively uncommon in United States—1-7:100,000 annually; up to 160:100,000 in parts of Asia and Africa
b. Four to five times more frequent in males
2. Etiology
a. Cirrhosis
   (1) Viral hepatitis—Hepatitis B (carriers have 220 times increased risk of cirrhosis), hepatitis C
   (2) Alcohol consumption—Promotes cirrhosis; 15% of HCC in the United States may be attributable to alcohol
   (3) Inheritable liver diseases that progress to cirrhosis—α_1-Antitrypsin deficiency, hemochromatosis, and others
b. Chemical carcinogens—Aflatoxin, vinyl chloride, Thorotrast
c. Exogenous steroid hormones—3.2 times increased risk for women who have used oral contraceptives
d. Cigarette smoking—2.4 times increased risk for people who smoke
3. Pathology—Two distinct histologic subtypes
a. Nonfibrolamellar—Most frequent, often associated with hepatitis B and cirrhosis. Resectability rate is low; median survival of 22 months.
b. Fibrolamellar—Eosinophilic hepatocytes with marked perihepatocyte fibrosis. Often in younger patients with no association with hepatitis B or cirrhosis. Usually well differentiated, more often resectable, and associated with a median survival of 50 months.
4. Signs and symptoms
a. Weakness, malaise, upper abdominal or shoulder pain, and weight loss
b. Most common sign is hepatomegaly—Other signs include jaundice, ascites, and splenomegaly.
c. A few patients present with an acute abdominal event secondary to rupture of the tumor or hemorrhage.

d. In patients with stable cirrhosis, a sudden clinical worsening or sudden appearance of portal hypertension and variceal bleeding may herald the rapid growth of an HCC.

e. Paraneoplastic syndromes may be present—Parathyroid hormone, erythropoietin, carcinoid syndrome, or hypertrophic pulmonary osteodystrophy

5. Diagnosis

a. Tumor markers
  (1) α-Fetoprotein (AFP)
    (a) Useful as a screening tool in patients at risk (alcoholics, chronic liver disease, cirrhosis)
    (b) >70% of patients with hepatoma >3 cm have increased AFP.
    (c) A significant number of patients with acute or chronic hepatitis and cirrhosis, as well as some pregnant women, have elevated AFP without HCC.
  (2) Others with reduced sensitivity

b. Radiologic evaluation
  (1) Ultrasonography important in early diagnosis in combination with AFP
  (2) Angiography provides information about anatomic features of the tumor and its possible involvement in vascular structures.
  (3) Contrast CT detects >90% of lesions larger than 2-3 cm.
  (4) MRI, with greater sensitivity than CT

c. Laparoscopy—useful to detect occult metastases

6. Treatment

a. Surgery
  (1) Although liver resection is the only therapy that substantially increases survival, its overall role is limited because of the usual background of cirrhosis, poor condition of the patient, and advanced tumor.
  (2) Only 10% of patients have resectable tumors.
  (3) Intraoperative ultrasound has permitted limited resections in cirrhotic patients.
  (4) 5-year survival in resected patients is 24-50%, and 5-year survival in all patients is only 5%.
  (5) Preoperative assessment
    (a) Physical exam, chest radiograph, CT of abdomen to rule out extrahepatic sites of disease
    (b) Contrast CT/MRI/angiography to evaluate factors that determine extent of resection—Proximity to major vessels, tumor thrombus in major veins or biliary tree
    (c) Document adequate functional reserve capacity of the liver—Albumin, serum glutamic-oxaloacetic transaminase (SGOT), total bilirubin, and prothrombin time. Galactose elimination capacity is used in some centers.
    (d) Evidence of cirrhosis with portal hypertension is a major surgical risk factor, and Child's classification should be determined.

43

LIVER TUMORS

    (6) Resection should attain at least a 2-cm tumor-free margin to minimize recurrence.

    (7) Transplantation has been performed in selected subgroups (incidental tumors found at the time of transplant, small localized fibrolamellar tumors in patients with severe cirrhosis that precludes liver resection).

    (8) Overall recurrence rate—38-68%.

  b. Nonsurgical treatment

    (1) Chemotherapy—Recent trials with doxorubicin (Adriamycin) have shown some promise.

    (2) Radiation—Poor response overall

    (3) Others—Hepatic artery ligation, arterial embolization, and cryotherapy

B. HEPATOBLASTOMA
1. Most common primary hepatic liver tumor in children
2. Presents as an abdominal mass—>60% <2 years old
3. AFP elevated in >95% of cases
4. Usually relatively low grade
5. Up to 60% 5-year survival with resection
6. Newer protocols show promise using preoperative combination therapy with chemotherapy and radiation.

C. BILE DUCT CANCER (CHOLANGIOCARCINOMA)
1. General
a. Accounts for 5-20% of primary liver carcinomas
b. Intrahepatic and extrahepatic variants

2. Intrahepatic disease
a. Associated with chronic cholestasis, congenital cystic diseases of the liver, and infestation with *Clonorchis sinensis* (liver fluke)
b. Other associations—Chronic cholestasis, hemochromatosis, cirrhosis, and congenital cystic liver disease

3. Extrahepatic disease
a. 10% of primary hepatic malignancies
b. May arise anywhere along the hepatic ducts or bile ducts

4. Signs and symptoms
a. Symptoms—Pruritus, vague abdominal pain, mild cholangitis, and jaundice are the usual presenting symptoms.
b. Signs—Slight hepatomegaly possible; jaundice.

5. Treatment of choice remains surgical resection, but long-term survival rates remain poor.
a. Only 25% of tumors are resectable, with a 15-20% 5-year survival rate.
b. Unresectable patients should undergo palliation (bypass or intubation procedure) to increase survival.

D. SARCOMAS

1. Angiosarcoma—Associated with Thorotrast, vinyl chloride, and arsenic. Usually occurs as multiple nodules. No cure.
2. Leiomyosarcoma, fibrosarcoma, and rhabdomyosarcoma rarely occur.

E. EPITHELIOID HEMANGIOENDOTHELIOMA

1. Characteristic diffuse involvement of liver
2. High metastasis rate
3. Clinical course extremely variable

F. METASTASIS

1. By far the most common malignancy found in the liver—40% of patients with solid tumors develop liver metastases.
2. Bronchogenic carcinoma is the most common primary cause of hepatic metastasis. Next most common are prostate, colon, and breast.
3. Symptoms—Pain, ascites, jaundice, palpable mass, weight loss, anorexia
4. Most lesions favorable for resection have been found by early laboratory detection before the onset of symptoms or signs. For this reason, liver function tests and carcinoembryonic antigen are part of the recommended follow-up protocol for colorectal cancer.
5. Colorectal adenocarcinoma—Liver is the most common site of metastasis.
6. Carcinomas of the stomach, pancreas, gallbladder, ovary, breast, and head and neck have not responded favorably following resection of hepatic metastasis.
7. Major hepatic resections for palliation of symptoms from carcinoid tumors or insulinomas have been performed.
8. Need at least 2-cm tumor-free margins in resection to decrease the incidence of recurrence.
9. Chemotherapy or cryotherapy may be effective in the treatment of certain hepatic metastasis; hepatic artery infusion via implantable pump may be used in colorectal carcinoma metastasis.
10. Contraindications for resection—Total hepatic involvement, vena cava or portal vein invasion, extrahepatic tumor.

43

LIVER TUMORS

The Pancreas

Curtis J. Wray, MD

A. GENERAL CONSIDERATIONS

1. Transverse retroperitoneal location posterior to the stomach and lesser omentum at the level of L1 and L2
2. Anterior surface covered by peritoneum; posterior boundary includes the superior mesenteric vessels, portal vein, aorta, inferior mesenteric vein, and the splenic vein
3. Adult pancreas weighs 75-125 g and is 15-20 cm in length.
4. Divided into five anatomic segments

a. Head—Lies within confines of duodenal C-loop to the right of the superior mesenteric vessels

b. Uncinate process—Portion of the head that projects inferiorly behind superior mesenteric vessels and portal vein and anterior to inferior vena cava and aorta

c. Neck—Narrow segment overlying superior mesenteric vessels and portal vein

d. Body—Lies left of the neck and is superior and adjacent to fourth portion of duodenum, ligament of Treitz, and proximal jejunum; forms posterior floor of lesser sac

e. Tail—Lies left of the body and extends into the splenic hilum

B. PANCREATIC DUCT SYSTEM

1. Main pancreatic duct (duct of Wirsung)

a. Extends from the tail through the midportion of the gland, lies slightly closer to the posterior surface of the pancreas

b. In the head, descends inferiorly and joins the intrapancreatic portion of the common bile duct to form common pancreaticobiliary channel slightly proximal to the papilla of Vater

c. Diameter—3.0-4.8 mm in head, 2.0-3.5 mm in body, 0.9-2.4 mm in tail

2. Accessory pancreatic duct (duct of Santorini)

a. Located in the head in a more ventral plane; originates from the main pancreatic duct in the neck and terminates in the minor papilla at a point ≈2 cm proximal to the papilla of Vater

b. Drains the anterior portion of pancreatic head

3. Ampulla of Vater

a. Dilation on the posteromedial wall of second portion of duodenum where common pancreaticobiliary channel empties biliary and pancreatic secretions

b. Associated with a series of adjacent muscular coats at the pancreaticobiliary duct junction called the *sphincter of Oddi*

c. The ampulla is present in 90% of patients; in 10% the individual ducts empty separately into the duodenum and there is no ampulla.

44

C. VASCULATURE

1. Arterial supply

a. Gastroduodenal artery—Branch of the hepatic artery that gives rise to the anterior and posterosuperior pancreaticoduodenal arteries that form collaterals with branches of the superior mesenteric artery (SMA) to supply the head of the pancreas

b. SMA—Gives rise to inferoanterior and posterior pancreaticoduodenal arteries that join the above arcades

c. Blood supply to the neck, body, and tail is more variable and consists of the superior dorsal pancreatic artery, inferior transverse pancreatic artery, and multiple short branches of the splenic and left gastroepiploic arteries.

2. Venous drainage—Parallels arterial supply, but lies superficial to its arterial counterpart; drains into the portal system via the superior mesenteric and splenic veins

3. Lymphatic drainage—Follows venous drainage in all directions.
Superior nodes along the superior border of pancreas receive lymph from the anterior and superior upper half of the gland. *Inferior* nodes along the inferior border of the head and body drain the anterior and posterior lower portion of the pancreas. *Anterior* nodes are located beneath the pyloric channel and drain the anterior surface of the head. *Posterior* nodes are located in the posterior groove between the duodenum and pancreas; drainage is from the posterior surface of the head. *Splenic* nodes drain the tail of the pancreas.

II. ACUTE PANCREATITIS

A. GENERAL CONSIDERATIONS

1. Acute pancreatitis presents as a broad spectrum of pathologic changes in the pancreas that range in severity from mild parenchymal edema to fulminant hemorrhagic necrosis.

2. Pancreatitis is a nonbacterial inflammation caused by the activation, interstitial release, and digestion of the pancreas by its exocrine secretions.

3. Most patients (80-95%) experience only mild to moderate symptoms with a self-limiting course and recover fully with only supportive care.

4. However, 10-15% of patients develop acute hemorrhagic or necrotizing pancreatitis, with considerable associated morbidity and mortality despite maximal intensive supportive care.

5. Over the past several decades, mortality from acute pancreatitis has decreased from 25% to 5%. This change most likely reflects improved supportive care as well as better awareness and earlier recognition of potentially life-threatening complications.

B. ETIOLOGY

Gallstones and alcohol are by far the most common etiologies, accounting for >90% of cases of acute pancreatitis.

1. Gallstones
a. May be related to a transient obstruction of the main pancreatic duct by a stone passing through the common bile duct
b. Usual age of onset is mid-40s, with women more commonly affected than men
2. Alcohol
a. Exact mechanism of alcohol-related injury is unknown. Most recent evidence suggests that ethanol increases ductal permeability both by a toxic metabolic mechanism and by causing a small increase in ductal pressure.
b. This usually occurs in a patient with underlying pancreatic disease and insufficiency.
3. Hyperlipidemia—Types I, IV, and V have been implicated.
4. Hypercalcemia—Most commonly seen with hyperparathyroidism that could lead to intraductal precipitation of calcium
5. Trauma
a. External (penetrating or blunt)
b. Postoperative
   (1) Following surgery on the biliary tract, upper GI tract, pancreas, colon, and spleen
   (2) Occasionally after operations remote from the pancreas (e.g., cardiopulmonary bypass)
c. Endoscopic retrograde cholangiopancreatography (ERCP)
6. Pancreatic duct obstruction—Ampullary stenosis, tumor, pancreatic divisum, duodenal diverticulum, ascaris infestation
7. Ischemia—Circulatory shock, emboli, vasculitis, polyarteritis nodosum, aortic graft, hypothermia
8. Drugs—Azathioprine, estrogens, thiazides, furosemide, ethacrynic acid, sulfonamides, tetracycline, steroids
9. Infection—Viral (mumps, cytomegalovirus, hepatitis B), mycoplasmal
10. Others—Scorpion venom, posterior penetrating peptic ulcer, postrenal transplant
11. Familial
12. Idiopathic

C. CLINICAL PRESENTATION
1. Generally, the first episode of acute pancreatitis is the most severe.
2. Symptoms
a. Abdominal pain (>90% of patients), usually constant midepigastric pain with maximal intensity within several hours of onset. Usually occurs several hours after a heavy meal and is associated with nausea and persistent emesis. 50% with pain radiating to back. Alleviated by sitting up and aggravated by motion.
b. Nausea and vomiting usually accompany pain.
c. Anorexia

THE PANCREAS 44

3. Signs
a. Epigastric tenderness or, less commonly, diffuse abdominal tenderness with peritoneal signs. Right lower quadrant tenderness may be present due to fluid/inflammation tracking down the right paracolic gutter.
b. Abdominal distention with diminished or absent bowel sounds due to paralytic ileus
c. Fever, tachycardia
d. Palpable epigastric mass—May be secondary to pancreatic phlegmon
e. Left flank ecchymosis (Grey Turner's sign) and periumbilical ecchymosis (Cullen's sign) occur in 1-3% of cases and suggest severe hemorrhagic pancreatitis. They are the result of blood-stained peritoneal fluid dissecting through tissue planes of the abdominal wall to the flank or along the falciform ligament to the umbilical area. Associated with profound fluid losses.

D. DIAGNOSIS
1. Usually based on patient's history and clinical impression supported by appropriate laboratory and radiologic evaluation
2. Laboratory tests
a. CBC with differential, prothrombin time, partial thromboplastin time, electrolytes, Ca^{2+}, Mg^{2+}, glucose, blood urea nitrogen (BUN), creatinine, amylase, lipase, alkaline phosphatase, bilirubin, aspartate transaminase (AST), alanine transaminase (ALT), triglycerides, urinalysis (excretion >5000 IU/day is abnormal)
b. ECG—Exclude myocardial infarction
c. Serum amylase
   (1) Elevated in 90% of cases
   (2) Increase occurs within hours of onset of symptoms and gradually returns to normal range within 5-7 days.
   (3) Degree of initial elevation does not correlate with severity of attack, nor does it predict clinical outcome. Values >1000 IU/dL are suggestive of gallstone pancreatitis.
   (4) Hyperamylasemia is not specific for pancreatitis. Other causes include the following.
      (a) Pancreatic—Trauma, carcinoma, pseudocyst, ascites, abscess
      (b) Intra-abdominal—Gangrenous cholecystitis, intestinal obstruction, mesenteric ischemia or infarction, ruptured aortic aneurysm, perforated peptic ulcer, peritonitis, acute appendicitis, afferent loop syndrome, ruptured ectopic pregnancy, ruptured graafian follicle, salpingitis
      (c) Salivary gland disorders—Mumps, parotitis, trauma, impacted calculi, irradiation sialadenitis
      (d) Impaired amylase excretion—Renal failure, macroamylasemia
      (e) Miscellaneous—Severe burns, diabetic ketoacidosis, pregnancy, head trauma, pneumonia, liver disease, drugs

d. Amylase isoenzymes—Can differentiate between s-type (salivary) and p-type (pancreatic) amylase; may be useful to determine if hyperamylasemia is of nonpancreatic origin; not widely used

e. Serum lipase
(1) Remains elevated longer than serum amylase
(2) More specific but less sensitive than serum amylase
(3) May be elevated in intestinal ischemia, perforated peptic ulcer, or acute cholecystitis

3. Radiologic procedures

a. Chest radiograph
(1) Findings suggestive of but not specific for acute pancreatitis include left pleural effusion, elevated left hemidiaphragm, or basilar atelectasis.
(2) As baseline in the event of respiratory deterioration
(3) To rule out pneumoperitoneum or pneumonia

b. Abdominal radiograph (nonspecific findings)
(1) Most frequent finding is air in dilated loop of intestine adjacent to pancreas
(2) "Sentinel loop sign"—Dilated proximal jejunal loop
(3) "Colon cut-off sign"—Distended colon from ascending to mid-transverse with no air distally
(4) Nonspecific ileus pattern
(5) Others—Cholelithiasis, loss of psoas margins, pancreatic calcifications

c. Ultrasound—Useful in initial evaluation of pancreas to rule out cholelithiasis and pseudocyst

d. CT scan
(1) More sensitive and specific than ultrasound for evaluation of pancreatic abnormalities
(2) Dynamic CT scan (contrast-enhanced) is preferred because it can identify pancreatic perfusion, ischemia, and necrosis. A viable pancreas "enhances" as contrast agent perfuses the gland.

e. ERCP—Contraindicated for diagnosis of acute pancreatitis; indicated after resolution for recurrent disease, or if anatomic abnormality is suspected

E. PROGNOSIS

1. Approximately 10-15% of patients with acute pancreatitis develop severe prolonged illness with significant morbidity and mortality.
2. Ranson's criteria—11 prognostic signs for identifying high-risk patients

a. Present at admission
(1) Age >55 years
(2) White blood cell (WBC) count >16,000 cells/mm^3
(3) Glucose >200 mg/dL
(4) Lactate dehydrogenase >350 IU/L
(5) AST >250 IU/dL

44

THE PANCREAS

  b. During the initial 48 hours
      (1) Hematocrit decrease >10%
      (2) BUN increases >5 mg/dL
      (3) Serum Ca^{2+} <8 mg/dL
      (4) Arterial Po_2 <60 mm Hg
      (5) Base deficit >4 mEq/L
      (6) Fluid sequestration >6 L
  c. Mortality—Correlates with Ranson's criteria
      (1) 0-2 signs—2%
      (2) 3-4 signs—15%
      (3) 5-6 signs—40%
      (4) 7-8 signs—≈100%

F. THERAPY
  1. IV fluids and electrolyte replacement—Cornerstone of therapy; use of lactated Ringer's solution or normal saline to maintain urine output of 0.5-1 mL/kg/h
  2. Foley catheter—Facilitates accurate measurement of intake and output; indirect assessment of tissue perfusion
  3. Nasogastric suction—Indicated if vomiting present or persists; has not been shown to alter clinical course in mild cases by randomized, prospective trials
  4. NPO until abdominal pain, tenderness, and ileus have resolved and amylase is normal or near normal
  5. Parenteral nutrition—Indicated in severe, complicated cases of pancreatitis or when the patient is expected to be NPO >7 days. Incidence rates of severe complications and overall mortality are not affected. Administration of lipid preparations is safe.
  6. Analgesia—Meperidine preferred to morphine because it is thought to have less potential for sphincter of Oddi spasm
  7. Respiratory monitoring—Respiratory complications occur in 15-55% of cases. May require careful monitoring if Pao_2 <70 mm Hg and supplemental oxygenation. Severe cases of acute pancreatitis may lead to acute respiratory distress syndrome and require mechanical ventilation.
  8. Antibiotics—Not indicated in uncomplicated cases, but may be indicated in the presence of pancreatic necrosis. Imipenem has recently been shown to be more effective in decreasing septic complications; however, overall morbidity is unchanged.
  9. Serial lab studies—Close monitoring of CBC, electrolytes (including Ca^{2+} and Mg^{2+}), and amylase
  10. Alcohol withdrawal prophylaxis for selected patients with alcohol-induced pancreatitis. Scheduled dose of a benzodiazepine; thiamine 100 mg q.d. x 3 days; folate 1 mg q.d. x 3 days; multivitamins q.d.

11. Histamine (H_2) blockers—No proven benefit in acute pancreatitis; may be indicated in critically ill patients as ulcer prophylaxis or in treatment of associated upper GI disease

12. ICU monitoring—Indicated in moderate to severe cases or in patients at high risk as determined by Ranson's criteria. Endotracheal intubation and positive end-expiratory pressure ventilation may be indicated in the presence of progressive respiratory insufficiency unresponsive to other treatment.

13. Surgical management—Specific indications included the following.
   a. Uncertainty of diagnosis is such that life-threatening intra-abdominal processes cannot be ruled out.
   b. Progressive deterioration despite optimal supportive care
   c. Complications of pancreatitis (abscess, pseudocyst), abdominal compartment syndrome from fluid sequestration
   d. Treatment of gallstone pancreatitis
      (1) Current recommendations—Surgery (cholecystectomy with intraoperative cholangiogram) after the acute attack has subsided but during the same hospitalization period (4-6 days)
      (2) 30% recurrence rate if surgery delayed 4 to 6 weeks

G. COMPLICATIONS

1. Pancreatic necrosis
   a. Diagnosed by dynamic CT or elevated serum acute-phase reactants (e.g., C-reactive protein, α_2-macroglobulin, complement C3 and C4)
   b. ≈40% of patients requiring an operation for pancreatic necrosis have positive bacterial tissue cultures at laparotomy.
   c. Decreased rate of pancreatic and nonpancreatic sepsis has been demonstrated by prophylactic use of imipenem/cilastatin in sterile pancreatic necrosis.[1] In a recent study[2] of patients with necrotizing pancreatitis, 68% of patients treated with prophylactic antibiotics continued to have sterile pancreatic tissue, whereas in 32%, infection occurred.
   d. Surgical débridement and serial open packing indicated for clinical deterioration or evidence of pancreatic sepsis

2. Pancreatic sepsis/abscess
   a. A serious and life-threatening complication of acute pancreatitis
   b. Occurs in 2-5% of patients and in >50% of those with ≥six Ranson's prognostic signs
   c. Characterized by extensive necrosis of retroperitoneal fat, mesentery, and mesocolon, while the pancreas remains relatively intact but inflamed.
   d. Most deaths occur after 7-10 days and result from septic complications, usually infected necrotic tissue.
   e. Pathogens—Most commonly enteric organisms; includes *Klebsiella* spp, *Escherichia coli*, *Proteus* spp, *Enterobacter* spp, *Enterococcus* spp, *Serratia* spp, *Pseudomonas* spp, anaerobic species, *Staphylococcus* spp,

44

THE PANCREAS

Bacteroides spp, and *Candida* spp; 50% are polymicrobial. Fungal infection seen in up to 25% of patients with infected pancreatic tissue.
f. Multiresistant organisms can be expected in up to 10% of patients with infected necrotizing pancreatitis
g. Diagnosis—Usually occurs 1-4 weeks after onset of pancreatitis
  (1) Fever, abdominal pain, tenderness/distention, paralytic ileus, and leukocytosis
  (2) Persistent hyperamylasemia and nonspecific liver function tests in 50% of cases
  (3) CT scan—Most accurate mode for diagnosis; finding of air bubbles in a peripancreatic fluid collection or areas of liquefactive necrosis; CT-guided percutaneous needle aspiration is helpful to differentiate infected vs. sterile fluid collection
h. Treatment
  (1) Broad-spectrum antibiotics
  (2) Surgical drainage consisting of either laparotomy with wide débridement and drainage, or laparotomy with débridement and serial open packing

3. Pseudocyst
a. Definition—Collection of pancreatic secretions within a cyst lacking a true epithelium; consists of surrounding tissues walling off a pancreatic duct disruption
b. Most common complication of pancreatitis (2-10% of patients)—Appears 2-3 weeks after initial attack; frequently found in the lesser peritoneal sac posterior to the stomach
c. Signs and symptoms—Early satiety, abdominal pain, nausea, vomiting, epigastric tenderness, abdominal mass, and persistent hyperamylasemia
d. Diagnosis—CT and ultrasound each 90% accuracy; ERCP may demonstrate site of duct disruption, multiple cysts (seen in 20% of patients), and/or ductal anatomy
e. Complication rate—If untreated, 20% by 6 weeks and 67% if cyst persists for 12 weeks; includes secondary infection, hemorrhage, or rupture
f. Treatment
  (1) 50% resolve spontaneously by 4-6 weeks.
  (2) Expectant, supportive management for 4-6 weeks until a thick, fibrous, reactive wall has formed and the cyst remains unchanged.
  (3) Then internal drainage via a cystogastrostomy, cystojejunostomy, or cystoduodenostomy; *always* biopsy a pseudocyst wall to rule out malignant cystic neoplasm.
  (4) External drainage for infected pseudocysts or one with immature walls

4. Pancreatic ascites
a. Secondary to pseudocyst disruption (more common) or direct pancreatic duct disruption; usually seen in alcoholics with chronic pancreatitis
b. Painless, massive ascites may be associated with a left pleural effusion

c. Diagnosis—Made by paracentesis; high amylase (>1000 U/L) and high protein (>3.0 g/dL)

d. Treatment—NPO, parenteral nutrition for 4-6 weeks. Somatostatin has been shown to lead to resolution of pancreatic ascites. If does not resolve, ERCP to delineate ductal anatomy and then surgical internal drainage or resection.

5. Pancreatic fistulas

a. Secondary to complicated acute pancreatitis, pancreatic surgery, or abdominal trauma

b. Treatment—NPO, parenteral nutrition for 4-6 weeks. Somatostatin has been shown to be effective in accelerating the closure rate of pancreatic fistulas. If does not resolve, ERCP to evaluate anatomy and then surgical internal drainage or distal resection.

6. Hemorrhage

a. Usually due to erosion of arterial pseudoaneurysm secondary to pseudocyst, abscess, or necrotizing pancreatitis. Hemorrhage may be gastrointestinal, intraperitoneal, or retroperitoneal. 6% incidence of bleeding associated with pseudocysts.

b. Signs and symptoms—Abdominal pain, increasing size of abdominal mass, hypotension, falling hematocrit

c. Diagnosis—Angiography to localize if patient stable

d. Treatment—Immediate surgery if patient is unstable or bleeding is uncontrolled. Selective embolization may be possible if the patient is stable.

III. CHRONIC PANCREATITIS

A. GENERAL CONSIDERATIONS

Chronic pancreatitis is characterized by recurrent or persistent abdominal pain that is generally associated with evidence of exocrine and endocrine pancreatic insufficiency. It is the result of irreversible destruction and fibrosis of pancreatic parenchyma.

B. ETIOLOGY

Chronic pancreatitis is most commonly associated with history of alcohol abuse; it is also seen with hyperparathyroidism, pancreatic trauma, and pancreas divisum.

C. CLINICAL MANIFESTATIONS

1. Recurrent or chronic abdominal pain—Seen in 95% of patients with chronic pancreatitis. Described as dull, aching, or boring pain that is typically epigastric and radiates to the back.

2. Anorexia and weight loss—Are common in 75% of patients

3. Steatorrhea and malabsorption

4. Insulin-dependent diabetes mellitus (IDDM)—Occurs in up to 30%

5. History of narcotic analgesic abuse frequently seen

D. DIAGNOSIS

1. Suspected based on clinical findings. Routine laboratory tests not generally helpful; amylase may be normal or only mildly elevated.
2. Radiologic evaluation
a. Abdominal radiograph—Pancreatic calcifications (95% specific for chronic pancreatitis)
b. CT scan—Useful for evaluation of both parenchymal and ductal disease
c. ERCP—Vitally important role for planning surgical management because it provides a "road map" of pancreatic ductal system
   (1) Early changes—Dilated duct with filling of secondary and tertiary branches
   (2) Later changes—Ductal strictures and calculi; pseudocyst may be present; characteristic "chain of lakes" due to areas of alternating ductal dilation and stricture (less frequently observed than uniform ductal dilation)
d. CT and ERCP are mandatory prior to consideration of surgical management.

E. NONOPERATIVE MANAGEMENT

1. Control of abdominal pain
a. Abstinence from alcohol
b. Frequent, small-volume, low-fat meals
2. Treatment of IDDM
3. Exogenous pancreatic enzyme supplementation to treat steatorrhea and malabsorption

F. INDICATIONS FOR SURGERY

1. Abdominal pain
2. Common bile duct obstruction
3. Duodenal obstruction
4. Persistent pseudocyst
5. Pancreatic fistula and/or pancreatic ascites
6. Variceal hemorrhage secondary to splenic vein obstruction—Treated by splenectomy
7. Rule out pancreatic carcinoma
8. Colon obstruction

G. SURGICAL MANAGEMENT

1. Goal—To relieve debilitating pain while attempting to preserve pancreatic exocrine and endocrine function
2. Pancreatic duct drainage
a. Duval procedure—Distal pancreatectomy with end-to-end pancreaticojejunostomy
   (1) Originally used to relieve proximal duct obstruction by allowing simple retrograde drainage of the pancreas via its tail

     (2) Does not adequately decompress the ductal system in cases of widespread ductal disease

     (3) Currently, applicable to the rare case of isolated proximal ductal stenosis not involving the ampulla

b. Puestow procedure—Lateral side-to-side pancreaticojejunostomy

     (1) Most widely used and preferred surgical treatment

     (2) Involves unroofing and incising the pancreatic duct along its entire length from a point adjacent to the duodenum to the distal portion of the pancreatic tail (with or without removal of the spleen or mobilization of the pancreas) and side-to-side anastomosis to an overlying Roux-en-Y limb of jejunum

     (3) Allows for decompression of the entire pancreatic duct

     (4) A pancreatic duct >10 mm in diameter, an anastomosis >6 cm in length, and pancreatic calcifications are determinants of a successful Puestow procedure.

     (5) Provides substantial pain relief in ≈65-85% of patients

3. Pancreatic resection

a. Indicated for pain relief when pancreatic duct is narrow or normal in diameter

b. Limited distal pancreatectomy—Resection of 40-80% of gland extending no farther than to pancreatic neck; applicable only for true focal disease in distal pancreas

c. Subtotal distal pancreatectomy—Resection of 80-95% of gland including inferior portion of head and uncinate process, but leaving intrapancreatic portion of common bile duct in continuity

d. Pancreaticoduodenectomy (Whipple's procedure)

     (1) Involves resection of head of pancreas to the level of the superior mesenteric vein (SMV), as well as duodenum, pylorus, distal stomach, gallbladder, and distal common bile duct

     (2) Restoration of GI continuity involves bringing up the proximal jejunum through the transverse mesocolon and creating a pancreaticojejunostomy, choledochojejunostomy, and gastrojejunostomy.

     (3) Considered in patients with chronic pancreatitis who have parenchymal disease primarily restricted to pancreatic head

     (4) Also useful in cases associated with biliary or duodenal obstruction

     (5) Preserves endocrine function of pancreas

     (6) With proper patient selection, up to 80% of patients can obtain satisfactory pain relief.

e. Pyloric-preserving pancreaticoduodenectomy (modified Whipple's procedure)

     (1) Same as standard Whipple except for preservation of entire stomach, pylorus, and first portion of duodenum

     (2) Re-establishment of GI continuity involves a duodenojejunostomy as well as pancreaticojejunostomy and choledochojejunostomy.

      (3) Leaves motor, secretory, and reservoir functions of stomach intact and thus reduces the risk of dumping syndrome

  f. Duodenum-preserving resections of the pancreatic head

    (1) Beger procedure—Proposed as alternative to standard Whipple's for patients with disease localized to head and uncinate process. Involves duodenum-preserving subtotal resection of pancreatic head combined with Roux-en-Y drainage of the retained proximal and distal portions of the pancreatic duct.

    (2) Frey procedure—Consists of a nonanatomic resection ("coring out") of the pancreatic head, leaving the posterior pancreatic capsule and a rim of pancreatic tissue intact along the duodenal C-loop. Proximal pancreatic duct is ligated and distal duct is opened widely. Drainage is via a Roux-en-Y side-to-side pancreaticojejunostomy.

  g. Total pancreatectomy—Option for patients with continued pain despite previous lesser resections; patients manifest endocrine as well as exocrine insufficiencies

4. Pancreatic denervation—Lumbodorsal sympathectomy and splanchnicectomy; high failure rate with only short-term relief seen

5. Islet cell transplantation—Currently performed for type I diabetes mellitus

a. May be performed percutaneously through liver and is repeatable

b. 1-2 mL of packed islet cells can be injected into the portal vein under angiographic guidance.

c. Major factors limiting islet transplantation

    (1) Low percentage of patients reach insulin independence and normalization of glucose homeostasis

    (2) Limited survival of fully functional grafts

d. Most patients recover partial function and a reduction in pretransplant insulin requirements.

e. Most patients have fasting C-peptide concentrations but abnormal fasting glucose and hemoglobin A1c values.

f. Patients with partially functioning grafts may not be insulin free; however, a recent study[3] showed that 81% of patients with partially functioning grafts had near-normal protein and lipid metabolism. Only 16% had normal protein and lipid metabolism at 4 years.

H. ENDOSCOPIC MANAGEMENT

Endoscopic management involves endoscopic pancreatic duct stone removal, sphincterotomy, and placement of a common bile duct stent.

IV. PANCREATIC CANCER

A. EPIDEMIOLOGY

1. Fourth most common cause of cancer death in men and fifth most common cause of cancer death in women in the United States

2. Incidence of 28,000 cases per year, with death rate closely paralleling incidence

3. Overall survival rate—10% at 1 year and <2% at 5 years
4. Mean survival for unresectable disease is 6 months.
5. Rarely develops before 50 years of age; incidence increases steadily with increasing age; median age of presentation is 69 years, with ≈3/4 of all patients ≥60 years
6. Male-to-female ratio—1.7 to 1
7. Incidence in black males—30-40% higher than white males
8. At the time of diagnosis—90% of patients have disease extending beyond the pancreas and 50% have distant metastasis

B. ETIOLOGY

1. Cigarette smoking—Most clearly established risk factor (twofold to fivefold increased relative risk with heavy smoking)
2. Other suggested (but not proven) risk factors
a. Specific occupations—Chemists, metal workers, coke and gas plant workers
b. Long-term exposure to benzidine and β naphthylamine
c. Heavy alcohol consumption
d. High-fat diet
e. Diabetes mellitus
f. Chronic pancreatitis
g. Familial pancreatitis
h. Mutations found in K-*ras* genes in >85% of human pancreatic cancer specimens
i. Mutation also found in *p16^{ink4}* gene, located on chromosome 9p21 (a gene also associated with melanoma)

C. HISTOPATHOLOGIC CLASSIFICATION

1. Ductal adenocarcinoma—90% (most common type)
2. Giant cell carcinoma—4%
3. Adenosquamous carcinoma—3%
4. Mucinous carcinoma—2%
5. Mucinous cystadenocarcinoma—1%
6. Acinar cell adenocarcinoma—1%

D. ANATOMIC DISTRIBUTION

1. Pancreatic head—75%
2. Pancreatic body—20%
3. Pancreatic tail—5%

E. CLINICAL PRESENTATION

The early signs and symptoms of pancreatic cancer are vague and nonspecific, and thus most patients present with disease advanced beyond the scope of potentially curative treatment.
1. Abdominal pain
a. Occurs in 80-90% of patients and is the presenting symptom in 65% of cases

44

THE PANCREAS

b. Typically located in the midepigastrium and is characterized as a deep-seated, dull ache or boring pain that is progressive and often worse at night; pain may radiate to the low thoracic or upper lumbar back

c. Severe pain is slightly more common with carcinoma of body and tail.

d. Unrelenting back pain usually is caused by retroperitoneal invasion.

2. Weight loss—60%; average weight loss, 20 pounds

3. Anorexia—60%. A feature of anorexia associated with pancreatic cancer is that patients may feel hungry until they begin to eat, at which time they rapidly lose appetite.

4. Jaundice

a. Only presenting symptom in up to 30% of cases

b. Much more commonly associated with carcinoma of head (75%) than with carcinoma of body and tail

c. May signify a better prognosis because small tumors still confined to the pancreas can present with obstruction of intrapancreatic common bile duct

d. *Painless* jaundice (13%) is *not* common in pancreatic cancer but occurs more often with ampullary or primary bile duct tumors.

e. Courvoisier's sign—A palpable, dilated gallbladder in the presence of painless jaundice; seen in <20% of patients

5. Other signs and symptoms

a. Weakness, fatigue—30%

b. Diarrhea or constipation—25% or 10%, respectively

c. Steatorrhea—10%

d. Cholangitis—10%. Indicates ascending infection secondary to bile duct obstruction

e. Recent onset of diabetes mellitus—20%

f. Hematemesis and/or melena—8%; may be caused by direct invasion of the stomach or duodenum

g. Trousseau's sign—6%; migratory thrombophlebitis

Note: A surgical dictum is that *vague abdominal pain with weight loss,* with or without jaundice, in an older patient (>50 years old) *is pancreatic cancer until proven otherwise.*

F. DIAGNOSTIC STUDIES

1. Ultrasound

a. Useful as screening method and for evaluating biliary ducts

b. Sensitivity approaches 70%; specificity, 95%

c. Nondiagnostic in 20% of patients owing to bowel gas interference and overall patient size

d. Role for endoscopic ultrasound not yet fully recognized

2. Abdominal CT scan

a. Mainstay of both diagnosis and evaluation of disease spread

b. Sensitivity, 85%; specificity, 95%

c. CT-guided percutaneous needle aspirate of mass may be helpful in tissue diagnosis.

d. Allows visualization of liver and status of abdominal lymph nodes

3. ERCP

a. Most sensitive imaging technique to diagnose pancreatic cancer; sensitivity, 95%; specificity, 85%

b. Can be combined with cytologic analysis of pancreatic or duodenal secretions or brush cytology

c. Findings suggestive of pancreatic cancer
   (1) Pancreatic duct obstruction
   (2) Double-duct sign constriction of both pancreatic and bile ducts in the head of the pancreas
   (3) Necrotic cavity formation secondary to diffuse or focal disease

d. Associated with a small but significant risk of serious complications (e.g., pancreatitis, hemorrhage)

e. Provides opportunity to place a stent to relieve obstruction

4. Percutaneous transhepatic cholangiography

a. Largely replaced by ERCP owing to lower complication rate

b. Useful in evaluation of patient suspected of having pancreatic cancer when there is no visualization of common bile duct by ERCP

5. Selective angiography

a. Sensitivity 70-94%

b. Largely replaced as primary diagnostic study by less invasive imaging techniques

c. Used to determine presence of abnormal vasculature, such as right hepatic artery arising from SMA, and to determine unresectability based on encasement of the SMA, SMV, hepatic artery, or portal vein

6. Laparoscopy

a. Invasive and of no value or benefit in patient with obstruction who requires surgical bypass for relief of symptoms

b. May be helpful tool in staging pancreatic cancer because it can detect hepatic and peritoneal metastases missed on CT in up to 20% of patients

7. Serum chemistries—Generally nonspecific and of little use in diagnosis

a. Hepatic profile—Elevated bilirubin, alkaline phosphatase; sometimes slight increase in transaminases

b. Glucose intolerance

c. Occasional elevation of amylase, lipase, or elastase

8. Serologic tumor markers

a. CA 19-9—Sensitivity, 83%; specificity, 82%

b. CEA—Sensitivity, 56%; specificity, 75%

c. Not useful as screening test but may be useful for follow-up to monitor for recurrent disease after resection or response to adjuvant therapy

44

THE PANCREAS

G. TREATMENT

1. A number of patients presenting with pancreatic cancer are candidates for resection or palliative surgical treatment, although most patients present with advanced disease.
2. Nonoperative management
a. Potential option for documented distal metastases, unresectable local disease, and in patients with associated acute or chronic debilitating illnesses
b. Attempt tissue diagnosis by percutaneous needle biopsy of primary tumor, cytologic determination at ERCP or percutaneous trans-hepatic cholecystostomy, or biopsy of distant metastases
c. Palliation of pain—Analgesics or percutaneous celiac ganglion block
d. Palliation of biliary obstruction—Percutaneous trans-hepatic drainage catheter or endoscopically placed stent
e. Palliation of duodenal obstruction—External-beam radiation therapy (EBRT) (minimal success); percutaneous endoscopic gastrostomy
3. Resectional surgical therapy
a. At operation the abdomen and pelvis are thoroughly explored for extrapancreatic disease (e.g., liver, omentum, serosal implants, mesentery, and lymph node metastases outside the potential resection margins) before proceeding with pancreatic dissection. The next step is determination of resectability. Encasement of the hepatic artery, superior mesenteric vessels, or portal vein by tumor is indicative of nonresectability.
b. For all patients explored with curative intent, only 20% of cancers of the head of the pancreas are candidates for resection.
c. Pancreaticoduodenectomy (Whipple's procedure)
   (1) The traditional resection procedure for pancreatic cancer
   (2) See section III. G. 3. d for details.
   (3) Overall operative mortality is ≈5% in experienced centers.
   (4) Most common postoperative complication is pancreatic fistula in 5-20% of patients.
   (5) Recent support for aggressive curative resection procedures involving extended regional lymph node dissection. Resection of arterial and portal vein segments as well as involved neighboring organs may be indicated in some cases.
d. Pyloric-preserving pancreaticoduodenectomy (modified Whipple's procedure)
   (1) See section III. G. 3. e for details.
   (2) No compromise in survival compared with standard Whipple's procedure
e. Total pancreatectomy
   (1) Possible indication due to multicentricity in 30-40% of pancreatic cancers
   (2) No advantage over pancreaticoduodenectomy, but higher morbidity including very brittle diabetes mellitus

(3) May be indicated when invasive carcinoma present at resection line or when the friable texture of the pancreatic remnant prohibits creating a safe pancreaticojejunal anastomosis

f. Distal pancreatectomy and en bloc splenectomy

    (1) For rare patient with potentially resectable pancreatic cancer of body and tail

    (2) Prognosis still poor but serves as good palliation of tumor-associated pain

4. Palliative surgery

a. Performed on patients with unresectable disease discovered at time of laparotomy

b. Goal is to alleviate biliary obstruction, duodenal obstruction, and tumor-associated pain

c. Biliary obstruction—Treated by choledochojejunostomy or cholecystojejunostomy

d. Duodenal obstruction—Treated by gastrojejunostomy

e. Pain—Treated by intraoperative chemical splanchnicectomy (injection of 50 mL of either 50% alcohol or 6% phenol along both sides of celiac axis). May be done percutaneously.

f. Some surgeons advocate cytoreduction/resection for palliation.

5. Adjuvant therapy

a. Chemotherapy

    (1) Most commonly used agents are 5-fluorouracil (5-FU), gemcitabine, mitomycin C, streptozocin, doxorubicin, and lomustine (methyl-CCNU).

    (2) Gemcitabine has a low response rate but an overall improvement in survival in comparison with 5-FU.

    (3) 5-FU has potentiating effect on radiation therapy.

b. Radiation therapy

    (1) Modalities—EBRT, intraoperative radiation therapy, and interstitial implants (brachytherapy)

    (2) Positive responses reported with radiation therapy for both resectable and unresectable disease

    (3) Beneficial in relieving pain from pancreatic cancer

c. Multimodality therapy (chemotherapy plus radiation therapy)

    (1) Combination chemotherapy and radiation therapy with EBRT and 5-FU following surgical resection can significantly improve median survival.

    (2) Preoperative chemotherapy and radiation therapy presently undergoing prospective analysis to determine whether this may be better tolerated and possibly "downstage" previously unresectable tumors

V. PRIMARY CYSTIC NEOPLASMS OF THE PANCREAS

A. GENERAL CONSIDERATIONS

1. Important to distinguish these neoplasms from the more routine and mundane inflammatory pancreatic pseudocysts because their respective managements differ so radically

44

THE PANCREAS

2. Patients with primary cystic neoplasms tend to be older (>50 years), are more commonly female (≈80%), have no history of pancreatic abnormalities, and are seen at diagnosis with signs and symptoms related to the mass effect of the lesion. The lesions are truly asymptomatic in up to 40% of patients, with discovery of the cystic mass at the time of evaluation for an unrelated disorder.
3. CT scan generally shows multiple cysts without other pancreatic or peripancreatic inflammatory changes, and ERCP generally shows a normal pancreatic duct without communication with the cystic mass.

B. HISTOPATHOLOGIC CLASSIFICATION

1. Serous cystadenoma

a. Most common benign tumor of exocrine pancreas with little tendency for malignant transformation
b. Composed of a honeycomb of multiple (>6) small-diameter, sometimes "microscopic cysts" (<2 cm) lined by a glycogen rich, low-cuboidal epithelium
c. Cysts generally 6-10 cm in overall gross size, of equal frequency throughout the pancreas, and contain clear cyst fluid
d. Resection generally advocated but can be managed by close observation in frail or elderly patients or patients with high operative risks

2. Mucinous cystadenoma/cystadenocarcinoma spectrum

a. Represent a diverse, heterogenous spectrum of related neoplasms, ranging from benign mucinous cystadenoma to overt malignant cystadenocarcinoma
b. Mucinous cystadenomas have tremendous latent malignant potential (>80%) and are more common in women (8:1).
c. Composed of a tall columnar epithelium that expresses mucin that can have papillary invaginations with multiple areas of atypia, dysplasia, carcinoma in situ, and overtly invasive carcinoma
d. Generally appear as "macroscopic cysts" (>2 cm) with <6 cysts, are 8-10 cm in overall gross size, and are more often located in the body and tail of the pancreas
e. All mucinous neoplasms should be considered malignant and managed by potential curative resection.
f. 5-year survival is >50% for mucinous cystadenocarcinoma resected for cure.

3. Unusual cystic neoplasms

a. Acinar cell cystadenocarcinoma
b. Cystic choriocarcinoma
c. Cystic teratoma
d. Angiomatous cystic neoplasms

VI. CLINICAL STAGING

1. Staging system for pancreatic carcinoma is based on the extent of primary tumor (defined by extension through the pancreatic capsule), the status of regional lymph nodes, and the presence of metastatic disease.
2. TNM classification
a. Primary tumor (T)

  Tx—Primary tumor cannot be assessed
  T0—No evidence of primary tumor
  T1a—Tumor limited to pancreas, ≤2 cm in diameter
  T1b—Tumor limited to pancreas, >2 cm in diameter
  T2—Tumor extends to duodenum, bile duct, or peripancreatic tissues
  T3—Tumor extends directly to stomach, spleen, colon, or adjacent large vessels

b. Regional lymph nodes (N)

  Nx—Regional lymph nodes cannot be assessed
  N0—Regional lymph nodes not involved
  N1—Regional lymph nodes involved

c. Distant metastases (M)

  Mx—Presence of distant metastasis cannot be assessed
  M0—No distant metastasis
  M1—Distant metastasis present

3. TNM staging system

  Stage I—T1, T2, N0, M0; no direct extension beyond duodenum, bile duct, or peripancreatic tissues without regional nodal involvement
  Stage II—T3, N0, M0; direct extension into adjacent tissues without regional nodal involvement
  Stage III—Any T, N1, M0; regional lymph node involvement with or without direct tumor extension
  Stage IV—Any T, Any N, M1; distant metastatic disease present

4. R classification—To indicate presence or absence of residual tumor following surgical intervention

  R0—No residual tumor
  R1—Microscopic residual tumor
  R2—Macroscopic residual tumor
  R0 corresponds to curative resection, R1 and R2 to noncurative resection

5. Radiographic staging

  Stage 1—Resectable (T1-T2, selected T3, Nx, M0); no encasement of celiac axis or SMA; patent SMV confluence; no extrapancreatic disease
  Stage 2—Locally advanced (T3, Nx-1, M0); arterial encasement (celiac or SMA) or venous occlusion (SMV or portal); no extrapancreatic disease

44

THE PANCREAS

Stage 3—Metastatic (T1-3, Nx-1, M1); metastasis to liver, peritoneum, and others

VII. PROGNOSIS

1. Surgical resection remains the sole curative treatment of pancreatic carcinoma. In the past, 5-year survival after pancreatic resection was rare (<5%). However, several recent reports have 5-year survival at 20-25%.
a. Patients with tumors <2 cm—5-year survival approaches 30%
b. Patients with no lymph node metastasis even higher survival
c. Study by Sohn and associates[4] of 616 patients undergoing surgical resection—Overall survival at 1 year, 63%; 5-year survival, 17%; median survival, 17 months. Right-sided tumors have 1-year and 5-year survival rates of 64% and 17%, respectively, compared with left-sided lesions, which have 1-year and 5-year survival rates of 50% and 15%, respectively.
   (1) Other favorable prognostic signs—Negative resection margins, tumor size < 3 cm, blood loss <750 mL, well-differentiated to moderately differentiated tumor

REFERENCES

1. Perdozoli P, Bassi C, Vesentini S, Campedilli A: A randomized multicenter clinical trial of antibiotic prophylaxis of septic complications in acute necrotizing pancreatitis with imipenem. Surg Gynecol Obstet 176: 480-483, 1993.
2. Gloor B, Muller CA, Worni M, et al: Pancreatic infection in severe pancreatitis: The role of fungus and multiresistant organisms. Arch Surg 136:592-596, 2001.
3. Luzi L, Perseghin G, Brendel MD, et al: Metabolic effects of restoring partial beta-cell function after islet allotransplantation in type 1 diabetic patients. Diabetes 50:277-282, 2001.
4. Sohn TA, Yeo CJ, Cameron JL, et al: Resected adenocarcinoma of the pancreas—616 patients: Results, outcomes, and prognostic indicators. J Gastrointest Surg 4:567-579, 2000.

RECOMMENDED READINGS

Dimagno EP, Reber HA, Tempero MA: AGA technical review on the epidemiology, diagnosis, and treatment of pancreatic ductal adenocarcinoma. American Gastroenterological Association. Gastroenterology 117:1464-1484, 1999.

Hunt GC, Faigel DO: Assessment of EUS for diagnosing, staging, and determining resectability of pancreatic cancer: A review. Gastrointest Endosc 55:232-237, 2002.

Martin RF, Rossi RL: Multidisciplinary considerations for the patients with cancer of the pancreas or biliary tract. Surg Clin North Am 80:709-728, 2000.

Stojadinovic A, Brooks A, Hoos A, et al: An evidence-based approach to the surgical management of resectable pancreatic adenocarcinoma. J Am Coll Surgeons 196:954-964, 2003.

Wagman R, Grann A: Adjuvant therapy for pancreatic cancer: Current treatment approaches and future challenges. Surg Clin North Am 81:667-681, 2001.

44

THE PANCREAS

Surgical Diseases of the Spleen

Joseph Kim, MD

I. ANATOMY AND FUNCTION

A. ADULT ANATOMY
1. Average adult spleen—Size of a fist and weighs 75-175 g
2. Splenic pedicle—Hilum contains the splenic artery, vein, lymphatics, and tail of the pancreas
3. Microanatomy
a. White pulp—Reticular framework surrounding the trabecular arteries occupied by lymphocytes
b. Red pulp—Network of sinuses bounded by cords, scaffolding for macrophages, through which red blood cells (RBCs) must pass to enter the sinuses
c. Marginal zone—Between white and red pulps; consists of ill-defined vascular space

B. FUNCTION
1. Organ of the reticuloendothelial system
2. Filtration of senescent RBCs (4% of blood volume per minute) and encapsulated microorganisms
3. Pitting function (opsonization) carried out by properdin and tuftsin
4. Immunologic response (primarily IgM production) to bacterial sequestration

II. INDICATIONS FOR SPLENECTOMY

A. GENERAL
Indications for splenectomy have changed in recent years owing to improved treatment for underlying disorders. Mortality rate of splenectomy for hematologic disease is <1%, with a morbidity rate of 10%.

B. TRAUMA
See Chapter 14.

C. CYSTS
1. Congenital
2. Acquired
a. Enlargement may lead to pain and/or compression of surrounding organs.

D. CONGENITAL HEMOLYTIC ANEMIAS
1. Hereditary spherocytosis
a. Abnormal RBC membrane caused by defect in spectrin, predisposing the cell to sequestration in the spleen

b. Splenectomy is indicated for anemia, cholelithiasis (from increased hemoglobin catabolism and bile pigment production), recurrent virus-induced aplastic crisis, and intractable leg ulcers.

c. Most common hemolytic anemia to be indicated for splenectomy

2. Hereditary elliptocytosis

a. Abnormal RBC membrane caused by dimerization of spectrin from its normal tetrameric form

b. Similar indications for splenectomy as hereditary spherocytosis

3. Thalassemia

a. Decreased production of β-globin chains leads to excess of α chains.

b. Accumulation leads to precipitation on cell membrane, causing a distortion in the shape of the cell, leading to sequestration and hemolysis in the spleen.

c. Indicated for massive splenomegaly, painful splenic infarct, and increased transfusion requirements

E. AUTOIMMUNE

1. Immune thrombocytopenic purpura (ITP)

a. Average age 36 years, usually female. ITP associated with AIDS is more common in males.

b. Symptoms of bruising, petechiae, mucosal hemorrhage, menorrhagia, or prolonged bleeding are common.

c. Characterized by increased platelet production (four or five times normal) and higher megakaryocyte mass on bone marrow biopsy

d. Thrombocytopenia due to IgG antibodies directed at a platelet antigen IIb/IIIa

e. The spleen is usually small or normal in size.

f. Medical treatment—Achieves remission in 15% of adult patients
   (1) Platelet transfusions for active bleeding or severe risk of life-threatening hemorrhage
   (2) Corticosteroids—Shown to increase platelet production in 3-7 days; usually a 2-week course is given
   (3) IV gamma globulin
   (4) In childhood, most cases follow a viral illness and are self-limited, with resolution within 1 year.

g. Most common hematologic indication for splenectomy

h. Splenectomy is indicated when medical management fails or for recurrence of disease.
   (1) Preoperative steroids or gamma globulin to increase platelets to acceptable level may be used.
   (2) Complete remission following splenectomy occurs in 70-80% and is more likely in persons responsive to steroids preoperatively.
   (3) A thorough search should be performed intraoperatively for accessory splenic tissue.
   (4) Patients who are thrombocytopenic after splenectomy require further therapy with danazol, cyclophosphamide, vinca alkaloids, or IV gamma globulin.

2. Autoimmune hemolytic anemia (AIHA)
a. Acquired hemolytic anemia from anti-RBC antibodies directed against Rh locus.
b. Hemolysis, fluctuating jaundice, splenomegaly, and reticulocytosis
c. Positive direct Coombs' test—Warm (IgG).
d. IgG-coated cells are sequestered in the spleen.
e. Disease can be associated with certain drugs (penicillin, cephalothin, streptomycin, methyldopa, quinidine, and sulfonamides).
f. Blood transfusions and steroids are the primary treatment, resulting in improvement in 80% of patients.
g. Splenectomy indicated in warm reactive AIHA (not helpful in IgM AIHA) not responsive to medical management or requiring large steroid doses for maintenance.

F. SPLENECTOMY FOR SYMPTOMS
1. Hypersplenism
a. Divided into primary hypersplenism, in which underlying disease is unknown, and secondary hypersplenism, in which the primary disease accounts for the increased splenic function.

2. Splenic vein thrombosis
a. 50% are caused by pancreatitis, but pancreatic carcinoma, pseudocyst, and penetrating gastric ulcer are other causes.
b. Causes gastric varices that can be the etiology of upper GI hemorrhage.
c. Splenectomy resolves both problems and should be done once other causes of portal hypertension are ruled out.

3. Infectious mononucleosis
a. Splenomegaly common in Epstein-Barr virus infection
b. "Spontaneous" rupture probably just susceptibility to injury with minor trauma
c. May require splenectomy

G. HEMATOLOGIC MALIGNANCIES
1. Hairy cell leukemia
a. Most patients with hematologic malignancies are not considered for early splenectomy, with the exception of hairy cell leukemia.
b. Splenectomy is the first treatment.
c. Secondary therapy consists of α interferon and 2′-deoxycoformycin if splenectomy fails to improve the cytopenia.
d. Chemotherapy is first if bone marrow cellularity is >85%.

2. Hodgkin's disease
a. A malignant lymphoma characterized by Reed-Sternberg cells
b. Incidence peaks in late 20s and again begins increasing over the age of 45 years; more common in males
c. Commonly presents as asymptomatic lymphadenopathy, and constitutional symptoms (B symptoms) of fever, night sweats, and

weight loss usually indicate widespread disease and a less favorable prognosis

d. Treatment and ultimate survival depend on disease distribution, the presence or absence of B symptoms, and histologic subtype.

e. Staging laparotomy

(1) Consists of exploratory laparotomy with liver biopsy, splenectomy, para-aortic node sampling, and bone marrow biopsy

(2) Indications are stages I and II disease, for which treatment is usually radiation therapy alone. Patients with stages III and IV, for which chemotherapy or combined modality therapy will be used, are not candidates for staging laparotomy.

(3) A change in clinical stage occurs in 35-40% of patients.

(a) 25-35% are up-staged (higher stage) after staging laparotomy.

(b) 5-15% are down-staged.

H. THROMBOTIC THROMBOCYTOPENIC PURPURA

1. Condition of thrombocytopenia, microangiopathic hemolytic anemia, neurologic abnormalities, fever, and renal failure secondary to platelet microthrombi

2. 90% idiopathic, female > male, with peak in 3rd decade

3. Poor prognosis, with 10% 1-year survival

4. Treatment focuses on plasmapheresis, high-dose steroids, and antiplatelet drugs; splenectomy may be performed for poor response to these treatments, with few reports of improvement.

III. OTHER SPLENIC DISORDERS OF SURGICAL SIGNIFICANCE

A. SPLENIC ARTERY ANEURYSM

1. Rare, but occurs more in women than in men

2. Medial dysplasia is the usual cause in women, and atherosclerosis is the usual cause in men.

3. May cause vague abdominal pain

4. Occasionally ruptures with early containment by lesser sac or exsanguinating hemorrhage into peritoneal cavity; <10% rupture, and of these, 20% are during pregnancy

5. Elective aneurysm excision should be performed in good-surgical-risk patients or women of childbearing age.

6. Splenic function should be preserved.

B. SPLENIC ABSCESS

1. Rare and usually occurs with a primary focus, such as other abscesses or endocarditis

2. Fever, chills, left upper quadrant (LUQ) tenderness, and splenomegaly

3. Diagnosed by CT or sonogram

4. Splenectomy is the preferred treatment unless the abscess is unilocular and subcapsular, in which case percutaneous drainage may be effective.

C. SPLENIC CYSTS
1. Pseudocysts—50-75%, related to previous injury
2. Epithelial (nonparasitic)—10% of cysts, prone to rupture if >10 cm in size. May be lymphangiomas, dermoid cysts, or cystic hemangiomas. Symptomatic cysts are treated with aspiration; splenectomy is indicated if cysts are very large or diagnosis is uncertain.
3. Parasitic—Echinococcal most common; should not be aspirated

D. ECTOPIC SPLEEN
1. Normal spleen found in the lower abdomen
2. Most common in young, multiparous women
3. Elongated splenic pedicle predisposes to splenic torsion. If splenic torsion occurs, splenectomy is required.
4. When recurrent vague symptoms are present or found incidentally, splenopexy may be performed.

IV. OPERATIVE APPROACH

A. OPEN SPLENECTOMY

B. LAPAROSCOPIC SPLENECTOMY
1. First successful case reported by Delaitre and Maignien in 1991[1]
2. Indications same as for open splenectomy
3. Contraindications
a. Severe cardiopulmonary disease
b. Cirrhosis with portal hypertension
c. Pregnancy
4. Preoperative preparation
a. Administer polyvalent pneumococcal vaccine 2 weeks prior to surgery.
b. Children receive *Haemophilus influenzae* type B vaccination 2 weeks prior to surgery.
5. Laparoscopic technique
a. Nasogastric tube, Foley catheter, sequential compression devices (SCDs), beanbag, axillary roll
b. Right lateral decubitus position at 60 degrees
c. 15-degree reverse Trendelenburg position to gravity-weight the spleen
d. Three 10-mm port sites
e. Search for accessory spleens—Hilum is most common
f. Dissection
   (1) Division of short gastric vessels
   (2) Division of splenocolic ligament

      (3) Ligation of the inferior pole vessels
      (4) Hilar control
      (5) Division of phrenic attachments
  g. Placement of spleen into retrieval bag—May introduce ring forceps to morcellate the spleen
  h. May enlarge middle incision, or use hand-assisted technique to remove the whole spleen

6. Results
a. Increased operating time
b. Decreased blood loss
c. Decreased requirement for narcotics postoperatively
d. Decreased length of hospitalization
e. No difference in complication rates compared with open method

V. COMPLICATIONS OF SPLENECTOMY

A. IMMEDIATELY POSTOPERATIVELY
1. Peripheral blood changes
a. Leukocytosis
b. Thrombocytosis
c. Presence of Howell-Jolly bodies
2. Hemorrhage—From splenic pedicle or short gastric vessels. Many advocate nasogastric tube postoperatively to decompress the stomach and decrease potential bleeding from the short gastric vessels.
3. Atelectasis (usually left lower lobe)—Most common complication
4. Subphrenic abscess or hematoma—Presents as fever and LUQ pain or left shoulder pain, usually about 5 days after surgery. This may require re-exploration or percutaneous drainage.
5. Pancreatitis or pancreatic fistula resulting from parenchymal manipulation

B. POSTSPLENECTOMY SEPSIS
1. Overwhelming sepsis usually with an encapsulated organism such as *Pneumococcus* sp or *Haemophilus* sp. Incidence in splenectomized patients is 40 times that of the general population.
2. Occurs in 4.25% of splenectomized patients, with a higher rate associated with hematologic disease. Rates for trauma splenectomies are <1%.
3. Fatal 50% of the time.
4. Vaccinations for *Streptococcus pneumoniae* and *H. influenzae* should be given to all splenectomy patients. Vaccines are more effective if given 10-14 days before surgery.
5. Prophylactic penicillin is given to children <18 years of age and reduces the incidence significantly.

REFERENCE

1. Delaitre B, Maignien B: Splenectomy by the laparoscopic approach: Report of a case. Presse Med 20:2263, 1991.

Laparoscopic Inguinal Hernia Repair

Grace Z. Mak, MD

More than 500,000 inguinal hernias are repaired every year, making hernia repair one of the most common surgical procedures in the United States. To date, there exists no "perfect" inguinal hernia repair. Traditional repairs using autologous tissue to close the hernia have a recurrence rate of 5-10%. Hernia repair using prosthetic mesh and tension-free suture lines appears to have a lower recurrence rate. Laparoscopic hernia repair is a recently developed alternative to traditional and mesh herniorrhaphy. Potential advantages of laparoscopic hernia repair include faster postoperative recovery rates and, potentially, lower recurrence rates. Disadvantages include the need for general anesthesia; the use of a posterior, buttressed repair with mesh; undefined recurrence rates; and potentially higher in-hospital costs.

46

I. GENERAL

A. APPROACHES
1. Transabdominal preperitoneal (TAPP)
2. Extraperitoneal laparoscopic repair with mesh (ELM) or total extraperitoneal placement of mesh (TEPP)
3. Intraperitoneal laparoscopic onlay mesh (IPOM)

B. ANATOMY OF THE PREPERITONEAL SPACE
1. Laparoscopic approaches require understanding of the inguinal anatomy in the preperitoneal space. In Figure 46-1, the key anatomic landmarks in the preperitoneal space are identified, along with typical locations of a direct, indirect, and femoral hernia.
2. In both TAPP and ELM repairs, the herniated contents are reduced from within the abdomen, and the defect in the abdominal wall is identified. The defect is closed with mesh stapled to the posterior surface of the abdominal wall, reinforcing the floor of all three hernia spaces. The mesh is tacked medially to the rectus sheath, inferiorly to the iliopubic tract beginning at Cooper's ligament, and superiorly and laterally to transversalis fascia, thus buttressing the myopectineal orifice. To avoid the femoral blood vessels medially and the genitofemoral and lateral femoral cutaneous nerves laterally, it is important not to staple below the iliopubic tract.
3. Care must also be taken to avoid the "triangle of doom," whose apex is formed by the spermatic vessels and vas deferens. The external iliac vessels lie within this triangle hidden by peritoneum. No dissection should be done in this area, and stapling should be done only medial to the vas deferens and lateral to the spermatic vessels.

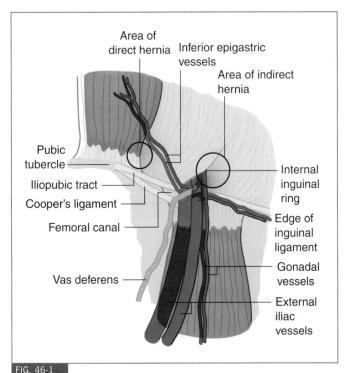

FIG. 46-1
Key landmarks of the inguinal anatomy in the preperitoneal space and typical locations of direct, indirect, and femoral hernias. *(From Geis WP, Crafton WB, Novak MJ, Malago M: Laparoscopic herniorrhaphy: Results and technical aspects in 458 consecutive procedures. Surgery 114:765, 1993.)*

C. PREOPERATIVE PREPARATION

1. History and physical exam

a. In older patients with new hernia, consider the etiology of the straining (i.e., prostate cancer, colon cancer, pulmonary disease).

b. Preoperative antibiotic (i.e., second-generation cephalosporin)

2. Relative contraindications to laparoscopic hernia repair

a. Previous lower abdominal operation

b. Known sliding or inguinal-scrotal hernia—Reduction of the hernia can be difficult.

c. Poor candidate for general anesthesia.

II. DETAILS OF SPECIFIC PROCEDURES

A. TAPP
1. Operative procedure
a. Intra-abdominal laparoscopy using three ports—A 10-mm infraumbilical camera port, a 10-mm dissection port placed lateral to the rectus abdominis on the contralateral side to the hernia, and a 5-mm ipsilateral dissection port

b. Reduction of herniated abdominal contents and the peritoneum from the inguinal canal into the abdominal cavity

c. Incision of peritoneum high over hernia defect and entry into preperitoneal space

d. Dissection within the preperitoneal space exposing the abdominal wall defect. Cooper's ligament, the inferior epigastric vessels, the gonadal vessels, the vas deferens, and the internal inguinal ring should be identified.

e. Reinforcement of the posterior abdominal wall with mesh, thus closing the abdominal wall defect. The mesh should cover all points of weakness, including the deep inguinal ring, femoral ring, and Hesselbach's triangle, size ≈15 × 10 cm. The mesh is secured with staples medially to the symphysis pubis, Cooper's ligament, and conjoint tendon and the rectus sheath extending laterally to the transversalis fascia. The mesh should then be tested to ensure that there is no tension.

f. Reapproximation of the peritoneum, thus preventing direct contact between the abdominal viscera and the prosthetic mesh

g. Closure of laparoscopy ports

2. Advantages
a. Best established laparoscopic approach

b. Reduction of herniated abdominal contents is easier than with ELM, and viability of the contents in a strangulated hernia may be determined under direct visualization.

c. Easier to unroll and place mesh

d. Preferred for recurrent hernias repaired by either open or laparoscopic approach

3. Disadvantages
a. If the peritoneum is not adequately closed, there will be direct contact between mesh and abdominal contents—This may increase risk for small bowel adhesions.

b. Intra-abdominal procedure with the attendant risks of perforation of intra-abdominal viscus and blood vessels on trocar placement

B. ELM
1. Operative procedure
a. Incision of the infraumbilical anterior fascia, placement of a dissecting balloon below the rectus abdominis muscle, anterior to the posterior fascia. The dissecting balloon is advanced in this plane to the pubis and

46

LAPAROSCOPIC INGUINAL HERNIA REPAIR

inflated, developing the preperitoneal space. Low pressure (10 mm Hg) CO_2 insufflation maintains the preperitoneal cavity.
b. A 10-mm infraumbilical camera port, a 10-mm port between pubis and umbilicus, and a 5-mm port just above pubis; all ports placed in the midline
c. Reduction of herniated contents including peritoneum from within the preperitoneal space
d. The dissection of the abdominal wall defect and its repair with mesh is similar to the TAPP procedure.

2. **Advantages**
a. Ideally, because the peritoneum is never violated, the risk of contact between intra-abdominal contents and mesh is minimized.
b. Dissection of the abdominal wall defect can be easier than the TAPP.
c. Avoids intra-abdominal cavity
d. Can be performed under regional anesthesia

3. **Disadvantages**
a. In comparison with the TAPP repair, reduction of a large hernia sac can be difficult.
b. If the peritoneum is accidentally entered, pneumoperitoneum can reduce the preperitoneal space, making the dissection difficult.

C. IPOM
1. Operative procedure
a. Entrance into abdominal cavity similar to TAPP
b. Hernia is cleared of intestine and adhesions
c. Hernial orifice is then covered with mesh and secured with staples to peritoneum, pubic tubercle, and Cooper's ligament

2. Advantages
a. Can be performed with low-pressure pneumoperitoneum, thus making it possible to be performed with local anesthesia
b. Hernia defect is easily recognized and cleared with minimal dissection

3. Disadvantages
a. Not effective for medial defects because staples are placed medially to peritoneum, allowing migration into defect only of peritoneum and mesh
b. Structures beneath peritoneum are not seen accurately and are thus at risk of damage
c. Increased risk of bowel obstruction and fistula formation
d. Conversion to open repair—0-7%

III. RESULTS

A. RETROSPECTIVE STUDIES
1. Results suggest that laparoscopic approach is viable with low complication rates and faster return to activity.
2. Major limitation is short-term follow-up in all of the studies (maximum of 65 months). Studies of open repair have shown that a large percentage of hernia recurrences occur 5-10 years after surgery.

B. PROSPECTIVE STUDIES

1. Several small prospective, randomized trials
2. Results indicate that patients repaired laparoscopically return to work faster with less postoperative pain. Medical cost may be higher, but the societal benefit of early return to work is significant.
3. Lack of follow-up is a limitation of all the studies.

C. POSSIBLE ADVANTAGES

1. Decreased risk of graft infection owing to small size of incisions and great distance between graft and wound
2. High closure of peritoneal sac
3. Diagnosis and treatment of bilateral hernias without extensive dissection
4. Placement of mesh in preperitoneal space counteracts the forces of intra-abdominal pressure on mesh
5. Better visualization of inguinal anatomy, including nerve and vascular structures

D. POSSIBLE DISADVANTAGES

1. Increased cost, though this could decrease with reusable equipment and decreased operative time
2. Requires general anesthesia

E. COMPLICATIONS

1. Mortality—0.1%
2. Morbidity—0-6%
a. Urinary retention
b. Neuralgia most commonly due to lateral cutaneous nerve injury (minimized by use of helical titanium tacks rather than staples)
c. Port hernia
d. Bladder injury
3. Recurrence—1-3%
a. Early recurrence most commonly due to mesh of inadequate size
b. Owing to significant learning curve with laparoscopic repair, recurrence rate is higher with initial repairs.

IV. CONCLUSIONS

The exact role of laparoscopic herniorrhaphy remains to be determined. Laparoscopic hernia repair is a viable alternative to standard repairs. Patients with bilateral and recurrent hernias appear to be the best candidates for this type of approach. Large prospective, randomized studies with long follow-up are needed to validate the use of laparoscopic herniorrhaphy.

46

LAPAROSCOPIC INGUINAL HERNIA REPAIR

Abdominal Wall Hernias

Grace Z. Mak, MD

It has been only within the past century, with an improved understanding of inguinal anatomy, aseptic technique, and improvements in suture material, that significant improvements in hernia management have occurred.

I. TERMINOLOGY

47

A. HERNIA
Hernia is the protrusion of a part or structure through tissues normally containing it.

B. REDUCIBILITY
Reducibility means that the contents can be restored to their anatomic location.

C. INCARCERATION
Incarceration is an irreducible hernia, which may be acute and painful or chronic and asymptomatic.

D. STRANGULATION
Strangulated hernia is an incarcerated hernia with vascular compromise of the herniated contents. It usually occurs in indirect, femoral, and umbilical hernias.

E. SLIDING HERNIA (Fig. 47-1)
Sliding hernia is a portion of the hernial sac that is composed of a wall of a viscus (frequently cecum or sigmoid colon).

F. RICHTER'S HERNIA (Fig. 47-2)
Richter's hernia is a condition in which only one sidewall of a viscus lies within the hernial sac (i.e., a "knuckle" of small bowel). It may incarcerate or strangulate without obstructing, then spontaneously reduce, resulting in gangrenous bowel with perforation.

II. INCIDENCE

A. GENDER
1. Male-to-female ratio—7:1

B. GENERAL
1. Lifetime risk of developing a hernia—Males 5%, females 1%
2. Most common surgical disease of males
3. Most common groin hernia in either sex is indirect inguinal hernia; however, femoral hernias are more common in females
4. Aging increases the incidence of groin hernias.

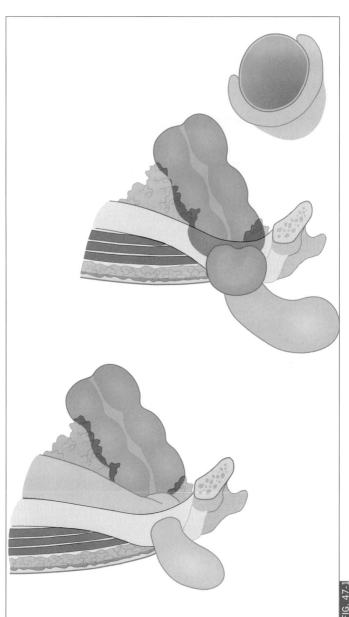

FIG. 47-1

Sliding hernia.

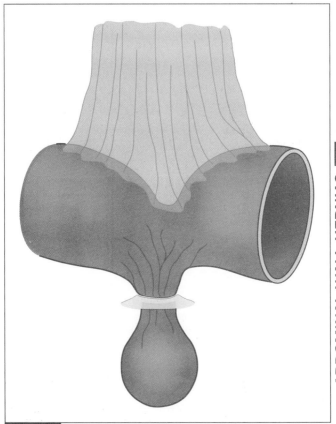

FIG. 47-2

Richter's hernia.

III. ANATOMIC CONSIDERATIONS

A. LAYERS OF THE ABDOMINAL WALL
The layers of the abdominal wall are skin, subcutaneous fat, Scarpa's fascia, external oblique muscle, internal oblique muscle, transversus abdominis muscle, transversalis fascia, and peritoneum.

B. HESSELBACH'S TRIANGLE
Hesselbach's triangle is bordered by the lateral edge of the rectus sheath, inferior epigastric vessels, and inguinal ligament. **Note:** *These tissues are not in the same plane.*

C. INGUINAL LIGAMENT

The inguinal ligament runs from the anterior superior iliac spine to the pubic tubercle. It is formed from the external oblique aponeurosis.

D. LACUNAR LIGAMENT

The lacunar ligament is that part of the inguinal ligament reflected from the pubic tubercle onto the iliopectineal line of the pubic ramus.

E. COOPER'S LIGAMENT

Cooper's ligament is a strong fibrous band on the iliopectineal line of the superior pubic ramus.

F. EXTERNAL RING

The external ring is an opening in the external oblique aponeurosis through which the ilioinguinal nerve and spermatic cord or round ligament pass.

G. INTERNAL RING

The internal ring is bordered superiorly by internal oblique muscle and inferomedially by inferior epigastric vessels and transversalis fascia.

H. PROCESSUS VAGINALIS

The processus vaginalis is a diverticulum of parietal peritoneum that descends from the abdomen along with the testicle and comes to lie adjacent to the spermatic cord. There is subsequent obliteration of its lumen in normal individuals during development.

I. FEMORAL CANAL

The femoral canal is bordered by the inguinal ligament, lacunar ligament, Cooper's ligament, and femoral sheath.

J. INFERIOR LUMBAR TRIANGLE

The inferior lumbar triangle is an upright triangle bordered posteriorly by the latissimus dorsi muscle, inferiorly by the iliac crest, and anteriorly by the external oblique muscle with a floor formed by the internal oblique muscle and transversus abdominis.

IV. CLASSIFICATION OF HERNIAS

A. GROIN HERNIAS (Fig. 47-3)

1. Indirect inguinal hernia—Sac lies anteromedial to cord, exiting through the internal ring; lateral to the inferior epigastric artery
2. Direct inguinal hernia—Sac passes through Hesselbach's triangle (medial to the inferior epigastric artery)
3. Pantaloon hernia—Components of both direct and indirect inguinal hernias straddle the inferior epigastric vessels

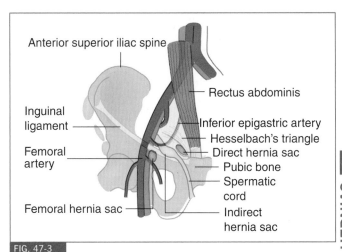

FIG. 47-3

Groin hernias. Inf. epig. art. = inferior epigastric artery.

4. Femoral hernia—Sac passes through the femoral canal, medial to the femoral vein

B. VENTRAL HERNIAS
1. Umbilical hernia—Congenital or acquired
2. Incisional hernia—Develops in previous fascial closure
3. Epigastric hernia—Defect in linea alba above the umbilicus

C. MISCELLANEOUS HERNIAS
1. Littre's hernia—Inguinal hernia sac that contains a Meckel's diverticulum
2. Spigelian hernia
a. Ventral hernia occurring at the semilunar line (lateral edge of rectus)
b. Usually occurs where semilunar line and semicircular line intersect and rectus sheath becomes completely anterior
3. Parastomal hernia—Hernia at ostomy site
a. Occurs more frequently at colostomy sites than at ileostomy sites
b. More likely to occur if stoma site is through the semilunar line rather than the rectus sheath
c. Usually occurs lateral to ostomy
4. Petit's hernia—Sac exits through the inferior lumbar triangle
5. Obturator hernia—Sac exits through the obturator foramen
6. Perineal hernia—Defect occurs in the muscular floor of the pelvis anteroposterior to superficial transverse perineal muscle, or complete rectal prolapse

7. Sciatic hernia—Rarest of all hernias; sac exits through the greater or lesser sacrosciatic foramen

V. ETIOLOGY

A. INDIRECT INGUINAL HERNIA
Caused by a congenital patency of the processus vaginalis, indirect inguinal hernia refers to herniation through internal ring facilitated by a weak inguinal floor.

B. DIRECT INGUINAL HERNIA
Direct inguinal hernia is an acquired weakness in the floor of Hesselbach's triangle.

C. CONTRIBUTING FACTORS
Contributing factors include obesity, chronic cough, chronic obstructive pulmonary disease, pregnancy, constipation, straining on urination, ascites, and previous hernia repair.

VI. DIAGNOSIS

A. HISTORY
1. History of a palpable, soft mass that increases with straining
2. May reduce spontaneously or manually
3. May be pain with straining

B. EXAMINATION
Exam reveals a palpable mass that increases in size while the patient strains. Examine patients when they are upright and supine.
1. Femoral hernia may reflect superiorly over the inguinal ligament, presenting in the inguinal region.
2. Obesity may make identification of small hernias difficult.
3. Obturator, lumbar, sciatic, and even femoral hernias may be easily missed by physical exam.
4. Abdominal radiographs or CT scan may demonstrate hernias not detectable by physical exam.

C. SMALL BOWEL OBSTRUCTION
Intestinal obstruction may be the first manifestation of a hernia.

VII. REPAIR OF HERNIAS

A. INGUINAL HERNIAS
For an inguinal hernia, the defect in the transversalis fascia needs to be repaired.

1. Cord lipoma—Preperitoneal fat found on the cord that has been pushed in by the hernia sac that should be resected if possible.
2. High ligation of sac—In children, if the only defect is a patent processus vaginalis, no further repair is needed.
3. Bassini—Transversalis fascia and transversus abdominis arch (conjoined tendon) are approximated to the shelving edge of inguinal ligament. Can be done in two layers, as follows.
   a. Transversalis repair
   b. Transversus abdominis arch to inguinal ligament
4. McVay (Cooper's ligament repair)—Transversus abdominis arch approximated to Cooper's ligament; must use relaxing incision in rectus sheath or mesh.
5. Halsted I—Bassini-type repair, except the imbricated external oblique reinforces the repair beneath the spermatic cord that lies in the subcutaneous tissue. Rarely used.
6. Ferguson—Bassini-type repair; however, spermatic cord lies beneath reconstructed inguinal floor.
7. Preperitoneal—Expose hernial defect from beneath abdominal wall fascia in the preperitoneal space. Useful approach for repair of recurrent hernia.
8. Shouldice—Two-layer running overlapping repair of transversalis fascia, reinforced by a two-layer running overlapping approximation of transversus abdominis arch to inguinal ligament.
9. Lichtenstein repair—Marlex (polypropylene) mesh, tension-free repair. Lowest recurrence rate, but infection risk of foreign body.
10. Laparoscopic repair—Preperitoneal or transperitoneal repair using synthetic material.

B. FEMORAL HERNIAS

Femoral hernias require a Cooper's ligament repair (McVay), Shouldice repair, or preperitoneal repair. Many large direct hernias are also repaired in this manner.

C. VENTRAL HERNIAS

Ventral hernias require wide mobilization, primary repair of fascial defect if possible; often require synthetic material, e.g., polypropylene or polytetrafluoroethylene (PTFE).

VIII. POSTOPERATIVE COMPLICATIONS

A. SCROTAL HEMATOMA

A scrotal hematoma may result from blunt dissection and inadequate hemostasis.

47

ABDOMINAL WALL HERNIAS

B. HEMORRHAGE
Deep bleeding enters the retroperitoneal space and may not be apparent initially. Suspect this with hypotension, orthostasis, or tachycardia.

C. DIFFICULTY VOIDING
Difficulty in voiding is more common in elderly males.

D. PAIN
Painful scrotal swelling results from compromised venous return of testes.

E. NEUROMA/NEURITIS
Neuroma or neuritis results from an entrapment or severance of nerves at the repair site that usually resolves spontaneously.

IX. RECURRENCE

A. RATE
1. 2-3% with indirect inguinal hernias; some "recurrences" are direct hernias that were missed at the initial operation.
2. Lowest for Shouldice or Lichtenstein procedure
3. Higher with direct hernias and when the underlying process (chronic cough, constipation, urinary obstruction) causing increased intra-abdominal pressure has not been corrected

B. TECHNICAL ERRORS
1. Excessive tension on suture line
2. Internal ring too loose
3. Indirect hernia sac not identified at the time of operation
4. Inadequate tissue strength despite adequate reconstruction (requires Marlex or other reinforcement)
5. Failure to identify concomitant femoral hernia at time of repair of inguinal hernia
6. Failure to repair "prehernia" laxity in floor

X. MISCELLANEOUS

A. GENERAL REMARKS
1. Marlex mesh placed over the fascial defect may be used if the defect cannot be closed owing to inadequate tissue or excessive tension. Often used to reinforce repairs.
2. Repair of bilateral inguinal hernias is recommended in children.
3. Consider orchiectomy in elderly males with multiple recurrences.

B. REDUCTION OF INCARCERATED HERNIA
1. Trendelenburg position, sedation, and gentle continuous compression may allow reduction of a recently incarcerated hernia.

2. Significant tenderness, induration, erythema, or leukocytosis suggests possible strangulation and necessitates immediate surgical exploration.
   Note: *No reduction should be attempted!*
3. Use of a truss can result in distortion of anatomy, owing to fibrosis of the inguinal canal, complicating and delaying the required surgery; a truss should be avoided in all but extremely high-risk patients.
4. Reduction en masse—Reduction of hernia sac and contents from the extracavitary position with persistent entrapment of the contents within the sac. Patients should be observed postreduction for signs and symptoms of strangulation.

Endovascular Surgery

Jaime R. Este-McDonald, MD

With the advent of balloon angioplasty, mechanical arthrectomy, stents, and endografts (the use of covered stents for endoluminal bypassing), the multidisciplinary specialty of endovascular surgery has emerged. This specialty currently encompasses the use of angiography, intravascular ultrasound, and/or angioscopy via catheter-based systems through a remote vascular site to remove, remodel, stent, or bypass vascular stenoses, blockages, dissections, aneurysms, and injuries. This field is beyond the scope of this handbook, but there are some concepts that are important in the care of these patients on a vascular service. This chapter outlines angiography and endovascular interventions such as endoluminal angioplasty and stenting/grafting.

Endovascular surgery is invasive and therefore has inherent risks. The indications, risks, and benefits have to be clear, as with any other invasive procedure.

48

I. ANGIOGRAPHY

A. DEFINITION
1. *Angiography* is the evaluation of arteries and veins through imaging that allows characterization of disease by looking at intraluminal anatomy and flow.
2. This usually includes the infusion of a contrast agent that passes intraluminally, allowing blood vessels to stand out against the background of other soft tissues and the use of serial film or digital imaging systems.
3. In general, angiography is indicated in patients for whom an intervention is planned that requires information that cannot be obtained by noninvasive means.
4. The angiographer is usually prepared to proceed with an endovascular intervention, depending on the diagnostic findings during angiography.

B. COMMON INDICATIONS FOR DIAGNOSTIC ANGIOGRAPHY
1. Evaluation of the aorta prior to endovascular repair
2. Evaluation of mesenteric vessels for visceral ischemia or preoperatively for cancer resection (pancreatic cancer)
3. Evaluation of renal arteries for renovascular hypertension or renal donor anatomy
4. Evaluation of extremities for acute or chronic ischemia
5. Evaluation of cerebral vasculature for etiology of neurologic symptoms
6. Evaluation of traumatic arterial injuries
7. Evaluation and treatment of pulmonary embolus

C. RISKS
The risks for angiography depend on the vascular bed to be imaged, the contrast agent being used, and the preprocedural diagnosis. These are related to the following.
1. Access site
a. Bleeding/hematomas at access site
b. Arteriovenous fistulas
c. Pseudoaneurysms
d. Retroperitoneal hematomas
e. Perforation of a vessel by catheters or balloons (increased in arterial tortuosity and calcification)
2. Embolization or occlusion of the vascular bed distal to the access or catheterization site (e.g., stroke for carotid or kidney infarct for renal catheterization)
3. Contrast induced
a. Allergic reactions
  (1) Urticaria
  (2) Anaphylactic reactions
  (3) May be ameliorated by diphenhydramine and steroids administered prior to contrast agent
b. Renal failure
  (1) May be dose related
  (2) Increased risk in prior renal failure/insufficiency, proteinuria, diabetes, advanced age, and dehydration
  (3) Prehydration is recommended
  (4) Mannitol and/or furosemide are used but with no confirmed benefit
  (5) Usually transient and resolves spontaneously in 7 days but can be progressive
c. Cardiac
  (1) Congestive heart failure
    (a) Usually in patients with renal failure
    (b) Increased risk during pulmonary artery injections and in patients with preexisting cardiac dysfunction
  (2) Can affect intracardiac conduction, myocardial function, or coronary artery tone induced by the hyperosmolality of the contrast agents (decreased by the use of low-osmolality agents)
d. Nausea and vomiting
e. Burning in the distribution of the vascular bed being infused with contrast agent

D. PREOPERATIVE EVALUATION
1. Complete history
a. Reactions to seafood, iodine, anesthetics, contrast agents, or sedatives/narcotics
  (1) Contrast is iodinated.
  (2) Seafood usually contains iodine.

(3) Lidocaine or similar drugs are used for local anesthesia.

(4) Sedation with narcotics or other sedatives is common.

b. Documented evidence or review of systems that suggests renal, cardiac, pulmonary, diabetic, or bleeding diseases

c. Family history of any of the above

d. Medications

(1) Diuretics

(a) Suggest chronic dehydration

(b) May need preoperative hydration

(2) Metformin

(a) Can increase renal failure

(b) Should be avoided for 24 hours before and 48 hours after operation

2. Complete physical

a. Preoperative vascular and neurologic exam is *extremely* important.

(1) Any neurologic deficits need to be documented.

(2) Pulse/Doppler status needs to be documented for all extremities.

(3) Preoperative blood pressure measurements in both arms should be recorded.

3. Laboratory data

a. CBC

b. Renal chemistries (Na, K, Cl, CO_2, creatine, blood urea nitrogen [BUN], and glucose)

4. All patients are potential candidates for an intervention such as thrombolytics and should have the following.

a. 18-gauge IV catheter—At least one, preferably two

b. No arterial punctures just prior to procedure

c. No attempted central venous access just prior to procedure unless there is no other access and is approved by the surgeon

d. No IM injections

e. Type and screen

f. Foley catheter

II. ENDOVASCULAR INTERVENTIONS

Endovascular interventions include angioplasty, stenting, endoluminal grafting, thrombectomy, and catheter-directed thrombolysis. The details of these procedures are beyond the scope of this handbook, but the risks, benefits, and preoperative evaluations are important to understand while caring for these patients.

A. PREOPERATIVE CONSIDERATIONS

1. Preoperative evaluation and preparation are the same as for diagnostic angiography.

a. All patients undergoing angiography should also consent to possible percutaneous transluminal angioplasty (PTA) and stenting to avoid

48

ENDOVASCULAR SURGERY

having to come back for another procedure that could have been completed at the time of the initial angiogram.

b. Special historical facts are important to risk analysis, especially in regard to thrombolytic therapy. These are not all absolute contraindications but may increase patient risks and include the following.

    (1) Recent fall and/or trauma
    (2) Recent surgery or recent obstetric delivery
    (3) History of intracranial pathology—Recent stroke, subdural hematoma, or aneurysm
    (4) History of metastatic cancer
    (5) Active bleeding from any source
    (6) Recent CPR
    (7) Hemorrhagic retinopathy
    (8) Pregnancy
    (9) Peptic ulcer disease
    (10) Uncontrolled hypertension
    (11) Left-sided heart thrombus
    (12) Bacterial endocarditis
    (13) Atrial fibrillation with mitral valve disease

2. Patients undergoing continuous thrombolytic infusions should have the following.

a. Serial CBC, prothrombin and partial thromboplastin times, and fibrinogen levels checked no less frequently than q 8 h, usually q 6 h

b. Serial evaluations for local or remote site bleeding such as hematuria, GI, strokes, pericatheter bleeding, or retroperitoneal hematomas

    (1) Medical adjuncts to thrombolytic therapy that increase the risk of bleeding complications
        (a) Heparin
        (b) Clopidogrel
        (c) Glycoprotein IIb/IIIa antagonist—Eptifibatide (Integrilin), abciximab
    (2) Bleeding risk can last for up to 36 hours with current agents
    (3) Overall bleeding risk

c. Serial evaluations for clot embolization into distal circulation

3. Postprocedural care includes assessment of the following.

a. End-organ ischemia after stenting or angioplasty secondary to dissection, thrombosis, or embolus

b. Renal function, especially in high-risk patients

c. Bleeding

B. GENERAL RISKS AND BENEFITS OF INTERVENTION OR DIAGNOSTICS IN SPECIFIC VASCULAR BEDS

1. Cerebral

a. Angiogram carries a 1-2% risk of stroke.

b. Intervention

  (1) 4-7% stroke risk for atherosclerosis; may be less for other indications such as vasculitis or trauma
  (2) Technical success rate—>95%
  (3) Long-term results not available
  (4) Reserved for study protocols or for patients who are high surgical risks

2. Renal
a. Overall complication rate—17%, including puncture site (4.5%)
b. Complications related to catheterization of renal artery
  (1) Direct injury, spasm, occlusion, or infarction—≈10%
  (2) Decrease in renal function—≈3%
  (3) New dialysis requirement—<0.5%
  (4) Requiring surgery—≈2%
  (5) 30-day mortality—≈1.3%
c. PTA alone
  (1) Restenosis rate—≈18% at 1-2 years
d. PTA and stent
  (1) Renal function benefit—≈66%
  (2) Hypertension benefit—≈68%
  (3) Restenosis rate—≈18% at 1-2 years
  (4) Major complications (requiring additional therapy or change in treatment plan)—≈7%

3. Lower extremity interventions
a. Iliac arteries
  (1) Primary patency—87% at 1 year and 72% at 5 years
  (2) Secondary patency—87% at 5 years
  (3) Major complications—≈10%
b. Femoropopliteal vessels
  (1) Primary patency—60% at 2 years
  (2) Secondary patency—78% at 2 years
  (3) Major complications—≈10%

48

ENDOVASCULAR SURGERY

The Diabetic Foot

Robert M. Cavagnol, MD

There are ≈10 million diabetic patients in the United States (20% type I and 80% type II). Lower extremity disease is the most common reason for hospital admission. Approximately two thirds of all nontraumatic lower extremity amputations are performed on patients with diabetes.

I. ETIOLOGY

A. ATHEROSCLEROSIS
1. Peripheral vascular disease tends to be bilateral and involve the larger vessels.
2. Small-vessel disease in diabetic patients can play a role in causing tissue ischemia secondary to thickening of the intima and basement membrane. Palpable distal pulses are a good indication that ulcer healing may occur.

B. PERIPHERAL NEUROPATHY
1. Occurs in diabetic patients who have had the disease ≥10 years.
2. May be related to deposition of sorbitol metabolites in nerves.
3. Loss of sensation allows minor injuries to go unrecognized.
4. Structural deformities (hammer toes, hallux valgus, Charcot joints) and improper weight bearing exacerbate the lesions.

C. IMPAIRED IMMUNITY
1. Abnormal polymorphonuclear leukocyte function at blood glucose levels >250 mg/dL
2. Decreased leukocyte chemotaxis
3. Impaired phagocytosis and intracellular killing

D. CHARCOT JOINTS
1. Abnormal weight bearing leads to painless osteoarthritis and to joint deformities.
2. Resultant inflammation may mimic infection.
3. Can precipitate mal perforans ulcers

II. PATHOLOGY

A. FOOT OR TOE ULCER
1. Results from injury, ischemia, or foreign body
2. Poorly fitting shoes and improper weight bearing lead to callus formation.
3. Neuropathy prevents the patient from noticing trauma, exacerbating the injury.

49

B. INFECTION
1. Begins with minor foot trauma or trivial break in the skin.
2. Inadequate circulation and impaired host defense permit spread of infection.
3. Continued ambulation causes spread of infection along fascial planes.
4. Infections are polymicrobial, with *Peptococcus* spp, *Proteus* spp, *and Bacteroides fragilis* being the most common. Consider *Pseudomonas* spp in patients from chronic care facilities.

III. TREATMENT

A. NONINFECTED FOOT ULCERS
1. Assess extent and severity.
2. Assess degree of neuropathy and vascular insufficiency.
3. Control hyperglycemia.
4. Judicious débridement of necrotic tissue and calluses
5. Local wound care and wet-to-dry dressings
6. Improve circulation, revascularization if indicated
7. Careful follow-up and podiatric appliances

B. INFECTED DIABETIC FOOT
1. Determine the extent of spread of the infection.
2. Assess distal circulation by pulse exam, Doppler, noninvasive studies.
3. Radiographs—Rule out soft tissue gas or foreign body.
4. Consider bone scan to evaluate for osteomyelitis.
5. Broad-spectrum antibiotics—Ampicillin/sulbactam or piperacillin/tazobactam
6. Operative intervention to drain abscesses and débride nonviable tissue
7. Aggressive wound care and whirlpool therapy
8. May require skin graft or tissue flap for wound closure
9. Absolute non-weight bearing
10. Control hyperglycemia
11. Becaplermin (Regranex) 0.01% gel shown to accelerate healing once infection is eliminated
12. Revascularization may be indicated once infection has cleared.
13. Consider amputation for nonviable limb.

C. PREVENTIVE ASPECTS
1. Most important component of diabetic foot care
2. Proper-fitting footwear—Instruct patient to never ambulate barefoot
3. Nail care, treat mycotic nail infections
4. Keep web spaces clean and dry.
5. Daily examinations of plantar surface, with mirror, for injury or foreign bodies

Acute Limb Ischemia

Robert M. Cavagnol, MD

I. ETIOLOGY

A. ARTERIAL EMBOLISM

1. Cardiac—Most common source of peripheral emboli. Usually causes occlusion of large-diameter vessels.
a. Mural thrombus—Previous myocardial infarction, atrial fibrillation, rheumatic heart disease, mitral stenosis, aneurysm, cardiomyopathy
b. Endocarditis
c. Atrial myxoma
2. Aorta and proximal arteries; more commonly embolize to smaller digital blood vessels
a. Aneurysmal source, in order of decreasing frequency—Aortic, popliteal, femoral
b. Atheroembolism ("blue toe syndrome") from an ulcerating atherosclerotic plaque in a large proximal artery
c. Paradoxical embolus—Venous embolic source that passes through an intracardiac shunt (atrial or ventricular septal defect); rare
3. Location of emboli
a. Axial limbs—70-80% of sites
b. Generally lodges at bifurcations of vessels
   (1) Common femoral—≈34%
   (2) Aortoiliac—≈22%
   (3) Popliteal trifurcation—≈14%
   (4) Upper extremity—≈15%
c. Mortality is higher with more proximal location—Aorta > iliac > femoral > popliteal
4. Distinction between embolization and thrombosis is critical because operative management is vastly different. Loss of pulses in one limb with preservation of palpable pulses in the contralateral limb suggests embolism.

B. ARTERIAL THROMBOSIS

1. Atherosclerosis—Clot on the surface of a plaque, hemorrhage beneath a plaque, stenosis, aneurysm
2. Congenital anomaly
a. Popliteal entrapment
b. Adventitial cystic disease
3. Infection
4. Hematologic disorders—Polycythemia, hypercoagulable state
5. Flow-related disorders—Congestive heart failure, shock, dehydration

C. ARTERIAL TRAUMA

Arterial trauma can be iatrogenic or incidental.

1. Blunt—Posterior knee dislocation and others
2. Penetrating—Direct injury to vessel, indirect through "blast effect" of a missile, long bone fracture
3. Iatrogenic—Arterial monitor, angiography, cardiac catheterization, arterial blood sample

D. DRUG-INDUCED VASOSPASM
Drug-induced vasospasm may result from illicit drug use, inadvertent arterial injection, and extravasation of vaopressors.

E. AORTIC DISSECTION

F. SEVERE VENOUS THROMBOPHLEBITIS (PHLEGMASIA ALBA DOLENS)

G. PROLONGED IMMOBILIZATION

H. IDIOPATHIC

II. INITIAL ASSESSMENT

A. HISTORY
1. Pain—Onset, location, duration
2. History of previous claudication, rest pain, tissue loss
3. Cardiac disease—Valvular heart disease, atrial fibrillation, cardiomyopathy, myocardial infarction
4. Recent trauma
5. History of hypertension, chest or back pain, pulsatile abdominal mass
6. Drugs—Ergotamines, dopamine, or history of IV drug use
7. Low-flow states—Septic shock, dehydration, hemorrhage, congestive heart failure

B. EXAMINATION
1. 6 Ps of acute arterial insufficiency
   *P*ain
   *P*aralysis
   *P*aresthesias
   *P*allor
   *P*ulseless
   *P*oikiothermia
2. Hair loss, trophic skin and nail changes consistent with long-standing arterial insufficiency
3. Complete bilateral pulse examination including auscultation for bruits and portable Doppler exam when unable to appreciate pulses by palpation
4. Assessment of limb viability
   a. Muscle turgor—Soft = viable; "doughy" = ischemic; stiff = nonviable

b. Neurologic status—Paralysis and anesthesia generally indicate a nonviable limb.
5. Cardiac examination—Rhythm, murmurs, rub
6. Chest radiograph and kidney, ureter, and bladder study—Look for wide mediastinum and vascular calcifications.
7. ECG—Look for evidence of myocardial infarction, atrial fibrillation

III. SECONDARY ASSESSMENT

A. DURATION
1. "Golden period" of 6 hours before ischemia and myonecrosis may become irreversible
2. Noninvasive studies can be helpful but must not delay definitive therapy

B. INDICATIONS FOR ARTERIOGRAPHY
1. Not necessary if diagnosis is readily apparent
2. Determine site of vascular obstruction, and identify inflow.
3. Suspected thrombosis
4. Suspected aortic dissection
5. Suspected multiple emboli

C. OPERATIVE RISK
1. Most patients have underlying heart disease. The need for an emergent operation, combined with potential cardiac disease, makes the operative risk high.
2. Embolectomy under local anesthesia carries a lower operative risk than amputation or attempted revascularization.

D. PRECAUTIONS
1. Attempts should not be made to restore blood flow to nonviable limbs.
2. High incidence of mortality secondary to reperfusion injury
3. Expedient amputation at the lowest viable level

IV. MANAGEMENT OF ACUTE ARTERIAL INSUFFICIENCY

A. IMMEDIATE
1. In all cases, immediate heparinization to prevent further propagation of thrombus
2. Bolus with heparin 80 units/kg, then 18 units/kg/h and adjust to maintain partial thromboplastin time (PTT) at 1.5 to 2 times normal.

B. ARTERIAL EMBOLIZATION
1. After heparinization, emergent surgical embolectomy is the treatment of choice.
a. Local anesthesia

50

ACUTE LIMB ISCHEMIA

b. Isolation of artery (usually common femoral) with proximal and distal control

c. A Fogarty balloon-tipped catheter is introduced through an arteriotomy and passed beyond the area of clot. The balloon is inflated and the catheter withdrawn, bringing the clot out in front of it. It may be necessary to "milk" the lower leg to remove small vessel clots—Separate popliteal arteriotomy may be useful in some cases.

d. Examine clot—An irregular leading edge suggests retained fragments may still exist.

2. Need completion angiography after removal of embolus

a. Back bleeding and clinical examination are poor indicators of success.

b. 20% of patients have a good functional result after embolectomy despite absent distal pulses.

C. ARTERIAL THROMBOSIS

1. Generally suspected from history and exam—Claudication, trophic skin changes, lack of palpable pulses on opposite side

2. Previous collateralization secondary to chronic occlusive disease may prevent development of myonecrosis.

3. Arteriography is key for identifying optimal surgical approach.

4. Patients usually have long-standing arterial insufficiency and require a bypass procedure.

D. ATHEROEMBOLISM (BLUE TOE SYNDROME)

Atheroembolism is caused by an occlusion of small digital vessels with palpable pulses in the major peripheral arteries.

1. Heparinization acutely—Long-term anticoagulation is of no value

2. Elective angiography to search for treatable embolic causes

3. Thromboendarterectomy or complete arterial replacement with prosthetic graft if the source is identified

E. ARTERIAL TRAUMA

1. Generally results from intimal flap with resultant thrombosis

2. Penetrating injuries—Most common, e.g., missile, blast, fracture, severe ligament tears and dislocation at the knee

3. Arteriography mandatory—Embolectomy and repair or bypass of damaged vessel

F. VENOUS THROMBOSIS (see Chap. 12)

1. Major venous thrombosis involving the deep venous system of the thigh and pelvis produces a characteristic clinical picture of pain, extensive edema, and blanching (termed *phlegmasia alba dolens*).

2. As impedance of venous return from the extremity progresses, there is danger of limb loss from cessation of arterial flow leading to congestion, cyanosis, and distended veins (termed *phlegmasia cerulea dolens*).

3. Risk of venous gangrene if pulses are absent mandates heparinization and venous embolectomy with protective distal arteriovenous fistula.

G. DRUG-INDUCED VASOSPASM
Treat drug-induced vasospasm by discontinuing the drug; occasionally, the use of IV nitroprusside drip (vasodilation), phentolamine (α blockade), or topical transdermal nitroglycerin ointment (Nitropaste) is of value.

H. AORTIC DISSECTION
1. Identify by history (hypertension, back/chest pain) and exam (absent pulses throughout).
2. Aortography (including thoracic arch) if suspected

I. THROMBOLYTIC THERAPY
1. Lysis of clot by continuous arterial infusion of streptokinase or tissue plasminogen activator
2. Should be considered when the morbidity and mortality of the surgical alternative are higher than the anticipated risks of thrombolytic therapy (i.e., acute myocardial infarction)
3. May be of use with occlusion of tibial and popliteal vessels, where surgical results are less successful
4. Patients with blue toe syndrome or "trash foot" may also be candidates.
5. Use in patients with thrombosis of previous bypass grafts may be particularly effective.
6. May only be used when limb is clearly viable because it may take 24-36 hours for circulation to be restored

J. POSTOPERATIVE MANAGEMENT
1. Continue heparin after surgery; begin warfarin when PTT stable on heparin, continue until patient no longer at risk for further emboli; discontinue heparin when patient is adequately anticoagulated on warfarin
2. Hourly neurologic and vascular exams
3. Monitor electrolytes, urinary output, and others.
4. Watch for reperfusion injury.
a. Ischemic muscle converts to anaerobic metabolism, with paralysis of the cellular Na^+,K^+ pump. The pH falls while concentrations of K^+, lactic acid, muscle enzymes, myoglobin, and oxygen free radicals all rise dramatically. Once the threatened muscle is reperfused, these toxic metabolites circulate throughout the body and can cause renal failure as well as multiorgan system failure.
b. Myoglobin precipitates in the renal tubules (acidic environment), leading to necrosis with a worsening spiral of oliguria, hyperkalemia, and metabolic acidosis.
c. Treatment—When myoglobin is present

50

ACUTE LIMB ISCHEMIA

(1) Check serum creatine phosphokinase, electrolytes, and urine myoglobin.
(2) Correct hyperkalemia.
(3) Alkalinize urine with IV NaHCO$_3$ and provide adequate volume resuscitation.
(4) Give osmotic diuretic—Mannitol, 1 g/kg IV
(5) Fasciotomy to decompress compromised muscle
(6) Hemodialysis if necessary
d. Mortality with this syndrome can be quite high.
5. Identify and treat the underlying etiology—Atrial fibrillation, mitral stenosis, myocardial infarction

K. COMPARTMENT SYNDROME
1. Caused by severe ischemia for an extended period
2. Ischemia causes cell membrane damage and leakage of fluid into the interstitium.
3. Tissue swelling within a closed fascial compartment causes muscle necrosis and nerve ischemia.
4. If suspected, compartment pressures should be measured immediately. If >40 mm Hg, perform fasciotomy.
5. Fasciotomies allow muscles to expand and relieve high pressure.

V. PROGNOSIS

A. GENERAL
1. Mortality rate for arterial occlusion is 10-20%.
2. 5-15% of patients with arterial embolism require amputation.

B. COMPLICATONS
1. Amputation is the procedure of choice in patients with irreversible ischemia or those unable to tolerate extensive reconstruction.
2. The major factor in mortality is underlying cardiac disease.

Abdominal Aortic Aneurysm

Curtis J. Wray, MD

I. EPIDEMIOLOGY

A. GENERAL
1. Abdominal aortic aneurysm (AAA) is the most common type of aneurysm for which people present for treatment.
2. Found in up to 14% of men 65-74 years of age and 4% of women 65-74 years of age
3. Males predominate with 4:1 ratio.
4. Familial tendency (sex-linked and autosomal inheritance)—Relative risk for first-degree relatives of affected individuals is 11.6 times higher than non-first-degree relatives of similar age and sex.

B. RISK FACTORS
1. Current study by Singh and associates[1] noted that duration of cigarette smoking, hypertension, use of antihypertensive medication, total cholesterol, and high plasma fibrinogen were risk factors for AAA.
2. Inheritable connective tissue disorders, such as Marfan and type IV Ehlers-Danlos syndromes, can lead to aneurysm formation.

II. ANATOMY

A. ABDOMINAL
AAA refers to the abdominal aorta from the diaphragmatic hiatus at T12 to the bifurcation at L4.

B. OTHER
1. Celiac axis at the upper portion of L1, superior mesenteric artery (SMA) at the lower one third of L1, inferior mesenteric artery (IMA) at L3, and renal arteries at the upper portion of L2
2. Normal diameter of aorta—$\approx$2 cm

III. PATHOLOGY

A. LOCATION
1. Infrarenal, below origin of renal arteries in 95% of cases
2. May extend to involve common iliac arteries, rarely beyond

B. SIZE
The size of AAAs is 3-15 cm, usually fusiform aortic dilation. Mycotic aneurysms are typically saccular.

C. OTHER MANIFESTATIONS
Other manifestations of diffuse atherosclerosis associated with AAA include the following.

1. Coronary artery disease—30%
2. Hypertension—40%
3. Associated occlusive arterial disease
a. Carotid arteries—7%
b. Renal arteries—2%
c. Iliac arteries—16%
4. Associated with other clinically significant aneurysms
a. Thoracic aorta—4%
b. Femoral artery—3%
c. Popliteal artery—2%

IV. NATURAL HISTORY

A. STATISTICS
1. 5-year rate of rupture of untreated AAA
a. ≥7 cm—75%
b. 6 cm—35%
c. 5-6 cm—25%
2. 5-year survival rate of untreated AAA
a. <6 cm—48%
b. >6 cm—6%
3. Autopsy studies showed that 9.5% of aneurysms <4 cm had ruptured, 25% of aneurysms 4-7 cm had ruptured, and 65% of aneurysms >7 cm had ruptured.

B. OTHER DESCRIPTORS
1. Increased size = increased risk of rupture
2. Grow an average of 0.4 cm/yr

V. CLINICAL PRESENTATION

A. COMMON CHARACTERISTICS
Most aneurysms are asymptomatic, and 75% are found on routine abdominal examination or ultrasound/CT scan done for other reasons.

B. ACTIVE LEAKAGE
1. Actively leaking AAA may present with abdominal, back, or flank pain due to tension on the peritoneum from the aneurysm or blood. Complaints may be mild or severe and require a high index of suspicion. A leaking AAA may rapidly result in exsanguination due to free intraperitoneal rupture.
2. With leakage or free rupture, patients may present in shock.

VI. PHYSICAL EXAMINATION

A. PALPATION
1. Presence of pulsatile mass on deep palpation—5-cm aneurysm palpable in most patients
2. Tortuous aorta may mimic AAA, presenting as a pulsating, expansile abdominal mass different from other abdominal masses that merely transmit aortic pulsations (e.g., pseudocyst, pancreatic carcinoma).
3. In thin individuals, aortic pulsations may be unusually prominent; however, careful bimanual palpation should confirm normal diameter.

B. OTHER PULSES
It is important to evaluate other peripheral arteries for associated occlusive disease (pulses and bruits) or further aneurysmal disease.

VII. DIAGNOSTIC STUDIES

A. ABDOMINAL PLAIN FILMS
1. Often diagnostic
2. Calcific rim ("egg shell") is often visible projecting anterior to the spine on cross-table lateral view.

B. ULTRASOUND (B-MODE)
1. Simplest, least expensive method of detecting and following aortic aneurysms
2. Can also evaluate blood flow in renal and visceral arteries

C. CT SCAN
1. Can provide accurate characterization of entire aorta
2. Can also provide information about wall thickness, renal and iliac artery anatomy
3. New three-dimensional CT scan can be used for more detailed measurements.

D. AORTOGRAPHY
1. Poor study for diagnosis or assessment of size, as mural thrombus within AAA can obscure actual aneurysm size. Aortography provides important information regarding associated vascular lesions.
2. Indications for aortography
a. Hypertension—To rule out renal vascular causes
b. Unexplained impairment of renal function
c. Aneurysm near renal arteries
d. Symptoms compatible with mesenteric ischemia
e. Evidence of peripheral artery occlusive disease
f. Evidence of "horseshoe" kidney

51

ABDOMINAL AORTIC ANEURYSM

VIII. CARDIAC WORK-UP OF ELECTIVE AAA REPAIR

Owing to the high incidence of concomitant coronary artery disease and postoperative cardiac complications, the cardiac work-up is an essential part of the preoperative evaluation. The diagram shown in Figure 51-1 may be useful:

IX. OPERATIVE INDICATIONS

A. PRINCIPLES

Patients with aneurysms >4-5 cm are candidates for elective operation unless concomitant medical problems increase the operative risk or a second pathologic process markedly reduces the patient's life expectancy.

1. Size increase of >0.5 cm in 6 months
2. When the aneurysm becomes symptomatic, operation becomes imperative regardless of aneurysm size.

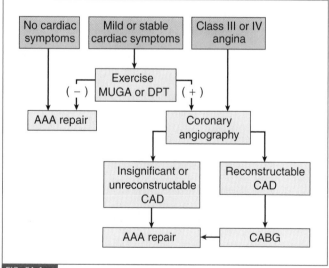

FIG. 51-1

Cardiac work-up in the preoperative phase. AAA = abdominal aortic aneurysm; MUGA = multigated equilibrium radionuclide angiography; DPT = dipyridamole thallium 201 [imaging]; CAD = coronary artery disease; CABG = coronary artery bypass graft.

X. MANAGEMENT OF RUPTURED AAA

A. DIAGNOSIS
1. Abdominal pain—May be associated with back or flank pain and shock of varying degree (may be very mild)
2. Pulsatile mass—May be palpable in 50%; may be absent owing to hypotension
3. Rupture—Contained vs. free. Free rupture is usually associated with hemodynamic instability.
4. Clinical exam is most important—Hemodynamically unstable patients go directly to the OR. Stable patients with questionable presence of AAA may undergo emergent abdominal CT scan or ultrasound.
5. May simulate other intra-abdominal or medical conditions, e.g., renal colic, pancreatitis, myocardial infarction, muscular backache—High index of suspicion is needed.

B. THERAPY
1. Rapid and maintained replacement of blood loss with crystalloid and blood transfusion to correct hypotension
2. Midline approach used with rapid isolation of the aorta just below diaphragm for proximal control (approach via the gastrohepatic omentum); clamping for ≈30 minutes is possible without significant visceral ischemia
3. Infrarenal clamp placed after aneurysm is incised and surrounding hematoma evacuated, providing better visualization and avoiding damage to renal vasculature
4. Low-porosity woven or polytetrafluoroethylene graft should be used with ruptured AAA, because preclotting is not possible.
5. Renal insufficiency most common complication postoperatively. May be prevented in part by mannitol (12.5 g) or furosemide (40 mg) infusion prior to anesthesia induction.
6. Mortality rate—≈50%

XI. ELECTIVE MANAGEMENT OF AAA

A. PREOPERATIVE PREPARATION
1. Optimize cardiovascular function and fluid volume.
2. Mechanical ± antibiotic bowel preparation. Paregoric given PO preoperatively reduces size of small bowel.
3. Establish water diuresis with adequate IV hydration before anesthesia and maintain during surgery. A thermodilution pulmonary artery (Swan-Ganz) catheter may be helpful during preoperative hydration and perioperative maintenance of adequate filling pressures and cardiac output. Mannitol

51

ABDOMINAL AORTIC ANEURYSM

(50 g) IV prior to cross-clamping aorta helps maintain adequate glomerular filtration rate.
4. Perioperative parenteral antibiotics

B. VIA MIDLINE OR TRANSVERSE INCISION
1. Aorta is mobilized
2. Infrarenal clamp is placed for proximal control

C. ILIAC ARTERIES
The iliac arteries are clamped for distal control.

D. IMA
1. Ligated from within the aneurysm to avoid injury to collateral vessels to the left colon
2. In patients with decreased visceral blood supply and patent IMA, it may be necessary to reimplant artery into graft

E. ANTERIOR PORTION OF ANEURYSM WALL
The anterior aneurysm wall is opened and the thrombus is removed.

F. POSTERIOR WALL
1. Left in place
2. Lumbar vessels are suture ligated.

G. PROSTHETIC GRAFT
1. Sewn in place
2. Tube graft if iliac arteries are normal
3. Bifurcation graft if iliac arteries are aneurysmal

H. NONRESECTIVE SURGICAL THERAPY
1. In a high-risk patient, axillary-bifemoral graft with induced aortic aneurysm thrombosis via catheter deposition of thrombogenic material or coil is a *rarely* used option
2. High complication rate, including thrombus extension into renal or mesenteric arteries and rupture of aorta, has caused most surgeons to abandon this form of therapy

XII. COMPLICATIONS

A. ATHEROEMBOLISM ("TRASH FOOT")
1. Results from occlusion of small distal lower extremity arteries from embolization of aneurysmal sac fragments, or from thrombosis due to extended aortic clamp time
2. Large emboli above the ankle can be removed with an embolectomy catheter.

B. MYOCARDIAL ISCHEMIA, ARRHYTHMIA, AND INFARCTION
1. Arrhythmias—Common
2. Fatal myocardial infarction in 3% of elective patients, 10% of symptomatic patients, and 16% of ruptured-AAA patients
3. Coronary artery disease is responsible for 50-60% of all deaths secondary to AAA repair.

C. RENAL INSUFFICIENCY
1. Causes
a. Hypovolemia
    (1) Preoperative dehydration
    (2) Blood loss from leaking or ruptured aneurysms
    (3) Intraoperatively when aortic cross-clamp is removed; can be prevented by adequate hydration
    (4) Inadequate operative fluid replacements
b. Atheromatous debris or thrombus dislodged during the procedure and embolizing to the kidney (renal atheroembolism)
c. Renal artery occlusion from aortic cross-clamping must be considered.
2. Oliguric renal failure—<3%, but >20% of patients with ruptured aneurysms. Mortality rate of patients with renal failure and ruptured AAA is ≈50%.

D. STROKE
Stroke associated with AAA can be embolic or secondary to hypotension.

E. COLON ISCHEMIA
1. Occurs in 2-6% of patients undergoing repair of AAA
2. Normally there are two prominent collaterals between the SMA and the IMA, (1) the marginal artery of Drummond and (2) the meandering mesenteric artery (not normally present in the absence of SMA or IMA stenosis). These may be stenosed or occluded by the general atherosclerotic process.
3. Prevent ischemia and ensure adequate perfusion by several intraoperative maneuvers.
a. Palpate the root of the SMA—pulsatile or not?
b. Examine the IMA orifice from within the opened aneurysm sac—Open (retrograde bleeding) or not? A large, wide-open IMA suggests the need to reimplant the artery.
c. Doppler ultrasound—Presence of audible Doppler flow over the base of the large bowel mesentery and serosal surface appears to imply a higher risk of ischemic colitis
d. Fluorescein—Ultraviolet luminescence should show bowel viability.
4. Suspect ischemia if patient has bowel movement during the first 24-72 hours after surgery. Stool is usually positive for blood (grossly or by Heme test).

a. Mucosal ischemia most common and usually manifested by mucosal sloughing; resolves spontaneously in most cases
b. Requires immediate flexible sigmoidoscopy for diagnosis
c. Transmural involvement requires re-exploration and colonic resection with colostomy.
d. Broad-spectrum antibiotic therapy is controversial.

F. SPINAL CORD ISCHEMIA
Spinal cord ischemia is rare after AAA repair (2%); it is more common with thoracic aneurysm repair.
1. **Syndrome**—Paraplegia with loss of light touch and pain sensation and loss of sphincter control. Proprioception and temperature sensation are spared.
2. **Pathology**
a. Anterior spinal artery is formed in the neck and supplies the spinal cord.
b. Several "anterior radicular arteries" feed into the anterior spinal artery.
c. The lowest (and largest) anterior radicular artery usually arises at the T8-L1 level, but occasionally the origin is lower, leading to obliteration with abdominal aortic surgery (0.5% of cases).

G. CHYLOUS ASCITES
Chylous ascites can occur as a result of inadequate ligation of lymphatics during proximal aortic dissection.

H. LATE COMPLICATIONS
1. **Aortoenteric fistula**
a. De novo or more commonly from proximal suture line of aortic graft
b. Distal portion of duodenum most common location—82% duodenum, 8% small bowel, 6% large bowel, 5% stomach
c. Presentation—GI bleeding with associated abdominal and back pain; may have "herald bleed" of more minor degree followed by exsanguinating hemorrhage
d. Diagnosis—Endoscopy to rule out other source; if no definitive site is found, graft–enteric fistula must be assumed
e. Treatment—Remove graft, oversew aorta, repair enteric defect; drain retroperitoneum (with or without antibiotic irrigation); extra-anatomic bypass (axillary-bifemoral)
2. **Late infection of prosthetic graft material requires extra-anatomic bypass and removal of infected graft material and oversewing the aortic stump.**
3. **Sexual dysfunction**
a. Retrograde ejaculation and/or inability to maintain erection in 30-40% of men due to aortoiliac surgery
b. Caused by injury to sympathetic plexus around the aorta and failure to maintain hypogastric perfusion

XIII. PROGNOSIS

A. SURGICAL REPAIR
Surgical repair has been shown to double the survival time of patients with AAA.
1. Operative mortality for elective repair is 1-2%.
2. Mortality for emergent repair of ruptured AAA ranges from 20-80% (mean, 50%), depending on the condition of the patient at presentation.

XIV. ENDOVASCULAR REPAIR OF AAA

A. GENERAL
1. ≈40,000 elective repairs of AAA are performed each year.
2. First repair of an AAA using a transfemoral insertion of a prosthetic graft reported by Parodi and associates[2] in 1991
3. First U.S. Food and Drug Administration–approved device (Endovascular Technologies) implanted in 1993

B. OUTCOME
1. Long-term outcome of this method remains uncertain. Recent studies have compared endovascular repair with that of traditional open repair.
2. Study by Dattilo and colleagues[3] evaluated 7-year experience with 362 AAA endografts. Death occurred in 1.6%, all elderly and high-risk—1.4% required early conversion (<2 days); 2.2% underwent late conversion for a variety of problems. Rupture occurred in 0.8%, and AAA sac growth >5 mm was observed in 5.6%. Overall, 10.7% needed catheter-based or limited surgical reintervention.
3. Study by Aquino and coworkers[4] investigated quality of life following endovascular repair using the standard SF-36 Health Survey. Patients receiving endoluminal repair demonstrated better physical and functional scores as early as 1 week after discharge. These patients also returned to baseline status significantly earlier than patients receiving traditional open repair.

51

ABDOMINAL AORTIC ANEURYSM

REFERENCES

1. Singh K, Bonaa KH, Jacobsen BK, et al: Prevalence of and risk factors for abdominal aortic aneurysms in a population-based study: The Tromso study. Am J Epidemiol 154:236-244, 2001.
2. Parodi JC, Palmaz JC, Barone HD: Transfemoral intraluminal graft implantation for abdominal aortic aneurysms. Ann Vasc Surg 5:491-499, 1991.
3. Dattilo JB, Brewster DC, Fan CM, et al: Clinical features of endovascular abdominal aortic aneurysm repair: Incidence, causes, and management. J Vasc Surg 35:1137-1144, 2002.
4. Aquino RV, Jones MA, Zullo TG, et al: Quality of life assessment in patients undergoing endovascular or conventional AAA repair. J Endovasc Ther 8:521-528, 2001.

Mesenteric Ischemia

Donn H. Spight, MD

Mesenteric ischemia is an uncommon entity that carries a high mortality rate, usually owing to delay in diagnosis. It is defined by a state of perfusion insufficient to meet the metabolic needs of the end organs supplied by the mesenteric circulation. These organs can include the colon, stomach, liver, gallbladder, and spleen. Successful treatment requires a high index of suspicion and recognition of both the chronic and acute forms.

I. ANATOMY AND PHYSIOLOGY

A. GI TRACT
Circulation deficits in the GI tract are uncommon owing to abundant collateral circulation between the following.
1. Celiac axis
2. Superior mesenteric artery (SMA)
3. Inferior mesenteric artery (IMA)

B. COLLATERAL VESSELS
1. Pancreaticoduodenal arcade (celiac and SMA)
2. Branch of left colic artery (SMA and IMA)
3. Marginal artery of Drummond—often small, not continuous, especially at splenic flexure (SMA and IMA)
4. Arc of Riolan (SMA and IMA)

C. PHYSIOLOGY
1. Occlusive—Macrovascular acute or chronic interruption of segmental blood flow
2. Nonocclusive—Microvascular vasospasm in response to systemic physiologic stress
a. Sympathetic stimulation
b. Decreased blood flow
c. Drugs—Digitalis and others

II. ACUTE MESENTERIC ISCHEMIA

A. RISK FACTORS
Risk factors include cardiac arrhythmia, advanced age, low cardiac output states, valvular heart disease, myocardial infarction, and malignancy.

B. CLINICAL PRESENTATION
The hallmark of mesenteric ischemia is severe, acute midabdominal pain *out of proportion* to physical findings.
1. Early—Prominent symptoms of GI emptying (i.e., nausea, vomiting, diarrhea); diffuse abdominal tenderness without peritoneal signs; active bowel sounds may be present

2. Late—Symptoms of intestinal infarction. Hypotension and acidosis eventually lead to shock. Fever, bloody diarrhea, and peritonitis develop late and are ominous findings. There is an 80-85% mortality rate at this point despite intervention.
3. Early diagnosis improves survival.

C. ETIOLOGY

1. Embolization of SMA—40%; one third of patients have antecedent embolic episodes (lower extremity embolus, cerebrovascular accident). Most emboli commonly lodge 3-10 cm distal to SMA origin, proximal to middle colic artery.
2. Thrombosis of SMA—40%; thrombus formation on atherosclerotic plaque or stenotic lesion. Often preceded by symptoms of chronic mesenteric ischemia, e.g., postprandial pain, weight loss, bloating, diarrhea.
3. Nonocclusive ischemia—20%; vasoconstriction of mesenteric vasculature due to low cardiac output (low-flow state). Common predisposing conditions include myocardial infarction, congestive heart failure, renal or hepatic disease, medications (e.g., digoxin), trauma, and hypovolemia or hypotension.

D. DIAGNOSIS

1. Mesenteric angiography (with lateral views of aorta) is the *definitive* diagnostic test.
2. Laboratory derangements include the following.
a. Increased hematocrit consistent with hemoconcentration
b. Leukocytosis with left shift
c. Increase in amylase, lactate dehydrogenase, creatine phosphokinase, or alkaline phosphatase
d. Evidence of marked metabolic acidosis with persistent base deficit.

E. MANAGEMENT

1. Simultaneous fluid and electrolyte resuscitation and evaluation should be conducted *expeditiously*.
2. Nasogastric tube, Foley catheter
3. If peritonitis is present or if there is evidence of intestinal infarction, immediate abdominal exploration should be performed.
4. Embolus—Arteriography shows occlusion of SMA, with embolus lodged just beyond inferior pancreaticoduodenal and middle colic arteries (meniscus sign).
a. Systemic heparinization should be initiated.
b. Angiography catheter may be used to infuse papaverine both preoperatively and postoperatively.
c. Following adequate resuscitation, immediate exploration should be performed. Embolectomy is performed via transverse

arteriotomy in the SMA. Arteriotomy may be closed with or without a vein patch.

d. Assess bowel viability by direct inspection and/or fluorescein examination. Administer sodium fluorescein (1 g IV) and inspect the bowel under ultraviolet (Wood's) lamp. Viable bowel has a smooth, uniform fluorescence.

e. Consider second-look operation to reinspect bowel if there is questionable viability.

5. Thrombosis—Arteriogram shows complete occlusion of SMA at origin, with infrequent collateralization.

a. *Immediate* operation is necessary. Diagnosis is often made late, and extensive bowel necrosis is present. At exploration, bowel is often gray and pulseless.

b. Revascularization should be attempted with aortomesenteric bypass graft (prosthetic or saphenous vein).

c. Resect nonviable bowel *after* revascularization. Consider a second-look operation.

6. Nonocclusive—Arteriography shows marked narrowing and "pruning" of distal mesenteric vessels but not of large vessels.

a. Treatment is primarily nonoperative. Patients are often extremely ill and are poor surgical risks.

b. Optimize cardiac output (if possible).

c. Angiographic catheter should be left in place in the SMA and papaverine infused.

d. Repeat angiography is performed after 24 hours.

e. Laparotomy indicated if peritoneal signs present

52

MESENTERIC ISCHEMIA

III. CHRONIC MESENTERIC ISCHEMIA

Chronic mesenteric ischemia is atherosclerotic involvement of two of three main visceral arteries supported by a large number of collaterals.

A. DIAGNOSIS

Symptoms are often applicable to multiple etiologies, e.g., gallbladder disease and occult GI cancer.

1. Chronic epigastric abdominal pain, colicky in nature, occurring 30-60 minutes after meal. May be relieved by defecation.

2. Involuntary weight loss ("food fear")

3. Presence of abdominal bruit

4. Angiography—Used after other disease entities ruled out. Should include lateral view of aorta and take-off vessels.

B. TREATMENT

Surgical revascularization is indicated.

1. Nutritional repletion

2. Bypass grafting

a. Two-vessel aortomesenteric graft (saphenous vein or prosthetic)

b. Combined infrarenal-aortic implant and aortomesenteric graft
3. Transaortic endarterectomy—For multivessel disease

C. PROGNOSIS
There is a relief of pain in 90% of cases.
1. Best long-term results with multivessel revascularization
2. Recurrence—10-30% with multivessel revascularization vs. 50% for single-vessel revascularization

IV. MESENTERIC VENOUS THROMBOSIS

A. CLINICAL PRESENTATION
In contrast with that of acute arterial ischemia, the onset of symptoms with mesenteric venous thrombosis is usually insidious. Life-threatening complications are the result of bowel wall edema, systemic hypovolemia, and hemoconcentration that eventually compromise arterial inflow.
1. Acute abdominal pain, *out of proportion* to physical findings
2. May show the following
a. Signs of hypovolemia
b. Low-grade fever
c. Active bowel sounds
d. Abdominal distention
e. Localized tenderness (if infarction has occurred)
f. Heme-positive stools

B. ETIOLOGY
1. Association with another pathologic process—Malignancy, visceral infection, pancreatitis, portal hypertension, trauma
2. Hypercoagulable states due to coagulation disorders
3. Idiopathic

C. DIAGNOSIS
1. Leukocytosis.
2. Radiographs—May show distended small bowel loops, portal venous gas, or gas in bowel wall. Normal in 25% of cases.
3. Barium enema—Thumbprinting and luminal narrowing. May limit angiographic evaluation.
4. Angiography—Prolonged arterial phase; nonvisualization of the venous phase, reflux of contrast into the aorta
5. CT scanning—Visualization of intraluminal thrombus, enlargement of thrombosed vein, focal or segmental bowel wall thickening
6. Duplex ultrasound scanning of the mesenteric and portal veins has also been used. Often limited by distended bowel gas pattern.

D. TREATMENT
Treatment begins with fluid and electrolyte resuscitation and management, including a nasogastric tube and a Foley catheter.
1. **Early heparinization for suspected thrombosis**
2. **Antibiotics**
3. **Laparotomy for peritonitis or suspected infarction**
a. Wide resection followed by reanastomosis usually recommended
b. Thrombectomy considered for large segments of compromised bowel
c. Consider second-look operation
4. **Postoperative care—Continue anticoagulation, possibly for life.**
5. **Evaluate the etiology of thrombosis, including a work-up for hypercoagulable state.**

52

MESENTERIC ISCHEMIA

Urologic Surgery

James B. Colombo, MD, and Nancy Y. Kim, MD

I. UROLOGIC INFECTIONS

A. CYSTITIS

1. Clinical presentation—Dysuria, urgency, frequency, incontinence, hematuria, low back and suprapubic pain
2. Etiology—Coliform bacteria cause most acute uncomplicated cases. Nosocomial infections are caused by more resistant pathogens; gram-negative organisms predominate (*Escherichia coli, Proteus* spp, *Enterobacter* spp, *Klebsiella* spp, *Pseudomonas* spp). Occasionally *Streptococcus faecalis* and *Staphylococcus* species are cultured.
3. Female cystitis is typically an ascending bacterial infection (fecal-perineal-urethra) associated with sexual activity, pregnancy, and the postpartum period.
4. Male cystitis is usually associated with urologic pathology such as obstruction (benign prostatic hyperplasia, stricture, cancer), urine stasis (neurogenic bladder), foreign body (calculus, indwelling catheter), and inadequate treatment of persistent urinary pathogens (chronic bacterial prostatitis).
5. Laboratory findings—A catheterized urine specimen from the female and a clean-catch midstream-voided specimen from the male are equivalent. Urinalysis shows at least 5-10 white blood cells per high-power field, often with hematuria and bacteriuria. Other nonspecific features include urine nitrate and leukocyte esterase. Urine culture is required for conformation; typically grows >100,000 colony-forming units (CFU)/mL
6. Treatment consists of empiric use of broad-spectrum oral antibiotics with gram-negative organism coverage. Organism-specific antibiotics can begin once culture results are obtained. Uncomplicated cases can be treated with a 3-5 day course.
a. Trimethoprim 160 mg/sulfamethoxazole 800 mg PO b.i.d.
b. Nitrofurantoin 50 mg PO q.i.d.
c. Ciprofloxacin 500 mg PO b.i.d.
7. If symptoms and cultures clear on antibiotics in sexually active females, no further work-up is necessary. Males require further urologic evaluation to rule out urologic pathology.
8. Children with cystitis require a thorough urologic evaluation including a renal ultrasound and a voiding cystourethrogram (VCUG). A VCUG should be obtained 4-6 weeks after an acute infection.
9. Patients with chronic indwelling urinary catheters or those on self-catheterization have urine colonized with bacteria, typically two or more pathogens. If these patients are asymptomatic, treatment is not necessary and is rarely successful in clearing bacteria.

53

Adequate hydration and good bladder emptying are essential in preventing the progression of colonization to infection.

B. ACUTE BACTERIAL PROSTATITIS
1. Clinical presentation—Acute onset of fever; chills; urgency; frequency; low back, perineal, or rectal pain. Rectal examination reveals an exquisitely tender, firm, and indurated prostate. Vigorous rectal exam or massage should be *avoided* because of the risk of causing bacteremia and septicemia. Diagnosis is often based on symptoms and physical examination.
2. Etiology—Primarily caused by aerobic gram-negative organisms similar to the species that cause cystitis
3. Laboratory findings—Leukocytosis with differential left shift. Urinalysis shows pyuria, microscopic hematuria, and bacteriuria.
4. Urethral instrumentation should be avoided. Patients may require placement of suprapubic catheter in acute urinary retention.
5. Complications—Acute bacterial cystitis, acute urinary retention, prostatic abscess, pyelonephritis, epididymo-orchitis, bacteremia, and septic shock
6. Treatment—Empiric therapy should be started immediately with broad-spectrum antibiotics against gram-negative rods and enterococci. In stable patients, oral antibiotics should be used for a total of 4-6 weeks. Trimethoprim/sulfamethoxazole attains adequate prostate tissue levels as well as the quinolones (ciprofloxacin, levofloxacin) do. In the unstable patient showing signs of sepsis, combination therapy with IV aminoglycoside and ampicillin is indicated.

C. ACUTE EPIDIDYMO-ORCHITIS
1. Clinical presentations—Painful, swollen, tender epididymis and testicle. Overlying scrotal skin may be red, swollen, and warm. A tense, reactive hydrocele may be present, which makes testicular palpation difficult. The spermatic cord is often thickened and painful, with radiation to the ipsilateral flank.
2. Etiology—Usually acquired by a retrograde spread from the urethra or bladder. In sexually active males (<35 years) *Chlamydia trachomatis* and *Neisseria gonorrhoeae* are the most common organisms. In children and males >35 years of age, commonly found organisms include *E. coli, Proteus* spp, *Klebsiella* spp, *Enterobacter* spp, and *Pseudomonas* spp. Associated with concomitant urinary tract infection and urinary tract obstruction.
3. Laboratory findings—Leukocytosis with differential left shift. Urinalysis may show pyuria and bacteriuria. Urine culture may grow gram-negative bacilli listed in section I. C. 2. Special cultures (often unsuccessful) are required for isolation of *Chlamydia* and *Neisseria* organisms from urethral discharge.

4. Testicular torsion must be ruled out. Doppler ultrasonography or radionuclide scanning can diagnose this condition.
5. Complications—May cause abscess formation, testicular infarction or infertility
6. Treatment
   a. Bedrest during acute phase
   b. Scrotal elevation—Athletic support, ice pack to scrotum
   c. Avoidance of sexual activity and physical activity
   d. Analgesia, antipyretics, and antibiotics
      (1) Sexually transmitted organisms—Ceftriaxone 1 g IM followed by a 2-3 week course of doxycycline 100 mg PO b.i.d. Both patient and partner should be treated. Use of a condom during sexual activity is encouraged.
      (2) Nonsexually transmitted organisms—Trimethoprim 160 mg/sulfamethoxazole 800 mg PO b.i.d. for 4 weeks is appropriate initial therapy. Specific antibiotics are determined by urine culture and sensitivity results.

D. ACUTE PYELONEPHRITIS

1. Clinical presentation—Fever, chills, severe costovertebral angle pain and tenderness, frequency, urgency, dysuria, nausea, and vomiting
2. Etiology—Acute bacterial infection of the renal parenchyma initiated by ascending bacteria (reflux) and, far less commonly, by hematogenous and lymphatic routes of infection. Associated gram-negative enteric organisms are *E. coli, Klebsiella* sp, *Proteus* sp, *Pseudomonas* sp, *Serratia* sp, *Enterobacter* sp, and *Citrobacter* sp. Occasionally *Staphylococcus aureus* and enterococci are isolated.
3. Laboratory findings—Significant leukocytosis with left shift. Urinalysis is significant for pyuria, bacteriuria, occasional hematuria, and leukocyte or granular casts. Urine culture is typically positive for >100,000 CFU/mL.
4. Imaging techniques—IV urography, CT scan, radionuclide studies, or Doppler ultrasonography
5. Differential diagnosis—Includes pancreatitis, basal pneumonia, appendicitis, cholecystitis, diverticulitis, pelvic inflammatory disease, and renal or perirenal abscess
6. Treatment—Minimally symptomatic patients who are tolerating their diet can be treated expectantly with oral broad-spectrum antibiotics against gram-negative bacilli. In the severely ill patient, prompt treatment is essential to prevent sepsis, renal scarring, and loss of renal function. Initial empiric treatment should consist of IV aminoglycoside and ampicillin. Antibiotics should be guided by urine culture results, and IV therapy is continued for at least 7-10 days or until the patient is afebrile for 24 hours. Conversion to appropriate oral antibiotics can be initiated and is usually continued for at least 2 weeks.

53

UROLOGIC SURGERY

7. If symptoms and fever persist after 72 hours of appropriate antibiotics and fluid therapy, urologic evaluation is required to investigate other pathology such as renal abscess, stones, or obstruction.

II. UROLOGIC EMERGENCIES

A. TRAUMA

1. Hematuria following trauma

a. Degree of hematuria does not correlate with severity of injury.

b. All pediatric trauma, gross hematuria, microhematuria associated with systolic blood pressure <90 mm Hg, rapid deceleration injuries, and penetrating injuries should undergo radiologic evaluation. Up to 20% of patients with significant upper tract injuries have no hematuria.

c. Rapid renal evaluation can be done by bolus injection of IV contrast material (2 mL/kg) followed by a plain kidney, ureter, bladder (KUB) radiographic study.

2. Renal trauma

a. Etiology

    (1) Blunt renal trauma—Usually motor vehicle accidents. Accounts for 80-85% of renal injuries. Patients with injuries to the flank, abdomen or lower chest are suspicious for renal injury.

    (2) Penetrating renal trauma—Usually knife or gunshot wounds; 80% involve other organ systems

b. Classification

    (1) Minor injuries—≈85%

        (a) Renal contusion—Bruising of renal parenchyma

        (b) Cortical laceration—Superficial laceration of parenchyma not involving the collecting system

    (2) Major injuries—≈15%; deep laceration involving corticomedullary laceration with extension into collecting system. Associated with retroperitoneal and perinephric hematomas.

    (3) Vascular—≈1%; involves renal vascular pedicle

    (4) Staging

    Grade I: Contusion, contained subcapsular hematoma

    Grade II: Nonexpanding, confined perirenal hematoma or cortical laceration <1 cm without urinary extravasation

    Grade III: Parenchymal laceration extending <1 cm into cortex without urinary extravasation

    Grade IV: Parenchymal laceration through corticomedullary junction and into collecting system or segmental vessel thrombosis

    Grade V: Pedicle injury; shattered kidney

c. Diagnosis

    (1) CT scan—Delineates parenchymal lacerations, urinary extravasation, retroperitoneal hematomas, nonviable parenchyma, and surrounding organ damage

(2) IV pyelogram (IVP)—Failure to visualize kidney suggests hypotension, pedicle injury, or congenital absence of kidney. Can indicate urinary extravasation. Prompt function without extravasation suggests minor injury such as renal contusion or a cortical laceration.

(3) Angiography—Useful for renal pedicle injury detection as long as patient is hemodynamically stable

d. Treatment

    (1) Prior to any operative attempt at renal exploration, the function of the uninjured kidney must be known.

    (2) Penetrating renal trauma often requires exploration.

    (3) Blunt renal trauma

        (a) 85% of cases can be managed nonsurgically with bedrest, hemodynamic monitoring, and hydration.

        (b) Renal pedicle injuries always require surgical exploration and repair or nephrectomy.

        (c) Intermediate injuries may involve eventual surgical intervention depending on the clinical course and injury severity. Operative indications include persistent retroperitoneal bleeding, urinary extravasation, and evidence of nonviable parenchyma. Penetrating injuries should be explored. In 80% of cases, there is associated organ injury, and renal exploration becomes part of the explorative laparotomy.

e. Complications—Urinomas, hydronephrosis, arteriovenous fistulas, renovascular hypertension, hemorrhage

3. Ureteral trauma

a. Ureters are rarely injured due to blunt trauma; however the blast effect from projectiles can injure the ureter even in the absence of actual transection. Most injuries are iatrogenic from pelvic surgery with transection or ligation of the ureter.

b. Treatment depends on the mechanism of injury and location (lower, middle, or upper ureter). Excretory urograms, retrograde pyelograms, and CT scans define the injury.

    (1) Simple ureteral ligation—Prompt recognition may be treated by release of ligature. Late recognition may require partial ureterectomy and ureteral reimplantation.

    (2) Simple surgical transection—Requires immediate ureteroureterostomy and stent placement

    (3) Gunshot wound—Requires exploration and wide débridement of injured segment because of the potential blast effect. Ureteroureterostomy or transureteroureterostomy may be required.

4. Bladder trauma

a. Etiology—External blunt trauma, pelvic fracture (90%), penetrating injury, iatrogenic (pelvic or gynecologic surgery)

b. Presentation—Bony pelvis generally protects the bladder from external violence. Nevertheless, 10-15% of patients with pelvic fracture have a bladder or urethral injury. Bladder rupture may present as an acute

53

UROLOGIC SURGERY

abdomen with urinary extravasation into the peritoneal cavity (intraperitoneal rupture). Bone fragments from a pelvic fracture may penetrate the bladder with pelvic urinary extravasation (extraperitoneal rupture).

c. Diagnostic evaluation
   (1) History of lower abdominal trauma or pelvic fracture. Significant bladder injury in the absence of a pelvic fracture is highly unlikely in blunt trauma.
   (2) Patients may exhibit lower abdominal pain, urinary retention, suprapubic tenderness, gross hematuria, or signs of pelvic hematoma.
   (3) Radiographic evaluation
      (a) KUB—Examine for pelvic fractures, soft tissue masses, or deviated bowel gas patterns that suggest pelvic hematoma or urinoma.
      (b) IVP—Documents function of kidneys and ureters. Inadequate to rule out bladder extravasation.
      (c) Cystogram—Urethral injury in males must be ruled out with a retrograde urethrogram prior to the insertion of a urethral catheter. Cystogram is performed after bladder catheterization. Fill the bladder with 75 mL of contrast material and examine the radiograph for signs of gross extravasation. Add additional contrast material for a total of 300 mL to fully distend the bladder. Obtain films with the bladder filled and empty (drainage by gravity). The postdrainage film is crucial in identifying extravasation. Anteroposterior and oblique views are helpful. Extraperitoneal ruptures are seen as flamelike extensions in the pelvis. Intraperitoneal ruptures show contrast agent outlining bowel loops.

d. Treatment
   (1) Penetrating injuries—Usually require prompt exploration, débridement, and repair. Patients are at high risk for concomitant rectal injury.
   (2) Blunt injuries
      (a) Small extraperitoneal bladder ruptures with sterile urine and no associated intra-abdominal injuries can be managed with catheter drainage.
      (b) Intraperitoneal bladder ruptures require immediate exploration, repair, and drainage.
      (c) Manipulation of pelvic hematoma is discouraged owing to the risk of increased bleeding and infection.

e. Complications—Pelvic abscess, peritonitis, partial incontinence when laceration involves bladder neck

5. Urethral trauma
a. Anatomy—Male urethra is divided into anterior (bulbous and pendulous) and posterior (prostatic and membranous) parts. Anterior urethra is

located distal to the urogenital diaphragm. Anterior injuries are associated with straddle-like injury to the perineum and urethral instrumentation. Posterior urethra is located from the bladder neck to the urogenital diaphragm. Posterior urethral injuries are associated with pelvic fractures. Female urethral injuries are uncommon.

b. Anterior urethral injuries may extravasate blood along fascial planes. An injury limited to Buck's fascia results in blood extravasation along the penile shaft. An injury through Buck's fascia demonstrates blood extravasating along abdominal fascial planes (Scarpa's fascia) and the scrotum and perineum (Colles' fascia).

c. Posterior urethral injuries usually occur with pelvic fractures and are associated with pelvic hematomas. Blood at the meatus, urinary retention, and a high-riding prostate on digital rectal exam suggest posterior injury.

d. Diagnostic procedures—All suspected urethral injuries in males must be evaluated by a retrograde urethrogram prior to urethral catheter insertion. Catherization can convert a partial tear into a complete disruption. A 12-Fr catheter is placed into the urethral meatus; 3 mL is injected into the balloon port to hold the catheter in place. Retrograde injection of 25 mL of contrast medium is performed to document urethral extravasation. If no extravasation is seen, a catheter is then inserted. If there is any difficulty in passing the catheter, a urology consult should be obtained.

e. Treatment
   (1) Minor anterior urethral lacerations can be managed by suprapubic cystotomy drainage. Penetrating injuries require exploration, débridement, and repair.
   (2) More severe anterior urethral injuries (e.g., straddle injuries) require exploration.
   (3) Management of posterior urethral injuries is controversial.
      (a) Immediate repair involves exploration with primary reanastomosis.
      (b) Delayed repair consists of suprapubic catheter placement for urinary diversion with delayed repair in 3 months. This approach is preferred when the patient has concomitant severe injury to other organ systems.

f. Complications—Urethral stricture, impotence, incontinence

B. ACUTE SCROTUM

1. Definition—Swollen, tender scrotum associated with a testicular, epididymal, or spermatic cord abnormality. Common in the pediatric population.
2. Differential diagnosis—Testicular torsion, testicular or epididymal appendix torsion, epididymo-orchitis, tense hydrocele, or incarcerated inguinal hernia. Correct diagnosis and expedient intervention are keys to prevent organ loss.

a. Testicular torsion is the spontaneous twisting of the testicular pedicle producing acute ischemia. Presents as the acute onset of severe testicular or unilateral scrotal pain, swelling, and tenderness in the 10- to 18-year-old population. Urinalysis is normal. The testicle is elevated in the scrotum and assumes a horizontal lie. Cremasteric reflex is usually absent in testicular torsion. A color Doppler ultrasound or radionuclide scan can be used when the diagnosis is in doubt. Expedient diagnosis and action are essential because delay in treatment for >6 hours can result in irreversible testicular damage. Surgical treatment consists of exploration, detorsion, and orchiopexy. Orchiectomy is used for nonviable testes. Orchiopexy of the contralateral testicle is performed at the same time to prevent future torsion.

b. Acute epididymo-orchitis occurs in patients along the entire age range. Onset of pain is gradual and may be accompanied by irritation with voiding. Urinalysis often shows pyuria. Scrotal elevation may relieve the pain. The contralateral testicle is normal on palpation. Treatment consists of symptomatic relief and appropriate antibiotics.

c. Torsion of testicular and epididymal appendages (appendices)—Small, pedunculated appendages of the testicle and epididymis can spontaneously twist on their pedicles. This acute ischemia can cause severe pain mimicking a testicular torsion. Patients are usually prepubertal and have no voiding complaints. Urinalysis is normal. Examination reveals a tender, pea-sized mass near the epididymal head. The actual testicle is nontender. A "blue dot" sign is sometimes seen on scrotal illumination. Treatment is supportive and consists of bedrest, ice packs, scrotal elevation, and analgesics. Scrotal exploration may be needed to rule out testicular torsion.

d. Incarcerated inguinal hernia—Usually confused with testicular torsion only in young male patients. Acute onset, severe pain, scrotal swelling, and hyperemia may be seen. Nausea and vomiting often accompany the clinical picture. Urinalysis is normal.

III. URINARY RETENTION

A. ETIOLOGY

Bladder emptying is a coordinated event, consisting of bladder contraction with sphincter relaxation in the absence of bladder outlet obstruction. Acute urinary retention is commonly the result of a previous partial bladder outlet obstruction with an acute decrease in detrusor pressure or increase in outlet resistance. Retention is frequently caused by acute infection, bleeding, overdistention of the bladder, and drugs (α agonists, anticholinergics, antihistamines, and anesthetics).

1. Factors that inhibit a coordinated bladder contraction

a. Neurogenic dysfunction—A neurologic process that results in a hyporeflexic ("flaccid") neurogenic bladder and, commonly, injury to the sacral spinal cord, cauda equina, or pelvic nerves. Can be present in the acute phase of any spinal cord injury (spinal shock).

b. Decompensated bladder—Overdistention of the bladder can overstretch the detrusor muscle and inhibit its ability to contract (e.g., long-term diabetes, prolonged use of antipsychotics or anticholinergics)

2. Factors that cause bladder outlet obstruction

a. Male—Benign prostatic hypertrophy, prostate cancer, urethral stricture, bladder neck contracture, bladder calculi

b. Female—Urethral stenosis, urethra trauma, urethral diverticulum, cystocele, urethrocele, urethral carcinoma

B. PRESENTATION AND DIAGNOSIS

1. Acute symptoms—Urgency, suprapubic pain, decreased urine output
2. Chronic symptoms—Progressive obstructive voiding symptoms leading eventually to anuria or overflow incontinence
3. An asymptomatic patient can present with an abdominal mass, renal insufficiency, or bilateral hydronephrosis.
4. Diagnosis is usually confirmed by placement of a Foley catheter with return of a large quantity of urine or a bladder ultrasound showing bladder distension.

C. TREATMENT

Urinary drainage must be provided by the least invasive method available. Definitive treatment can be addressed at a later date.

1. Attempt is made to pass an 18-Fr Foley catheter.

a. Common causes for inability to pass a Foley catheter
   (1) Inadequate lubrication (lubrication can be inserted into the urethra with small syringe or 2% lidocaine urojet applicator)
   (2) Young male patient who forcefully contracts the external sphincter (will fatigue after ≈30 seconds)
   (3) Urethral strictures (scar tissue occluding urethral lumen)
   (4) Enlarged median lobe of the prostate or defect from a previous transurethral resection of the prostate (TURP) can create an acute angulation in the prostatic urethra. A coudé catheter may be placed successfully because of its angulated tip.

b. If initial attempts at passing an 18-Fr Foley or coudé-tip catheter are unsuccessful, a urologist should be consulted. The use of filiforms and followers, percutaneous cystotomy, or formal cystoscopy may be required.

2. Definitive treatment of urinary retention varies with the causative factors.

a. Benign prostatic hypertrophy—Can be treated medically with tamsulosin 0.4 mg PO q.d. or doxazosin 1 mg PO q.h.s. Surgical intervention includes TURP or open prostatectomy (removal of only in the inner adenoma of the prostate through a surgical incision).

b. Prostate cancer—Usually has metastasized to bone or lymph nodes when obstruction occurs. Treatment at this point is hormonal

53

UROLOGIC SURGERY

(orchiectomy vs. luteinizing hormone–releasing hormone agonist). Prostate cancer can also cause urinary retention by spinal cord compression from vertebral metastasis (neurogenic hyporeflexic bladder).

c. Bladder neck contracture—Caused by scarring at the bladder neck, usually following TURP. Managed by transurethral incision of the bladder neck.

d. Urethral stricture—Managed by transurethral incision or urethroplasty

e. Hyporeflexic neurogenic bladder—Usually managed with intermittent straight catheterization (ISC)

f. Decompensated bladder—Managed by ISC

3. Postobstructive diuresis—Following relief of urinary retention (>200 mL/h)

a. Primarily due to excess water and solute retained during period of urinary retention (physiologic diuresis)

b. Rarely, a diuresis occurs due to a tubular defect with loss of the kidney's ability to concentrate urine. A hypovolemic state can result from this pathologic diuresis. The patient's vital signs should be closely monitored for orthostatic changes, and IV fluid replacement should be administered as needed. Serum and urine electrolyte monitoring is also helpful.

IV. UROLITHIASIS

A. ETIOLOGY

1. Calcium-containing stones (calcium oxalate and calcium phosphate)

a. Account for 70-80% of urolithiasis

b. Patients usually present at 30-50 years of age.

c. More common in men

d. Risk of stone recurrence—50% in 5 years

e. Hypercalciuria can be classified as absorptive (due to high intestinal absorption), renal (renal leak of calcium), or resorptive (due to hyperparathyroidism).

f. Renal tubular acidosis type I and medullary sponge kidney are associated with calcium phosphate stones.

g. Hyperoxaluric calcium nephrolithiasis is seen in association with increased urinary oxalate levels. Seen in inflammatory bowel disease and fat malabsorption conditions.

h. Radiopaque

2. Struvite (infection) stones

a. Account for 15% of urolithiasis

b. Contain magnesium, ammonium, and phosphate

c. More common in women

d. Urease-producing bacteria such as *Proteus, Klebsiella, Pseudomonas,* and *Staphylococcus* produce an alkaline urine (pH >7).

e. Less radiopaque than calcium stones

f. Can produce staghorn stones with stone components filling various renal calyces

3. Uric acid stones

a. Account for 5% of urolithiasis
b. May be associated with gout, myeloproliferative disease, rapid weight loss, and treatment with cytotoxic drugs
c. Radiolucent
d. Most patients do not have elevated serum uric acid levels.
e. Urinary pH <5.5

4. Cystine stones

a. Due to an inborn error of metabolism resulting in abnormal intestinal mucosal and renal tubular absorption of cystine, ornithine, lysine, and arginine
b. Urinalysis reveals hexagonal crystals.
c. Sodium cyanide nitroprusside urine test is purple when positive.
d. Stones precipitate when urinary cystine level >250 mg/d.

B. PRESENTATION

1. May be asymptomatic or may cause symptoms from obstruction of the ureteropelvic junction or along the course of the ureter
2. Renal colic is caused by stretching of the collecting system or ureter.
3. Noncolicky renal pain is caused by distention of the renal capsule.
4. Pain can be referred to the flank, abdomen, or genitalia.
5. Distal stones can cause irritating voiding symptoms.
6. Bladder stones can cause irritating symptoms—dysuria, urgency, frequency; rarely, can cause complete bladder outlet obstruction
7. Differential diagnoses include appendicitis, small bowel obstruction, diverticulitis, ovarian torsion, and ectopic pregnancy.
8. Obstructing calculi with infected urine causing pyonephrosis is an emergency. Pyelovenous and pyelolymphatic backflow can cause systemic sepsis. Prompt drainage by percutaneous (nephrostomy tube) or endoscopic (retrograde stent) means is warranted.

C. DIAGNOSIS

1. Urinalysis with microscopic hematuria and occasionally pyuria. Urinary pH and urinary crystals are also important indicators of stone type.
2. Radiographic studies—Noncontrast CT scan, IVP, retrograde pyelograms
3. Metabolic work-up with serum studies and 24-hour urine done after acute event is resolved
4. Strain urine for stone passage.

D. TREATMENT

1. Small (<4 mm), uncomplicated stones can be managed with oral analgesics and fluid hydration as outpatients.
2. Patients with obstructing calculi in a solitary kidney, persistent nausea and vomiting, fever, urinary tract infection, or pain uncontrolled by oral analgesics should be treated as inpatients.

53

UROLOGIC SURGERY

3. Obstructing calculi in an infected urinary system need emergent intervention by either antegrade or retrograde relief of obstruction.
4. Endoscopic treatments include ureteroscopy with stone manipulations, extracorporeal shock wave lithotripsy, and percutaneous nephrolithotomy.
5. Open surgical intervention includes pyelolithotomy, anatrophic nephrolithotomy, radial nephrotomy, ureterolithotomy, partial nephrectomy, and nephrectomy.

RECOMMENDED READINGS

Tanagho EA, McAninch (eds): Smith's General Urology, 16th ed. New York, Lange Medical Books/McGraw-Hill, 2004.

Walsh PC, Retik AB, Vaughan ED, Wein AJ (eds): Campbell's Urology, 8th ed. Philadelphia, WB Saunders, 2002.

Wessells H: Evaluation and management of renal trauma in the 21st century. *In* AUA Update Series, Vol XXI, Lesson 30. Houston, American Urological Association, 2002.

Renovascular Hypertension

Thaddeus P. O'Neill, MD

I. DEFINITION

Renovascular hypertension is systemic hypertension resulting from decreased renal blood flow and subsequent activation of the renin-angiotensin system.

A. ETIOLOGY
1. Most common cause of surgically correctable hypertension
2. Other surgical causes—Primary aldosteronism, pheochromocytoma, coarctation of the aorta, abdominal coarctation, Takayasu's disease, Cushing's syndrome, renal parenchymal disease

B. GENERAL
1. Found in <5% of individuals with hypertension
2. Activation of the renin-angiotensin system is protective to prevent renal parenchymal injury during times of inadequate perfusion.

II. PHYSIOLOGY (Fig. 54-1)

A. GENERAL
Renovascular hypertension was originally described by Goldblatt 50 years ago. He demonstrated that hypertension could be produced by 70% narrowing of the renal artery.

B. SPECIFIC FUNCTIONS
1. Renin is released from the juxtaglomerular apparatus in response to a decrease in Na^+ concentration or decreased perfusion.
2. Renin proteolytically cleaves angiotensinogen to angiotensin I.
3. Angiotensin-converting enzyme (ACE) causes cleavage of angiotensin I (a decapeptide) to angiotensin II (an octapeptide) in the lung.
4. Angiotensin II is the most potent vasoconstrictor known and causes contraction of smooth muscle in all vascular beds. Angiotensin II causes hypertension and stimulation of aldosterone secretion from the adrenal gland. Angiotensin II is cleaved to form angiotensin III, which also causes aldosterone release.
5. Aldosterone is produced by the zona glomerulosa of the adrenal gland. It contributes to hypertension by stimulating active absorption of sodium in the distal tubules of the kidney, leading to increased intravascular volume.

C. HYPERTENSION AND OTHERS
1. Renovascular hypertension can be either renin or volume dependent.
2. Renin-dependent disease occurs with unilateral renal artery stenosis. Activation of the renin-angiotensin system results in a compensatory

54

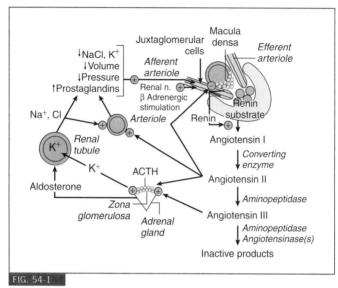

Renin-angiotensin-aldosterone system. ACTH = adrenocorticotropic hormone.

natriuresis by the unaffected kidney. The patient remains euvolemic; thus, the hypertension is caused only by vasoconstriction.
3. Volume-dependent disease occurs with bilateral renal artery stenosis. Compensatory diuresis is lost, so the hypertension is driven primarily by volume expansion.

III. PATHOLOGY

A. ATHEROSCLEROSIS
1. Represents 75% of renovascular hypertension
2. 85% of atheromatous plaques occur at the renal artery ostia and most are contiguous with aortic lesions.
3. Primarily occurs in elderly males (in their 6th decade of life)
4. The left renal artery is more commonly affected.
5. 30-50% are bilateral.

B. FIBROMUSCULAR DYSPLASIA
Fibromuscular dysplasia is an idiopathic disorder with several different histologic subtypes; it accounts for 20% of renovascular hypertension.
1. Medial fibroplasia
a. Accounts for 85% of dysplastic lesions
b. Occurs primarily in young (30-50 years of age) multiparous women

c. Forms focal stenosis surrounded by microaneurysms in the midrenal artery and distal renal artery, which resemble a "string of beads" on angiogram

d. 85% involve the right renal artery; 50% are bilateral.

e. Etiology may be related to changes in smooth muscle cells under the influence of estrogens or damage caused by stretching during pregnancy.

f. Other arteries, such as the internal carotids and iliacs, can be affected.

2. Intimal fibrodysplasia

a. Accounts for 5% of dysplastic disease

b. Occurs primarily in children and adolescents, with no gender predominance

c. Most common cause of renovascular hypertension in the pediatric population

d. Results in smooth focal or tubular stenosis of the renal artery

e. Etiology is thought to be related to persistence of embryonic myointimal cushions, trauma, or abnormal flow patterns.

3. Perimedial fibrodysplasia

a. Accounts for 10% of dysplastic lesions, usually affects young women

b. More progressive than medial fibrodysplasia

c. Solitary or multiple areas of stenosis without dilations in the distal renal artery

C. DEVELOPMENTAL RENAL ARTERY DISEASE

1. Rare cause of renovascular hypertension
2. Found equally in males and females
3. Accounts for 40% of renovascular hypertension in children
4. Arteries are hypoplastic at their origin from the aorta with an hourglass shape.
5. Etiology may result from abnormal fusion of the dorsal aorta during development. Can be associated with coarctation of the abdominal aorta or aortic hypoplasia.

D. OTHER CAUSES OF RENOVASCULAR HYPERTENSION

Other causes include aneurysms, arteriovenous malformations, dissections, renal artery thrombosis, and emboli from arterial plaques.

IV. CLINICAL MANIFESTATIONS

A. ABDOMINAL BRUIT (50-80% OF PATIENTS)

B. HYPERTENSION

1. Onset <35 or >50 years of age
2. Hypertension refractory to triple-drug therapy
3. Sudden worsening of stable hypertension, especially in patients with known atherosclerosis
4. Malignant hypertension

54

RENOVASCULAR HYPERTENSION

C. DECREASED RENAL FUNCTION
There is decreased renal function after starting an ACE inhibitor.

D. UNILATERAL SMALL KIDNEY

V. DIAGNOSIS

A. SCREENING STUDIES
1. Laboratory studies
a. Captopril challenge test—Plasma renin levels measured before and after administration of captopril accurately discriminate between renovascular and essential hypertension.
b. Plasma renin activity profile—Plasma renin plotted against 24-hour urine sodium excretion can identify right ventricular hypertrophy; however, plasma renin levels can be normal in up to 25% of patients with the disease.
c. Obtain necessary serum and urine chemistries to rule out other potential causes of hypertension, e.g., primary hyperaldosteronism (sodium, potassium), pheochromocytoma (urine catecholamines), hyperthyroidism (thyroid-stimulating hormone, thyroxine), and hyperparathyroidism (calcium).
2. Duplex ultrasound—Reliable, noninvasive method to detect renal artery stenosis
a. Peak systolic velocity is measured in the pararenal aorta and in each renal artery.
b. A ratio of renal-to-aortic peak systolic velocities >3.5 correlates with a significant (>60%) stenosis.
c. Obesity, bowel gas, or recent surgery often prevents a technically adequate study.
3. IV pyelogram—A widely used but highly inaccurate screening test
a. Renovascular hypertension is suspected if there is a difference of ≥1.5 cm in renal length or if there is a delay in the appearance of contrast material on one side.
b. Up to 30% of patients with renovascular hypertension demonstrate no abnormal findings.

B. FUNCTIONAL STUDIES
1. Captopril renal scan
a. Baseline radionuclide scintigraphy is performed, after which 25-50 mg of captopril is administered PO. The scan is then repeated after 1 hour.
b. A drop in glomerular filtration rate after the administration of captopril is specific for hemodynamically significant renal artery stenosis.
c. Asymmetry of appearance and excretion of the radioisotope are also suggestive of renal artery disease.
d. Less accurate study when bilateral renal artery stenosis is present

e. ACE inhibitors must be withheld 1 week prior to study for accurate results. Other antihypertensive agents may be continued.

2. Selective renal vein renin assay

a. The test is performed by cannulating each renal vein and sampling blood renin levels.

b. A positive test is indicated by an increase in renin from the affected kidney by a ratio of ≥1.5 compared to the normal kidney.

c. Test has limited value in patients with bilateral renal artery stenosis

d. Patients should be fluid and salt restricted and off all antihypertensive medications for accurate results, further limiting its usefulness.

C. ARTERIAL STUDIES

1. Contrast angiography

a. The gold standard in the diagnosis of renal artery stenosis

b. If functional studies are positive, angiography is performed to confirm anatomic stenosis and to plan appropriate interventions.

c. CO_2 angiography can be used to reduce the contrast load for patients with impaired renal function.

2. Magnetic resonance angiography

a. A high-quality, noninvasive imaging modality that may eventually replace conventional angiography

b. Ideal for patients with impaired renal function or contrast agent allergies

c. Limited to centers with appropriate equipment and experienced radiologists

VI. TREATMENT

A. MEDICAL THERAPY

1. Requires close follow-up, compliant patients, and life-long medications—Even with control of hypertension, renal mass and function can be lost in up to 40% of patients.

2. Pharmacologic management of renovascular hypertension is restricted to patients not amenable to interventional therapies.

a. Operative therapy has proven to be safer than long-term medical management.

b. Reported mortality from surgical and medical therapy—30% and 70%, respectively

3. ACE inhibitors are the most effective therapy.

a. Can be associated with a substantial decrease in renal excretory function, especially in patients with atherosclerotic disease

b. Should be avoided if bilateral renal artery stenosis is present

4. Calcium channel blockers and β blockers are second-line agents.

B. ENDOVASCULAR THERAPY

1. Percutaneous transluminal renal angiplasty (PTA).

a. Involves a controlled disruption of the vessel wall via balloon dilation

b. Treatment of choice for medial fibromuscular dysplasia, short segments of stenosis in the main renal artery, and nonostial atherosclerotic lesions
c. Plaque lesions, especially ones involving the ostia and aorta, have a high rate of technical failure and restenosis.
d. >90% of patients improve, but long-term results are still unclear.

2. PTA with stent placement
a. Intraluminal stents have improved patency rates of ostial lesions and other renal lesions refractory to traditional balloon angioplasty.
b. Treatment of choice for patients at high risk for surgical intervention with ostial lesions

C. SURGICAL THERAPY
1. Renal artery revascularization
a. An aortorenal bypass using autogenous saphenous vein is the procedure of choice when the aorta is relatively spared of atherosclerotic change.
b. Prosthetic grafts with polytetrafluoroethylene Gore-Tex or Dacron are acceptable alternatives with similar patency rates.
c. Saphenous vein should be avoided in children because it is prone to aneurysmal degeneration. Autogenous hypogastric artery is the conduit of choice in the pediatric population.
d. Initial revascularization is critical; reoperation is associated with a high nephrectomy rate (50%).
e. Renal artery bypass often accompanies aortic repairs for occlusive or aneurysmal disease.
f. Effective only if initiated prior to irreversible parenchymal loss

2. Renal endarterectomy
a. Appropriate for atherosclerotic disease and the treatment of choice for bilateral ostial lesions
b. Can be performed either through a longitudinal aortotomy with primary closure or through a transverse aortotomy extending into each renal artery with patch closure

3. Hepatorenal/splenorenal bypass
a. Extra-anatomic bypass is a useful alternative in high-risk patients or patients who have had prior aortic surgery.
b. Bypass procedures avoid cross-clamping of the aorta and are associated with less cardiac and pulmonary morbidity.
c. Hepatorenal bypass using the gastroduodenal artery or saphenous graft is used for right renal revascularization.
d. Splenorenal bypass is used for revascularization of the left kidney.

4. Nephrectomy (<10% of patients)
a. Indicated in unilateral renovascular disease in a small (<8 cm) kidney with minimal excretory function and persistent hypertension
b. Atrophic kidneys do not contribute to creatinine clearance but continue to produce renin and hypertension.
c. Also indicated for patients who have failed revascularization

5. Surgical outcomes

a. Mortality—1-2%

b. Overall, 80-90% are better or cured in carefully selected patient groups
    (1) Pediatric fibrodysplasia—97%
    (2) Adult fibrodysplasia—94%
    (3) Adult focal atherosclerosis—91%
    (4) Adult diffuse atherosclerosis—72%, but only 24% cured

c. Patients with fibrodysplastic disease and lateralizing renins do better. Older patients with atherosclerosis do worse.

d. Nephrectomy is uniformly successful.

Pediatric Surgery

Philip K. Frykman, MD, PhD

Children are not simply little adults. They have their own particular diseases and physiologic responses. In general, however, the surgical philosophy and the approach to surgical diseases are similar.

I. FLUID AND ELECTROLYTE REQUIREMENTS

A. MAINTENANCE FLUIDS
1. Body weight method

Body Weight (kg)	Free Water/Hour	Free Water/Day
0-10	4 mL/kg/h	100 mL/kg/d
11-20	40 mL for 1st 10 kg + 2 mL/kg/h for each kg >10 kg	1000 mL + 50 mL/kg/d for each kg >10 kg
>20	60 mL for 1st 20 kg + 1 mL/kg/h for each kg >20 kg	1500 mL + 20 mL/kg/d for each kg >20 kg

2. Body surface area method—2000 mL/m^2/24 h (not accurate for infants <10 kg body weight; requires calculation of body surface area from nomogram using height and weight)

B. MAINTENANCE ELECTROLYTES
1. Na^+—3-5 mEq/kg/24 h
2. K^+—2-3 mEq/kg/24 h
3. Ca^{2+}—2 mEq/kg/24 h
4. Mg^{2+}—0.15-1 mEq/kg/24 h

C. RESUSCITATION FLUIDS
1. Crystalloid—Lactated Ringer's or normal saline, 10-20 mL/kg
2. Blood products
a. Whole blood—10-20 mL/kg
b. Packed red blood cells—5-10 mL/kg
c. Plasma—10-20 mL/kg
d. 5% albumin—10-20 mL/kg
e. 25% albumin—2-4 mL/kg

II. TOTAL PARENTERAL NUTRITION

Total parenteral nutrition (TPN) is indicated in states of prolonged ileus, GI fistulas, supplementation of oral feeds (short bowel syndrome, malabsorption states), and catabolic wasting states (malignancy or sepsis) and in the treatment of necrotizing enterocolitis. Children, particularly neonates, have little nutritional reserve, so TPN must be considered early.

A. GENERAL

1. In general, total maintenance rates for IV fluids are calculated first, then the concentration of nutrients in the TPN is gradually increased daily.
2. Estimate maintenance water requirements as in section I. A.

B. SPECIFIC REQUIREMENTS

1. Caloric requirements (include allowance for stress, growth)
   a. 0-1 years—90-120 kcal/kg/d
   b. 1-7 years—75-90 kcal/kg/d
   c. 7-12 years—60-75 kcal/kg/d
   d. 12-18 years—30-60 kcal/kg/d
2. Protein calories (≈15% of total calories)
   a. 0-1 years—2-3.5 g/kg/d
   b. 1-7 years—2-2.5 g/kg/d
   c. 7-12 years—2 g/kg/d
   d. 12-18 years—1.5 g/kg/d
3. Lipid calories (≈30-40% total calories, should not exceed 50%)
   a. Lipid formulations
      (1) 10% = 10 g/100 mL = 1.1 kcal/mL
      (2) 20% = 20 g/100 mL = 2.0 kcal/mL
   b. Begin with 0.5 g of lipid/kg/day and increase by 0.5 g/kg/d to a maximum of 3 g/kg/d.
4. Carbohydrate calories (≈50% total calories)—Minimum glucose infusion rate of 4-6 mg/kg/min for neonates

III. TRAUMA

See Chapter 14.

IV. LESIONS OF THE HEAD AND NECK

A. BRANCHIAL CLEFT ANOMALIES

1. Branchial sinuses and cysts are remnants of embryologic structures.
2. Most common anomaly arises from second branchial cleft (fistula from tonsillar fossa to anterior border sternocleidomastoid)
3. Fistulas are usually discovered in childhood; cysts frequently present along the anterior border of the sternocleidomastoid and are not seen until adulthood.
4. Fistulas present with mucoid discharge; cysts present as mass anterior and deep to the upper third of the sternocleidomastoid. May become infected; 10% are bilateral; risk of in situ carcinoma in adults.
5. Diagnosis is aided by ultrasonography to identify the cystic nature of a mass, if not apparent by physical exam.
6. Treatment—If infected, require incision and drainage; otherwise, excised during formal neck dissection under general anesthesia

B. THYROGLOSSAL DUCT REMNANTS

1. Thyroid develops from an evagination in the base of the tongue (foramen cecum) to the anterior larynx. If thyroglossal duct persists, the tract forms a cyst, which may become enlarged and symptomatic.
2. Most frequently occurs as a rounded, cystic mass of varying size in midline of the neck inferior to the hyoid that moves with swallowing and protrusion of the tongue
3. Document the presence of remaining normal thyroid tissue separate from the cyst prior to excision. Preoperative thyroid scanning can be helpful.
4. Symptoms include dysphagia, pain, or simple mass; may become infected. Symptoms of hypothyroidism may be present. Rarely is a site for adult carcinoma (<1% of patients).
5. Treatment involves total excision of the cyst, the central body of the hyoid bone, and the tract to the foramen cecum. If total excision of all thyroid tissue is unavoidable, thyroxine supplementation will be required.

C. CYSTIC HYGROMA

1. Benign tumor of lymphatic origin; occurring in 1:12,000 births
2. Most often located in the posterior triangle of the neck with predilection to the left side. Can cause respiratory insufficiency in infancy or when glottic structures are involved.
3. 90% diagnosed by second year of life
4. Translumination can help distinguish cystic hygroma from solid masses. Ultrasonography can be helpful in confirming diagnosis, especially superficial lesions.
5. Sudden enlargement usually due to hemorrhage in the lesion
6. Treatment is by excision, although radical surgery, i.e., excising involved blood vessels and nerves, is contraindicated. Sclerotherapy with multiple agents such as bleomycin, doxycycline, and fibrin glue has been used with mixed results.

V. THORACIC DISORDERS

A. PULMONARY SEQUESTRATION

1. Lung tissue with absent or abnormal bronchial communication to the normal tracheobronchial tree; blood supply derived from systemic arterial source
2. Extralobar—66% diagnosed in infancy
a. 90% located in left posterior costophrenic sulcus
b. Rarely, manifests as respiratory insufficiency. Most frequently is asymptomatic and found incidentally on chest radiograph. Sequestration may become infected by hematogenous spread of bacteria despite lack of communication with airway or lung tissue.

c. Arterial supply usually low thoracic or abdominal aorta; venous drainage into azygos or hemiazygos system

d. Commonly have coexisting congenital anomalies (15-40%), especially diaphragmatic hernia

e. Invested in visceral pleura

3. Intralobar—Majority diagnosed after age 1 year, often in adulthood

a. Should suspect in patients with recurrent pneumonias within the same bronchopulmonary segment

b. 60% in left hemithorax; communicates with normal lung only via the pores of Kohn; become infected due to inadequate drainage

c. Arterial supply similar to extralobar; venous drainage via pulmonary vein of affected lobe causing a left-to-right shunt that can progress to congestive heart failure

d. Incorporated within normal pulmonary parenchyma

4. Diagnosis by plain radiograph ranging from opacification to cystic parenchymal lesions with air-fluid levels. Color ultrasonography with Doppler-flow analysis is highly sensitive and specific. Chest CT scan with three-dimensional reconstruction is also valuable for diagnosis; angiography is infrequently used.

5. Symptomatic sequestrations require resection; extralobar by simple excision; intralobar frequently requires formal lobectomy; life-threatening hemorrhage possible if systemic vascular supply not recognized and controlled intraoperatively.

B. BRONCHOGENIC CYSTS

1. Derived from abnormal budding of the primitive tracheobronchial tube; most commonly seen in mediastinum or pulmonary parenchyma

2. Produces symptoms of bronchial or esophageal obstruction but may also be asymptomatic with incidental discovery on chest radiograph

3. Has mucoid central core surrounded by wall of cartilage and smooth muscle; lined with ciliated columnar epithelium

4. 70% located within lung tissue; 30% located within mediastinum, extrinsic to lung

5. Should be excised regardless of symptoms, usually by simple excision, although formal lobectomy may be required

C. CYSTIC ADENOMATOID MALFORMATION

1. Results from focal pulmonary dysplasia rather than hamartomatous change

2. May present from asymptomatic mass to fetal hydrops (fatal), but most common presentation is respiratory distress in the newborn. Can present in later life due to recurrent pulmonary infection.

3. Symptoms produced by progressive air trapping with enlargement of mass and compression of normal lung and airways; may have associated pulmonary hypoplasia and pulmonary hypertension

4. Treatment is formal lobectomy; rarely, systemic arterial supply may be present as in pulmonary sequestration. Pulmonary hypertension and lung hypoplasia can occur in patients with large lesions. Extracorporeal membrane oxygenation (ECMO) may be required in severe cases.

D. CONGENITAL LOBAR EMPHYSEMA

1. Progressive obstructive emphysema leading to massive distention of the involved lobe, often mimicking a tension pneumothorax
2. Affects left upper lobe and right upper and middle lobes most commonly, unusually lower lobes
3. Two thirds of patients are male; rare in blacks and premature infants
4. >50% develop symptoms within first few days of life, which include dyspnea, wheezing, cough, tachypnea, and cyanosis. Neonates often trap fetal lung fluid in lobe, so chest radiograph may look like pneumonia until fluid clears.
5. Caused by partial airway obstruction due to abnormal cartilaginous support of the bronchial wall (ball-valve effect); leads to progressive air trapping with compression of normal lung and mediastinal shift
6. First, must perform bronchoscopy to rule out external compression of bronchus by anomalous pulmonary vein or artery or large patent ductus arteriosus
7. Primary treatment is lobectomy.

E. CONGENITAL DIAPHRAGMATIC HERNIA (BOCHDALEK)

1. Occurs as result of failure of fusion of the transverse septum and the pleuroperitoneal folds during the 8th week of development
2. Incidence up to 1:2000 live births; posterolateral defects account for 75-85%; most on left side
3. Excluding malrotation and patent ductus arteriosus, incidence of associated congenital defects between 10-20%
4. Pathophysiology related to development of ipsilateral (and to varying degrees contralateral) pulmonary hypoplasia and to the development of persistent fetal circulation is also called *persistent pulmonary hypertension of the newborn;* this produces right-to-left shunting with failure of oxygenation and ventilation. Prognosis depends on the severity of pulmonary hypoplasia.
5. Present with respiratory distress (dyspnea, cyanosis, hypoxemia); scaphoid abdomen, decreased breath sounds, cardiac dextroposition. Symptoms may develop immediately or several hours after birth ("honeymoon period"), the latter of which is associated with better prognosis.
6. Chest radiograph—Usually confirms diagnosis by findings of loops of gas-filled bowel within chest (may be confused with cystic adenomatoid malformation); may require GI contrast study in the stable patient to confirm diagnosis

7. Preoperative preparation—Patient must first be stabilized.

a. Decompress stomach—10-Fr Replogle nasogastric tube

b. Intubate; mechanical ventilation maintaining high Pao_2 and moderate hypocapnia ($Paco_2 \approx 30$ mm Hg) using low airway pressures; high-frequency oscillatory, inhaled nitric oxide. Avoid mask ventilation of patient.

c. Correct acidosis with $NaHCO_3$ and maintain tissue perfusion. Many authors advocate alkalinization; however, recently permissive hypercapnia looks promising for improved survival.

d. Place monitoring catheters—Postductal arterial line, adequate venous access

e. Echocardiography performed early to assess cardiac anomalies and evaluate presence and severity of pulmonary hypertension and shunting. Cardiac malformations account for $\approx 60\%$ of associated anomalies.

8. Surgical repair after infant has been stabilized medically using transabdominal primary closure of diaphragmatic defect or patch closure with prosthetic material

9. If patient remains unstable, ECMO has been shown to improve survival in infants with congenital diaphragmatic hernia and reversible pulmonary hypertension. Repair may then occur in 3-6 days or at completion of ECMO.

10. Inhaled nitric oxide to reverse pulmonary hypertension may be useful.

F. **ESOPHAGEAL ATRESIA AND TRACHEOESOPHAGEAL FISTULA**

1. Embryonic failure of separation of the trachea from the esophagus

2. Usually present in the neonatal period with excessive salivation, feeding intolerance, drooling, or gagging; maternal polyhydramnios. H-type fistula may present at later age with recurrent pneumonias.

3. Diagnosis

a. Clinical suspicion in newborn with findings enumerated in section V. F. 2

b. Inability to pass catheter beyond proximal esophagus

c. Obtain upright chest radiograph; absence or presence of gas in stomach and GI tract (determines esophageal atresia vs. tracheoesophageal fistula, respectively)

d. Obtain ultrasound to determine position of aortic arch and presence of associated cardiac (>30%) and genitourinary (12%) anomalies.

4. Types of atresias and tracheoesophageal fistulas (Fig. 55-1)

Type A (6-7%)—Isolated esophageal atresia without fistula; gasless abdomen on radiograph

Type B (1%)—Esophageal atresia with proximal tracheoesophageal fistula

Type C (86%)—Esophageal atresia with distal tracheoesophageal fistula

Type D (1-5%)—Esophageal atresia with proximal and distal tracheoesophageal fistula

Type E (5%)—Tracheoesophageal fistula without atresia (H type)

Type F (1%)—Esophageal stenosis without fistula

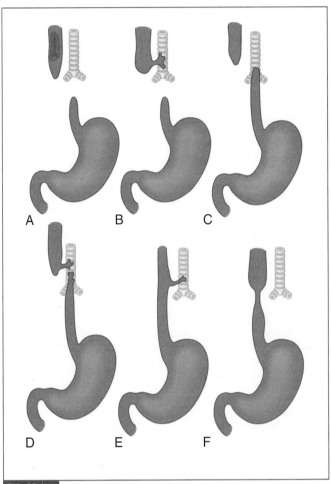

FIG. 55-1

A to F, Types of tracheoesophageal fistulas. See text (section V. F. 4) for descriptions of each type.

5. Preoperative preparation

a. 10-Fr Replogle catheter into proximal segment to prevent aspiration

b. Elevate head of bed

c. Avoid mask or pressure ventilation

d. Supportive fluid, electrolyte, and nutritional therapy; broad-spectrum antibiotics

6. Surgical treatment—Depends on cardiopulmonary stability of patient

a. Stable patient, no life-threatening anomaly, weight >2500 g
   (1) Immediate primary extrapleural thoracotomy, ligation/division of fistula, primary repair of esophageal atresia
   (2) Extrapleural chest drainage, with or without gastrostomy

b. Unstable patient, life-threatening anomaly, weight <1500 g
   (1) Decompressive gastrostomy
   (2) Delayed primary repair (1-2 weeks) when stable

c. Unstable patient, persistent pulmonary distress (usually due to continued aspiration) and need for ventilatory support
   (1) Decompressive gastrostomy
   (2) Staged repair—Extrapleural ligation/division of fistula, followed by transpleural primary repair of atresia when stable

d. Isolated atresia without fistula—Lower esophageal segment frequently too short for primary repair; initially requires cervical esophagostomy with a stomach, colon, or small bowel interposition later (≈1 year of age)

7. Outcome

a. Anastomotic leak occurs in 11% of patients, and anastomotic stricture occurs in 26%.

b. Survival is largely dependent on associated congenital defects.

c. High incidence of gastroesophageal reflux (44%); may require eventual fundoplication

G. MEDIASTINAL MASSES

Masses in the mediastinum are categorized into four anatomic subdivisions.

1. Superior—Thymoma, thymic cyst, lymphoma, thyroid mass, parathyroid mass

2. Anterior—Thymoma, thymic cyst, teratoma, dermoid, lymphangioma, hemangioma, lipoma, fibroma

3. Middle—Pericardial cyst, bronchogenic cyst, lymphoma, granuloma

4. Posterior—Neurogenic tumors (neuroblastoma, ganglioneuroma), foregut duplications and cysts

VI. GI TRACT

A. HYPERTROPHIC PYLORIC STENOSIS

1. Gastric outlet obstruction due to hypertrophied pyloric muscle

2. Affects 3 in 1000 infants; male-to-female ratio is 5:1

3. Occurs in first 2 months of life, with average age of clinical presentation 3-6 weeks. Nonbilious vomiting that increases in volume and frequency is seen. Dehydration is present with classic electrolyte picture of "contraction" alkalosis (hypokalemia, hypochloremia, and metabolic alkalosis). Unconjugated hyperbilirubinemia is also present.

4. 90% have palpable pyloric tumor ("olive") in the midepigastrium to right upper quadrant (RUQ); examination is facilitated by nasogastric decompression and sedation.

5. Contrast upper GI study and/or ultrasound useful for confirming diagnosis when pyloric tumor not palpable or equivocal; should not be routinely obtained if symptoms and palpable mass present

6. Preoperative management

a. Operation is never an emergency, and adequate preoperative preparation is necessary for low morbidity.

b. Nasogastric decompression

c. Fluid resuscitation and electrolyte correction including potassium repletion (once urine output ensured) are mandatory before operative repair. Correct HCO_3 to <30.

7. Surgical treatment—Classic operation is Fredet-Ramstedt pyloromyotomy (reported mortality ≈0.3%) via RUQ, periumbilical, or laparoscopic approach

8. Postoperative management

a. Nasogastric tube removed in OR

b. Continued IV hydration

c. Oral fluids (electrolyte solution) begun 6-12 hours postoperatively, gradually advanced over 1-2 days to full-volume formula feeds

B. INTESTINAL OBSTRUCTION IN THE NEONATE

1. Should suspect with history of maternal polyhydramnios, bilious emesis, abdominal distention, or failure to pass meconium within first 24 hours of life

2. *Bilious vomiting in an infant is a surgical emergency and requires emergent evaluation to rule out malrotation and midgut volvulus.*

3. Intrinsic duodenal obstruction

a. Frequent association with other anomalies

b. May be due to duodenal web, atresia, or stenosis

c. Presents with bilious vomiting, minimal abdominal distention

d. Abdominal radiographs reveal "double-bubble" sign.

e. Surgical treatment includes excision of webs or duodenostomy for atresia and evaluation of distal bowel for other atresias.

4. Extrinsic duodenal obstruction—Malrotation

a. Malrotation of the midgut results in a narrow base for the small bowel mesentery, with predisposition to volvulus and intestinal infarction.

b. Presents with sudden onset of bilious vomiting as newborn

c. Volvulus frequently results in significant vascular compromise and intestinal obstruction.

d. Most reliably diagnosed by upper GI to visualize malpositioned ligament of Treitz

e. Treatment includes emergent laparotomy and Ladd's procedure. This consists of evisceration, reduction of volvulus by counterclockwise rotation, division of "Ladd's bands" thereby widening the mesenteric base between the duodenum and the colon, appendectomy, and placement of the small bowel in the right side and the colon in the left side of the peritoneal cavity.

55

PEDIATRIC SURGERY

f. Nonviable bowel should be resected; questionably viable bowel should remain with a planned 24-hour second-look laparotomy.

5. Jejunoileal obstruction—Atresia and stenosis

a. Result of late mesenteric vascular accidents in utero
b. Abdominal radiographs show dilated loops of small bowel; contrast enema usually demonstrates small unused "microcolon," although it may be normal.
c. Martin-Zerella classification

    Type I—Single mucosal atresia, bowel wall and mesentery in continuity, and normal bowel length

    Type II (most common)—Single atresia with discontinuity of bowel and gap in mesentery

    Type III—Multiple atresias

    Type IV—"Apple peel" or "Christmas tree" deformity with markedly decreased bowel length

d. Operative management is individualized, depending on number and length of atresias; includes resection with anastomosis, tapering enteroplasty, and exteriorization in the presence of compromised bowel

6. Meconium ileus

a. Obstruction of the distal ileum from inspissated meconium—Associated with cystic fibrosis
b. Simple meconium ileus—Bowel is impacted with pellets of meconium, with proximally dilated ileum packed with thick, tarlike meconium
c. Complicated meconium ileus—Associated with meconium cysts, atresia, perforation, or meconium peritonitis
d. Presents with progressive abdominal distention and failure to pass meconium; abdominal radiograph obstruction shows no air-fluid levels; "soap bubble" appearance in proximal colon; contrast enema shows microcolon with inspissated plugs of meconium
e. May respond to nonoperative therapy with Gastrografin enemas
f. Operative intervention indicated for complicated cases and where nonoperative therapy fails; ranges from simple enterotomy and irrigation of bowel with N-acetylcysteine (Mucomyst) to bowel resection with primary anastomosis or temporary diverting colostomy
g. Survival predominantly based on associated pulmonary complications of cystic fibrosis

7. Hirschsprung's disease

a. Absence of parasympathetic ganglion cells in the affected segment of intestine; rectum and rectosigmoid most common
b. Familial forms of Hirschsprung's disease associated with mutations in *RET* proto-oncogene, endothelin receptor B (*ENDRB*), and endothelin 3 (*ET3*) genes
c. Suspected in any infant who does not pass meconium in the first 24 hours of life, has newborn intestinal obstruction, or has chronic constipation during the first year of life

d. Diagnosis obtained from barium enema (rectum of small to normal size with proximal colorectal dilation) and suction rectal biopsy (absence of ganglion cells in Meissner's (submucosal) and Auerbach's (intermuscular) plexus; increase in acetylcholinesterase staining)

e. Currently, most infants with a new diagnosis of Hirschsprung's disease are treated with a one-stage pull-through operation. Previously, the standard was a multiple-stage approach starting with diverting colostomy proximal to the aganglionic segment, followed by a definitive pull-through procedure at 9-12 months of age.

f. Laparoscopic one-stage pull-through procedures are becoming more frequently used.

g. Complications include enterocolitis (10-30%), anastomotic leak (1-5%), and stricture (3-5%).

C. INTESTINAL OBSTRUCTION IN THE INFANT (2 MONTHS-2 YEARS)

1. Intussusception

a. Most common cause of bowel obstruction in 2-month-old to 2-year-old age range; >50% have documented recent viral infection.

b. Due to telescoping of one segment of bowel (intussusceptum) into another (intussuscipiens). Ileo-cecal occurs most commonly.

c. Sudden onset of recurring severe, cramping abdominal pain; vomiting; drawing up of legs; 60% have bloody ("currant jelly") stools. An elongated mass may be palpable in RUQ with an "empty" right lower quadrant.

d. Diagnosis by air or barium enema—"Coiled spring" appearance

e. Initial treatment by attempted hydrostatic reduction during air enema if peritonitis or free air has been ruled out first (70-80% success rate)

f. Requires surgical exploration if air enema reduction is unsuccessful or if peritonitis is present; manual reduction is performed distal to proximal, followed by appendectomy if bowel remains viable. If manual reduction is not possible or if lead point is identified, resection is indicated.

2. Incarcerated hernia (see Chap. 47)

D. NECROTIZING ENTEROCOLITIS

1. Most common GI emergency in the premature neonate

2. >90% in premature or low-birth-weight infants

3. Etiology not known—Appears to be related to ischemic intestinal damage, bacterial colonization, and intraluminal substrate (feedings)

4. Early clinical findings—Ileus, gastric retention, bilious vomiting, and bloody stools. Progressive findings include lethargy, apnea, bradycardia, hypothermia, shock, acidosis, and neutropenia.

5. Radiographic findings—Pneumatosis intestinalis. Late findings include "fixed" loop of bowel (suggests gangrenous changes) and portal vein air or free air.

6. Medical management

a. Gastric decompression, NPO

b. Systemic antibiotics

c. Fluid resuscitation, correction of acidosis, parenteral nutrition

d. Close monitoring—Serial CBC, platelet count, and upright abdominal films (q 6 hours)

7. Indications for surgery

a. Free air or portal vein air on radiograph (absolute indication)

b. Clinical deterioration—Persistent acidosis, thrombocytopenia, leukopenia

c. Diffuse peritonitis, abdominal wall erythema or induration

d. Paracentesis suggestive of nonviable bowel if fluid brown and cloudy, extracellular bacteria on Gram stain, large number of white blood cells with differential >80% neutrophils

E. MECKEL'S DIVERTICULUM

1. The most common form of persistent vitelline duct remnant; less commonly persistent vitelline duct with sinus, persistent omphalomesenteric band, and vitelline duct cyst

2. Occurs on antimesenteric border of ileum within 60 cm of ileocecal valve

3. Complications

a. Bleeding—22%; usually painless, due to ulceration of adjacent tissue from ectopic gastric mucosa; usually stops spontaneously, but can be massive

b. Obstruction—13%; secondary to internal hernia around persistent omphalomesenteric band

c. Inflammation—2%; mimics acute appendicitis

d. Intussusception—1%

4. Diagnosis—High degree of suspicion, confirmed by ^{99m}technetium-pertechnate scan; can have false-positive results with enteric duplications or false-negative results with H_2 blockers if ectopic gastric mucosa present

5. Treatment by wedge resection of diverticulum or segmental ileal resection with primary anastomosis; include appendectomy

6. Incidental Meckel's diverticulum—Generally recommend resection in patient <18 years of age, particularly if heterotopic tissue present; not indicated in asymptomatic adults

7. Remember the "rule of 2s"—Occurs in 2% of the population, symptomatic in 2% of cases, approximately 2 feet from the ileocecal valve, 2 inches in length, 2 types of mucosa (gastric/pancreatic), twice as many males as females, 2 presentations (bleeding, obstruction)

F. APPENDICITIS

1. Most common emergent abdominal operation in children

2. Ruptured in 30-50% of children at presentation

3. See Chapter 34.

G. GASTROESOPHAGEAL REFLUX

1. See Chapter 30.
2. Differs from adult gastroesophageal reflux
a. Emesis is the most common presentation; malnutrition and failure to thrive; aspiration pneumonia and asthma; esophagitis; laryngospasm
b. Frequently associated with mental retardation
c. Preoperative evaluation
   (1) Upper GI to exclude gastric outlet obstruction and malrotation
   (2) Esophagogastroduodenoscopy to rule out Barrett's and to grade esophagitis
   (3) pH probe is most sensitive and specific for pathologic reflux (pH <4 for >4% of the time).
   (4) Obtain technetium gastric emptying scan to rule out delayed gastric emptying or outlet obstruction.
d. Initial treatment is nonoperative for 6-8 weeks—Has a 80% response rate
   (1) Upright position, thickened feedings, metoclopramide, H_2 blockers
   (2) Frequently resolves spontaneously
   (3) Contraindicated in patients with esophageal stricture or near-miss sudden infant death syndrome
e. Operative therapy
   (1) Usually not performed in children <6 months of age
   (2) Indications—Failed medical therapy, severe esophagitis, Barrett's metaplasia, stricture, bleeding, neurologically impaired patient that needs a gastrostomy tube
   (3) Two most common repairs—Nissen (360 degree) and Thal (270 degree); 10% and 20% recurrence, respectively. Laparoscopic approach is frequently used.
   (4) Pyloroplasty in patients with delayed gastric emptying

VII. ABDOMINAL WALL DEFECTS

A. OMPHALOCELE

1. A covered defect of the umbilical ring into which abdominal contents herniate; sac composed of an outer layer of amnion and an inner layer of peritoneum
2. >50% of infants have serious associated congenital defects (GU, cardiac, GI); always associated with malrotation
3. Sac may contain only intestine, but usually contains liver as well; may be associated with loss of abdominal domain, with contracted abdominal cavity
4. Management includes covering sac with sterile dressing; protection from hypothermia; gastric decompression; parenteral nutrition; and broad-spectrum antibiotics.
5. Surgical treatment—Small defects can be closed primarily; moderate defects can have the skin closed with the subsequent hernia being

repaired later; larger defects require staged closure using Silastic silo.

6. Overall survival depends on the size of the defect as well as the severity of associated congenital defects; mortality averages 30-35%.

B. GASTROSCHISIS

1. Defect of the anterior abdominal wall just lateral and usually to the right of the umbilicus.

2. No peritoneal sac, with resulting antenatal evisceration of bowel through the defect; resulting chemical irritation of bowel wall leads to thick edematous membrane on bowel surface, foreshortened bowel.

3. Always associated with nonrotation; 15% associated with intestinal atresias; other congenital defects unusual

4. Management
   a. Prevention of excessive insensible fluid and heat loss through exposed bowel; gastric decompression
   b. Large amounts of IV fluids needed to maintain perfusion; initiation of total parenteral nutrition; broad-spectrum antibiotics
   c. Primary repair successful in 70% of cases; if not possible, is treated with gradual decompression using a Silastic silo

C. UMBILICAL HERNIA

1. Defect of the umbilical ring; more common in females and blacks

2. Spontaneous closure in 80% of patients, usually if <2 cm in diameter; if >2 cm, less chance of spontaneous closure

3. Observation recommended until child is 3 to 4 years of age; if persistent, undergo elective repair; large defects are repaired earlier

D. INGUINAL HERNIA

1. Due to persistence of the embryonic processus vaginalis

2. Incidence varies with gestational age (9-11% in premature infants, 3.5-5% in term infants).

3. ≈10% bilateral; contralateral exploration indicated if patient is <1 year old (60% bilateral). Laparoscopy through the hernia sac can be used to perform exploration of contralateral side.

4. Most are indirect.

5. Examination reveals immobile, tender mass in groin, with mass extending along spermatic cord up to the internal ring.

6. Major complication is bowel incarceration with strangulation and possible infarction; significantly higher in preterm infant (31%) and in infants in first year of life (15%).

7. High ligation of sac is adequate repair; may repair bilateral hernias simultaneously

8. Incarcerated hernia—In the absence of signs of compromised bowel (fever, peritonitis, leukocytosis) or obstruction, attempt reduction when diagnosed; achieved by placing firm pressure in the direction of the

inguinal canal; facilitated by sedation and elevation of the legs and torso. If irreducible, or if strangulation is suspected, urgent repair is indicated.

VIII. NEOPLASMS

A. NEUROBLASTOMA
1. Usually in children <4 years of age
2. Origin—Neural crest tissue and pathologically classified as a small, round, blue cell tumor of childhood
3. Metabolically active—Catecholamines (90%)
4. Wide range of biologic behavior from highly malignant to benign ganglioneuroma or spontaneously regression
5. Presentation—70% disseminated at presentation
a. Abdominal mass—Retroperitoneal, adrenal medulla, or paraspinal ganglia
b. A large thoracic primary may present with respiratory distress. Spinal cord compression. Symptoms of catecholamine or vasoactive intestinal polypeptide excess.
c. Horner's syndrome may result from a cervical primary tumor.
6. Diagnosis
a. Urinary catecholamine breakdown products—Vanillylmandelic acid and homovanillyic acid screening 92% accurate
b. CT or MRI—May demonstrate spinal involvement more accurately
c. Bone scan and bone marrow aspiration
d. MIBG nuclear scan shows bone involvement and primary tumor
7. Treatment—Based on assessment of biologic features (karyotype, N-*myc* amplification) and clinical stage
a. Stage 1 or 2—Operative resection with node removal
b. Stage 3 or 4—Primary or delayed operative resection, chemotherapy and radiation therapy
8. Prognosis—Inversely related to age
a. Tumor stage and location
b. N-*myc* gene amplification, stroma-poor or nodular-rich pathology, elevated serum ferritin or lactate dehydrogenase associated with poor prognosis

B. NEPHROBLASTOMA (WILMS' TUMOR)
1. Embryonal renal neoplasm—Mesenchymal origin. Two related but separate tumors are clear cell sarcoma and malignant rhabdoid tumor.
2. The *WT1* tumor suppressor gene is responsible for inherited forms of Wilms' tumors.
3. Presentation
a. Maximal incidence—1-5 years of age
b. 10% associated with congenital abnormalities—WAGR (*W*ilms' tumor, *a*nidria, *g*enitourinary malformations, mental *r*etardation) syndrome, Beckwith-Wiedemann syndrome, Denys-Dash syndrome

55

PEDIATRIC SURGERY

    c. Symptoms—Fever; abdominal pain; firm, irregular, painless abdominal
       mass; hematuria; hypertension

    d. Diagnosis—Ultrasound (cystic vs. solid, invasion of vena cava), CT or
       MRI, chest radiograph to screen for pulmonary metastases

4. Treatment

    a. Operative—Tumor removal even with distant metastases, 4.4-7.0% of
       cases have bilateral involvement

    b. Solitary lung metastases may be excised.

    c. Adjuvant chemotherapy and radiation therapy beneficial. Preoperative
       chemotherapy and radiation therapy may enable operative therapy for
       tumors initially too large for resection, those with intravascular extension
       of tumor thrombus proximal to intrahepatic vena cava, and those with
       bilateral Wilms' tumors.

**5. Prognosis—Worse with anaplasia, sarcomatous changes, positive nodes,
    higher staging, older age**

    a. Favorable histology syndrome—>80% survival for 4 years

    b. Unfavorable histology—50-70% survival for 4 years

RECOMMENDED READING

Rowe MI, O'Neill JA, Grosfeld JL, et al (eds): Pediatric Surgery.
   St. Louis, Mosby, 1998.

Cardiac Surgery

Sara J. Pereira, MD

I. PREOPERATIVE EVALUATION

A. HISTORY AND PHYSICAL EXAMINATION
1. Signs or symptoms of congestive heart failure
a. Jugular venous distention
b. Rales
c. S_3 gallop
2. Arrhythmias, presence of a pacemaker and/or defibrillator
3. Neurologic symptoms, syncope
4. Vascular examination
a. Claudication, pain at rest
b. Documentation of peripheral pulses—Radial, ulnar, femoral, dorsalis pedis
c. Evaluation of carotid disease, bruits
5. Evaluation of neck for potential internal jugular cannulation

B. MEDICATIONS
1. A comprehensive list of both preadmission and preoperative medications should be included in the preoperative note.
2. In general, medications are continued until surgery, especially antianginal agents, antihypertensive agents, nitroglycerine and heparin drips, and antiarrhythmic agents.
3. Perioperative steroid and insulin coverage is per routine.

C. PREOPERATIVE TESTING
1. Electrocardiogram—Arrhythmias, ischemic changes, conduction delays, chamber enlargement
2. Laboratory—CBC, electrolytes, type and crossmatch for 2 units of packed red blood cells
3. Posteroanterior and lateral chest radiograph
4. Nuclear perfusion testing
a. Myocardial reserve
b. Functional significance of coronary lesion
5. Review of cardiac catheterization and echocardiogram results
a. Distribution of coronary artery disease
b. Evaluation of ventricular wall motion and ejection fraction
c. Presence of valvular dysfunction

D. PREOPERATIVE ORDERS
1. Accurate height and weight recorded in chart to calculate body surface area
2. Hibiclens scrub the night before surgery
3. NPO after midnight

4. Antibiotics on call—Cefuroxime 1.5 g IV piggyback or use vancomycin 1 g IV piggyback for reoperative patients

II. OPERATIVE PROCEDURES

A. CORONARY ARTERY BYPASS GRAFTING (CABG)

1. Indications
a. Chronic stable angina, unrelieved by medication
b. Unstable angina, despite treatment
c. Acute myocardial infarction—If significant coronary disease exists beyond the area of infarction, ongoing angina postinfarction, or unstable hemodynamic status. Controversy exists on the timing of surgical intervention.
d. Ventricular arrhythmias with coronary disease
e. Failed percutaneous transluminal coronary angioplasty (PTCA)
2. CABG shown to be superior to medical treatment of coronary disease in the following situations
a. In patients with asymptomatic or mild angina and the following
    (1) Significant left main disease
    (2) Three-vessel coronary artery disease with proximal left anterior descending disease and/or decreased left ventricular function
b. In patients with chronic moderate to severe angina
c. Unstable angina despite full medical therapy
d. Failed PTCA
e. Persistent ventricular arrhythmias in patients with coronary artery disease
3. No difference in rates of myocardial infarction in CABG and medically treated patients
4. Internal mammary artery grafts conduit of choice due to superior patency rates compared to saphenous vein grafts (in situ and free grafts) (90-95% vs. 50-60% at 10 years)

B. VALVE REPLACEMENT OR REPAIR

1. Aortic stenosis
a. Commonly due to bicuspid valve, rheumatic disease, or calcific aortic stenosis
b. Symptoms include triad of dyspnea, angina, and syncope
c. Indications for surgery include symptomatic patients with valve gradient of >50 mm Hg or valve area <0.8 cm^2/m^2. Asymptomatic patients with significant stenosis and left ventricular hypertrophy should additionally be considered.
d. Coronary angiography is performed owing to high rate of concomitant coronary artery disease.
2. Aortic insufficiency
a. Etiologies include rheumatic disease, annular ectasia, endocarditis, and aortitis.

b. Frequently asymptomatic, but symptoms of congestive heart failure may be present

c. Indications for surgery—Symptomatic patients and patients with cardiomegaly or deteriorating systolic function as assessed by echocardiography

3. Mitral stenosis

a. Primarily rheumatic in origin

b. Symptoms—Dyspnea, orthopnea, and paroxysmal nocturnal dyspnea. Radiographs may demonstrate left atrial enlargement and pulmonary venous hypertension.

c. Indications for surgery—Presence of chronic symptoms or acute episodes of pulmonary venous hypertension.

d. Chronic atrial fibrillation—A complication of progressive left atrial enlargement.

4. Mitral regurgitation

a. Etiologies—Rheumatic disease, myxomatous valve structure, endocarditis, ischemia or papillary muscle dysfunction, and congenital structural defects

b. Severity and development of symptoms—Varies with etiology; rheumatic disease is more insidious in onset, whereas ischemic mitral regurgitation is often acute in onset

c. As with mitral stenosis, indications for surgery depend on the severity of symptoms.

d. Ischemic mitral regurgitation is usually corrected at the time of coronary bypass, with either valve replacement or annuloplasty. Often mild ischemic mitral regurgitation may improve by coronary bypass only. Depending on the structural defect present, rheumatic or myxomatous valve disease may be corrected by valve repair or replacement. The advantages of repair vs. replacement are the low rate of endocarditis and lack of need for long-term anticoagulation.

C. AORTIC DISSECTION

1. Etiology—Hypertension, atherosclerosis, cystic medial necrosis (e.g., Marfan syndrome), infections, trauma, pregnancy

2. Clinical considerations

a. Dissections diagnosed within 2 weeks from onset of symptoms are *acute*

b. Mortality secondary to *acute* dissection ranges from 57-89%

3. DeBakey classification

Type I—Intimal disruption of ascending aorta that extends to involve the entire descending thoracic aorta and abdominal aorta

Type II—Involves the ascending aorta only (stops at the innominate artery)

Type III—Involves the descending thoracic and abdominal aorta only (distal to left subclavian artery)

4. Stanford classification

Type A—Any dissection that involves the ascending aorta

56

CARDIAC SURGERY

      Type B—Any dissection that involves only the descending aorta,
      distal to the left subclavian artery

5. Diagnosis is usually made by aortogram or chest CT scan.
Preoperative control of hypertension with nitroprusside and β blockers
is an essential part of management.

6. Dissection may advance proximally, disrupting coronary blood flow or
inducing aortic valve incompetence; or distally, causing stroke,
renal failure, paraplegia, or intestinal ischemia.

7. Indications for emergent operative repair

a. Acute type A dissection

b. Type B dissection with failed medical therapy such as hypertension,
inadequate pain control, progressive dissection by radiographic studies,
impaired organ perfusion, or impending aortic rupture

8. Operative repair involves replacement of the affected aorta with a
prosthetic graft. Cardiopulmonary bypass is required for repair of
type A dissections, and hypothermic circulatory arrest is often used for
transverse arch dissections. Aortic valve replacement and coronary
reimplantation may be required for type A aneurysms that involve
the aortic root. Type B dissections can be medically managed unless
expansion, rupture, or compromise of branch arteries develops or
hypertension becomes refractory.

9. Postoperative complications include renal failure, intestinal ischemia,
stroke, and paraplegia. Mortality with surgical intervention currently
ranges from 6-16%.

D. TRAUMATIC AORTIC DISRUPTION

1. This injury results from deceleration injury and usually occurs just distal
to the left subclavian artery, at the level of the ligamentum arteriosum.

2. Chest radiograph findings include widened mediastinum,
pleural capping, associated first and second rib fractures, loss of the
aortic knob, hemothorax, deviation of the trachea or nasogastric tube,
and associated thoracic injuries (scapular and clavicular fractures).

3. Definitive diagnosis is made by aortogram, but chest CT and
transesophageal echocardiography also aid in the diagnosis.

4. Imperative that immediate life-threatening injuries (e.g., positive
diagnostic peritoneal lavage) be treated prior to repair

E. CONGENITAL HEART SURGERY

Numerous congenital anomalies have been described, but in general most
congenital heart disease can be broken down according to the physiologic
disturbances.

1. Obstructive lesions—Include valvular stenoses and coarctation of the
aorta. Long-term sequelae include concentric cardiac hypertrophy and
subsequent failure due to ventricular pressure overload. Repair or
replacement of the involved valve or segment is the mainstay of
operative treatment.

2. Left-to-right shunts (acyanotic)—Atrial and ventricular septal defects make up most patients in this group. Also included are patent ductus arteriosus and truncus arteriosus. Symptoms are due to chronic volume overload of the pulmonary circulation, which eventually leads to pulmonary hypertension. Cyanosis is a late finding in these anomalies, due to right-sided heart pressures exceeding left-sided heart pressures (Eisenmenger's syndrome). Operative repair involves patch closure of the septal defect or ductal ligation.

3. Right-to-left shunts (cyanotic)—These defects include tetralogy of Fallot, transposition of the great arteries, tricuspid atresia, total anomalous pulmonary venous drainage, and Ebstein's anomaly. These defects involve complex repairs that are usually performed during infancy. Palliative procedures include Blalock-Taussig shunts (subclavian artery to pulmonary artery) and aortopulmonary artery shunts.

56

CARDIAC SURGERY

III. POSTOPERATIVE CARE

A. HEMODYNAMICS

1. Invasive monitors include arterial lines, pulmonary artery catheters, and occasionally left atrial catheters.
2. Every effort should be made to optimize ventricular filling pressures and systemic blood pressures. In general, up to 2 L of crystalloid is used; after that, blood or colloid is used to increase filling pressures. Hypertension aggravates bleeding along suture lines and is controlled by a nitroprusside drip. Lower blood pressures are preferred as long as a mean blood pressure >60 mm Hg is maintained. There are numerous causes for hypotension postoperatively; before beginning specific treatment, know the filling pressures, cardiac rhythm, cardiac index, and systemic vascular resistance.

B. ANTIARRHYTHMICS

1. Digoxin is given prophylactically to most CABG and valve repair patients. Contraindications include preexisting conduction defects or bradycardia.
2. Atenolol has been shown to be a useful adjunct to digoxin. Contraindications include conduction defects, recent myocardial infarction, poor ventricular function, and diabetes mellitus.

C. ANTICOAGULATION

1. Antiplatelet agents and aspirin are given to all CABG patients.
2. Patients with mechanical valve replacements are given warfarin starting postoperative day 1, and the dosage is adjusted to maintain international normalized ratio (INR) between 2.5 and 3.5.

D. HARDWARE

1. Mediastinal tubes are discontinued when drainage is <200 mL/8 h and no air leak is present.

2. Antibiotics are discontinued after the mediastinal tubes are removed or at 24 hours.
3. Pacing wires are by convention atrial on right side and ventricular on left side. They are removed at 3 days or the day prior to discharge.

IV. POSTOPERATIVE COMPLICATIONS

A. ARRHYTHMIAS

1. Ventricular ectopy—Most common
a. For frequent (>6-10/min) or multifocal premature ventricular complexes, treat with lidocaine bolus of 1 mg/kg, followed by drip at 2-4 mg/min.
b. Cardioversion needed if progresses to symptomatic ventricular tachycardia or if patient develops ventricular fibrillation
c. Atrial or atrioventricular pacing at a slightly higher rate may suppress ectopy.

2. Nodal or junctional rhythm
a. May not need treatment for asymptomatic, normotensive patient
b. Rule out digoxin toxicity; make certain serum K^+ >4.5; rule out hypomagnesemia.
c. May require atrioventricular sequential pacing if loss of atrial kick has significant hemodynamic sequelae.

3. Supraventricular tachycardia (SVT)—Includes atrial fibrillation and flutter
a. Onset may be preceded by multiple premature atrial contractions
b. Atrial ECG using atrial pacing leads often helpful in distinguishing fibrillation from flutter during rapid rates
c. Atrial fibrillation—Digoxin used to control rate
d. Atrial flutter may be treated by the following
   (1) Rapid atrial pacing >400 beats/min
   (2) Digitalization followed by IV β blocker
   (3) IV verapamil followed by digitalization. Calcium-channel blockers must be given judiciously as wide complex SVT can mimic ventricular tachycardia.
e. In both instances, if any significant drop in blood pressure or cardiac output occurs, the arrhythmia should be treated with synchronous DC cardioversion at 25-50 joules. This should be done prior to digitalization, however, to prevent onset of ventricular arrhythmias.
f. Adenosine can be used initially as a diagnostic and therapeutic intervention. Transient bradycardia/asystole allows interpretation of rhythm and may be therapeutic.
g. Diltiazem may also be used if adenosine fails to convert. Load with 15-25 mg initially (may repeat if no effect in 15-20 minutes), and start drip at 5-10 mg/h.

B. BLEEDING

1. Etiology—Includes medications, clotting deficits, reoperation, prolonged operation, technical factors, hypothermia, and transfusion reactions

2. Treatment
a. Ensure normothermia.
b. Measurement of clotting factors—Prothrombin time, partial thromboplastin time, fibrinogen, platelet count, activated clotting time
c. Correction
    (1) Fresh frozen plasma, cryoprecipitate, platelets
    (2) Protamine for prolonged heparinization
d. Transfusion reaction protocol if suspected
3. Exploration for postoperative hemorrhage—Indications include mediastinal tube output of >300 mL/h despite correction of clotting factors. Technical factors found as etiology >50% of time.

C. RENAL FAILURE
1. Incidence—1-30%
2. Diagnosis—Renal vs. prerenal azotemia
3. Management
a. Optimize volume status and cardiac output.
b. Discontinue nephrotoxic drugs.
c. Maintain urine output >30 mL/h (low-dose dopamine, furosemide, ethacrynic acid as indicated; furosemide (Lasix) or furosemide/chlorothiazide (Diuril) drips for persistent oliguria.
d. Dialysis—Either continuous venovenous or hemodialysis may be used.
e. Outcome—Mortality rates 0.3-23% depending on the degree of azotemia; if dialysis is required, mortality ranges from 27-53%

D. RESPIRATORY FAILURE
1. Mechanical—Mucus plugging, malpositioned endotracheal tube, pneumothorax
2. Intrinsic—Volume overload, pulmonary edema, atelectasis, pneumonia, pulmonary embolus (uncommon)

E. LOW CARDIAC OUTPUT SYNDROME (CARDIAC INDEX <2.0 L/min/m²)
1. Signs—Decreased urine output, acidosis, hypothermia, altered sensorium
2. Assessment—Heart rate and rhythm (ECG: possible acute myocardial infarction), preload and afterload states (pulmonary artery catheter readings), measurement of cardiac output
3. Treatment
a. Stabilize rate and rhythm.
b. Optimize volume status and systemic vascular resistance.
c. Correct acidosis, hypoxemia if present (chest radiograph for pneumothorax).
d. Inotropic agents, e.g., dobutamine or milrinone drips
e. Persistent low cardiac output despite inotropic support requires placement of intra-aortic balloon pump.

56

CARDIAC SURGERY

F. CARDIAC TAMPONADE

1. Onset—Suggested by increasing filling pressures with decreased cardiac output; decreasing urine output, and hypotension; quiet, distant heart sounds, and eventual equalization of right- and left-sided atrial pressures
2. High degree of suspicion that coincides with excessive postoperative bleeding
3. Chest radiograph may demonstrate wide mediastinum; echocardiogram if readily available or diagnosis uncertain
4. Treatment—Emergent re-exploration is treatment of choice and may be needed at bedside for sudden hemodynamic decompensation. Transfusion to optimize volume status and inotropic support; avoid increased positive end-expiratory pressure.

G. PERIOPERATIVE MYOCARDIAL INFARCTION

1. Incidence—5-20%
2. Diagnosis—New-onset Q waves postoperative; serial isoenzymes, increased MB fractions; segmental wall motion abnormalities by transthoracic or transesophageal echocardiogram
3. Treatment—Vasodilation (IV nitroglycerine is preferred to nitroprusside). Continued hemodynamic deterioration should be treated with immediate intra-aortic balloon counterpulsation. This "unloads" the ventricle and may preserve nonischemic adjacent myocardium.
4. Outcome—Associated with increased morbidity and mortality, as well as poorer long-term results.

H. POSTOPERATIVE FEVER

1. Common in the first 24 hours postoperatively; most commonly atelectasis, however may be associated with pyrogens introduced during cardiopulmonary bypass. Treat pyrexia with acetaminophen and cooling blankets, because associated hypermetabolism and vasodilation can be detrimental to hemodynamic status and increase myocardial work.
2. Postoperative fevers in valve patients should be followed closely with cultures. CABG patients should have full fever work-up on 5th postoperative day if still febrile, because most postoperative fevers are due to atelectasis.
3. Special attention should be paid to invasive monitors, and lines in place >3 days should be changed.
4. Perioperative antibiotics should be continued until all invasive monitors and drainage tubes have been removed.
5. Sternal wound—Daily inspection for drainage and stability. Sternal infections are disastrous in the cardiac patient, and early evidence of postoperative infection should be treated with operative débridement.

6. Postpericardiotomy syndrome—Characterized by low-grade fever, leukocytosis, chest pain, malaise, and pericardial rub on auscultation. Usually occurs 2-3 weeks following surgery and is treated with nonsteroidal anti-inflammatory agents. Steroids are necessary for some cases.

I. CNS COMPLICATIONS

1. Etiologies—Preexisting cerebrovascular disease, prolonged cardiopulmonary bypass, intraoperative hypotension, and emboli (either air or particulate matter)
2. Transient neurologic deficit—Occurs in up to 12% of patients. Improvement usually occurs within several days.
3. Permanent deficit—Suspect in patients with delayed awakening postoperatively; may have pathologic reflexes present
4. Postcardiotomy psychosis syndrome—Incidence of 10-24%. Starts around postoperative day 2 with anxiety and confusion; may progress to disorientation and hallucinations. Treat with rest and quiet environment; antipsychotics may be given as necessary. It is essential to rule out organic cause of delirium, e.g., substance withdrawal, hypoxemia, hypoglycemia, and electrolyte abnormality.
5. CT scan early for suspected localized lesions; electroencephalogram in patients with extensive dysfunction
6. Treatment—Optimize cerebral blood flow and avoid hypercapnia.
a. Postoperative seizures treated with lorazepam and phenytoin
b. Mannitol may be needed in presence of increased intracranial pressure, depending on hemodynamic status.

RECOMMENDED READINGS

Booth DC, Deupree RH, Hultgren HN, et al: Quality of life after bypass surgery for unstable angina: Five-year follow up results of a Veterans Affairs Cooperative Study. Circulation 83:87, 1991.

DeBakey ME, McCollum CH, Crawford ES, et al: Dissection and dissecting aneurysm of the aorta: Twenty-year follow up of five hundred twenty-seven patients treated surgically. Surgery 92:1118, 1982.

Emergency Cardiac Care Committee and Subcommittees, American Heart Association: Guidelines for resuscitation and emergency cardiac care. JAMA 268:2171, 1992.

Gersh BJ, Califf RM, Loop FD, et al: Coronary bypass surgery in chronic stable angina. Circulation 79 (Suppl I):46, 1989.

56

CARDIAC SURGERY

Carcinoma of the Lung

Sara J. Pereira, MD

I. EPIDEMIOLOGY

A. GENERAL
1. Most common cancer in highly industrialized nations
2. Male-to-female ratio—1.15:1
3. 171,900 new cases in the United States each year
4. <5% of patients with lung cancer are <40 years of age

B. MORTALITY
1. Leading cause of cancer deaths in men and women
2. Cancer deaths reached plateau in women in 1990, decreasing in men since 1984

57

II. ETIOLOGY

A. CIGARETTE SMOKING
1. Overall risk of lung cancer in smokers is 10-25 times that of nonsmokers
2. Risk of lung cancer is directly related to number of cigarettes smoked, duration of use, depth of inhalation, and amount of tar and nicotine in cigarettes
3. Association of lung cancer with exposure to passive smoking is secondary to nitrosamines and oxides in tobacco smoke
4. Cigarette smoke acts synergistically with environmental pollutants in carcinogenesis.
5. Only 10-15% of patients with lung cancer are nonsmokers.

B. OCCUPATIONAL EXPOSURE
1. Asbestos—Workers have 50-90% increased risk of lung cancer
2. Ionizing radiation
3. Arsenic
4. Nickel
5. Chromium
6. Chloromethyl ethers
7. Mustard gas

C. ATMOSPHERIC POLLUTION (DUE TO INDUSTRIAL EXPANSION)

D. GENETIC PREDISPOSITION

III. PATHOLOGY

A. HISTOLOGIC CLASSIFICATION
The following is the histologic classification of malignant epithelial lung tumors according to World Health Organization (1981).

1. Small cell carcinoma—20%
a. Oat cell carcinoma
b. Intermediate cell type
c. Combined oat cell carcinoma
2. Non–small cell carcinoma—80%
a. Adenocarcinoma—40%
   (1) Acinar adenocarcinoma
   (2) Papillary adenocarcinoma
   (3) Bronchogenic adenocarcinoma
   (4) Solid carcinoma with mucus formation
b. Squamous cell carcinoma—30-50%
c. Large cell carcinoma—10%
   (1) Giant cell carcinoma
   (2) Clear cell carcinoma
d. Carcinoid tumor—3-5%

B. LOCATION OF PRIMARY TUMORS
1. "Central" tumors—Squamous and small cell carcinomas
2. "Peripheral" tumors—Adenocarcinoma and large cell carcinomas

C. METHOD OF SPREAD
1. Invades lymphatics and blood vessels, resulting in early metastasis
2. Small cell carcinoma is most aggressive
3. 30-50% of patients with lung cancer have lymphatic or hematogenous spread at initial presentation.
4. Metastases in order of preference—Regional lymph nodes, liver, adrenals, brain, bone, and kidneys
5. Contralateral pulmonary metastases at postmortem examination—10-14%

IV. FOUR MAJOR TYPES OF MALIGNANT EPITHELIAL LUNG TUMORS

A. SQUAMOUS CELL CARCINOMA
1. Most common primary malignant epithelial lung tumor
2. Occurs in the segmental, lobar, or main stem bronchi in 90% of cases
3. Relatively slow growing and late to metastasize
4. Spread pattern
a. Endobronchial growth and invasion of peribronchial lung parenchyma, soft tissue, and lymph nodes
b. Peripheral tumors commonly invade chest wall
5. Microscopically
a. Well-differentiated tumors produce keratin, epithelial pearls, and squamous pattern
b. Poorly differentiated tumors with less obvious keratinization
6. Diagnose with bronchoscopy and brushings.

7. Commonly associated with obstructive pneumonitis, collapse, or consolidation

B. SMALL CELL CARCINOMA
1. 20% of malignant epithelial lung tumors
2. Originates in the bronchial mucosa and grows into the walls of bronchi, peribronchial spaces, and lung parenchyma
3. Most appear as hilar abnormalities with wide mediastinum.
4. Noted for its rapid growth and early metastasis, with clinical features commonly due to metastases
5. Invasion of the superior vena cava is common.
6. Staging (based on TNM)—Includes imaging of brain and bone marrow biopsy
a. Limited—Disease limited to one radiation field
b. Extensive—Spread beyond one radiation field
7. Precise diagnosis is required because treatment and prognosis of small cell carcinoma differ considerably from that of non–small cell carcinoma.

C. ADENOCARCINOMA
1. 40% of malignant epithelial lung tumors
2. Increasing in both men and women
3. Most common lung cancer histology
4. Often a peripheral tumor
a. Arises mostly in the periphery of lung parenchyma
b. May be related to focal scars or regions of fibrosis
5. Grow rapidly and metastasize early to mediastinal, periaortic, supraclavicular, and cervical lymph nodes
6. Present with metastases to adrenals, liver, bone, and brain.
7. Diagnose with CT-guided fine-needle aspiration or video-assisted thoracoscopic surgery (VATS) with wedge biopsy.

D. LARGE CELL CARCINOMA
1. 10% of malignant epithelial lung tumors
2. Most tumors occur in a peripheral and subpleural location.
3. Histologic features
a. Do not show definitive squamous or glandular differentiation
b. Grow in sheets without organization or pattern
c. Necrosis and hemorrhage are dominant features of these tumors.
4. Rapid growth and early metastasis
5. Very poor prognosis
6. ≈10% have mediastinal widening on chest radiograph.

E. CARCINOID TUMORS
1. 3-5% of lung cancers
2. Not associated with smoking

3. No sex difference
4. Originate from neuroendocrine (Kulchitsky) cells of bronchial mucosa
5. 90% are central and arise in main, lobar, or segmental bronchi.
6. Grow slowly and metastasize late
7. 5% of tumors between 2 and 4 cm metastasize to regional lymph node at diagnosis.
8. Excellent prognosis with resection (94-100% survival)
9. Carcinoid syndrome occurs in <5%.

V. METASTATIC TUMORS IN THE CHEST

A. GENERAL
1. Lungs are one of the most frequent sites for metastases.
2. Lungs are first organ to filter many venous-borne metastases.
3. May present as diffuse pulmonary involvement or SPN

B. METASTATIC MALIGNANCIES
1. Common malignancies metastatic to lung—Breast, melanoma, renal cell, prostate, thyroid, pancreatic, soft tissue sarcoma, and osteosarcoma

VI. CLINICAL FEATURES

A. LOCAL MANIFESTATIONS
Local manifestations may be nonspecific, because most patients also suffer from chronic bronchitis and emphysema due to cigarette smoking.
1. Cough and sputum
a. Evaluate for change of an established cough
b. Evaluate for change in quality or quantity of sputum
2. Dyspnea—Sudden onset may indicate obstruction of a main bronchus.
3. Hemoptysis
4. Wheezing
5. Chest pain—Constant, debilitating, and localizing pain may be due to metastatic bony erosion.

B. METASTATIC MANIFESTATIONS
1. Intrathoracic manifestations
a. Pleural effusion
b. Pleuritic pain
c. Superior vena cava syndrome
   (1) Compression or direct invasion of great veins of the thoracic outlet
   (2) Dyspnea, severe headaches, and periorbital, facial, and neck edema
d. Pericardial effusion
2. Extrathoracic manifestations
a. Brachial neuritis—Tumor invading the brachial plexus
b. Horner's syndrome

(1) Tumor invading cervical and first thoracic segment of sympathetic trunk

(2) Ptosis, myosis, and anhidrosis on affected side

c. Hoarseness—Tumor spread involving the ipsilateral recurrent laryngeal nerve

d. Metastases to liver, adrenals, brain, bones, and kidneys

e. Bone metastases usually osteolytic; most frequently ribs and vertebrae involved

C. NONMETASTATIC SYSTEMIC MANIFESTATIONS
1. Endocrine-related syndromes
2. Metabolic (weight loss)
3. Thrombophlebitis

VII. DIAGNOSIS

A. RADIOLOGY
1. Chest radiograph—Abnormalities suspicious of malignancy include the following

a. Atelectasis or lobar emphysema

b. Enlarged hilum or hilar mass

c. Atelectasis or lobar emphysema

d. Enlarged upper or middle mediastinum

e. Evidence of bony erosion due to metastases

2. CT scan

a. May reveal additional pulmonary nodules

b. Evaluate spread to pleural and mediastinal structures.

c. Direct percutaneous transthoracic needle biopsy

d. Use of CT scanning for screening of SPN is being studied.

3. Positron emission tomography (PET) scanning

a. May differentiate benign from malignant lung tumor and evaluate metastatic mediastinal lymph node

b. Based on high rate of glycolysis by uptake of fluorodeoxyglucose in malignant tumors

B. SPUTUM CYTOLOGY
1. 70-80% sensitive with multiple specimens and central tumors
2. May perform bronchial brushings to improve yield in peripheral tumors
3. Cytology most diagnostic for squamous cell carcinoma, intermediate for adenocarcinoma, least for small cell carcinoma

C. BRONCHOSCOPY
1. Flexible bronchoscopy performed in all patients with lung tumor
2. Higher yield in patients with central tumors
3. Complications—Rare
4. Allows transbronchial biopsies, brush cytology, and bronchial washings for cytology

D. MEDIASTINOSCOPY
1. 50% of patients have involved mediastinal lymph nodes at initial presentation.
2. Mediastinoscopy is used in patients with mediastinal nodes >1 cm prior to thoracotomy to evaluate resectability and staging.
3. May access anterior superior mediastinal or subcarinal lymph nodes for biopsy
4. Lymph nodes are positive for metastatic disease in 50-65% of patients.

E. PERCUTANEOUS NEEDLE BIOPSY
1. False-negative result in 10% of patients
2. May be performed transbronchoscopically or via percutaneous approach with CT guidance
a. Transbronchoscopic approach is indicated for extrabronchial tumors without bronchial wall abnormalities
b. CT guidance is used for peripheral lesions >1 cm.
3. Contraindications
a. Bleeding disorders or anticoagulation
b. Bullous disease near the lesion
4. Complications
a. Pneumothorax—20-25%; only 10% require chest tube placement
b. Minor hemoptysis—6%

F. VIDEO-ASSISTED THORACOSCOPIC SURGERY
1. May excise peripheral nodule, biopsy lymph nodes, and evaluate effusion
2. Proceed directly to VATS for wedge biopsy of peripheral lesion for diagnosis.

VIII. TNM CLASSIFICATION AND STAGING

A. TNM CLASSIFICATION FOR LUNG CARCINOMA (1986 INTERNATIONAL STAGING SYSTEM)
1. Primary tumor (T)
   - T0: No tumor
   - Tx: Positive cytology
   - Tis: Carcinoma in situ
   - T1: <3 cm, no main bronchial invasion
   - T2: >3 cm or any size that invades hilum, visceral pleura, or main bronchus
   - T3: Invades parietal pleura, chest wall, diaphragm, mediastinum, or pericardium
   - T4: Invades mediastinum, great vessels, trachea, esophagus, carina, vertebral body, or malignant effusion

2. Regional lymph nodes (N)

N0: No nodes

N1: Ipsilateral nodes (peribronchial or hilar)

N2: Ipsilateral nodes (mediastinal) or subcarinal nodes

N3: Contralateral nodes (mediastinal) or hilar; ipsilateral or contralateral scalene or supraclavicular nodes

3. Distant metastases (M)

M0: No metastasis

M1: Metastasis

B. STAGING FOR LUNG CANCER

Occult carcinoma: Tx N0 M0

Stage Ia: T1 N0 M0

Stage Ib: T2 N0 M0

Stage IIa: T1 N1 M0

Stage IIb: T2 N1 M0, T3 N0 M0

Stage IIIa: T3 N1 M0, T1-3 N2 M0

Stage IIIb: any T N3 M0, T4 any N M0

Stage IV: any T, any N, M1

C. REGIONAL LYMPH NODE STATIONS (AMERICAN THORACIC SOCIETY)

2R: Right upper paratracheal (suprainnominate) nodes

2L: Left upper paratracheal (supra-aortic) nodes

4R: Right lower paratracheal nodes

4L: Left lower paratracheal nodes

5: Aortopulmonary nodes

6: Anterior mediastinal nodes

7: Subcarinal nodes

8: Paraesophageal nodes

9: Pulmonary ligament nodes

10R: Right main bronchial nodes

10L: Left main bronchial nodes

11: Intrapulmonary nodes

IX. TREATMENT OF NON–SMALL CELL CARCINOMA

A. SURGICAL

1. Assessment of pulmonary reserves

a. Pulmonary function test

b. Clinical assessment by stair climbing at a normal rate without significant increase in pulse or respiratory rate

(1) One flight—Tolerate thoracotomy

(2) Two flights—Tolerate lobectomy

(3) Three flights—Tolerate pneumonectomy

57

CARCINOMA OF THE LUNG

Resection	Pneumonectomy	Lobectomy	Wedge/Segmental
MVV	>55% predicted	>40%	>35%
FEV₁	>2.0 L/min or >80% predicted	>1.0 L/min	>0.6 L/min

FEV_1 = forced expiratory volume in 1 second; MVV = maximum voluntary ventilation.

2. Surgical resection of tumor for non–small cell carcinoma stages I-III

a. Of non–small cell carcinomas cases
   (1) 65% inoperable at time of diagnosis
   (2) 15% inoperable at thoracotomy
   (3) 20% undergo resection (of these, 15% of patients die within 2-3 years after surgery from local or distant metastases)
b. Wedge resection or segmentectomy
   (1) Indications—Peripheral tumor <3 cm, patients with marginal pulmonary reserve that would not tolerate thoracotomy, or patients with metachronous or synchronous tumors
   (2) High local recurrence rate reported in some series, especially with adenocarcinoma
c. Lobectomy
   (1) Procedure of choice for disease confined to one lobe
   (2) Includes entire first-level lobar lymphatics
   (3) Mortality rate—0-8%
   (4) Sleeve lobectomy for peribronchial tumor or lymph node involvement at resection site
d. Pneumonectomy
   (1) Indications—Hilar involvement or tumor extension across oblique fissure
   (2) Can result in poor pulmonary reserve with *significant* change in lifestyle
   (3) Mortality rate—5-10%
e. Chest wall resection with reconstruction en bloc for stage III disease
f. Stage IV disease with "single brain metastasis-only" group that benefits from surgical resection

3. Mediastinal lymph node sampling dissection is routinely performed for curative resection.

B. NONSURGICAL THERAPY

1. Radiation

a. Palliation—Often helpful in relieving symptoms of superior vena cava obstruction and mediastinal invasion, as well as cough, hemoptysis, and pain (especially bone pain)
b. Preoperative irradiation
   (1) No improvement in survival, but increased postoperative complications
   (2) Exception is superior sulcus tumor (Pancoast); improved survival (45% vs. 30%) with preoperative irradiation and en bloc resection
   (3) May increase survival with chemotherapy in stage IIIA
c. Postoperative irradiation—Controversial, under study

2. Chemotherapy—Used to treat patients with advanced disease
a. Response rates to single-agent and combined-drug chemotherapy are low.
b. May improve survival for stage IIIa disease in preliminary studies
c. Improves survival used postoperatively (adjuvant) after complete resection in stages IB–IIIA
3. Immunotherapy—Has not demonstrated survival advantage; may improve locoregional recurrence
4. Laser therapy—May be useful to relieve endobronchial obstruction in unresectable tumors

X. TREATMENT OF SMALL CELL CARCINOMA

A. GENERAL
1. Surgical intervention is rarely indicated.
2. Multidrug regimens are more effective than a single agent.
3. Many combinations have been shown to extend survival.
4. Side effects are worse with multiple agents.

B. TUMOR RESPONSE
1. Tumor response is seen in 75-95% of patients.
2. 50% of patients with limited disease (disease limited to one radiation field) see complete response.
3. 20% of patients with widespread disease see complete response.

XI. PROGNOSIS

A. OVERALL SURVIVAL
Overall 5-year survival rates for patients with non–small cell carcinoma of the lung are the following.
1. Stage I, resected—75%
2. Stage II, resected—45%
3. Stage III, resected—25%; nonresected, <10%

XII. WORK-UP OF SOLITARY PULMONARY NODULE

A. DEFINITION AND INCIDENCE
1. SPN is a peripheral pulmonary nodule <6 cm in diameter.
2. Incidence of SPN representing metastatic disease from an asymptomatic primary malignancy is exceedingly low. Extensive metastatic work-up is unnecessary.
3. Consider SPN to be metastatic if it occurs in a patient with current or previous extrapulmonary primary malignant tumor.
4. Incidence of diseases that may present as SPN
a. Malignant nodules—40% (depends on age of patient at presentation)
   (1) Bronchogenic carcinoma—30%

      (2) Solitary metastatic lesions—8%
      (3) Bronchial adenoma (mainly carcinoid)—2%
  b. Benign nodules—60%
      (1) Infectious granulomas—50%
      (2) Noninfectious granulomas—3%
      (3) Benign tumors—3%
      (4) Miscellaneous—4%

B. RADIOGRAPHIC CHARACTERISTICS OF BENIGN NODULES
1. Small, smooth, with sharply circumscribed margins
2. Calcification—Only 0.5% malignant
3. No increase in size in 2 years—Doubling time is 20 to 400 days for malignant tumors

C. MANAGEMENT OF SOLITARY PULMONARY NODULE
1. Further radiographic evaluation of the nodule, and evaluation for other pulmonary nodules (chest CT, PET scans)
2. Radiographic suspicion for benign nodule—Follow with yearly chest radiograph
3. Suspected malignancy
a. Attempt needle biopsy for diagnosis.
b. Bronchoscopy
c. Evaluate for thoracoscopy or thoracotomy with nodule resection.

Cardiac Risk Stratification for Noncardiac Surgery

Gyu Il Gang, MD

Cardiovascular disease accounts for more than 1 million deaths annually, half of all deaths in the United States.

The following is a statement from the American College of Cardiology (ACC) and the American Heart Association (AHA) made in 1996 (emphasis added)[1]:

58

> *The purpose of preoperative evaluation is not to give medical clearance but rather to perform an evaluation of the patient's current medical status; make recommendations concerning evaluation, management, and risk of cardiac problems over the entire perioperative period; and provide a clinical risk profile that the patient, primary physician, anesthesiologist, and surgeon can use in making treatment decisions that may influence short- and long-term cardiac outcomes.* No test should be performed unless it is likely to influence patient treatment.

I. MULTIVARIATE ANALYSIS OF CARDIAC RISK

A. GOLDMAN CRITERIA[2]

1. Nine variables associated with increased cardiovascular mortality or severe morbidity and assigned points are the following.

S3 gallop or jugular vein distention	11
Myocardial infarction within 6 months	10
Rhythm other than sinus, or premature atrial contraction on preoperative ECG	7
>5 premature ventricular complexes/min documented any time prior to OR	7
Intraperitoneal, intrathoracic, aortic operations	5
Age >70 years	4
Important aortic stenosis	3
Emergency operation	3
Poor general medical condition	3

   a. Pao_2 <60 mm Hg, $Paco_2$ >50 mm Hg
   b. K <3, HCO_3 <20, BUN >50, creatine >3
   c. Increased liver function tests, signs of chronic liver disease
   d. Bedridden from noncardiac disease

2. Table 58-1 shows the number of points in each Goldman class and the types of complications associated with each class.[2]

TABLE 58-1

GOLDMAN CRITERIA

Class (N)	Points	No or Minor Complications (N = 943)	Life-Threatening Complications (N = 39)	Cardiac Deaths (N = 19)
I (N = 537)	0-5	532 (99%)	4 (0.7%)	1 (0.2%)
II (N = 316)	6-12	295 (93%)	16 (5%)	5 (2%)
III (N = 130)	13-25	112 (86%)	15 (11%)	3 (2%)
IV (N = 18)	>25	4 (22%)	4 (22%)	10 (56%)

B. LEE CRITERIA[3]

1. The six variables associated with increased major cardiac complications in elective operations include the following.

a. High-risk type of surgery (intraperitoneal, intrathoracic, suprainguinal vascular)

b. Ischemic heart disease

c. History of congestive heart failure

d. History of cerebrovascular disease

e. Insulin therapy for diabetes

f. Preoperative creatinine >2.0

2. Table 58-2 shows the rates of major complications based on the number of Lee criteria present.[3]

II. CLINICAL PREDICTORS OF CARDIAC RISKS (see section V)

A. MAJOR

Major clinical predictors must be addressed and corrected prior to elective operation.

1. Unstable coronary syndromes
2. Decompensated congestive heart failure
3. Significant arrhythmias
4. Severe valvular disease

B. INTERMEDIATE

1. Mild angina pectoris
2. Prior myocardial infarction

TABLE 58-2

RATES OF MAJOR CARDIAC COMPLICATIONS ASSOCIATED WITH NUMBER OF LEE CRITERIA RISK FACTORS

Type of Study Group[3]	No. of Risk Factors			
	0	1	2	≥3
Derivation Group (%)	0.5	1.3	4	9
Validation Group (%)	0.4	0.9	7	11

3. Compensated or prior congestive heart failure
4. Diabetes mellitus
5. Renal insufficiency

C. MINOR
1. Advanced age
2. Abnormal ECG
3. Rhythm other than sinus
4. Low functional capacity
5. History of stroke
6. Uncontrolled systemic hypertension

III. RISKS IN SPECIFIC SURGICAL PROCEDURES

A. HIGH (CARDIAC RISK >5%)
1. Emergent major operations, especially in elderly
2. Aortic and peripheral vascular surgery
3. Anticipated prolonged procedures with large fluid shifts and/or blood loss

B. INTERMEDIATE (CARDIAC RISK 1-4%)
1. Carotid endarterectomy
2. Head and neck surgery
3. Intraperitoneal and intrathoracic surgery
4. Orthopedic surgery
5. Prostate surgery

C. LOW (CARDIAC RISK <1%)
1. Endoscopic procedures
2. Superficial surgeries
3. Cataract surgery
4. Breast surgery

IV. FUNCTIONAL STATUS

Metabolic equivalent unit (MET) is oxygen consumption (Vo_2) of a 70-kg 40-year-old man in the resting state. MET can be directly measured or estimated.

A. POOR
Functional status is poor if the patient is unable to walk four blocks or climb two flights of stairs without difficulty (4 METs).

B. INDETERMINATE
Indeterminate functional status is one that cannot be assessed because of confounding variables, e.g., claudication and primary pulmonary disease.

58

CARDIAC RISK STRATIFICATION

V. ALGORITHM RECOMMENDED BY THE ACC/AHA

Figure 58-1 shows an algorithm recommended by the ACC/AHA[1] to evaluate cardiac risk for noncardiac surgery (see *www.medcalc.com/periop.html* for additional details).

VI. MODIFICATION OF CARDIAC RISK

A. CORONARY REVASCULARIZATION

1. Coronary artery bypass graft (CABG)—Coronary Artery Surgery Study (CASS) registry data show that CABG is superior to medical management of coronary artery disease in reducing perioperative cardiac events.
2. Percutaneous transluminal coronary angioplasty (PTCA)—Bypass Angioplasty Revascularization Investigation (BARI) showed rates of perioperative myocardial infarction and death low for both PTCA and CABG (1.6%)

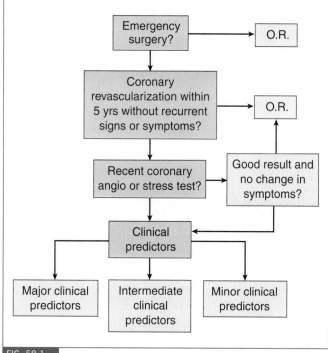

FIG. 58-1

Algorithm for determining cardiac risk in noncardiac surgery based on clinical predictors.

3. Perioperative risk reduction is maintained for ≈5 years, at which risk rises from <1% to >3.5%.

B. β BLOCKADE
1. Multicenter Study of Perioperative Ischemia Research Group
a. β Blockade decreased perioperative ischemia and long-term cardiac mortality.
b. No difference in perioperative mortality
2. Dutch Echocardiographic Cardiac Risk Evaluation Applying Stress Echocardiography Study Group
a. Cohort restricted to highest-risk patients undergoing elective surgery, i.e., abdominal aortic aneurysm and infrainguinal arterial reconstruction
b. Decreased perioperative cardiac events (ischemia and deaths) from 34% to 3.4%
3. Target heart rate <60 beats/min while keeping systolic blood pressure >100 mm Hg

58

REFERENCES

1. Eagle KA, Brundage BH, Chaitman BR, et al: Guidelines for perioperative cardiovascular evaluation for noncardiac surgery: Report of the American College of Cardiology/American Heart Association Task Force on Practice Guidelines (Committee on Perioperative Cardiovascular Evaluation for Noncardiac Surgery). J Am Coll Cardiol 27:910-948, 1996; Circulation 93:1278-1317, 1996.
2. Goldman L, Caldera DL, Nussbaum SR, et al: Multifactorial index of cardiac risk in noncardiac surgical procedures. N Engl J Med 297: 845-850, 1977.
3. Lee TH, Marcantonio ER, Mangione CM, et al: Derivation and prospective validation of a simple index for prediction of cardiac risk of major noncardiac surgery. Circulation 100:1043-1049, 1999.

CARDIAC RISK STRATIFICATION

Thoracoscopy

David P. O'Brien, MD

Hans Jacobaeus proposed thoracoscopy in 1910 and in 1913 performed the first thoracoscopic procedure. By inserting a cystoscope into the pleural cavity, he was able to perform pneumolysis as a therapy for pulmonary tuberculosis. With the introduction of streptomycin in 1945, interest in therapeutic thoracoscopy waned. However, its usefulness in the investigation of pleural disease and the diagnosis of intrathoracic tumors persisted. With the advent of video-assisted thoracoscopy (VATS) and refinement of lighting and instrumentation, a new age in thoracoscopy was launched. Today, VATS is routinely used not only to diagnose pleural and pulmonary disease but also to permit direct therapy for a wide variety of benign and malignant thoracic and mediastinal diseases.

59

I. DIAGNOSTIC THORACOSCOPY

A. DIAGNOSIS OF PLEURAL DISEASE
1. Definitive diagnosis of pleural effusion
2. Determination of pleural involvement in lung cancer
3. Diagnosis of malignant pleural effusion

B. LUNG BIOPSY FOR DIAGNOSIS OF DIFFUSE LUNG DISEASE
1. Greater visibility and accessibility to different areas of lung vs. traditional limited open thoracotomy
2. Traditional open lung biopsy is still preferred in critically ill, ventilator-dependent patients

C. PERIPHERAL INDETERMINATE PULMONARY NODULE
1. Noncalcified nodule <3 cm in diameter
2. Indeterminate etiology after appropriate work-up
3. Location in outer third of lung parenchyma
4. Absence of endobronchial extension

D. EVALUATION OF MEDIASTINAL DISEASE
1. Resection or biopsy of mediastinal mass
2. Adjunctive measure in staging of primary lung cancer—Usually in combination with cervical mediastinoscopy. Allows assessment of subcarinal, aortopulmonary window, lower mediastinal levels 8 and 9, and para-aortic lymph nodes. Has essentially replaced the Chamberlain procedure (mediastinotomy) in some institutions.

II. THERAPEUTIC THORACOSCOPY

A. PRIMARY SPONTANEOUS PNEUMOTHORAX
1. Indications

a. Persistent air leak >72 hours after chest tube insertion for initial spontaneous pneumothorax
b. First recurrence of a spontaneous pneumothorax
c. Initial pneumothorax in patients with history of pneumothorax on contralateral side
d. Initial pneumothorax in patients whose geographic distance from medical care or occupation (i.e., pilots, scuba divers) places them at extreme risk
2. Allows for bleb and bullae resection with endoscopic stapler, apical pleurectomy, mechanical pleural abrasion, and assessment of lung re-expansion

B. BULLOUS EMPHYSEMA
1. Performed with endoscopic stapling device if amendable. Otherwise, open bullectomy may be performed with buttressed staple lines and/or imbrication of the bullae and hand sewing after rupture.
2. Reserved for patients with large localized bulla with evidence of significant lung compression

C. PLEURAL DISEASE
1. Allows for adhesiolysis, breakdown of loculations, drainage of pleural fluid, and pleurodesis in the prevention of recurrent malignant effusion
2. Débridement and decortication during stage II (fibropurulent) of empyema
3. Evacuation of traumatic hemothorax
4. Ligation of thoracic duct following failure of conservative management in chylothorax

D. LUNG RESECTION
1. Indications
a. Indeterminate pulmonary nodule
b. Diagnosis of metastatic disease to lung
c. Wedge resection for early-stage T1 cancer or in patients with compromised pulmonary function
d. VATS lobectomy in selected patients (requires an experienced thoracoscopic surgeon)
   (1) Candidate tumors include peripheral stage I tumors <2 cm in diameter. Reduced operative morbidity and mortality and improved pulmonary function compared to open thoracotomy.
   (2) Hilar involvement with tumor or lymphadenopathy necessitates conversion to open procedure.

E. MEDIASTINAL DISEASE
1. Indications
a. Diagnosis of mediastinal mass
b. Staging of lung cancer prior to lobectomy

c. Resection of posterior mediastinal tumors without intraspinal extension

d. VATS thymectomy

e. Excision of symptomatic mediastinal cyst

F. PERICARDIECTOMY FOR EFFUSIVE DISEASE

1. Indications

a. Benign and malignant effusive disease

b. Purulent pericarditis

c. Radiation-induced pericarditis

2. Median sternotomy required for constrictive, noneffusive pericardial disease

G. ESOPHAGEAL DISEASE

1. Indications

a. Esophagomyotomy for achalasia

b. Resection of benign lesions

c. Staging of esophageal cancer

d. Resection of esophageal cancer

H. AUTONOMIC NERVOUS SYSTEM

1. VATS sympathectomy indications

a. Pain syndromes of the upper extremity, including reflex sympathetic dystrophy and causalgia

b. Hyperhidrosis

c. Vasospastic vascular disorders

2. Thoracic splanchnicectomy for pancreatic pain from cancer and chronic pancreatitis

I. APPLICATIONS IN TRAUMA

In trauma settings, use thoracoscopy only in hemodynamically stable patients.

1. Definitely helpful

a. To assess integrity of diaphragm

b. To control bleeding intercostals

c. To evacuate residual hemothorax

d. To evacuate empyema and decorticate

2. Potentially helpful

a. To assess mediastinal injury

b. To assess pericardial injury

c. To treat lung and bronchial lacerations

d. To treat esophageal injury (rare)

III. CONTRAINDICATIONS

A. ABSOLUTE

1. Inability of patient to tolerate single-lung ventilation (rare). Intubated patients requiring high concentrations of inspired oxygen and positive

59

THORACOSCOPY

end-expiratory pressures and increased peak airway pressures should be excluded.
2. Fused lung
3. Shock or cardiac arrest
4. Hemodynamically unstable

B. RELATIVE
1. Patients with ipsilateral prior thoracotomy or history of extensive pleural disease
2. Coagulopathy

IV. TECHNIQUE

A. ANESTHESIA
1. General anesthesia with single-lung ventilation using double-lumen endotracheal tube or bronchial blocker mechanism incorporated into single-lumen endotracheal tube allowing for ipsilateral lung collapse
2. Position patient in lateral decubitus position as for posterolateral thoracotomy with appropriate padding of pressure points

B. EQUIPMENT
1. Visualization performed with the use of a 5-mm thoracoscope. Zero-degree scope typically used, but 30-degree-angled scope provides superior visualization of dome and lateral recesses of the diaphragm.
2. Standard endoscopic dissecting and retracting instruments are used. Specialized endoscopic staplers are available.
3. Be prepared for conversion to open thoracotomy.

C. POSITIONING
1. Patient placed in full lateral position and prepared for open thoracotomy
2. Upper arm should be elevated and prepped in a sterile manner.
3. Sterile skin preparation should extend posteriorly from the spine, the shoulder superiorly, the sternum medially, and iliac crest inferiorly.

D. INSTRUMENT AND CAMERA ORIENTATION
1. Inject proposed port sites with local anesthetic with epinephrine to decrease perioperative pain.
2. Placement of port sites depends on procedure performed. At least three ports are usually required for full exploration. Optimal position of the camera and accessory ports often described with reference to a baseball diamond. Camera site generally at "home plate" in 6th or 7th intercostal space between midaxillary lines vertically aligned with iliac crest. Area of interest is at "second base," and additional ports are at "first and third bases."
3. Do not place instruments too close to site of pathology.

V. COMPLICATIONS

A. GENERAL
1. Overall incidence of complications—10%
2. Need for conversion to open thoracotomy

B. SPECIFIC
1. Prolonged air leak—Most common complication
2. Respiratory failure
3. Wound infection
4. Bleeding
5. Arrhythmia

VI. FUTURE OF THORACOSCOPY

As minimally invasive surgical technology is introduced into the field of thoracic surgery, a renewed enthusiasm for VATS has developed. Many therapeutic procedures are able to address both benign and malignant disease safely and without lengthy hospital stays. Additionally, evidence is mounting to suggest that hospital charges for patients undergoing the VATS procedure are lower than those undergoing open thoracotomy. Improved instrumentation, three-dimensional reconstruction, and robotics will continue to broaden this procedure's application and improve patient care.

RECOMMENDED READINGS

Chan P, Clarke P, Daniel FJ, et al: Efficacy study of video-assisted thoracoscopic surgery pleurodesis for spontaneous pneumothorax. Ann Thorac Surg 71:452-454, 2001.

Daniel TM, Kern JA, Tribble CG, et al: Thoracoscopic surgery for diseases of the lung and pleura. Ann Surg 217:566-574, 1993.

Kaseda S, Aoki T, Hangai N, et al: Better pulmonary function and prognosis with video-assisted thoracic surgery than with thoracotomy. Ann Thorac Surg 70:1644-1646, 2000.

Landreneau RJ, Mack MJ, Dowling RD, et al: The role of thoracoscopy in lung cancer management. Chest 113(1 Suppl):6S-12S, 1998.

59

THORACOSCOPY

Renal Transplantation

Scott R. Johnson, MD

I. PATIENT SELECTION

A. QUALIFICATIONS
1. Criteria
a. End-stage renal disease (ESRD) from a variety of causes
b. Patient life expectancy longer than graft half-life
2. Absolute contraindications
a. Malignancy
b. Current infection
c. Hepatitis
d. HIV
3. Relative contraindications
a. History of noncompliance
b. Malnutrition
c. Severe cardiovascular disease
d. Substance abuse
e. High likelihood of recurrent renal disease

B. PATIENT EVALUATION
1. History and physical exam
a. Original disease, previous transplant history
b. Transfusion history
c. Cardiovascular history, claudication, angina
d. Urinary tract dysfunction; obstruction, benign prostatic hypertrophy, chronic pyelonephritis
e. Malignancy
f. Chronic obstructive pulmonary disease, asthma, smoking
g. Diabetes mellitus
h. Liver disease, jaundice, biliary colic
i. Alcohol or substance abuse
j. HIV positive
2. Pretransplant studies
a. Routine screening lab studies; renal, hepatic, complete blood cell count (CBC), coagulation screen, urinalysis, calcium, phosphorus, magnesium
b. Hepatitis screen, HIV, VDRL, viral titers (cytomegalovirus, Epstein-Barr virus [EBV], varicella), throat and urine cultures, tuberculin skin test
c. Chest radiograph, ECG
d. Blood typing, human leukocyte antigen (HLA), panel-reactive antibodies
3. Specific evaluations
a. Atherosclerosis—Dipyridamole thallium scan. Consider catheterization or coronary artery bypass graft.
b. Peptic ulcer disease—Esophagogastroduodenoscopy. Consider H_2 blockers or highly selective vagotomy.

60

c. Cholelithiasis—Cholecystectomy
d. Colonic disease—Barium enema, colonoscopy. Consider colectomy if diverticulosis present.
e. Voiding cystourethrogram

II. INDICATIONS

A. PRIMARY RENAL DISEASES
1. Focal and segmental glomerulosclerosis
a. Recurrence rate in graft—20-30%
b. High risk of recurrence in age <15 years, protracted malignant course from diagnosis to ESRD, or mesangial proliferation on biopsy
c. 40-50% of patients with recurrence lose the graft.
2. IgA nephropathy
a. Recurrence—50%
b. Up to 80% recurrence with living-related donor graft
c. Graft loss with recurrence—<10%.
3. Membranoproliferative glomerulonephritis (MPGN) type I
a. Recurrence—20-30%
b. Graft loss with recurrence—40%
4. MPGN type II
a. Recurrence—Up to 80%
b. Graft loss with recurrence—10-20%
5. Membranous glomerulonephritis
a. Recurrence is unusual—3-7%
b. Graft loss is rare.
6. Antiglomerular basement membrane disease
a. Histologic recurrence—50%
b. Clinical recurrence—25%
c. Graft loss is rare.

B. SYSTEMIC DISEASES
1. Systemic lupus erythematosus
a. Recurrence—<1%
b. May reflect burned-out disease when ESRD develops or use of immunosuppression
2. Hemolytic uremic syndrome
a. Recurrence—10-25%
b. Graft loss due to recurrence—50%
c. Risk factors for recurrence
   (1) Transplant <3 months from diagnosis
   (2) Use of antilymphocyte globulin (ALG) or muromonab CD-3 (OKT3)
3. Henoch-Schönlein purpura
a. Histologic recurrence—30% of adults and up to 75% of children
b. Clinical recurrence—<10%

c. Graft loss is rare.

4. Diabetes mellitus
a. Leading cause of ESRD leading to renal transplant
b. Histologic recurrence—Up to 100%
c. Graft loss due to diabetes mellitus—≈5%

5. Mixed cryoglobulinemia
a. Recurrence—≈50%
b. Graft loss may occur.

6. Multiple myeloma
a. Recurrence appears to be common.
b. Death due to underlying disease appears to precede graft loss.

7. Wegener's granulomatosis
a. Recurrence has been noted to occur in the graft.
b. Recurrence can be treated with cyclophosphamide and steroids.

8. Primary hyperoxaluria type I
a. Recurrence and graft loss are the usual clinical course.
b. Combined liver-kidney transplant provides the deficient enzyme and appears to be the therapy of choice.

9. Cystinosis
a. Recurrence histologically is common but graft dysfunction is unusual.
b. Cystine accumulation continues in other organ systems and leads to morbidity.

10. Fabry's disease—Recurrences have been reported.

11. Sickle cell disease

12. Progressive systemic sclerosis

13. Alport's syndrome
a. Defect in collagen assembly resulting in sensorineural deafness and renal dysfunction
b. Renal transplants have been performed with results matching those of controls.
c. Presence of new collagen antigen in graft has led to the development of anti-glomerular basement membrane disease in recipients, which may lead to graft loss.

III. DONOR SELECTION—ANTIGEN MATCHING

A. ABO ANTIGENS
1. Matching required for renal transplant, otherwise hyperacute rejection ensues
2. Isoagglutinins are present in sera of individuals to A or B antigens not present
3. Several successful A2 to O renal transplants have been performed.
4. ABO-incompatible transplants may be performed if isoagglutinins are removed by splenectomy and plasmapheresis.

60

RENAL TRANSPLANTATION

B. HLA CLASS I OR II ANTIGENS
1. Class I antigens consist of A, B, or C loci antigens located on the surface membranes of all nucleated cells.
2. Class II antigens consist of DP, DQ, and DR loci found primarily on immune, dendritic, and endothelial cells.

C. LIVING DONORS
1. "Six-antigen match, HLA identical" implies that both haplotypes for class I A and B loci and the DR loci of class II antigens are identical between donor and recipient.
2. Long-term graft survival in HLA-identical transplants—90%
3. As HLA antigen disparity increases and graft survival worsens, the use of cyclosporine and donor-specific transfusions improves the graft survival in HLA-disparate transplants.

D. CADAVERIC DONORS
1. HLA A and B antigen matching in cadaveric transplantation may provide a long-term benefit.
2. HLA-DR matching provides a greater benefit than class I antigen matching.
3. The use of cyclosporine-based regimens appears to be responsible for the success without strong antigen matching.

IV. TRANSPLANT PROCEDURE

A. DONOR NEPHRECTOMY
1. Left kidney is preferred due to longer renal vein and better access to arteries.
2. Oblique flank incision over the 12th rib from the rectus to the parasternal line
3. Muscle layers are divided, exposing the peritoneum, which is retracted, and Gerota's fascia is exposed.
4. Gerota's fascia is incised and the kidney is exposed. The ureter is followed to a point beyond the iliac vessels and divided. A cuff of areolar tissue surrounding the ureter is also removed to ensure a vascular supply.
5. The artery is divided at the aorta followed by the renal vein.
6. The kidney is flushed with preservation solution (UW or Euro-Collins), placed on ice, and transported to the recipient room.

B. TRANSPLANT
1. Oblique incision cranial to inguinal ligament—Muscles are divided, then the peritoneum is exposed and retracted medially to expose the iliac vessels.
2. Vascular anastomoses are performed as follows.
a. Renal artery to external iliac artery (end to side)

b. Renal artery to hypogastric artery (end to end)

c. Renal vein to external iliac vein (end to side)

d. Accessory renal arteries can be anastomosed end to side to the largest renal artery and then anastomosed to the recipient vessels. Usually done ex vivo on ice.

3. Ureteroneocystostomy

a. Requirements

(1) Tension-free repair

(2) Water-tight repair

(3) 1-cm submucosal tunnel to prevent reflux

b. Methods

(1) Leadbetter-Politano—Uses a transvesical approach. Bladder is entered and the distal donor ureter is sewn mucosa to mucosa from within the bladder.

(2) Litch-extravesical approach ureteropyelostomy—Recipient proximal ureter is anastomosed to the donor renal pelvis.

C. POSTOPERATIVE CARE

1. General postoperative care does not differ from that of the general surgical patient.

2. Beware of volume depletion due to post-transplant diuresis. This can be avoided by replacing urine output milliliter per milliliter q 4 h with IV fluid of similar electrolyte composition.

3. Sutures or wound clips are generally left in place for 21 days due to delayed wound healing in renal failure patients and immunosuppressed patients.

4. Foley catheters are left in place for 2-5 days postoperatively.

D. ASSESSMENT OF GRAFT FUNCTION

1. Urine output—Nonspecific, decreased urine output may indicate hypovolemia, urinary obstruction, ureteral compromise, vascular compromise, acute tubular necrosis, rejection

2. Creatinine (Cr) and BUN—As in section IV. D. 1, nonspecific

3. Ultrasound—Demonstrates patency of artery and vein, detects fluid collection and hydronephrosis

4. Radionucleotide imaging—Can image flow and function

5. Renal biopsy—May yield definitive pathologic diagnosis in cases of dysfunction; difficult to assess cyclosporine nephrotoxicity

V. IMMUNOSUPPRESSION

A. IMMUNOSUPPRESSIVE DRUGS

1. Azathioprine

a. Imidazole derivative of mercaptopurine

b. Inhibits lymphoid proliferation by blocking DNA/RNA synthesis

c. Initial dose—3-5 mg/kg and tapered to 1-3 mg/kg

60

RENAL TRANSPLANTATION

d. Complications—Leukopenia, nausea and vomiting, pancreatitis, hepatitis

2. Glucocorticoids
a. Inhibit interleukin (IL)-1 and IL-6 production by macrophages
b. High doses at induction and tapered to a maintenance dose
c. Complications—Cushing's disease, osteoporosis, cataracts, hyperlipidemia

3. Cyclosporine
a. Cyclic polypeptide
b. Prevents production of IL-2 by T-helper cells
c. Metabolized by hepatic cytochrome P-450, and levels are affected by many commonly prescribed medications
d. Complications—Renal toxicity, hypertension, tremors, paresthesia, hypertrichosis

4. Antithymocyte globulins
a. Minnesota antilymphocyte globulin (MALG), antithymocyte globulin (Atgam), ALG, rabbit antithymocyte serum (RATS)
b. Polyclonal sera to human lymphocytes/thymocytes produced in animals
c. Function to deplete these cells from the recipient (lysis or reticuloendothelial system uptake)
d. Complications—Fever, chills, anaphylaxis, serum sickness, and acute respiratory distress syndrome

5. Monoclonal antibodies (muromonab CD-3)
a. Murine monoclonal antibody to the pan T-cell receptor CD-3
b. Deplete CD-3 cells from circulation.
c. Complications—Fever, chills, pulmonary edema

6. FK-506 (Prograf)
a. Similar to cyclosporine
b. Also prevents IL-2 production by T-helper cells
c. Also metabolized by hepatic P-450 system
d. Complications are similar to cyclosporine, including nephrotoxicity and neurotoxicity.

B. THERAPEUTIC REGIMENS
1. Cyclosporine monotherapy—Cyclosporine alone
2. Cyclosporine dual therapy—Cyclosporine and glucocorticoids or azathioprine
3. Cyclosporine triple therapy—Cyclosporine, glucocorticoids, and azathioprine
4. Sequential therapy
a. Induction therapy with antilymphocyte preparation, azathioprine, and glucocorticoids
b. Cyclosporine administration is delayed until renal function improves
c. Allows recovery from preservation injury prior to cyclosporine introduction
d. Results in delayed time to first rejection and lower Cr level at 3 months

VI. REJECTION

A. HYPERACUTE REJECTION
1. Occurs promptly after revascularization of the graft
2. Due to presence of preformed antibodies—Repeated transfusions, pregnancy, previous transplants
3. Graft thrombosis follows, requiring transplant nephrectomy.
4. Usually identified by a positive crossmatch

B. ACCELERATED REJECTION
1. Occurs around day 3-5 post-transplant
2. Reflects recipient sensitization to donor
3. Can be treated with antilymphocyte preparations but represents a risk factor for graft loss

C. ACUTE REJECTION
1. Accounts for 85% of rejection episodes in first 3 months post-transplant
2. May be related to noncompliance or medications that reduce cyclosporine levels
3. Symptoms—Fever, malaise, oliguria, graft tenderness, elevated Cr
4. Treated with glucocorticoids and, if resistant, then antithymocyte preparations

D. CHRONIC REJECTION
1. Diagnosis is difficult; can be based on biopsy or Cr increase after 6 months
2. Biopsy demonstrates obliterative fibrosis of vasculature and tubules.
3. Risk factors for chronic rejection include acute rejection episodes, low cyclosporine dosage, and infection.
4. No effective therapy is currently available.

VII. COMPLICATIONS

A. SURGICAL COMPLICATIONS
1. Vascular complications
a. Renal artery thrombosis
   (1) Incidence—≈1%
   (2) Presents with a sudden decline in urine output
   (3) Diagnosis with ultrasound, technetium scan, angiogram
   (4) Emergent revascularization is mandatory to prevent graft loss.
   (5) Causes—Intimal dissection, kinking, hyperacute rejection, irreversible acute or accelerated rejection, and hypercoagulable states
b. Renal artery stenosis
   (1) Incidence—2-10%

60

RENAL TRANSPLANTATION

       (2) Presents with refractory hypertension, unexplained rise in Cr, or a change in graft bruit

       (3) Diagnosis with Doppler sonography or angiography

       (4) Management may include hypertension control, percutaneous transluminal angioplasty, resection and reanastomosis, or bypass graft

  c. Renal vein thrombosis

       (1) Incidence—0.3-4.2%

       (2) Symptoms—Oliguria, graft swelling and tenderness, hematuria

       (3) Diagnosis—Angiography, Doppler sonography, technetium scan

       (4) Attempts at thrombectomy are usually unsuccessful at salvaging the graft, but success with thrombolytics has been reported.

       (5) Causes include vessel kinking, compression due to hematoma, lymphocele, or urinoma.

  d. Hemorrhage

       (1) Rare occurrence

       (2) Often related to the development of a mycotic aneurysm

       (3) Nephrectomy is usually indicated.

2. Urinary tract complications

  a. Ureteral leakage

       (1) Incidence—3-10%

       (2) Related to ureteral ischemia, anastomotic tension

       (3) Usually in first month after transplant

       (4) Symptoms—Pain with graft swelling, fever, and sepsis

       (5) Urine fistula

          (a) Diagnosis

          (b) CT scan, ultrasonogram may demonstrate fluid collection

          (c) Nuclear renography is less sensitive.

       (6) Management

          (a) Percutaneous nephrostomy and stenting

          (b) Ureteroneocystostomy revision

          (c) Boari flap, donor-recipient pyeloureterostomy

  b. Ureteral obstruction

       (1) Most common urinary complication

       (2) Etiology includes hematoma, kinking, or edema.

       (3) Late-onset obstruction is related to fibrosis from ischemia.

       (4) Presentation depends on degree of obstruction.

       (5) Oliguria, elevated Cr, sepsis, anuria

       (6) Diagnosis by sonography, antegrade pyelography (most sensitive), renal venography (less sensitive)

       (7) Management

          (a) Percutaneous nephrostomy and surgical correction

          (b) Percutaneous transluminal dilation and stenting

  c. Urinary bladder

       (1) Occur early after transplant

       (2) Present with palpable mass, rise in Cr, pain in graft bed

(3) Usually related to extravasation from anterior cystotomy

(4) Diagnosis made with sonography (fluid collection), cystography

(5) Management—Exploration and primary repair with bladder decompression

3. Miscellaneous complications—Lymphoceles

a. Incidence—0.6-18%

b. Many are asymptomatic and eventually are resorbed; some present with mass effects (vascular compression), lymph fistula

c. Diagnosis is made with sonography (fluid collection).

d. Management

(1) Percutaneous drainage—High recurrence rate and potential for infection

(2) Intraperitoneal window permits lymph drainage into the peritoneal cavity.

B. MEDICAL COMPLICATIONS

1. Infections

a. General considerations

(1) Influenced by degree of immunosuppression

(2) 80% of transplant recipients develop infection.

(3) 40% of transplant deaths are due to infection.

b. 1st month

(1) Etiology related to surgical procedure

(2) Wound infections, urinary tract infection, infections related to indwelling catheters

(3) Pneumonia

(4) Also infections transmitted with graft (HIV, cytomegalovirus, hepatitis)

c. 1st-6th month—High mortality due to degree of immunosuppression. Viral infections are common.

d. >6 months—Risk is reduced due to reduced immunosuppression.

2. Malignancy

a. General considerations

(1) Immunosuppression predisposes to the development of malignancy.

(2) Incidence of de novo malignancy—1-16% in renal transplant recipients

b. Lymphoproliferative disease (LPD)

(1) Strong association with EBV infection

(2) Incidence in renal transplant recipients—1%

(3) 80% are non-Hodgkin's lymphomas

(4) B-cell origin

(5) Extranodal (graft and CNS are common)

(6) Usually appear in the first 4 months post-transplant

(7) Muromonab CD-3 appears to increase the risk of LPD.

(8) Reduction of immunosuppression is usually required.

60

RENAL TRANSPLANTATION

c. Skin cancer
   (1) Nonmelanoma forms predominate.
   (2) Squamous cell is most common.
   (3) More aggressive than in general population
   (4) Increased incidence of regional metastasis
   (5) Present about 5 years post-transplant
d. Cervical cancer
   (1) Third most common post-transplant malignancy
   (2) Herpes simplex virus type 2 and human papillomavirus have been implicated in pathogenesis.
   (3) Conventional therapy is appropriate.
   (4) Reduction of immunosuppression is not mandated.

Liver Transplantation

Amit D. Tevar, MD

I. GENERAL CONSIDERATIONS

A. HISTORY
1. 1967—Starzl performed the first successful liver transplant.
2. 1983—Venovenous bypass was introduced for use during anhepatic phase.
3. 1984—Broelsch and associates introduced the split-liver transplantation.

B. INDICATIONS AND LISTING PROCESS FOR TRANSPLANTATION
In order for a patient to be placed onto the waiting list, he or she must have a Child-Turcotte-Pugh score of 7 or greater. Organs in each geographic area are distributed by United Network for Organ Sharing (UNOS) based on the patient's MELD (model for end-stage liver disease) score. MELD score is based on the following.
> Creatinine
> Bilirubin
> International normalized ratio (INR)

C. SPECIFIC DISEASES NECESSITATING TRANSPLANTATION
1. Alcoholic cirrhosis—Most common etiology of liver failure in United States
2. Hepatitis—Virtually all patients with chronic hepatitis B or C ultimately become reinfected, with variable outcomes.
3. Acute fulminant hepatic failure—Secondary to drug toxicity, hepatitis, Wilson's disease, pregnancy, Budd-Chiari syndrome, mushroom intoxication, and others. Acetaminophen toxicity is the most common cause.
4. Inborn errors of metabolism—This category includes glycogen storage disease, Wilson's disease, α_1-antitrypsin deficiency, and protein S deficiency, among others.
5. Primary hepatic malignancy—Controversial indication, associated with high likelihood of recurrent disease

D. ORGAN SELECTION
In general, standard criteria apply, including a hemodynamically stable donor with no evidence of sepsis or non-CNS primary malignancy, and ABO compatibility.
1. Cadaveric whole organ
2. Cadaveric reduced-sized grafts—Full right, full left, or left lateral lobe graft. With a left lateral lobe, a size discrepancy of 10:1 can be overcome.
3. Living related liver donation—Increases the limited pool of pediatric-sized livers; graft and patient survival rates as high as 95%

II. SPECIFIC OPERATIVE CONSIDERATIONS

A. TRADITIONAL OPERATIVE TECHNIQUE (Fig. 61-1)

1. Bilateral subcostal incision with midline extension to xiphoid process
2. Mobilization of the native liver. Isolation of the suprahepatic and infrahepatic venae cavae. Skeletonization of the hilar structures: portal vein, bile duct, and hepatic artery.
3. Establishment of venous-venous bypass to decompress the splanchnic venous system; selectively used with intestinal edema, hypotension following test clamping of the vena cava, extensive portal hypertension bleeding, and difficult hepatectomy. Cannulas (percutaneous or cut-down) from the portal and femoral veins drain blood into the axillary vein.
4. Recipient hepatectomy
5. Vascular anastomoses—Suprahepatic vena cava, infrahepatic vena cava, hepatic artery, and portal vein

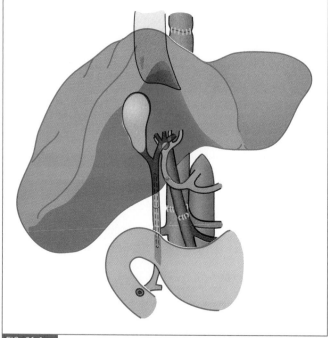

FIG. 61-1

Traditional hepatic transplantation.

6. Biliary anastomosis—End-to-end bile duct anastomosis or choledochojejunostomy
7. Abdominal fascial closure with nonabsorbable sutures

B. PIGGYBACK TECHNIQUE
1. Recipient hepatectomy altered to leave the recipient retrohepatic vena cava intact
2. Hilar dissection performed as in traditional technique
3. Recipient liver remains attached to vena cava only by hepatic veins
4. Recipient hepatectomy
5. Vascular anastomosis—Donor suprahepatic vena cava to recipient inferior vena cava in end-to-side fashion, donor infrahepatic vena cava ligated, hepatic artery and portal vein
6. Remainder of procedure done as in traditional technique

III. POSTOPERATIVE CONSIDERATIONS

A. POSTOPERATIVE CARE
1. Hemodynamic monitoring and resuscitation with the aid of pulmonary artery catheter
2. Ventilatory support often for 24 to 48 hours post-transplantation
3. Electrolyte management—Correction of glucose, calcium, potassium, magnesium, and phosphate are particularly important.
4. Infection surveillance and prophylaxis—Trimethoprim/ sulfamethoxazole, fluconazole, and ganciclovir
5. Immunosuppression—Protocols vary among institutions.
a. Anti-lymphocyte induction therapy available but has not been widely used
b. Calcineurin inhibitors remain the baseline postoperative immunosuppression. Prograf (FK506) (tacrolimus) is the most widely used agent. Renal toxicity is an important adverse effect.
c. Steroids are generally given as IV Solu-Medrol postoperatively, and patients are transitioned to oral prednisone as advancement of diet permits.
d. Mycophenolate mofetil (CellCept) is a commonly used third baseline immunosuppressive agent.

B. ASSESSMENT OF GRAFT FUNCTION
1. Routine laboratory tests—Transaminase levels, alkaline phosphatase, factor V level, serum bilirubin, and coagulation parameters are very nonspecific but are usually used to follow trends in graft function.
2. Radionuclide imaging can be used to assess hepatocellular function and continuity of biliary drainage.
3. Liver biopsy—Most specific for differentiating rejection from recurrent hepatitis, steatosis, ischemia, or other causes of graft dysfunction

C. COMPLICATIONS
1. Primary nonfunction—Has become relatively rare cause of graft dysfunction since the introduction of UW solution. Manifested by

failure to regain hepatic function in the early postoperative period. Urgent retransplantation is usually indicated.
2. Rejection—Occurs at some time in 60% of liver transplant patients. Diagnosis is made by biopsy of graft.
3. Hepatic artery thrombosis—Diagnosis is made by angiogram, after screening with ultrasound/Doppler examination
4. Portal vein thrombosis—Usually requires retransplantation but may respond to thrombolytic therapy. Less common than arterial complications.
5. Biliary complications—Manifested by fever and rising bilirubin and alkaline phosphatase levels; diagnosed by cholangiogram; biliary stricture managed by conversion to choledochojejunostomy or stent placement.
6. Vena caval obstruction
7. Renal dysfunction
8. Infection and immunosuppressive drug complications
9. Recurrence of native disease

D. RESULTS (2003 UNOS DATA[1])
1. Patient survival at 1 year—86%
2. Graft survival at 1 year—81%
3. Graft survival at 3 years—64%

REFERENCE

1. Cecka JM, Terasaki PI: The UNOS scientific renal transplant registry. United Network for Organ Sharing. Clin Transpl 1-18, 2003.

RECOMMENDED READINGS

Abecassis M, Blei A, Koffron A, et al: Liver transplantation. *In* Stuart FP, Abecassis MM, Kaufman DB (eds): Organ Transplantation, 12th ed. Georgetown, TX, Landes Bioscience, 2003, pp 205-243.

USTransplants.org. Scientific Registry of Transplant Recipients. Available at: http://www.ustransplant.org/. Accessed July 22, 2004.

Pancreas Transplantation

Donn H. Spight, MD

I. GENERAL CONSIDERATIONS

A. BACKGROUND
1. 1921—Banting and Best report the discovery of insulin.
2. 1966—Kelly and Lillehei perform the first pancreas transplant.
3. 1986—Corry and associates develop technique of urinary bladder diversion of exocrine secretions.
4. Today, >1000 pancreas transplants are performed yearly in the United States. 85% occur simultaneously with kidney transplant (simultaneous pancreas-kidney transplant [SPK]), 10% occur after kidney transplant (pancreas alone after kidney transplant [PAK]), and 5% occur alone (pancreas transplant alone [PTA]).

62

B. INDICATIONS FOR PANCREAS TRANSPLANTATION
Insulin-dependent diabetes mellitus (IDDM) is associated with increased risk of blindness (25 times), kidney disease (17 times), gangrene (20 times), and heart disease or stroke (2 times each) compared to nondiabetic patients. Pancreas transplant is performed in three categories of patients.
1. PAK—Patient with functioning renal transplant, to prevent the development of nephropathy in the transplanted kidney
2. SPK—Insulin-dependent diabetic with end-stage renal disease (ESRD) in need of simultaneous kidney-pancreas transplantation
3. PTA—Nonuremic, labile diabetic with hypoglycemic unawareness. Not as commonly performed. The risks of surgery and immunosuppression must be balanced against the likelihood of developing secondary complications of diabetes.

C. SPECIFIC INDICATIONS AND CONTRAINDICATIONS
1. IDDM documented by absence of circulating C peptide
2. Microalbuminuria with a creatinine clearance of <60 mL/min
3. Proteinuria with a projected dialysis requirement
4. Autonomic neuropathy
5. Retinopathy
6. Labile diabetes and failure of medical management
7. Absence of coronary artery disease
8. Absence of gangrene or ongoing sepsis
9. Age 18-50 years

D. ORGAN SELECTION
Most are performed from cadaveric donors. In addition to standard criteria for donor selection, specific contraindications to pancreas transplantation include the following.

1. Presence of diabetes mellitus
2. Chronic pancreatitis
3. Pancreatic damage secondary to trauma
4. History of alcohol abuse or relapsing pancreatitis (center-specific)

II. SPECIFIC OPERATIVE CONSIDERATIONS

A. OPERATIVE PROCEDURE (Fig. 62-1)

1. The recipient bed is prepared in the right iliac fossa.
2. Venous drainage is first established by portal vein–external iliac vein anastomosis.
3. Arterial inflow is determined by manner of donor harvest. With the whole graft, the celiac axis and superior mesenteric artery are preferentially removed together on an aortic patch that is anastomosed end to side to the recipient external iliac artery.
4. Management of exocrine secretions
   a. Diversion to the urinary bladder by anastomosis to second portion of duodenum, harvested en bloc with the pancreas. This most common technique is associated with the highest patient and graft survival and has the advantage of using urinary amylase to monitor graft function.
   b. Diversion into the bowel is more physiologic but is associated with fistula formation.
   c. Pancreatic duct occlusion with injectable synthetic polymer completely blocks exocrine secretion but can lead to severe inflammation and fibrosis.

B. POSTOPERATIVE CARE

1. Because vascular thrombosis is the most common cause of early graft loss, some form of perioperative anticoagulation is recommended. Suggested protocols include aspirin, systemic heparinization, and low-molecular-weight dextran.
2. Graft function can be monitored by urinary amylase levels and glucose homeostasis. Since 90% of the pancreas may be lost before glucose homeostasis is impaired, this is not very sensitive.
3. There is no reliable technique for the diagnosis of rejection. In the patient undergoing SPK, rejection is usually monitored by following serum creatinine levels. Rises in serum creatinine precede decrease in pancreatic exocrine function 90% of the time. Rejection demonstrated on biopsy of the renal allograft is also an indication of pancreatic rejection.
4. Immunosuppressive regimens vary, but most centers use induction with antilymphocyte globulin or muromonab CD-3 (OKT3) and maintenance with cyclosporine or FK506, prednisone, and azathioprine or mycophenolate mofetil. Rejection accounts for up to 32% of graft loss in the first year.
5. Radionuclide perfusion scans can be used to evaluate blood flow to the allograft.

62

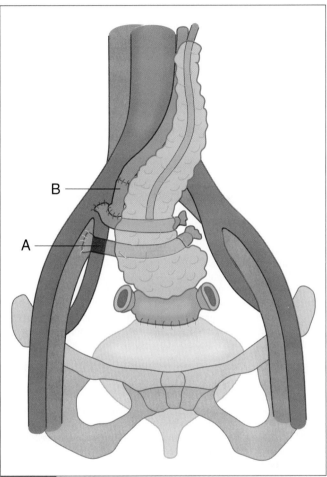

FIG. 62-1

Pancreas transplantation. A = venous anastomosis; B = arterial anastomosis.

C. COMPLICATIONS
1. Graft pancreatitis
a. Secondary to preservation injury and ischemia
b. Suggested by hyperamylasemia and local graft pain
c. May require drainage of peripancreatic collections or operative débridement of necrotic pancreas
2. Graft thrombosis

a. Most common cause of sudden early graft loss—10-20%

b. Attributed to the fact that the pancreas is a low-flow organ

c. If confirmed by radionuclide scan, the graft must be removed urgently to prevent septic or vascular complications.

3. Anastomotic failure

a. Presents with fever, leukocytosis, and drainage of clear fluid from the operative wound

b. Rare with bladder drainage of the exocrine pancreas, but can be fatal if not addressed early

4. Sepsis—Almost always related to the development of graft pancreatitis or anastomotic failure

5. Bleeding

a. Site is usually GI tract

b. Usually related to the use of anticoagulation in perioperative period

6. Peripheral hyperinsulinemia—Result of systemic venous delivery of insulin. Limited trials are under way to assess the viability of portal venous drainage.

D. RESULTS

1. Patient survival at 1 year—91%

2. Insulin independence at 1 year—SPK, 81%; PAK, 71%; PTA, 62%

3. Average graft survival at 3 years—65%

4. Insulin independence improves quality of life. Data support potential reversal of diabetic neuropathy, decreased recurrence of nephropathy in SPK for ESRD. Advanced, secondary diabetic complications such as retinopathy and vascular disease are unlikely to be improved.

III. ISLET CELL TRANSPLANTATION

A. BACKGROUND

1. Currently, PTA is performed rarely for diabetics with labile disease who fail to experience symptoms of life-threatening hypoglycemia.

2. PTA occurs less commonly than SPK and PAK due to the need for immunosuppression and high perioperative morbidity.

3. By isolating insulin-producing beta cells within the islets of Langerhans, organ transplantation may be obviated.

4. Enrollment in clinical trials is ongoing; however, it is limited by patient acceptance of low individual success compared with whole or partial organ transplant.

B. INDICATIONS

1. Autotransplantation after pancreatectomy for carcinoma or refractory pancreatitis

2. Allotransplantation in type I diabetics with hypoglycemic unawareness or inability to tolerate major transplant operation

C. TECHNIQUE

1. Pancreatic tissue obtained from pancreatectomy or cadaveric source is enzymatically digested.
2. Islet cells are extracted and purified via gradient separation.
3. Microencapsulation to decrease immunogenicity in allotransplant
4. Islet tissue infused into hepatic parenchyma via injection into portal vein
5. >300,000 islet cell equivalents required to attain insulin independence

D. RESULTS

Multiple challenges must be overcome before islet cell transplantation can become routinely successful. Paramount is the creation of an ideal microencapsulation vehicle that may ultimately facilitate further xenotransplantation efforts.

1. Insulin independence at 1 year—8-10%
2. 20% of patients obtain normal basal C peptide and improved glycemic regulation.

62

PANCREAS TRANSPLANTATION

The Hand

Jennifer L. Butterfield, MD

The first thing to do when evaluating any patient with a hand injury is to make sure that there are no serious or life-threatening problems that demand urgent attention. Once the patient has been found to be stable, a systematic examination of the patient's hand should be performed. After evaluating the hand, a decision should be made as to where to provide care, either in the emergency department or in the OR.

I. HAND EXAMINATION

A. HISTORY
1. Mechanism of injury—Laceration, crush, bite, and others
2. Time elapsed since injury or onset of infection
3. Associated injuries
4. Past medical history
5. Tetanus status
6. Hand dominance, preinjury function

B. PHYSICAL EXAMINATION
Because many hand injuries are work related or involve long-term disability, documentation of the injury is essential. To avoid confusion, standard terminology should be used. The hand has a dorsal and palmar surface and radial and ulnar borders (the terms *medial* and *lateral* are not used). The fingers have distal (DIP) and proximal (PIP) interphalangeal joints, whereas the thumb has a single interphalangeal joint (IP).

The components of a thorough examination include a vascular assessment, a neurologic assessment, and a motor assessment. Photographs should be taken if convenient.

1. **Vascular assessment**
a. Check for signs of arterial insufficiency—Pallor, pain, paresthesia, pulselessness
b. Assess brachial, radial, and ulnar pulses.
c. Assess capillary refill.

2. **Sensory assessment**
a. Assess radial, ulnar, and median nerves by their sensory distributions (Fig. 63-1).
b. Use pin-prick and two-point discrimination along longitudinal axis of each digit to rule out digital nerve injuries (should be no more than 6 mm distance at fingertip)
c. *Never* administer anesthetic before completing the sensory exam.

3. **Motor assessment**
The muscles that power the hand may be divided into extrinsic and intrinsic muscles. The extrinsic muscles have their muscle bellies

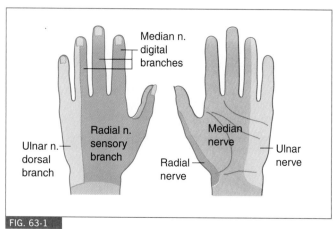

FIG. 63-1

Sensory areas of the left hand.

in the forearm and their tendon insertions in the hand. The intrinsic muscles have their origins and insertions in the hand.

a. Median nerve (Fig. 63-2)
   (1) Extrinsics
      (a) Wrist flexion with radial deviation—Flexor carpi radialis and palmaris longus
      (b) Wrist pronation—Pronator teres and pronator quadratus
      (c) Finger flexion at the PIP joints (flexor digitorum superficialis) and at the thumb IP joint (flexor pollicis longus) (Fig. 63-3)
      (d) Finger flexion at the DIP joints of 2nd and 3rd digits only (flexor digitorum profundus) (Fig. 63-4)
   (2) Intrinsics
      (a) Thumb opposition—Abductor pollicis brevis, flexor pollicis brevis, opponens pollicis (Fig. 63-5)
      (b) Finger flexion at metacarpophalangeal (MCP) joints of 2nd and 3rd digits only—Lumbricals
b. Ulnar nerve (Fig. 63-6)
   (1) Extrinsics
      (a) Wrist flexion with ulnar deviation—Flexor carpi ulnaris
      (b) Finger flexion at the DIP joints of ring and little fingers—Flexor digitorum profundus
   (2) Intrinsics
      (a) Ability to cross and abduct fingers (interossei) (Fig. 63-7)
      (b) Finger flexion at MCP joints of 4th and 5th digits only—Lumbricals
      (c) Adduction of the thumb—Adductor pollicis

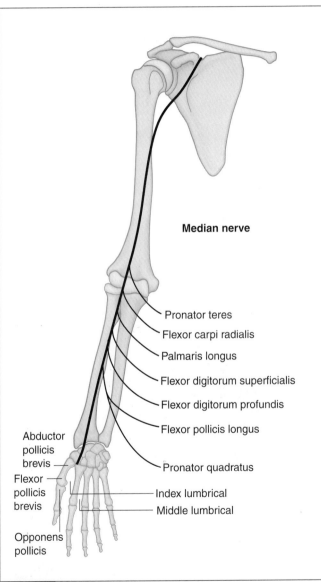

Median nerve

Pronator teres

Flexor carpi radialis

Palmaris longus

Flexor digitorum superficialis

Flexor digitorum profundis

Flexor pollicis longus

Pronator quadratus

Abductor pollicis brevis

Flexor pollicis brevis

Index lumbrical

Middle lumbrical

Opponens pollicis

FIG. 63-2

Motor distribution of the median nerve.

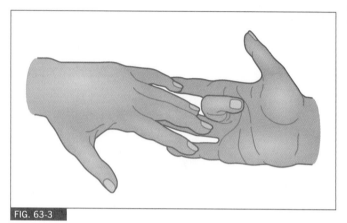

FIG. 63-3

Examination of the flexor digitorum superficialis.

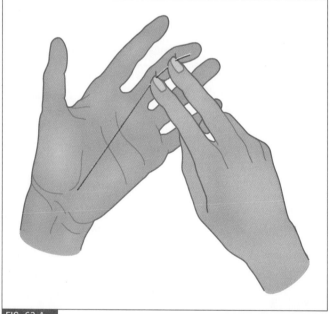

FIG. 63-4

Examination of the flexor digitorum profundus.

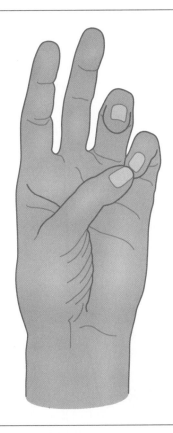

FIG. 63-5

Thumb opposition.

c. Radial nerve (Fig. 63-8)
   (1) The radial nerve innervates all of the finger and extensor muscles. There are no intrinsic extensor muscles.
      (a) Wrist extension—Extensor carpi radialis longus, extensor carpi radialis brevis, extensor carpi ulnaris
      (b) Finger extension—Test by having patient extend each finger independently. Extensor indicis proprius and extensor digiti minimi tendons can be tested by having patient make a fist and extending index and little finger independently (extensor indicis, extensor digitorum communis, extensor digiti minimi).
      (c) Thumb abduction—Abductor pollicis longus, extensor pollicis brevis, extensor pollicis longus

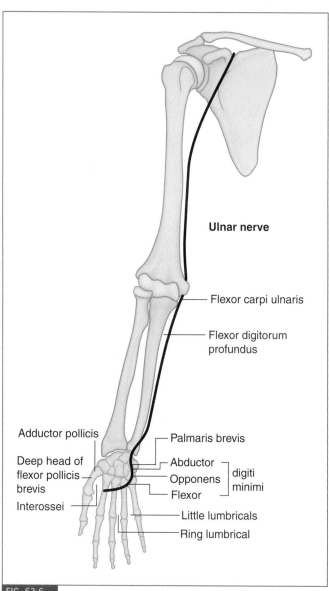

FIG. 63-6

Motor distribution of the ulnar nerve.

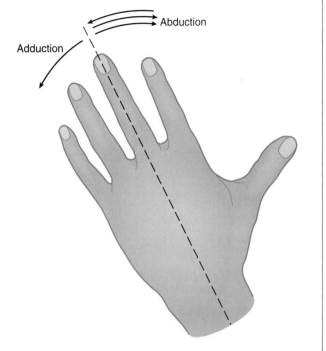

FIG. 63-7

Finger abduction.

C. DIAGNOSTIC TESTS

1. If there is *any* question about a foreign body, dislocation, or fracture, obtain radiographs. All injuries beyond the obviously superficial require radiographic examination.
2. Obtain anteroposterior, lateral, and oblique radiographs to avoid missing small fractures.
3. Beware of associated elbow and shoulder trauma, and obtain radiographs accordingly.

II. TREATMENT

A. DETERMINATION OF SITE OF CARE

1. The following can generally be handled in an emergency setting.

a. Superficial lacerations

b. Nail bed lacerations

c. Fingertip amputations

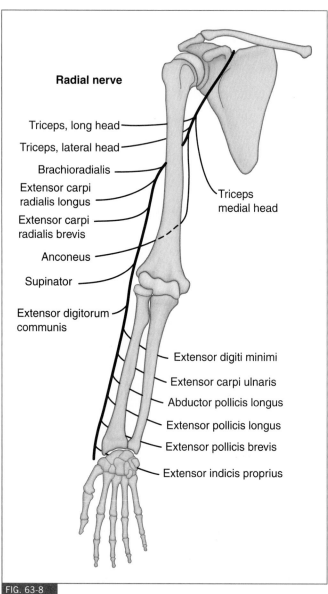

Radial nerve

Triceps, long head

Triceps, lateral head

Brachioradialis

Extensor carpi radialis longus

Extensor carpi radialis brevis

Anconeus

Supinator

Extensor digitorum communis

Triceps medial head

Extensor digiti minimi

Extensor carpi ulnaris

Abductor pollicis longus

Extensor pollicis longus

Extensor pollicis brevis

Extensor indicis proprius

FIG. 63-8

Motor distribution of the radial nerve.

d. Superficial foreign bodies

e. Closed fractures

f. Localized infections

2. The following should go to the OR.

a. Deep, extensive lacerations (e.g., from plate glass)

b. Open or irreducible fractures or dislocations

c. Vascular or nerve injuries. **Note:** *Never blindly clamp bleeding vessels.*

d. Major crush injuries

e. Deep infections

f. Proximal amputations

g. Compartment syndrome

B. GENERAL GUIDELINES FOR WOUND CARE

1. Irrigation and débridement of devitalized tissue

2. Control bleeding with pressure, and always elevate the extremity.

3. Antibiotics and tetanus prophylaxis as needed

4. Dressings and splints should be comfortable, conforming, and not circumferential.

5. In general, nonabsorbable monofilament sutures should be used for skin closure. The exception is in infants and children, in whom chromic sutures may be used to avoid the need for suture removal. Absorbable sutures are used for reapproximation of deeper tissues.

III. WOUNDS

A. PUNCTURE WOUNDS

1. Check for foreign body by radiography and exploration (if indicated).

2. Ellipse skin around wound to débride; avoid probing the wound

3. Leave open for drainage.

B. FLAP WOUNDS

1. Proximally based flaps usually have good blood supply. Distally based flaps have a greater risk of tip necrosis.

2. A flap sutured under tension is likely to become ischemic and should be allowed to retract and then should be sutured down.

C. AVULSED FLAP

1. May be sutured in place after defatting as a full-thickness skin graft

2. Usually does better with a formal split-thickness skin graft

D. FINGERTIP AVULSION

In young children, the avulsed tip may be defatted and sutured back on. Radiographs should be obtained to rule out epiphyseal plate injury.

However, in adults this injury requires surgical débridement and usually completion amputation.

E. BITE WOUNDS

1. Human or animal bites are prone to severe infection despite an innocuous appearance.
2. Most common pathogen—In human bites, *Eikenella corrodens;* in animal bites, *Pasteurella multocida;* both are sensitive to penicillin
3. Bites usually occur on the dorsal surface of MCP joints when due to punching in the mouth. Do not suture lacerations over MCP joints if human bite wound cannot be excluded.
4. Requires thorough wound débridement and irrigation
5. Leave wound open with wet dressing; splint and elevate
6. For human bites, admit patient for treatment with systemic antibiotics and hand soaks

F. NAIL BED INJURY

1. Drain subungual hematoma with needle-tip electrocautery. May need to remove nail plate if hematoma involves >30% of the matrix.
2. For a fractured nail or visible extension of laceration into matrix, remove loose nail and repair matrix with fine chromic suture and replace nail (with holes for drainage) as splint or pack edges of paronychia with nonadherent dressing.
3. Rule out growth plate injuries in children (see section V. B).

G. LACERATIONS

1. If the laceration is bleeding profusely, first try direct pressure for 10 to 15 minutes. Never blindly clamp in a bloody wound, because nerves are often closely associated with vessels and may be injured. If heavy bleeding persists, a blood pressure cuff can be used as a tourniquet (tourniquet pressure should be 100-150 mm Hg > systolic blood pressure) while waiting to go to the OR. The tourniquet should be released every 30 minutes.
2. Examine hand (see section I) to be sure that tendon and/or nerve injuries are not missed.
3. Knife lacerations generally cause less damage than glass. Glass tends to cause greater damage to underlying structures and may look deceptively superficial.

IV. INFECTIONS

Hand infections can have devastating sequelae if not treated properly. These infections require an aggressive approach of thorough débridement, irrigation, IV antibiotic, and splinting. Infections in diabetic patients are caused by mixed flora and require broad-spectrum antibiotics, e.g., amoxicillin (Augmentin) or ampicillin (Unasyn). Injuries that are treated in the emergency department require coverage only for gram-positive organisms, e.g., penicillin, erythromycin, oxacillin, or the cephalosporin groups. Immobilization is important in most hand injuries and infections. Most commonly the hand is splinted in the "position of safety," i.e., the wrist in dorsiflexion (30 degrees), the MCP joints at 70 degrees of flexion, the IP joints in full extension, and the thumb in abduction.

A. CELLULITIS
1. Presents with fever, swelling, lymphangitis
2. *Streptococcus* spp or *Staphylococcus* spp are the usual organisms.
3. Rule out a deep infection.
4. Treat with elevation and antibiotics.

B. PARONYCHIA
Paronychia is a localized infection at the base of the fingernail usually caused by nail biting or hangnails.
1. Clinical presentation consists of erythema, marked tenderness, and purulent drainage around the margins of the nail.
2. Treat with elevation of the nail fold. If this is inadequate therapy, then perform partial to total nail removal with antibiotics and nail elevation.
3. Bacteriology—*Staphylococcus* sp or mixed organisms
4. Chronic paronychia results from destruction of the nail matrix, usually as a result of infection. Nail fragments act as foreign bodies. Chronic drainage may be due to fungal infection or carcinoma.

C. FELON (DISTAL PULP SPACE INFECTION)
1. Tender, tense distal finger
2. Usually caused by *Staphylococcus aureus*
3. Treatment—Incision and drainage early; do not wait for fluctuance
4. Incise directly over the most superficial aspect of the infected area.
5. Late complications include osteomyelitis of the distal phalanx.

D. SUPPURATIVE TENOSYNOVITIS
1. Flexor tendon sheath infections are characterized by Kanavel's four cardinal signs.
a. Finger held in slight flexion
b. Finger uniformly swollen and red
c. Intense pain on passive extension
d. Tenderness to palpation along flexor sheath
2. Treat with incision and drainage of tendon sheath emergently in the OR; use antibiotics and elevation postoperatively.
3. If untreated, may spread to other tendon sheaths and the deep palmar space

E. HERPETIC INFECTIONS
1. Commonly found among health care personnel
2. Diagnosis is based on clinical findings of Tzanck smear of aspirate from vesicles. Immunofluorescent titers may be used for confirmation.

63

THE HAND

3. Clinical signs include erythema and painful swelling over the dorsum of affected fingers and the presence of small vesicles of clear fluid. Course usually is ≈2-3 weeks.

V. FRACTURES

Fractures of the bones of the hand are classified by the nature and site of the fracture line and whether the fracture is open or closed. An open fracture is one that communicates with the skin wound.

A. OPEN VS. CLOSED FRACTURES
1. Open fractures require irrigation and exploration of the wound and are a mandatory trip to the OR.
2. Closed fractures of the phalanges and metacarpals are treated conservatively in the emergency department with closed reduction and immobilization. The idea is to first block the digit with anesthetic, then exaggerate the deformity and manipulate the fragments back into anatomic alignment.
   Note: *Never use an epinephrine-containing local anesthetic in the hand.*

B. FRACTURES IN CHILDREN
1. The Salter classification system describes five types of growth (epiphyseal) plate injury in children.
2. Types I-III remodel well; however, types IV-V carry a poorer prognosis and may lead to shortening or angulation of the digit.

VI. DISLOCATIONS

The digit dislocates when it is subjected to significant deformational forces. The dislocation is named by the position of the distal segment in relation to the proximal segment. Most dislocations are reducible and may be either open or closed. In the presence of an open wound, the reduction should not be performed until the wound has been copiously irrigated (in the OR).

VII. TREATMENT OF THE PATIENT AND AMPUTATED PART FOR POSSIBLE REIMPLANTATION

Always obtain, at minimum, a phone consultation with a hand specialist prior to making any decisions regarding reimplantation.

A. STRONG CONTRAINDICATIONS
1. Associated injuries that make the patient too unstable for the prolonged initial reimplantation procedure and/or multiple subsequent procedures
2. Multilevel, crush, or degloving injury to the amputated part precluding functional recovery
3. Severe chronic illness

B. RELATIVE CONTRAINDICATIONS

1. Single-digit amputation, especially proximal to flexor digitorum superficialis insertion
2. Avulsion injuries, as evidenced by the following
a. Nerves and tendons dangling from the part
b. "Red streaks"—Bruising over the digital neurovascular bundles indicating vessel disruption
c. Previous injury or surgery to the part
d. Extreme contamination
e. Lengthy warm ischemia time—Applicable to macroreimplantation in which the part contains significant muscle mass
f. Age—Very advanced

C. HANDLING OF AN AMPUTATED PART

1. Cleanse gross debris with saline-moistened gauze.
2. Wrap in a moist saline sponge. Do *not* place directly in saline because desiccation and maceration of tissues will occur.
3. Place in plastic bag in iced-saline bath with several layers of gauze between the part and the ice.
4. Do *not* immerse part in ice or ice-cold saline—Freezing and thawing of cells can occur.

D. CARE OF THE PATIENT

1. Examine carefully for life-threatening associated injuries that can be overlooked, particularly in the macroreimplantation candidate.
2. Use direct pressure to control bleeding.

VIII. SUMMARY

Hand injuries are often associated with multiple other sites of injury, and it is essential that patients be evaluated for other life-threatening injuries (Advanced Trauma Life Support protocol). Once the patient is stable, a complete hand examination should be performed, including appropriate radiographs. After the examination, the site of care must be chosen and appropriate treatment instituted.

RECOMMENDED READINGS

Green DP: Operative Hand Surgery, 4th ed. New York, Churchill Livingstone, 1999.

Idler RS: The Hand: Examination and Diagnosis, 3rd ed. Philadelphia, Churchill Livingstone, 1990.

Lister G: The Hand: Diagnosis and Indications, 3rd ed. Edinburgh, Churchill Livingstone, 1993.

Masson JA: Hand: I. Fingernails, Infections, Tumors, and Soft-Tissue Reconstruction. Select Read Plast Surg 8(32):1-30, 1999.

Masson JA: Hand: III. Flexor Tendons. Select Read Plast Surg 8(34):1-40, 1999.

63

THE HAND

Masson JA: Hand: IV. Extensor Tendons, Rheumatoid Arthritis, and Dupuytren's Disease. Select Read Plast Surg 8(35):1-44, 1999.

Oishi SN: Hand: V. Fractures and Dislocations; The Wrist; and Congenital Anomalies. Select Read Plast Surg 8(36):1-35, 1999.

Rafols F, Orenstein H: Hand: II. Peripheral Nerves and Tendon Transfers. Select Read Plast Surg 8(33):1-46, 1999.

PART III

Procedures

Management of the Airway

Jefferson M. Lyons, MD

In the acutely injured or extremely ill patient, the ability to manage the airway correctly can be the difference between life and death. Although airway emergencies are not frequently encountered, all physicians should be adept at recognizing and initially treating them.

I. GENERAL PRINCIPLES

A. AIRWAY ASSESSMENT

1. **Is the airway patent, or is the airway compromised?**

a. Talking patients have a patent airway.

b. Compromise of the airway can be due to numerous reasons.
   (1) Complete or partial obstruction—Can be from an aspirated foreign body, vomitus, blood, extrinsic compression, or the tongue blocking the airway in an unconscious or sedated patient
   (2) Trauma—Tracheobronchial or bronchial disruption, fractured larynx, soft tissue edema secondary to significant facial and pharyngeal trauma, massive hematoma compressing the airway, or destruction of anatomy

2. **Patent airway—Must consider the patient's ability to maintain his or her airway**

a. If patient is able to maintain airway, proceed to assessment of breathing

b. If patient is unable to maintain airway, patient requires an artificial airway
   (1) Worsening mental status changes—CNS injury, oversedation, overdose, hypercarbia, hypoxemia, and others
   (2) Trauma—Increasing edema, hematoma, and loss of anatomy

3. **Nonpatent airway—Must establish a definitive airway to prevent impending death of the patient**

a. Obstruction—Must be relieved. Remove the foreign body either blindly or under direct visualization. Suction out vomitus, blood, and secretions. Remove foreign bodies with Magill forceps if visualized. Bypass the obstruction via a surgical airway if unable to remove it.

b. Trauma—Ultimately requires surgical repair, but a temporary, artificial airway is required

B. INDICATIONS FOR USE OF ARTIFICIAL AIRWAYS

1. **Absolute indications**

a. Inadequate ventilation
   (1) Apnea
   (2) Increasing $Paco_2$ (>50 mm Hg)

b. Inadequate oxygenation—Decreasing Pao_2 (<55 mm Hg on room air) unresponsive to supplemental O_2

c. Penetrating neck trauma with expanding hematoma

d. Acute airway obstruction

2. Strong relative indications

a. Inadequate airway protection—CNS disorders

b. Shock

c. Severe chest wall injury, e.g., flail segment, diaphragmatic rupture, open pneumothorax

d. Massive retroperitoneal hemorrhage

e. Severely injured, combative patient

3. Relative indications

a. Maxillofacial trauma

b. Pulmonary contusion

c. Inadequate pulmonary toilet

d. Augment work of breathing for patients with acutely elevated ventilatory workloads or decreased ventilatory capacity.

C. INITIAL MEASURES

1. Foreign body removal

a. Blind finger sweeps, Heimlich maneuver

b. Under direct visualization using Magill forceps or flexible bronchoscopy

2. Chin-lift, jaw-thrust—With in-line cervical traction for trauma patient

3. Oropharyngeal airway—Sized from corner of mouth to ear lobe; place in oropharynx by inserting with curve aimed superiorly and rotate into anatomic position after reaching posterior tongue

a. Relieves upper airway obstruction by elevating the base of the tongue off the posterior wall of the pharynx

b. May prevent inadvertent laceration of the tongue in the incoherent or seizing patient

c. Poorly tolerated in alert patient due to gag reflex

d. Can be used as a bite block with oral endotracheal tube

4. Nasopharyngeal airway—Lubricate and insert into the naris with bevel toward the septum and advance toward the lateral nasopharynx, allowing airway to slide into anatomic position

a. Used to relieve upper airway obstruction caused by tongue or soft palate falling against posterior wall of the pharynx

b. Suctioning via this airway is less traumatic than nasal suctioning.

c. Better tolerated than oropharyngeal airway

d. Alternate every 24 hours between right and left nares to minimize sinusitis, otitis media, and nasal necrosis

e. Avoid if coagulopathy present

II. DEFINITIVE AIRWAYS

A. ENDOTRACHEAL INTUBATION

1. Methods

a. Orotracheal intubation

    (1) Primarily for unconscious or anesthetized patients

    (2) Passed orally using direct laryngoscopy

    (3) Advantages—Rapid introduction, can accommodate larger endotracheal tube

    (4) Disadvantages—Patient discomfort, easily dislodged

b. Nasotracheal intubation

    (1) Passed via nasopharynx blindly or with laryngoscopy; more difficult to place

    (2) Method of choice in trauma patients with possible cervical spine injury

    (3) Advantages—Better tolerated, easier stabilization

    (4) Complications—Same as nasopharyngeal airway

2. Technique

a. Preparation

    (1) Obtain consent if patient's condition allows

    (2) Equipment—Ambu bag, laryngoscope, endotracheal tubes (various sizes), 10-mL syringe, lubricant, tube stylet placed in tube of choice, and anesthetic spray. Do not attempt endotracheal intubation without adequate suction set-up.

    (3) Select tube size (rule of thumb)—In adults, the diameter of fifth digit approximates tube size (usually 7-8). Tube size of ≥ 8 facilitates bronchoscopy.

        (a) 7.5 ID is an adequate size for most females.

        (b) 8 ID is adequate size for most males.

b. Orotracheal intubation

    (1) Preoxygenate patient with mask ventilation of 100% O_2 while monitoring oxygen saturation and arranging equipment

    (2) Place in sniffing position (neck flexed, head extended)—Contraindicated in patients with possible cervical spine injury

    (3) Anesthetize posterior pharynx with spray (time permitting)

    (4) Open mouth widely using crossed-finger technique with the right hand (thumb on lower incisors, index finger on upper incisors)

    (5) Insert laryngoscope using left hand in right-hand corner of mouth and advance, sweeping the tongue to the left

    (6) Have assistant apply cricoid pressure (Sellick's maneuver), especially in emergent intubation. Do not release until tube is in place and balloon is inflated, because aspiration risk is high.

    (7) When the epiglottis is visualized, the tip of the laryngoscope is placed above (for curved laryngoscope blades) or below (for straight blades) the epiglottis (Figs. 64-1 to 64-3)

        (a) Macintosh blades (curved blades)—The tip of the laryngoscope is placed superior to the epiglottis in the vallecula.

        (b) Miller blades (straight blades)—The tip of the laryngoscope is placed inferior to the epiglottis, actually lifting the epiglottis.

    (8) Operator lifts the laryngoscope by straightening the left arm to visualize cords. Take care not to tilt the laryngoscope back using the teeth as a fulcrum.

64

MANAGEMENT OF THE AIRWAY

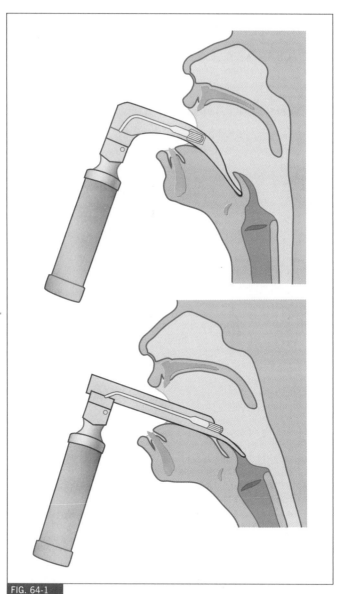

FIG. 64-1
Curved-blade (top) vs. straight-blade (bottom) laryngoscopy positioning.

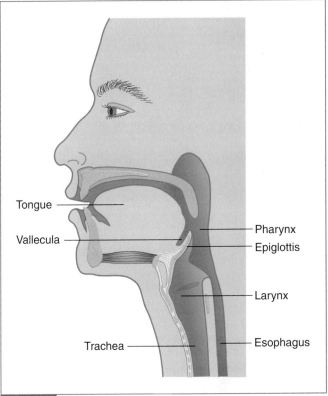

Tongue

Vallecula

Trachea

Pharynx

Epiglottis

Larynx

Esophagus

64

MANAGEMENT OF THE AIRWAY

FIG. 64-2

Cervical anatomy (sagittal view).

      (a) Pharynx may require suctioning for adequate visualization of cords. Suctioning should take no longer than 5 seconds.

      (b) Insert tracheal tube under direct vision *through* vocal cords. Time insertion with patient's inhalation. Inflate balloon with 3-4 mL air (see Figs. 64-2 and 64-3). After 15-30 seconds, if unsuccessful, remove laryngoscope and return to step (a).

c. Postintubation

    (1) Check for adequate and symmetrical ventilation by inspection and auscultation of the chest.

    (2) If cuff is present, inflate with minimal amount of air that will prevent leakage during ventilation. Cuff pressures ideally should be maintained at <20 mm Hg to prevent tracheal necrosis.

    (3) Secure tube with adhesive or tracheostomy tape

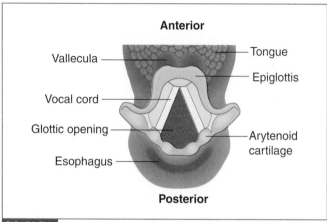

FIG. 64-3

Anatomy during direct laryngoscopy.

    (4) Check tube position by chest radiograph.
    (5) After 10-20 minutes, obtain arterial blood gas and adjust ventilator accordingly.
  d. Nasotracheal intubation
    (1) The patient should be breathing spontaneously for blind placement.
    (2) Should not be attempted in patients with suspected basilar skull fractures because intubation of the cranial vault is a devastating complication
    (3) Prepare and position patient as for orotracheal intubation
    (4) Anesthetize nasal mucosa with cocaine or lidocaine and small dose of phenylephrine for anesthesia and vasoconstriction to avoid epistaxis (time permitting)
    (5) Preoxygenate the patient.
    (6) Gently advance the tube through well-lubricated nares, going cephalad from nostril (to avoid the large inferior turbinate) and then posterior and caudad into the nasopharynx. Rotate the tube to facilitate passage.
    (7) Listen for patient breath sounds *through* the nasotracheal tube. Visualize mist from patient's exhalation in tube. Gently advance tube into trachea, during inspiration.
    (8) If unable to pass the tube, use laryngoscope and Magill forceps to introduce nasotracheal tube into the larynx under direct vision
    (9) Follow postintubation procedures as for orotracheal intubation.
3. Complications of intubation
a. Aspiration during attempted intubation

b. Malposition—Esophageal intubation, extubation, endobronchial intubation. Most common lethal error is esophageal placement; most common malposition is intubation of the right main stem bronchus.

c. Tube obstruction—Kinking, compression, foreign body, and secretions

d. Traumatic intubation, tracheal erosion due to long-term intubation

e. Tracheoesophageal fistula—Results from tracheal ischemia due to excessive cuff pressure

f. Spinal cord injuries from hyperextension of neck in patients with unstable cervical spine

g. If any question about tube placement, tube patency, or tube obstruction, remove tube and reintubate

B. CRICOTHYROTOMY

1. Definition—Surgical transtracheal intubation through the cricothyroid membrane

2. Indications—Urgent need for airway in a patient who cannot be intubated nasally or orally

3. Technique

a. Palpate thyroid and cricoid cartilage to define anatomy and identify cricothyroid membrane (Fig. 64-4).

b. Make a vertical midline incision and expose cricothyroid membrane. If no scalpel is available, a 14-gauge IV catheter attached to oxygen source may provide temporary oxygenation.

   Note: *Prolonged ventilation via the small catheter results in hypercarbia due to inadequate exhalation of CO_2.*

c. Incise cricothyroid membrane with scalpel (horizontal incision) and enlarge ostomy by turning scalpel handle 90 degrees

d. Insert appropriate size (usually 6 or 7 mm ID) tracheostomy or endotracheal tube through ostomy into the trachea

e. Check tube position by auscultation and obtain chest radiograph to confirm position

f. Consider converting cricothyrotomy to formal tracheostomy or endotracheal intubation when patient's condition allows. This should be performed within 24 hours due to risk of inadvertent loss of airway.

4. Complications

a. Early—Hemorrhage, creation of false passage, subcutaneous emphysema, perforation of esophagus, and mediastinal emphysema

b. Late—Tracheal stenosis, especially in pediatric age group. Consider converting to formal tracheostomy early in children.

C. TRACHEOSTOMY

1. Definition—Operative placement of an artificial airway through the anterior portion of the 2nd or 3rd tracheal ring

a. Techniques

   (1) Open operative procedure—Standard of care, minimal complication rate

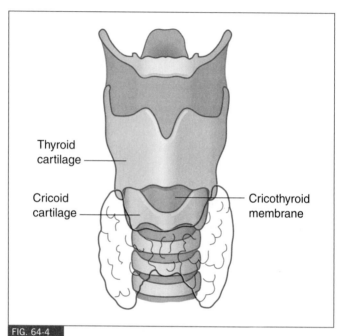

Anatomy of cricothyroid membrane.

    (2) Percutaneous tracheostomy—Newer technique; does not require OR (no travel); inexpensive, rapid, and comparable to open method for complication rate; has also been described to cause greater trauma to the airway and tracheal disruption

2. Indications

a. Perform electively (head and neck surgical patients) when operative procedure in upper airway may cause airway compromise.

b. Prolonged intubation

    (1) Tracheostomy is indicated if the patient remains intubated for 2-3 weeks. Tracheostomy should be postponed if high levels of positive end-expiratory pressure (PEEP) are required.

    (2) Early tracheostomy (<7 days of mechanical ventilation) is associated with shorter ICU stay and decreased hospital stay, duration of mechanical ventilation, and incidence of pneumonia.

    (3) Tracheostomy provides better patient comfort and mobility.

c. Upper airway obstruction

    (1) Not recommended for emergent airway control; better accomplished by a cricothyrotomy

(2) Anticipated obstruction or inability to perform elective intubation—A large goiter, pharyngeal or neck mass causing tracheal compression, laryngeal tumor, previous head and neck irradiation, and others

3. Complications

a. Hemorrhage—Early bleeding due to inadequate hemostasis usually managed with direct pressure. Late hemorrhage from erosion into major vessel, usually innominate artery. Temporary control of tracheoinnominate fistula can be obtained by placing a finger into the trachea through the tracheostomy incision and compressing the innominate artery against sternum while patient is returned to OR for emergent ligation via median sternotomy.

b. Pneumothorax, pneumomediastinum, and pneumoperitoneum

c. Accidental extubation—In the early postoperative period, it may be difficult to replace the tracheostomy tube since a mature tract has not yet developed. It is often preferable to place an oral endotracheal tube until the situation is stabilized. Intraoperative placement of "tag" sutures in the trachea facilitates replacement. Replacement may be facilitated by passing a small red rubber catheter through the skin incision into the trachea as a guide.

Note: *A clamp or a tracheostomy spreader can be used to hold soft tissues apart to allow air exchange.*

d. Tube malposition—Insertion into bronchi or mediastinum may occur. Confirm position with chest radiograph.

e. Obstruction—Foreign body, blood, inspissated secretions, and floppy cuffs

f. Swallowing dysfunction—Resolves with removal of tube or deflation of cuff

g. Tracheoesophageal fistula—Incidence as high as 0.5%, results from tracheal ischemia due to pressure from tracheostomy tube and cuff

h. Tracheomalacia—Due to cuff overinflation and high PEEP

i. In the obese patient, a standard tracheostomy tube becomes displaced into the pretracheal soft tissues. A spiral-flexible endotracheal tube (Anode tube) or custom-length tracheostomy tube may be required.

64

MANAGEMENT OF THE AIRWAY

III. INTUBATION METHODS

A. DIFFICULT INTUBATION

1. Patients known to be a difficult intubation should have anesthesia staff present for elective and emergent intubations.

2. Reasons can be acquired or congenital.

a. Congenital—Anatomic derangement, e.g., Treacher-Collins syndrome, micrognathia, anterior larynx, tracheoesophageal fistula, and spinal abnormalities

b. Acquired—Airway trauma, cervical spine injury, osteoarthritis, spinal fusion, and obesity

3. There must be a plan as to the sequence of alternative methods (i.e., bronchoscopy) to use in case standard techniques are unsuccessful. Have this equipment handy and ready to use.
4. Would have a tracheostomy tray at the bedside in case need for an emergent surgical airway arises
5. In elective intubations, if the patient is able to be ventilated with an Ambu bag and attempts are futile, then reverse induction agents and allow patient to breathe spontaneously.

B. ALTERNATIVE METHODS FOR INTUBATION

1. Digital intubation—Most efficacious in children because the distance from the epiglottis to the base of the tongue is shorter
   a. Place a bite block to prevent injury to finger, and insert gloved finger, most often middle, into posterior pharynx
   b. Palpate epiglottis and elevate it to expose the cords
   c. Slide endotracheal tube down finger as a guide into the trachea
   d. Check position and inflate balloon
2. Digital intubation with lighted stylet—Same technique as without, but lighted stylet allows transcutaneous visualization of placement
3. Laryngeal mask airway—Fits over the glottis and balloon fills dead space, allowing ventilation
4. Combitube—Airway composed of two tubes and is inserted blindly into oropharynx. If esophagus is intubated, may ventilate through esophageal lumen that is occluded distally, allowing tidal volumes to ventilate patient; if endotracheal intubation, may ventilate through tracheal tube just like endotracheal tube.
5. Percutaneous intubation—Percutaneously cannulate the trachea and using Seldinger technique, advance wire into oropharynx, use wire as a guide to insert endotracheal tube
6. Fiberoptic bronchoscopy—Place endotracheal tube over bronch, and then insert bronch past the cords. Slide endotracheal tube into place.

C. RAPID-SEQUENCE INDUCTION

1. Pharmacotherapy—Technique of sedating and paralyzing a patient to emergently place a definitive airway; numerous agents may be used, but usually an induction agent plus a neuromuscular blocker (NMB)
   a. Induction agents—Mainly used to place a patient in a state of sedation to allow airway placement
      (1) Barbiturates, e.g., thiopental—Act mainly on γ-aminobutyric acid receptors that cause a rapid depression of CNS activity
          (a) Rapidly equilibrate in the blood, allowing rapid onset, and are lipid soluble, so offset is also rapid and drug is redistributed to adipose tissue
          (b) Single dose of thiopental is 3 mg/kg—Causes loss of consciousness in ≈30 seconds, action peaks at 1 minute with a clinical duration of 5-8 minutes

       (c) Potent venodilators and negative inotropes. Use caution in patients with poor cardiac reserve or those who are hypotensive.

       (d) Thiopental causes histamine release. Avoid use in asthmatics.

   (2) Etomidate—Imidazole derivative with action similar to thiopental

       (a) Rapid onset, rapid peak, and brief duration

       (b) Has remarkable hemodynamic stability; drug of choice in hypotensive patients or those with poor cardiac reserve

       (c) Induction dose—0.3 mg/kg rapid IV push

       (d) Decreases intracranial pressure without dropping mean arterial pressure, making it an excellent choice for patients with head trauma

       (e) Has been shown to decrease cortisol activity after repetitive doses or infusion; not common after single dose

   (3) Benzodiazepines, e.g., midazolam—Similar to thiopental with rapid onset, peak, and duration

       (a) Loss of consciousness in ≈30-35 seconds with a 10-15 minute duration

       (b) Negative inotrope. Use caution with hypotensive or unstable patients.

       (c) Induction dose—0.1-0.3 mg/kg rapid IV push

   (4) Ketamine—Serves as an induction agent, paralytic, amnestic, and analgesic

       (a) Induction dose—1-2 mg/kg

       (b) Loss of consciousness in ≈30 seconds, peaks at 1 minute, duration of 10-15 minutes

       (c) Dissociative anesthetic causing a cataleptic state, provides profound analgesia

       (d) Provides great hemodynamic stability during induction, so good for tenuous patients

       (e) Causes bronchodilation and does not release histamine, so good agent for asthmatics

       (f) Major drawback—Causes hypnogogic (frightening) dreams, most often in the first 3 hours of use, which can be alleviated by pretreating with amnestic agents such as lorazepam (Ativan) or diazepam (Valium)

b. NMBs—Functionally paralyze patient to allow ease of intubation

   (1) Depolarizing agents—Compete with acetylcholine for receptor at motor endplate, causing depolarization and functional paralysis by preventing repolarization; only one in use is succinylcholine

       (a) Succinylcholine—Combination of two molecules of acetylcholine that is rapidly hydrolyzed by pseudocholinesterase in the circulation prior to reaching the motor endplate, which renders it a weak NMB

       (b) Maintains its activity until it diffuses out of motor endplate, i.e., no degradation at the endplate, so no reversal agent available

64

MANAGEMENT OF THE AIRWAY

(c) Activity is increased by states that decrease pseudocholinesterase activity, i.e., pregnancy, liver disease, cancer, and drugs such as metoclopramide (Reglan), which are cholinesterase inhibitors.

(d) Pseudocholinesterase deficiency—Genetic condition such that patient cannot degrade succinylcholine, thus delivering massive amounts to the endplate and potentiating its effect.

(e) Intubation level paralysis achieved in 1 minute, duration of 6-10 minutes, but patient may recover spontaneous respirations in ≈3 minutes

(f) Weak inotrope and chronotrope, with most common muscarinic side effect of bradycardia, which may be prevented with atropine prior to dose

(g) Has been associated with inducing ventricular fibrillation rarely

(h) Causes fasciculations, which may increase intracranial, intragastric, and intraocular pressures. Can be alleviated by a defasciculating dose of a nondepolarizing NMB.

(i) Exacerbates hyperkalemia associated with major crush injury, burns, and denervation syndromes

(j) Malignant hyperthermia has been shown to be related to succinylcholine's use; presents with rapid increase in temperature and rhabdomyolysis. Treat with hydration, diuretics, and dantrolene.

(2) Nondepolarizing NMBs—Pancuronium, vecuronium, and others

(a) Competitively inhibit the acetylcholine receptor at the motor endplate

(b) May be reversed with acetylcholinesterase inhibitors

(c) Older agents with slower onset and longer duration, newer agents being designed to work more quickly and have shorter half-life

(d) May be used in rapid-sequence intubation or as defasciculating agent for succinylcholine

2. Technique

a. Preparation—Important to have everything ready to handle all situations. Must have a plan as to choice and sequence of anesthetic agents, choice of tube size, and choice of equipment and technique for intubation. All monitors should be in place prior to induction including ECG, noninvasive blood pressure, and pulse oximetry. It is important to have adequate IV access and suction ready as well. It is preferential to preoxygenate patient with 100% O_2 while preparations are being made. This allows up to a 3-minute window of apnea before oxygen saturations begin to fall below 90% and ventilation is required.

b. Induction—Any pretreatments may be given prior to start of induction, i.e., defasciculating dose of NMB, lidocaine to prevent increased intracranial pressure, or β blocker to blunt sympathoadrenal response

(1) Administer induction agent of choice and immediately follow with NMB, usually succinylcholine.

(2) As patient loses consciousness, apply cricoid pressure (Sellick's maneuver) to prevent aspiration. If vomiting occurs, release cricoid pressure to prevent esophageal rupture and suction oropharynx, as patient is log-rolled to protect airway and clear airway of secretions. Once NMB takes effect, the patient will not functionally be able to vomit.

(3) Intubate patient with method of choice; confirm tube position with end-tidal CO_2 or auscultation.

(4) Secure airway and ventilate patient.

c. Postintubation—Chest radiograph to confirm position, sedation to keep patient comfortable on ventilator

Tube Thoracostomy

Lawrence E. Stern, MD

Tube thoracostomy is the insertion of a tube into the pleural space through a small incision.

I. DRAINAGE APPARATUS

A. THREE-BOTTLE SYSTEM (Fig. 65-1)
1. Bottle 1 (trap)—Pleural fluid collects in this bottle.
2. Bottle 2 (seal)—Positive intrapleural pressure forces air to pass through the water; however, air cannot reenter due to the "water seal."

3. Bottle 3 (suction)—Suction is regulated by the distance of the tube below the surface of the water (i.e., suction of −20 cm H_2O is achieved by placing the tip 20 cm below the water surface).
   Note: *The wall regulator should never be used to set the intensity of canister suction.*
4. Water seal is achieved by disconnecting bottle 3 from bottle 2 and leaving the short tube of bottle 2 open to the atmosphere.
5. Never close the system (i.e., turn off the wall suction and leave the system connected)—Analogous to clamping a chest tube

B. COMMERCIAL DRAINAGE SYSTEMS
Commercial drainage systems are equivalent to the bottles of the three-bottle system. Newer "dry" systems do not require water to set the suction intensity. Always have a drainage device set up prior to chest tube insertion.

II. CHEST TUBE INSERTION

A. INDICATIONS
Indications for tube thoracostomy include pneumothorax, hemothorax, pleural effusion, and instillation of intrapleural sclerosing agents.
1. Anticipated need helps determine the size of the thoracostomy tube.
a. Suspected hemothorax or empyema—Larger chest tubes (32-36 Fr)
b. Simple pneumothoraces or malignant pleural effusions—Smaller chest tubes (20-28 Fr)
2. Tube positioning
a. Pneumothoraces are best drained with a tube directed anteriorly and toward the apex.
b. Effusions are best drained with a tube directed posteriorly.
3. Tension pneumothorax should be decompressed by placement of a ≥16-gauge angiocatheter into the 2nd intercostal space at the midclavicular line prior to placement of a chest tube.

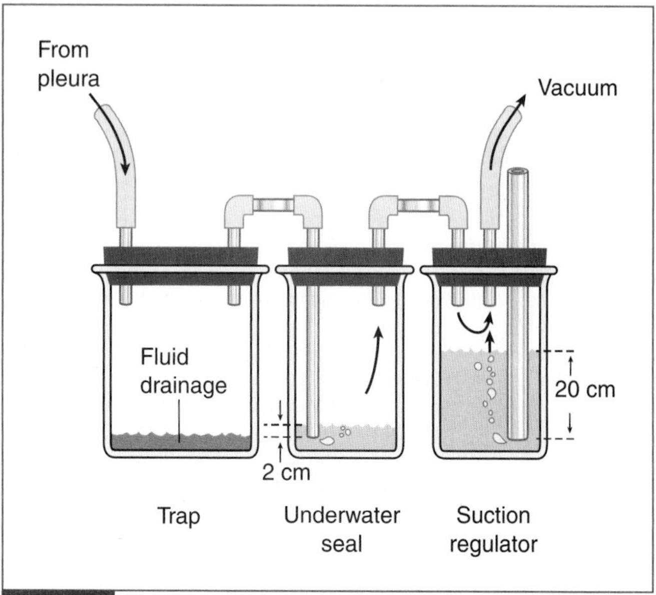

FIG. 65-1
Three-bottle drainage system.

B. TECHNIQUE

1. Position the patient by placing a folded towel beneath the scapula and abducting the arm, with the hand placed behind the head. A soft wrist restraint may be necessary to steady the arm in the proper position.
2. Chest tube placement should be as painless as possible. Sedation can be achieved with a combination of parenteral narcotics and benzodiazepines. Oxygen saturation should be monitored when employing conscious sedation.
3. Using sterile technique, prepare a wide operative field with bactericidal solution. When applying sterile drapes, be sure to leave landmarks exposed (i.e., nipple, scapula, costal margin).
4. Choose insertion site—Typically, a chest tube is inserted through the 4th or 5th intercostal space at the anterior axillary line. This position may need to be modified in certain circumstances (i.e., prior chest tube insertion, loculated effusion). In women, placement through breast tissue should be avoided whenever possible.
5. The incision will be placed at least one intercostal space below the planned level of insertion; therefore, infiltrate a wide area of skin and subcutaneous tissue over this site with local anesthetic.
6. Advance the needle to the rib below the planned insertion site and anesthetize the periosteum. Place the needle through the intercostal

space superior to the rib, thereby avoiding the neurovascular bundle, until the pleural space is entered. Aspiration of air or fluid confirms entry into the pleural space. Slowly withdraw the needle until it is out of the pleural space, then inject local anesthetic (10-20 mL) to provide pleural anesthesia.

7. Once adequate anesthetic has been infiltrated, make a skin incision large enough to admit the index finger.
8. Place a heavy suture (2-0 silk) through the center of the incision— This is used to secure the chest tube and to close the skin following chest tube removal.
9. Using a Kelly clamp, tunnel over the lower rib and into the intercostal space. Spread the intercostal muscles to the level of the pleura (Fig. 65-2).

   Note: *Stay on top of the rib to avoid damage to the neurovascular bundle.*
10. Once the pleura is reached, close the clamp and carefully push the tip through the pleura into the pleural space. A rush of air, blood, or other pleural fluid usually is encountered.

65

TUBE THORACOSTOMY

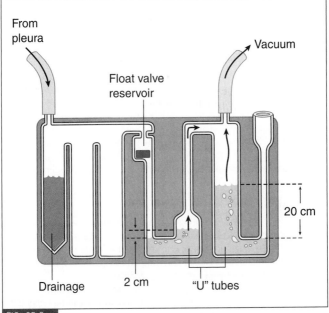

FIG. 65-2

Technique for chest tube insertion.

11. Spread the jaws of the clamp to create a passage large enough to admit the index finger. Insert the index finger into the pleural space and check for adhesions. The lung should be palpable during inspiration, confirming entrance into the pleural cavity.

12. Place one Kelly clamp on the end of the tube (to prevent spraying of pleural fluid) and grasp the chest tube at the tip with a second Kelly clamp. Guide the tube into the pleural space. Using the tip of the Kelly, direct the chest tube apically and either anterior or posterior (see section II. A. 2). The tube should be inserted to the level of the apex but should never be advanced against resistance.

    Note: *Ensure that the last hole in the chest tube (always located on the radiopaque marker line) is within the pleural cavity.*

13. Cinch the suture to the skin (do not tie a knot), thereby minimizing the gap around the chest tube. Tightly wrap the suture around the chest tube (leave adequate suture length for later usage), and tie the suture to the chest tube.

14. Remove the Kelly clamp on the end, and connect the tube to a drainage apparatus. Make sure a tight fit occurs (the end of the tube may need to be trimmed or a 3-in-1 adapter placed). The connection between the chest tube and the canister should always be secured using a banding gun or heavy adhesive tape. Intrapleural location of the chest tube can be confirmed by noticing the development of condensation on the inner surface of the tube during respiration and/or by noting the movement of fluid within the tubing during respiration.

15. A light dressing should be applied around the chest tube. If the skin edges are adequately approximated around the chest tube, an occlusive dressings is not required. If necessary, apply an occlusive dressing to the thoracostomy wound.

    Note: *The dressing should never be counted on to anchor a chest tube—the suture should always secure the chest tube position.*

16. Obtain a chest radiograph to document proper tube position, evacuation of air and/or fluid, and lung expansion. Posteroanterior and lateral radiographs are preferred instead of portable films whenever possible.

C. MAINTENANCE

1. Intensity of suction and timing of chest tube removal are controversial and vary according to the clinical indication for tube placement.

2. Daily chest radiographs are not necessary in a stable patient; however, a radiograph should be taken following discontinuation of suction or in a patient who experiences respiratory distress.

3. Change the dressing periodically to inspect the thoracostomy site.

4. Never clamp a chest tube! A tension pneumothorax can be created in a patient with a continued air leak.

D. COMPLICATIONS

1. Injury to intrathoracic and extrathoracic structures (intercostal vessels, pulmonary structures, diaphragm, great vessels, abdominal organs)—Can be minimized by digital exploration of the pleural cavity prior to tube insertion and avoiding the intercostal bundle
2. Tube malposition—Major or minor fissure, subcutaneous
3. Infection—Empyema
4. Tube displacement—Never readvance a chest tube; a new thoracostomy tube should be placed through a separate entrance site.
5. Hemorrhage—Intercostal vessels, lung parenchyma

III. CHEST TUBE REMOVAL

65

A. GENERAL

1. The exact timing of chest tube removal is ill defined and subject to multiple factors.
a. In general, when drainage is decreased to an acceptable amount (75-100 mL/24 h)
b. When "air leak" is not detectable
2. Iatrogenic pneumothorax is the most common complication.

B. PROCEDURE

1. Remove all dressings, cleanse the skin with bactericidal solution, and cut the knot of the anchoring suture. Unwind the suture from the chest tube (adequate suture length should remain to allow for skin closure).
2. Have an assistant pinch the skin around the chest tube.
3. Have the patient perform the Valsalva maneuver, and rapidly remove the chest tube while pinching the skin around the tube to avoid introduction of air.
4. Approximate the skin edges with the suture. An occlusive dressing is not required if the skin is adequately closed; otherwise, apply an occlusive dressing over the incision site. If the chest tube has been in place for a prolonged period, then an occlusive dressing should be used for added safety.
5. A postremoval chest radiograph is not required unless complications occur during removal.
6. The dressing should remain in place for 48 hours. The stitch can be removed and replaced with Steri-Strips at that time.

RECOMMENDED READING

Davis JW, Mackersie RC, Hoyt DB, Garcia J: Randomized study of algorithms for discontinuing tube thoracostomy drainage. J Am Coll Surg 179:553-557, 1994.

TUBE THORACOSTOMY

Thoracentesis

Marcus D. Jarboe, MD

I. GENERAL CONSIDERATIONS

A. INDICATIONS
1. Diagnostic evaluation of pleural fluid
2. Therapeutic aspiration of fluid or air to return lung volume

B. MATERIALS
1. Thoracentesis kit—Become familiar with the set available. Most are based on a catheter-over-needle design.
2. Without a kit
   a. Local anesthetic, sterile drapes, prep kit, gloves
   b. 25-gauge needle, 22-gauge 1½-inch needle, 5-mL syringe
   c. 16-18 gauge angiocatheter, 20-60 mL syringe
   d. Three-way stopcock
   e. IV pressure tubing, collection container, hemostat
3. 500-1000 mL vacuum bottle

C. PROCEDURE
1. Review upright chest radiograph, along with percussion of dullness to localize fluid. Blunting of the costophrenic angle on posteroanterior view indicates >250 mL is present. Decubitus film should be obtained to evaluate whether effusion is free flowing or loculated. Loculated effusions should be localized by ultrasound.
2. Obtain informed consent.
3. The patient should be sitting comfortably, leaning forward with arms resting over one or two pillows on a bedside table. In critically ill patients the lateral decubitus position is used.
4. Thoracentesis is generally performed along the posterior axillary line from the back. The correct site is one or two interspaces *below* the level of the effusion but *not* below the 8th intercostal space.
5. Using sterile technique, the area is prepped and draped. Local anesthetic is infiltrated intradermally over the superior margin of the rib below the chosen interspace. This is continued with the 1½-inch needle through the subcutaneous tissue to infiltrate the periosteum and is continued down until fluid is aspirated. Note this depth with a clamp on the needle at the level of the skin. Withdraw the syringe 0.5 cm, inject to anesthetize the pleura, and then remove the needle.
6. Insert a 16-18 gauge angiocatheter through the anesthetized area to the previous depth while continuously aspirating. Care must be taken to avoid the neurovascular bundle (by advancing *over* the superior portion of the rib). The pleura has been entered when fluid returns. Advance the angiocatheter over the needle and withdraw the needle. Occlude the catheter lumen with a finger to prevent a pneumothorax.

66

Interspace a three-way stopcock between the angiocatheter and the large syringe. The third lumen is directed to the collecting chamber.

7. Confirm the position of the needle by aspirating into the syringe with the stopcock "off" to the collection chamber. If good return is noted, turn the stopcock off to the patient and expel the contents of the syringe into the collection chamber. Repeat this procedure until the desired amount of fluid is removed or no further fluid is obtained. When an evacuated bottle is used, after confirming the position of the catheter, turn the stopcock off to the syringe and allow free aspiration.

8. Remove the angiocatheter and apply a sterile dressing.

9. Recommended pleural fluid studies

  a. Hematology—Cell count and differential
  b. Chemistry—Specific gravity, pH, lactate dehydrogenase, amylase, glucose, protein
  c. Microbiology—Gram stain; bacterial, fungal, and acid-fast bacillus cultures
  d. Pathology—Cell cytology to rule out malignancy (in heparinized bottle)

10. Obtain a chest radiograph to confirm the efficacy of the aspiration and to rule out a pneumothorax.

II. SPECIFIC CONSIDERATIONS

A. INTERPRETATION OF THE RESULTS

Table 66-1 shows the differences between transudate and exudate, based on lab findings.

B. DIFFERENTIAL DIAGNOSIS

1. Transudate—Cirrhosis, nephritic syndrome, congestive heart failure, lobar atelectasis, viral infection
2. Exudate—Empyema, malignant effusion, intra-abdominal infection, pancreatitis, tuberculosis, trauma, pulmonary infarction, chylothorax
3. Grossly bloody—Iatrogenic injury, pulmonary infarction, trauma, tumor, hepatic or splenic puncture

TABLE 66-1		
DETERMINATION OF TRANSUDATE VS. EXUDATE BASED ON LAB FINDINGS		
Lab Studies	Transudate	Exudate
Protein	<3 g/dL	>3 g/dL
Protein ratio (effusion to serum)	<0.6	>0.6
Specific gravity	<1.016	>1.016
LDH	Low	High
LDH ratio (effusion to serum)	<0.6	>0.9
Glucose	$2/3$ serum glucose	Low
Amylase	<200 IU/mL	>500 IU/mL
RBC	<10,000/mm^3	>100,000/mm^3
WBC	<1000/mm^3	>1000/mm^3

LDH = lactate dehydrogenase; RBC = red blood cell; WBC = white blood cell.

4. Extremely low glucose consistent with rheumatoid process

C. COMPLICATIONS
1. Pneumothorax
2. Hemothorax
3. Hepatic or splenic puncture
4. Parenchymal tear
5. Empyema

Notes: *(1) When the patient has positive-pressure ventilation, use ultrasound to mark the area of the fluid collection. In addition, use ultrasound in marginal patients to reduce the risk of tension pneumothorax; (2) may use triple-lumen central line set when aspirating large volumes; and (3) recheck diagnostic criteria with other sources.*

66

THORACENTESIS

Bladder Catheterization

David M. Kitchens, MD

I. URETHRAL CATHETERIZATION

A. INDICATIONS FOR CONTINUOUS CATHETERIZATION
1. Monitor urine output accurately.
2. Relieve urinary retention owing to infravesical obstruction or neuropathic/myopathic loss of bladder tone with the following possible complications.
   a. Postobstructive diuresis—If >200 mL/h, watch urinary output.
   b. Hemorrhage secondary to bladder mucosal disruption
   c. Hypotension with vasovagal response
3. Urinary incontinence—Temporary therapy, not long term
4. Perineal wounds—Burns, operative, traumatic, to prevent contamination
5. Remove clots with hematuria (24-28 Fr). A three-way catheter is sometimes placed to irrigate the bladder to prevent formation of clots during active bleeding.
6. Aid in healing after lower GU procedure; used as a stent
7. Medication-induced urinary retention—Seen commonly with antipsychotic drugs due to their anticholinergic properties
8. Make sure catheter is composed of silicone if it is to be left in place for >1 week because other materials may become encrusted and become a nidus for stone formation.

B. INDICATIONS FOR INTERMITTENT CATHETERIZATION (ROBINSON CATHETER)
1. If ultrasound is unavailable, then straight catheterization may be used to check postvoid residuals.
2. Sterile diagnostic urinalysis and cultures—This is used mainly for females because there is greater risk of contamination from skin flora than with males.
3. Management of neurogenic bladder and chronic urinary retention
4. Psychogenic urinary retention

C. CONTRAINDICATIONS
1. Psychogenic urinary retention (relative)
2. Trauma—≈10% of injuries seen in the emergency department
3. Posterior urethral disruption of concern in males more than females with pelvic fractures from deceleration accidents
4. Anterior urethral injury primarily caused by perineal or straddle trauma
5. Prostatic or urethral infection and epididymitis (relative)
6. Recent urethral or bladder neck surgery (variable)

D. MATERIALS (Figs. 67-1 and 67-2)
1. 16-20 Fr Foley catheter with 5-mL balloon—18 Fr most common, smaller in females

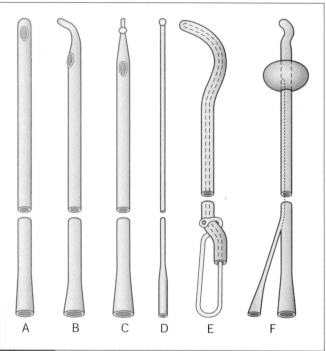

FIG. 67-1

Urethral catheters, including soft rubber *(A)*; coudé *(B)*; and Phillips *(C)*, which attaches to filiform *(D)*, which may be threaded over wire stylet *(E)*. *F*, Foley self-retaining urethral catheter.

2. 5-8 Fr pediatric feeding tube in infants (no balloon)—Do not use in adults secondary to coiling within urethra (1 Fr = 0.33 mm ED; luminal diameter may vary depending on how many ports are present in catheter).
3. Sterile catheterization kit with water-soluble lubricant, gloves, prep solution, cotton balls, drapes, and water for balloon inflation
4. Closed-drainage system
5. Normal saline irrigation and a catheter-tip syringe

II. TECHNIQUES

A. **MALES** (Figs. 67-3 and 67-4)
1. Position the patient in the supine position, legs spread slightly. Lay out equipment in a convenient array, using sterile gloves on both

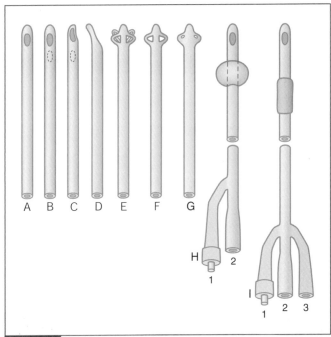

FIG. 67-2

Large-diameter catheters. *A*, Conical-tip urethral catheter; *B*, Robinson urethral
catheter; *C*, Whistle-tip urethral catheter; *D*, coudé hollow olive-tip catheter;
E, Malecot self-retaining, four-wing urethral catheter; *F*, Malecot self-retaining,
two-wing urethral catheter; *G*, Pezzer self-retaining drain, open-end head, used for
cystostomy drainage; *H*, Foley-type balloon catheter; *I*, Foley-type, three-way balloon
catheter, one limb of distal end for balloon inflation (1), one for drainage (2), and one
to infuse irrigating solution to prevent clot formation within the bladder (3).

hands. One should prepare the field as if a surgical procedure will be
taking place because the urinary tract is a sterile tract.

2. Grasp the penis with the nondominant hand on the dorsal end, taking
care not to occlude the urethra. If right-handed, stand on the patient's
right and hold the penis perpendicular to the body with the left hand
with modest tension (this hand is now contaminated and must remain
in place). Prep the glans, foreskin, and meatus using the sterile hand
with antiseptic solution. The foreskin is retracted in an uncircumcised
male to allow for an adequate prep.

3. Insert the well-lubricated catheter into the meatus while maintaining
slight stretching tension on the penis with gentle, constant pressure.

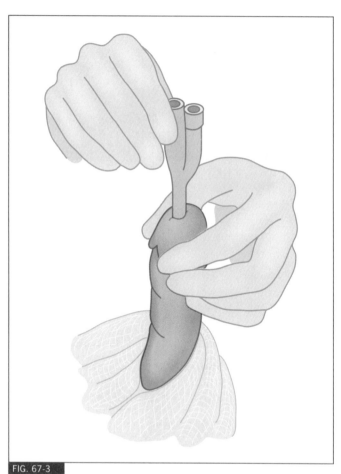

FIG. 67-3
Urethral catheterization in the male patient.

A second option is to instill ≈10 mL of 2% lidocaine jelly directly into the urethra prior to inserting the catheter. There will be some resistance as the catheter passes the external sphincter, then the prostate. Have the patient take slow, deep breaths to aid in passage. The catheter should be inserted to the balloon sidearm; urine return confirms that the catheter tip is within the bladder. If no urine is obtained, apply constant suprapubic tension and irrigate with 20-30 mL of normal saline to clear the ports. If there is free

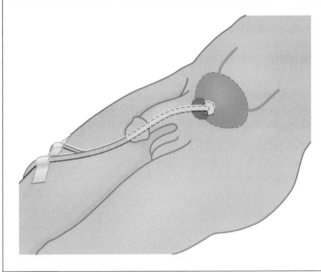

FIG. 67-4

Proper position of urethral catheter in the bladder.

return of irrigation, it is unlikely that the catheter resides in the bladder.

4. When you are confident that the balloon lies within the bladder, inflate the balloon with 10 mL of sterile water. Do not inflate the balloon with anything other than sterile water because precipitates could form and prevent deflation of the balloon. If excessive resistance exists, deflate the balloon and reattempt passage. Withdraw the catheter to seat the balloon against the bladder neck. Connect the catheter to a sterile closed-drainage system.

5. Advance the foreskin to prevent paraphimosis (the most common cause of paraphimosis is not advancing foreskin after catheter placement). Secure the catheter to the patient's thigh or abdomen with some slack to prevent accidental dislodgment and prevent catheter pull.

6. It is important to choose the smallest-diameter-size catheter to adequately drain the bladder (normally 16-18 Fr is adequate in an adult) to allow urethral secretions to escape around the catheter. This aids in preventing infection.

7. If any patient has a risk for endocarditis, it is always prudent to treat with appropriate systemic antibiotics prior to catheter insertion or removal.

B. FEMALES (Fig. 67-5)

1. Position the patient supine with knees flexed and legs fully abducted ("frog-leg" position) and drape the patient.
2. Spread the labia with the fingers of the nondominant hand to expose the urethral meatus (this hand is now contaminated and must remain in position). Prep the introitus from anterior to posterior. An assistant can help with retraction if necessary.
3. Sterilely insert a well-lubricated catheter (may lubricate catheter with 2% lidocaine jelly) into the urethral meatus. Return of urine confirms the position in the bladder. If no urine returns, apply suprapubic pressure, then irrigate as previously described for males.
4. Inflate the balloon with 10 mL of sterile water. Withdraw the catheter gently to seat it against the bladder neck. Tape it to the thigh with some slack and connect it to the sterile closed-drainage system.

C. DIFFICULT URETHRAL CATHETERIZATIONS

1. Causes—Meatal stricture, urethral stricture, prostatic enlargement, urethral disruption, urethral obstruction, and anxious patient. Obtaining a careful GU history can elicit most causes of a difficult urethral catheterization (sexually transmitted disease leads to urethral strictures, prostate surgery leads to bladder neck contracture, and so forth).
2. Possible solutions
   a. Ensure that the catheter is well lubricated, and repeat the attempt. If unsuccessful, try a larger-diameter catheter or coudé-tip catheter.
   b. If pain limits the procedure, instill 20 mL 2% lidocaine jelly and clamp for 5 minutes to allow the anesthetic to take effect in the urethra.
   c. If anxiety limits the procedure, use lorazepam (Ativan) or morphine sulfate administration and continual, gentle catheter pressure to bypass the external sphincter.
   d. Attempt intubation with larger catheters (20-24 Fr) because they are firmer than smaller-lumen catheters and may bypass the area of obstruction. Smaller catheters are less firm and can coil in the urethra.
   e. Meatal strictures can be dilated with a urethral sound or, less commonly, with a hemostat.
   f. Coudé catheter—Most useful
      (1) Tip forms an obtuse angle with the catheter body.
      (2) If the catheter is not passable, often the tip has become obstructed by the following.
         (a) The floor of the S-shaped bulbous urethra
         (b) A pocket formed by enlarged prostatic lobes
         (c) Urethral stricture
      (3) The coudé tip is directed against the roof of the urethra.
      (4) If the coudé tip becomes engaged in a pocket or fold, long-axis rotation causes disengagement.
      (5) Keeping the balloon port at the 12 o'clock position during placement ensures that the tip is being placed at the correct angle.

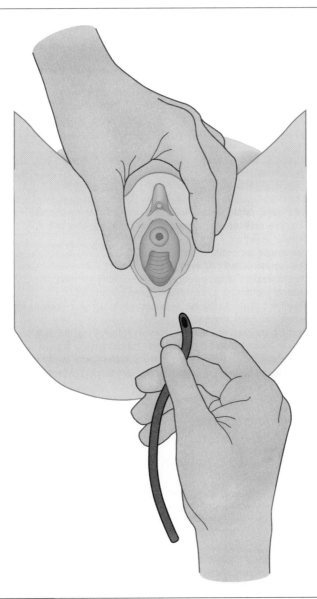

67

BLADDER CATHETERIZATION

FIG. 67-5

Urethral catheterization in the female patient.

g. The use of filiform and Phillips catheters may be necessary if a coudé catheter is impassable. This should always be attempted by a urologist.

h. If still unable to pass a catheter by these methods
   (1) Consider the possibility of urethral disruption and obtain a retrograde cystourethrogram.
   (2) Consider urologic placement of a catheter with cystoscopic aid or placement of a suprapubic catheter. Prior to inserting a suprapubic catheter one must always ensure that the patient does not have a coagulopathy or is not taking anticoagulating medications.

III. CATHETER CARE

A. CARE OF URETHRAL CATHETERS

1. Closed-drainage system is the primary concern. If necessary to open the system, sterile gloves should be employed with aseptic technique.
2. The urine collection bag should remain below the level of the catheter insertion.
3. Use aseptic technique during insertion
4. Remove the catheter as soon as feasible.
5. Careful washing of the meatus daily may inhibit infection.
6. Flush or replace the system if urine output decreases.
7. Tape the catheter to the medial aspect of the leg with flexibility for normal patient movement.
8. Restrain confused or agitated patients to prevent catheter removal with an intact balloon. If the catheter is inadvertently removed with the balloon intact, insert a new catheter under sterile conditions because this will likely tamponade any bleeding in the urethra.

B. COMPLICATIONS

1. Infection
   a. Primary source of nosocomial urinary tract infections—30-40% of patients have catheter-associated infection after 4 days of continuous catheterization.
   b. Possible causes
      (1) Contamination at the time of insertion due to a break in technique
      (2) Retrograde (ascending) infection, break in closed-drainage system
      (3) Bacterial colonization of meatus
      (4) Presence of foreign body
      (5) Sepsis secondary to inflation of the balloon in the prostatic urethra
      (6) Preexisting infection
2. False passage, urethral disruption
3. Hemorrhage and cystitis leading to hematuria
4. Urethral stricture
5. Obstructed catheter and urinary retention
6. Nidus for stone formation if left indwelling long term

7. Bladder spasms—This may lead to an extreme urge to void with incontinence of urine around the catheter; can be treated with anticholinergics while the catheter is in place
8. Squamous cell carcinoma of bladder (controversial) with long-term indwelling catheters over a period of years

C. CATHETER REMOVAL

1. Attach the syringe to a balloon port and allow the balloon to deflate completely.
2. If the balloon does not deflate completely, withdraw gently on the syringe.
3. If this does not work, several options exist to attempt to deflate balloon.

a. Cut the balloon port. Sometimes this allows the water to escape from the balloon.
b. If this is unsuccessful, then one can thread a Bentson guide wire through the balloon port.
c. If a Bentson guide wire is unsuccessful, then one may attempt to pass the firm end of a guide wire from a central line kit.

67

BLADDER CATHETERIZATION

GI Intubation

Parag Bhanot, MD

A. NASOGASTRIC (NG) TUBES

NG tubes are used for (1) gastric decompression, (2) gastric lavage, and (3) administration of oral contrast material. Pass the largest size tolerable to the patient.

1. **Levin tube**—A soft tube with a single lumen. Connect to low intermittent suction to prevent the gastric mucosa from occluding the tube.

2. Salem sump tube—Dual-lumen tube

a. The main lumen should be placed on low continuous suction. A side-port (blue) vents the tube to allow continuous sump suction without injury to the mucosa.

b. The vent should be flushed with 15 mL of air and the main lumen with 30 mL of saline q 3-4 hours to ensure patency. The vent is patent when it "whistles" continuously. The vent should never be flushed with liquid.

3. **Method of insertion**

a. Elevate the head of the patient at least 30 degrees, then flex the neck.

b. Lubricate the tube with water-soluble lubricant or viscous lidocaine.

c. Viscous lidocaine can be inserted into the nostril with cotton-tip applicators or syringe.

d. Insert the tube into a nostril and pass it into the nasopharynx (a small bend in the tip of the tube aids passage). The patient should swallow when the tube is felt in the back of the throat. Sips of water facilitate passage of the tube into the esophagus in an awake patient. To avoid tracheal intubation, do not force the tube.

e. Advance into the stomach.

f. A series of four black marks are on the main lumen. The proximal mark, at the nares, indicates insertion to the distal esophagus; the middle two marks indicate insertion to the body of the stomach; and the distal mark indicates insertion to the pylorus/duodenum.

g. Inadvertent nasotracheal intubation is confirmed by the patient's gasping for air, coughing, or inability to speak. Condensation may be visible in the tube. Immediately pull back the tube.

h. Confirm the tube position by instilling 20-30 mL of air while listening over the stomach with a stethoscope and by aspirating gastric contents. Aspiration of gastric contents is a more reliable method. Always confirm with a radiograph if the tube is to be used for feeding.

i. Secure the tube with tape. Tubes taped tightly to the nostril or nasal septum may lead to pressure necrosis (Fig. 68-1).

j. Patients with aberrant anatomy may need endoscopic guidance for safe insertion.

68

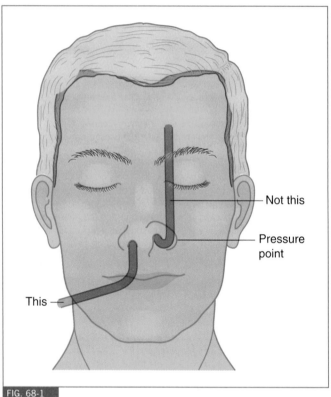

FIG. 68-1

Tube placement to avoid pressure necrosis.

B. OROGASTRIC TUBES
1. Preferred if NG intubation is contraindicated (anterior basilar skull fracture, nasopharyngeal trauma)
2. Ewald tube—Especially suited for lavage of the stomach and emergency evacuation of blood, toxic agents, medications, or other substances
a. Large (18-36 Fr) double-lumen tube
b. The 36 Fr lumen is connected to continuous suction; the 18 Fr lumen is used for irrigation.
c. Method of insertion—In patients with loss of consciousness or loss of the gag reflex, insertion of a cuffed endotracheal tube prior to orogastric tube insertion is preferred.
   (1) Lubricate the tube.
   (2) Insert the tube into the mouth and down the esophagus into the stomach. If the patient is conscious, have the patient sip water.

(3) Verify the position of the tube by aspiration of gastric contents and by auscultation.

(4) Connect to suction; begin irrigation when the stomach is empty. The amount of irrigant used should be monitored. The large bore of this tube may allow rapid overdistention of the stomach with the resultant risk of aspiration.

II. DUODENAL/SMALL BOWEL TUBES

A. NASODUODENAL FEEDING TUBES
1. Smaller in diameter, softer, and more flexible than NG tubes
2. Fluoroscopic placement preferred
3. Prior to institution of tube feedings, the tube position must be verified by radiograph.
4. Types of tubes
a. Corpak—Nonweighted, has a bullet at the tip to prevent passage of the tube into regions of the tracheobronchial tree that lack cartilaginous support; a wire stylet may be used to pass the tube into the duodenum under fluoroscopic guidance
b. Frederick-Miller—Has a stylet that allows for improved manipulation; must be placed under fluoroscopic guidance to prevent inadvertent tracheobronchial placement; preferred when postpyloric placement is necessary
5. Placement of the tube past the ligament of Treitz eliminates most of the potential for aspiration.
6. Nasoduodenal tubes allow for early institution of enteric feedings. This is important in the context of trophic feeds and in patients with unresolved ileus.
7. pH-guided nasointestinal feeding tubes—Advantages are decreased cost; rapid, easy placement; elimination of endoscopic/fluoroscopic requirements; decreased radiation exposure. Placement is similar to that for standard bedside feeding tube; pH monitor allows for continuous pH readings.
a. Flush the tube with 10 mL of water; insert guide wire; and lubricate tip with water-soluble lubricant.
b. Attach a temporary ground pad to the patient's skin; test the tube by attaching a monitor and placing the tip of the tube in contact with the tube's ground wire (pH reading of 0.5 indicates functioning sensor and monitor).
c. Attach the tube's ground wire to the ground electrode pad; care must be taken to ensure reference electrode does not become detached and that the electrode gel does not dry.
d. Gently push the tip of the nose superiorly as the tube is introduced; pass the tube through the nasopharynx and oropharynx and into the esophagus; initial readings average 6.5 to 6.6 (little variation).
e. The tube is advanced until gastric pH (<3.5) is observed.

68

GI INTUBATION

Note: *The stomach is the only viscus in continuity with the nasopharynx that routinely has a pH <5; if tube is advanced >45 cm without a drop in pH, then pulmonary placement or curling of tube in upper alimentary tract is likely.*

f. After observing gastric pH, cap the gastric decompression tube, if present, and insufflate 100-200 mL of air to distend the stomach; insufflate 10-mL air boluses every 3-5 cm of tube advancement. (These maneuvers lessen the tube's chance of gastric rugal fold entrapment.)

g. The tube is advanced until a sudden, rapid increase in pH readings is encountered, signifying transpyloric passage.

   Note: *When the rate of pH rise is gradual, the tube is likely to be curled in the stomach with the tip at the gastroesophageal junction.*

h. Obtain a plain radiograph of the abdomen after placement to confirm its position prior to use.

i. When the pH changes of initial-to-lowest and lowest-to-final are both >4 units, intestinal passage occurs in >90% of attempts.

j. Antiulcer regimens do not interfere with placement.

B. NASOINTESTINAL TUBES FOR DECOMPRESSION OF THE SMALL BOWEL

1. Used mainly for early postoperative bowel obstruction secondary to early adhesion formations or obstruction secondary to carcinomatosis

2. Cantor tube—Single-lumen tube with a mercury-filled balloon at the distal end

a. To prepare the balloon tip, inject 5 mL of mercury into the middle of the balloon tangentially with a 21-gauge needle, then withdraw all air from the balloon.

b. Lubricate the tube.

c. While the patient is sitting upright, use a cotton-tip applicator to help guide the balloon into the nasopharynx. When the tube falls into the back of the throat, have the patient swallow and the tube will travel by gravity into the stomach.

d. Once the tube is in the stomach, aspirate stomach contents, then place to gravity.

e. Tape the tube to the side of the face with a 4-6 inch loop. This permits the tube to advance by peristalsis.

f. Place the patient on the right side and advance the tube to the "P" position as marked on the outside of the tube. Have the patient remain in this position until the "D" mark is at the external naris, indicating passage into the duodenum.

g. Confirm duodenal position by radiograph. The tube may be positioned at the pylorus under fluoroscopic guidance.

h. Place the patient on the left side until the tube has advanced several inches. Allow the patient to resume activity and the tube to be drawn downward by peristalsis. Leave a 4-inch loop free. Pass the tube 3 inches q 4 hours. Irrigate with 15 mL of saline before advancing the tube.

i. When the tube no longer advances by peristalsis, place the tube on low intermittent suction.
j. To remove the tube, slow gentle withdrawal is necessary. The tube should be withdrawn ≈1 foot q 3-4 hours to prevent intussusception.
k. Abdominal radiographs should be obtained to demonstrate resolving obstruction.

3. **Miller-Abbott tube**—Dual lumen with one lumen for intermittent suction and the other to attach a balloon that can be filled with mercury or water once the tube enters the stomach.

C. TUBES FOR INTRAOPERATIVE INTESTINAL DECOMPRESSION
1. **Types**—Baker, Dennis, and Leonard tubes all have a suction port and a balloon to facilitate placement.
2. **Placement**
a. Introduce the tube into the stomach via the oral or nasogastric route.
b. Inflate the balloon and pass it manually through the duodenum into the small bowel.
c. May be placed through an enterotomy at the risk of intra-abdominal enteric spillage

68

GI INTUBATION

III. SENGSTAKEN-BLAKEMORE TUBE

A. DEFINITION
The Sengstaken-Blakemore tube is an oral gastric tube equipped with an esophageal and gastric balloon for tamponade and ports for aspiration.

B. ADVANTAGES
1. **Allows nonoperative direct control of the bleeding site**
2. **Causes immediate cessation of bleeding in >85% of patients**

C. DISADVANTAGES
1. **Frequent recurrence of hemorrhage after deflation of the balloon—25-55%**
2. **High incidence of complications—Aspiration, asphyxiation, esophageal perforation, ischemic necrosis**

D. INDICATION
The Sengstaken-Blakemore tube is used for acutely bleeding esophageal varices refractory to sclerotherapy and medical management.

E. INSERTION
1. **Test balloons for air leaks and proper inflation.**
2. **Measures to prevent aspiration**
a. Endotracheal intubation in virtually all patients
b. Gastric lavage to remove blood and clots
c. Have wall suction available.

   d. Pharynx is *not* anesthetized so as to maintain the gag reflex if the patient is not intubated.

3. Lubricate the tube and pass it into the stomach via the mouth.

4. The tube is advanced fully and air is injected into the suction lumen while auscultating over the stomach region.

5. Confirm the intragastric location of the gastric balloon by instilling small amount of water-soluble contrast into the balloon and obtaining a radiograph *before* inflating the balloon fully. Fluoroscopic visualization can be used also.

6. Suction is applied immediately to prevent regurgitation.

7. Inflate the gastric balloon with increments of 100 mL of air to a total of 450-500 mL. Double-clamp with rubber-shod surgical clamps. Stop air inflation *immediately* if the patient complains of epigastric pain or if insufflation of air is not audible over the epigastric region.

8. Apply gentle traction on the tube until resistance indicates that the balloon is at the esophagogastric junction.

9. Gastric lavage is performed through the gastric aspiration lumen using saline. The aspirate should become clear.

10. A second nasoesophageal tube is passed into the proximal esophagus to monitor continued bleeding above the gastric and/or esophageal balloons and to aspirate salivary secretions. The Minnesota tube is a modification that has an esophageal port to obviate the need for this extra tube.

11. If blood is detected continually in the gastric aspirate, the esophageal balloon should be inflated. Use the lowest pressure that stops bleeding. Double-clamp the balloon inlet with rubber-shod surgical clamps. Do not inflate the esophageal balloon >40 mm Hg.

12. If bleeding continues with esophageal tamponade, external traction should be initiated. Tape the tube to the facemask of a football helmet or attach to 1-2 pounds of traction to maintain gentle traction of the tube.

13. Gastric and esophageal lumina are connected to intermittent suction.

14. Tape scissors to the head of the bed in plain view in case urgent transection and removal of the tube are required.

15. Irrigate the gastric lumen tube frequently and record the appearance of the return fluid.

16. Both balloons are inflated for 24 hours, after which the esophageal balloon is slowly deflated and the patient is observed for signs of rebleeding. If rebleeding occurs, the esophageal balloon is reinflated.

17. If there is no rebleeding, the gastric balloon is deflated after 24 hours and the patient is observed.

18. If no further bleeding occurs 24 hours after the gastric balloon is deflated, mineral oil should be given prior to removal. The tube is

completely transected with scissors and removed. This ensures that balloons are deflated completely and that the tube is not reused.

19. The esophageal balloon is always deflated first to prevent the risk of migration, then asphyxiation.

20. After extubation, the mouth and posterior pharynx are suctioned to remove secretions.

68

GI INTUBATION

Paracentesis

Parag Bhanot, MD

I. GENERAL CONSIDERATIONS

A. INDICATIONS

1. Diagnostic
a. Etiology of ascites
b. Suspicion of spontaneous bacterial peritonitis—Fever, leukocytosis
c. Rapid increase in ascites previously controlled with medical therapy
2. Therapeutic—To relieve dyspnea and/or anorexia
a. Up to 2 L of ascitic fluid can be drawn off safely q 24 hours.
b. Colloid replacement is indicated with therapeutic paracentesis to prevent complications associated with rapid loss of volume—Give 100 mL of dextran 70 IV for each liter of fluid removed or 12.5 g of albumin per liter removed.
c. Consider peritoneovenous shunt if repeated paracentesis is required in a patient who is refractory to medical therapy.

B. TECHNIQUE

1. Ensure that a large-bore, functional IV is in place.
2. Position patient—Supine, slight reverse Trendelenburg, with a pillow under the opposite side
3. Empty the urinary bladder to decrease the incidence of bladder perforation.
4. Examine the abdomen and choose the site.
a. Ultrasound guidance may be needed in a scarred abdomen to avoid inadvertent bowel injury.
b. The preferred site is halfway between the anterior superior iliac spine and the umbilicus, lateral to the rectus abdominis muscle (Fig. 69-1).
5. Prep and drape sterilely.
6. Infiltrate with local anesthesia down to the peritoneum using a 25-gauge needle.
7. Switch to a 16-gauge angiocatheter, and while aspirating, advance until free fluid is encountered. (Make a Z-track when traversing the subcutaneous tissues and musculature to prevent an ascitic leak from a straight-entry track.)
8. Remove needle from catheter; attach three-way stopcock, and withdraw desired amount of fluid (50 mL of fluid is needed for a diagnostic tap). Connect IV tubing and a sterile bag or vacuum bottle if a large amount of fluid is to be withdrawn.
9. When finished, apply sterile dressing.

C. POTENTIAL COMPLICATIONS

1. Persistent leakage of ascites from paracentesis site
2. Intra-abdominal bleeding

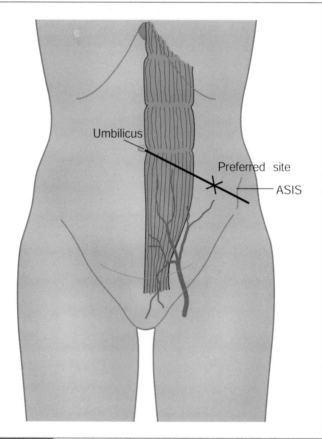

FIG. 69-1

Preferred site for paracentesis. ASIS = anterior superior iliac spine.

3. Infection of ascitic fluid
4. Perforated bowel
5. Perforated bladder—If index of suspicion is high, send urine sample. In contrast to ascitic fluid, urine should be negative for protein and glucose.
6. Hemodynamic instability—Hypotension secondary to fluid reaccumulation
7. Hepatorenal syndrome and/or worsening encephalopathy in cirrhotic patients
8. Electrolyte abnormalities—Hyponatremia

TABLE 69-1

LABORATORY DIAGNOSIS WITH ASCITIC FLUID

	Gross	Protein (g/dL)	Specific Gravity	RBC (>10⁴mm³)	WBC (mm³)	LDH Ascites: Serum	Other
Cirrhosis	Straw, bile stained	<2.5	<1.016	1%	<250	<0.6	—
Peritoneal neoplasm	Straw, bloody, mucinous, chylous	>2.5	>1.016	20%	>1000	>0.6	—*
Infection	Turbid, purulent, bloody, chylous	>2.5	>1.016	Variable	>1000	>0.6	pH < 7.3 Lymphs in TB
Pancreatic disease	Turbid, bloody, chylous	>2.5	>1.016	Variable	Variable	—	Amylase
CHF	Straw	Variable	<1.016	10%	<1000	<0.6	—
Nephrotic disease	Straw, chylous	<2.5	<1.016	—	<250	<0.6	—

*Malignant cells may be found in 50% of patients with cancer; however, ≈4% of patients with cirrhosis have malignant-appearing cells in their ascitic fluid.

RBC = red blood cell; WBC = white blood cell; LDH = lactate dehydrogenase; CHF = congestive heart failure; TB = tuberculosis.

69

PARACENTESIS

II. FLUID ANALYSIS

A. FLUID DETERMINATIONS
1. Cell count—Red blood cells, white blood cells
2. Gram stain, culture—Bacterial, fungal, acid-fast bacillus
3. Cytology
4. Chemical analysis—Specific gravity, total protein, amylase, lactate dehydrogenase, and pH

B. DIAGNOSIS
See Table 69-1.

Diagnostic Peritoneal Lavage

Jefferson M. Lyons, MD

I. GENERAL CONSIDERATIONS

A. INTRODUCTION
1. Mainstay evaluation of unstable patients with blunt abdominal trauma and selected cases of penetrating trauma
2. Ideally should be performed by the surgeon caring for the patient because it is a surgical procedure that alters subsequent examination of the patient
3. Unreliable in assessment of most retroperitoneal injuries
4. Usually performed early in patient evaluation, typically during secondary survey; if free intraperitoneal air suspected, perform abdominal films prior to diagnostic peritoneal lavage (DPL), which can introduce air
5. Nearly half of patients with hemoperitoneum do not have peritonitis on exam.
6. Also used for evaluating critically ill patients for suspected intraabdominal processes

B. INDICATIONS
1. DPL
a. Blunt abdominal trauma and manifestations of hypovolemia—Hypotension and tachycardia
b. Penetrating trauma with questionable involvement of the peritoneal cavity (controversial)
2. DPL and/or CT—Depends on the availability of CT and the time available for patient evaluation (Table 70-1). CT scan should be performed with both IV and GI contrast material. **Note:** *The patient must be hemodynamically stable!*
a. Depressed sensorium or altered pain response leading to possible false-negative physical examination—Ethanol intoxication, head injury, drug abuse, and spinal cord injury
b. Equivocal abdominal findings—Often a result of lower rib fractures, pelvic fractures, and lumbar spine fractures
c. Abdominal findings—Localized tenderness, guarding
d. Inability to perform serial exams—Patient undergoing general anesthetic for other injuries; DPL needed to definitively clear abdomen
e. Low rib fractures, particularly on left side
3. Controversial indications for DPL and/or CT
a. Penetrating injury to surrounding areas
  (1) Lower chest—Below nipples or 4th intercostal space
  (2) Flank
  (3) Buttocks and perineum
b. Stab wounds or low-caliber gunshot wounds with no significant physical findings

70

733

DPL VS. ULTRASOUND VS. CT IN BLUNT ABDOMINAL TRAUMA

	DPL	Ultrasound	CT Scan
Indication	Document bleeding if decreased blood pressure	Document fluid if decreased blood pressure	Document organ injury if blood pressure normal
Advantages	Early diagnosis and sensitive; 98% accurate	Early diagnosis; noninvasive and repeatable; 86-97% accurate	Most specific for injury; 92-98% accurate
Disadvantages	Invasive; misses injury to diaphragm or retroperitoneum	Operator dependent; bowel gas and subcutaneous air distortion; misses diaphragm, bowel, and some pancreatic injuries	Cost and time; misses diaphragm, bowel tract, and some pancreatic injuries

DPL = diagnostic peritoneal lavage.
From Advanced Trauma Life Support. Chicago, American College of Surgeons, 1997.

C. CONTRAINDICATIONS
1. Absolute contraindication—Obvious indications for exploratory laparotomy include free air, peritonitis, penetrating trauma
2. Relative contraindications
a. Multiple abdominal operations or midline scars—Appendectomy or Pfannenstiel's scar alone does not preclude DPL
b. Gravid uterus—Use supraumbilical open technique above fundus
c. Inability to decompress bladder—Use supraumbilical open technique
d. Inability to decompress stomach—Use infraumbilical open technique
e. Pelvic fracture with possible hematoma—Use supraumbilical open technique to avoid false-positive results obtained by entering retroperitoneal hematoma

II. TECHNIQUES

A. SEMI-OPEN
1. Insert nasogastric tube and urinary catheter—Stomach and bladder must be decompressed to avoid injury
2. Restrain patient, and sedate if necessary.
3. Shave periumbilical region—Above and below umbilicus
4. Prep region widely with povidone-iodine (Betadine), and drape with sterile towels.
5. Decide on supraumbilical or infraumbilical incision.
6. Infiltrate proposed site (skin and subcutaneous tissue) with 1% lidocaine with epinephrine—Enhances local hemostasis to minimize false-positive results; use even in comatose or anesthetized patient

7. Incise skin (1-3 cm vertical incision needed depending on body habitus) and subcutaneous tissue down to midline fascia.
8. Place towel clips on both sides of the fascial incision for traction.
9. Using a No. 11 scalpel blade, make a 2-3 mm stab incision in fascia.
10. With strong upward traction on the towel clips by the assistant, the operator places the trocar-catheter apparatus through the fascial opening and then pushes it through the peritoneum (and posterior fascia). This initial push should be done perpendicular to the skin and must stop after one feels the "pop" of the peritoneum. At this point, the trocar-catheter apparatus is tilted down, the catheter alone is advanced toward the pelvis, and the trocar is removed.
11. Attach the aspirating device and aspirate using a 12-mL syringe.
    a. If >10 mL of gross blood, positive
    b. If <10 mL of gross blood, then the aspirate is returned to the abdomen with the lavage fluid.
12. If aspirate is negative for blood, instill 1 L (10 mL/kg in children) lactated Ringer's solution or normal saline from a pressure bag. Shake the patient's abdomen periodically, or move the patient into and out of Trendelenburg. Use warm fluid in hypothermic patients.
13. When only a small level of fluid remains in the bag, drop the near-empty bag to the floor to drain the fluid. The fluid drains by siphon action; hence, if all the fluid is allowed to run in along with some air, the siphon is lost and must be restarted by applying suction via a needle and syringe to a port in the tubing. Tubing used must *not* have a one-way filter device.
14. While the fluid is draining, keep a sponge packed into the wound for hemostasis and constantly hold the catheter in place.
15. After the fluid has returned (300-500 mL minimum), clamp the tubing and withdraw the catheter (avoids siphoning blood from wound into bag).
16. Wound closure—A heavy suture may be placed to close the small fascial defect (optional), skin closure with skin staples (hold ends of wound taut with towel clips).

B. PERCUTANEOUS

The percutaneous approach is a closed (Seldinger) technique that uses a needle and trocar, guide wire, and advancing catheter.

C. OPEN TECHNIQUE

In the open technique, midline fascia is incised over 3-4 cm, the posterior fascia/peritoneum is held with hemostats and opened under direct vision, and a catheter without trocar is advanced into the peritoneal cavity. Fascial closure is required at completion.

70

DIAGNOSTIC PERITONEAL LAVAGE

III. SPECIFIC CONSIDERATIONS

A. TECHNICAL PROBLEMS
1. Poor fluid return—Adjust the catheter position, twist the catheter, place the patient in the reverse Trendelenburg position, apply manual pressure to the abdomen, instill an additional 500 mL of fluid, have patient take deep breaths, and make sure there is not a one-way valve in the IV tubing (fluid may exit the chest tube or Foley catheter).
2. Air in tubing—Check all connections; make certain the catheter is advanced far enough to avoid exposed side holes, re-establish siphon as described in section II. A. 13.
3. Infusion into abdominal wall—Recognize immediately and repeat the DPL.

B. COMPLICATIONS
1. Bowel injury
2. Bladder laceration
3. Injury to major blood vessels—Aorta, inferior vena cava
4. Hematoma
5. Wound infection

C. INTERPRETATION
1. Grossly positive—>10 mL of blood on initial aspirate
2. Microscopic/chemistry criteria—Positive on lavage (blunt trauma)
a. >100,000 red blood cells/mm^3—97% sensitivity, 99.6% specificity; >10,000-20,000 red blood cells/mm^3 for penetrating trauma (controversial)
b. >500 white blood cells/mm^3—>25-100 for penetrating trauma
c. Presence of particulate (fecal, vegetable) matter
d. Presence of bacteria on Gram stain
e. Elevated amylase, bilirubin
f. Fluid exiting the chest tube or Foley catheter

D. ALTERNATIVES
1. Focused assessment with sonography in trauma (FAST) in the trauma bay
a. Sensitivity, specificity, and accuracy comparable to CT and DPL in experienced hands
b. Rapid, noninvasive means to diagnose intra-abdominal injuries
c. May be repeated quickly at the bedside, allowing ongoing investigation.
d. Indications are the same as for DPL.
e. Complicating factors
   (1) Obesity
   (2) Subcutaneous air
   (3) Previous abdominal surgery
f. Technique—Same as that for formal ultrasound
   (1) Includes subxiphoid pericardial window, hepatorenal fossa (Morison's pouch), splenorenal fossa, and the bladder/pelvis

   (2) Perform a second control scan after 30 minutes, used to detect
       progressive hemoperitoneum.
2. CT scan. Note: *The patient must be hemodynamically stable.*
a. Time-consuming, used when no immediate need for celiotomy
b. Provides most specific information about individual organ injuries and
   their extent
c. May diagnose retroperitoneal and pelvic organ injuries, which may be
   missed by DPL or physical exam
d. Requires PO/IV contrast material
e. Relative contraindications
   (1) Delay time to use scanner if not immediately available
   (2) Uncooperative patient who cannot adequately be sedated
   (3) Inability to give IV contrast agent due to allergy or renal insufficiency
f. CT may miss some GI, diaphragmatic, and pancreatic injuries. Presence
   of free fluid in a patient with no liver or splenic injury mandates early
   exploration for suspected injury to the GI tract or its mesentery.

Principles of Abscess Drainage

Steven R. Allen, MD

May the sun never set on undrained pus.

I. SUPERFICIAL ABSCESSES

Superficial abscesses are usually subcutaneous and easily accessible. They include hydradenitis suppurativa, small breast abscesses, infected sebaceous cysts, and perianal abscesses.

A. TECHNIQUE

1. IV pain control (i.e., morphine, meperidine [Demerol]), and sedation (diazepam, midazolam). Naloxone (Narcan) should be available.
2. Localize the fluid collection by palpation—This may be difficult if extensive induration and edema are present.
3. Prep and drape in a sterile manner.
4. Field-block with appropriate local anesthetic.
5. Aspirate the fluctuant area with an 18-gauge needle to collect a sample for Gram stain and anaerobic and aerobic cultures. This may also help localize the fluid collection if a fluctuant mass is not readily palpable.
6. Adequately incise the fluctuant area. Follow the skin lines when possible. Excision of a small skin ellipse may aid in keeping the wound edges open, especially if outpatient packing and dressing will be needed. A linear or cruciate incision may be used.
7. Swab for culture if a sample was not previously obtained.
8. Break down loculations with finger or instrument. All collections must be drained adequately.
9. Irrigate liberally with saline.
10. Pack cavity with thin-strip gauze. Iodoform gauze can be used to help maintain hemostasis during the first 24 hours.
11. Leave packing intact for 24 hours, then remove and evaluate.

B. ANTIBIOTICS

Use of systemic antibiotics (PO or IV) depends on the degree of surrounding cellulitis and the condition of the patient.
1. Most superficial abscesses are caused by *Staphylococcus* spp.
2. Diabetic patients often have multiorganism infections and require broad-spectrum antibiotics. Narrow the coverage when the culture results return.

II. DEEP ABSCESSES

Deep abscesses include intra-abdominal, IM, deep breast, and perirectal types.

A. DRAINAGE

1. These require drainage in the OR for adequate exposure, analgesia, and equipment.
2. Drainage by interventional radiology may be feasible in specific cases, especially localized intra-abdominal collections.

a. CT guided
b. Ultrasound guided
c. Fluoroscopic guidance

B. ANTIBIOTICS

Antibiotic coverage should be provided perioperatively.

PART IV

Rapid References

Test	Units	Specimen Type	Norms
5-Nucleotidase	mIU/mL	Blood	3.0-11.0
Acid phosphatase, total	mIU/mL	Blood	0.0-6.0
Albumin	g/dL	Blood	3.5-5.0
Alkaline phosphatase	mIU/mL	Blood	35-95
Alpha$_1$-antitrypsin	mg/dL	Blood	85-213
Alpha-fetoprotein	ng/mL	Blood	<10
Ammonia	μmol/L	Blood	6-48
Amylase, serum	mIU/mL	Blood	0-88
Amylase, urine, fluid	U/Tvol	Urine	0-400
APTT	sec	Blood	22-32
Bilirubin, direct	mg/dL	Blood	0.0-0.4
Bilirubin, total	mg/dL	Blood	0.1-1.1
Bleeding time	min		≤9.5
BUN	mg/dL	Blood	5.0-20.0
CA-125	U/mL	Blood	0-35
C-Peptide	ng/mL	Blood	0.5-3.0
Calcitonin	pg/mL	Blood	Male: 4.4-31.6; Female: 3.0-14.8
Calcium, fluid	mg/Tvol	Urine	100-250
Calcium, ionized	mg/dL	Blood	4.5-5.3
Calcium, serum	mg/dL	Blood	8.5-10.5
Carbamazepine	μg/mL	Blood	4.0-12.0
Carboxyhemoglobin	%	Blood	0-2% (Nonsmoker); 0-8% (Smoker)
Carcinoembryonic antigen	ng/mL	Blood	0-3 (Nonsmoker); 0-5 (Smoker)
Chloride	mEq/mL	Blood	95-110
Cholesterol	mIU/mL	Blood	<200
Chromium, serum	μg/L	Blood	0.0-5.0
CO_2, total	mEq/L	Blood	21-33
CPK	mIU/mL	Blood	<250
CPK-MB%	%	Blood	0.0-5.0
Creatinine	mg/dL	Blood	0.7-1.4
Creatinine, urine, fluid	g/vol	Urine	1.0-1.8
CSF glucose	mg/dL	CSF	40-70
CSF protein	mg/dL	CSF	15-45
Cyanide	μg/mL	Blood	<0.1
Digoxin	ng/mL	Blood	0.5-2.2
Eosinophil count, blood	mm^3	Blood	0.0-450.0
Erythrocyte sedimentation rate	sec	Blood	<20
Ethanol	mg/dL	Blood	<100
Fecal fat	g/72 h	Stool	<15.0
Ferritin, serum	ng/mL	Blood	30-300
Fibrin degradation	Pμg/mL	Blood	<16
Fibrinogen	mg/dL	Blood	150-400

RAPID REFERENCES

Continued

NORMAL LAB VALUES AT THE UNIVERSITY OF CINCINNATI MEDICAL
CENTER—cont'd

Test	Units	Specimen Type	Norms
Folate level, serum	ng/mL	Blood	>3.0
Gamma GT	mIU/mL	Blood	8.0-40.0
Gastrin level, serum	pg/mL	Blood	<97.0 (fasting)
Glucose	mg/dL	Blood	60-100
Glycohemoglobin	%	Blood	4-8
Haptoglobin	mg/dL	Blood	27.0-139.0
Hematocrit	%	Blood	<u>Adult</u>: Male: 47 ± 7; Female: 42 ± 5
Hemoglobin	g/dL	Blood	<u>Adult</u>: Male: 16.0 ± 2.0; Female: 14.0 ± 2.0
IgA	mg/dL	Blood	48-348
IgD	mg/dL	Blood	0.0-14.0
IgE, total	IU/mL	Blood	<150
IgG	mg/dL	Blood	627-1465
IgM	mg/dL	Blood	66-277
IgM neonatal	mg/dL	Blood	<23
Lactic acid	mEq/L	Blood	0.0-2.0
Lactate dehydrogenase (LDH)	μ/mL	Blood	55-200
Lidocaine	μg/mL	Blood	1.2-5.0
Lipase, serum	U/L	Blood	25-170
Lithium	mEq/L	Blood	0.7-1.4
Magnesium, serum	mg/dL	Blood	1.5-2.5
N-Acetylprocainamide (NAPA)	μg/mL	Blood	<30
Osmolality, serum	mOsm/L	Blood	280-305
Osmolality, urine	mOsm/L	Urine	50-1200
Phenobarbital	μg/mL	Blood	15-40
Phenytoin	μg/mL	Blood	10-20
Phosphate, urine, fluid	mg/Tvol	Urine	0.0-1600.0
Phosphorus, serum	mg/dL	Blood	2.5-4.5
Platelet count	THOUS/CU	Blood	100-375
Porphobilinogen quantitative	mg/24 h	Urine	0.0-2.0
Potassium	mEq/L	Blood	3.5-5.0
Potassium, urine, fluid	mEq/Tvol	Urine	25-125
Procainamide	μg/mL	Stool	4.0-8.0
Prolactin	ng/mL	Blood	<20
Protein, total	g/dL	Blood	6.0-8.0
Protein, urine, 24 hours	mg/Tvol	Urine	0.0-150
Prothrombin time	sec	Blood	11.0-13.6
PTH mid-molecule	ng/mL	Blood	0.3-1.08
PTH, intact	μLEQ/mL	Blood	6.6-55.8
Reticulocyte count	%	Blood	0.2-2.0
Retinol binding protein	mg/dL	Blood	3.0-6.0
SGOT	mIU/mL	Blood	10.0-30.0

Continued

NORMAL LAB VALUES AT THE UNIVERSITY OF CINCINNATI MEDICAL
CENTER—cont'd

Test	Units	Specimen Type	Norms
SGPT	mIU/mL	Blood	7.0-35.0
Sodium	mEq/L	Blood	133-145
Sodium, urine, fluid	mEq/Tvol	Urine	40-220
T3 resin uptake	%	Blood	84-117
T3, reverse	pg/mL	Blood	100-500
T4	µg/dL	Blood	4.5-11.5
Theophylline	µg/mL	Blood	10.0-20.0
Thyroglobulin	ng/mL	Blood	<18
Thyroxine binding globulin	µg T4/dL	Blood	11.0-27.0
Tocainide	µg/mL	Blood	4.0-10.0
Transferrin	mg/dL	Blood	155-355
TSH	µIU/mL	Blood	0.5-6.0
Urea, urine or fluid	g/vol	Urine	7.0-16.0
Uric acid	mg/dL	Blood	4.0-8.0
Urine free cortisol	µg/24 h	Urine	29-140
Valproic acid	µg/mL	Blood	5-120
Vitamin B_{12} level	pg/mL	Blood	180-900
Vitamin B_1	µg/mL	Blood	1.6-4.0
Vitamin B_6	ng/mL	Blood	3.6-18.0
Vitamin D (25-OH)	ng/dL	Blood	12-68
Vitamin E	mg/dL	Blood	0.5-2.5
Zinc, serum	µg/L	Blood	700-1100

RAPID REFERENCES

CONVERSION DATA

Pounds to Kilograms
(1 kg = 2.2 lb; 1 lb = 0.45 kg)

Feet and Inches to Centimeters
(1 cm = 0.39 in; 1 in = 2.54 cm)

FAHRENHEIT/CELSIUS TEMPERATURE CONVERSION
(F = 9/5 C + 32; C = 5/9 [F − 32])

F		C	F		C	F		C
90	=	32.2	97	=	36.1	104	=	40
91	=	32.8	98	=	36.7	105	=	40.6
92	=	33.3	99	=	37.2	106	=	41.1
93	=	33.9	100	=	37.8	107	=	41.7
94	=	34.4	101	=	38.3	108	=	42.2
95	=	35	102	=	38.9	109	=	42.8
96	=	35.6	103	=	39.4			

METRIC SYSTEM PREFIXES (SMALL MEASUREMENT)

k	kilo-	10^3	n	nano-	10^{-9}
c	centi-	10^{-2}	p	pico-	10^{-12}
m	milli-	10^{-3}	f	fento-	10^{-15}
μ	micro-	10^{-6}	a	atto-	10^{-18}

NOMOGRAM FOR THE DETERMINATION OF BODY SURFACE AREA OF CHILDREN AND ADULTS

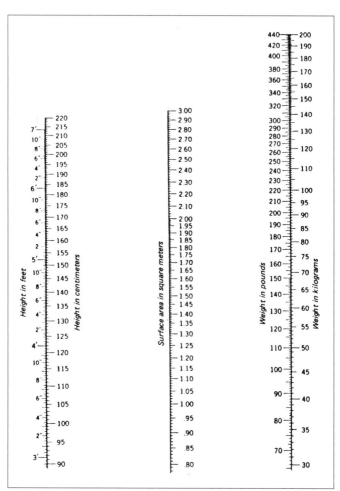

From Way LW (ed): Current Surgical Diagnosis and Treatment, 7th ed. Los Altos, CA, Lange Medical Publications, 1985, p 1188, with permission.

OXYHEMOGLOBIN DISSOCIATION CURVES FOR WHOLE BLOOD

$$\text{Hb saturation} = \frac{\text{Total blood } O_2 \text{ content (mL/100 mL)} - \text{Physically dissolved } O_2}{O_2 \text{ capacity of blood (mL/100 mL)} - \text{Physically dissolved } O_2}$$

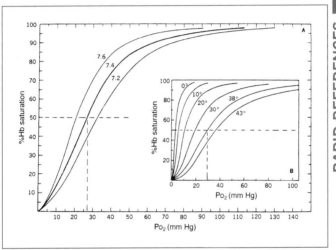

Large diagram indicates influence of change in acidity of blood on affinity of blood for O_2. Curves are based on studies by Dill and by Bock et al. on blood of one man (A.V. Bock). At a particular PO_2 (e.g., 40 mm Hg), acidification of blood results in release of O_2. Action of changes in PCO_2 appear due in part to their effect on pH and in part to formation of carbamino compounds, displacing 2,3-DPG from Hb. *Inset* shows, for blood of sheep, influence of temperature change on PO_2-% HbO_2 relationships; an increase in temperature (as in working muscle) aids in "unloading" O_2 from HbO_2; during hypothermia, hemoglobin has increased affinity for O_2. (From Lambertson CJ: Transport of oxygen, carbon dioxide, and inert gases by the blood. *In* Mountcastle VB [ed]: Medical Physiology, 14th ed. St. Louis, CV Mosby, 1980, p 1725.)

RAPID REFERENCES

Index

Note: Page numbers followed by the letter f refer to figures;
page numbers followed by the letter t refer to tables.

INDEX

Wound(s) *(Continued)*
  dehiscence of, 126
  drains from, 126–127
  dressings for, 124
  gunshot, 169
  hand, 679–680
  in burn patients
    care of, 212–214
    contracture of, 217
    infected, 215–217
      nonbacterial, 217
      nosocomial, 216
      prevention of, 216
      treatment of, 216
    outpatient treatment of, 218
  infection of, 137–138
    antibiotics for, 138–141
    care of, 125–126
    prevention of, 138
    surgical, treatment of, 133
  management of, for open fractures,
    194–195
  open, infection of, 137
  soft tissue
    infection of
      antibiotics for, 138–141
      postoperative fever and, 130
    management of, 123–125
  superficial, infection of, 137
  tetanus and rabies prophylaxis for,
    124–125
  traumatic
    care of, 123
    closure of, 123–124

Wound closure
  exceptions to, 124
  in soft tissue wounds, 123–124
  in wound healing, 122
Wound healing, 119–127
  cytokines and growth factors in,
    121–122
  factors influencing, 122–123
  physiology of, 119–121
  primary, by first intention, 122
  secondary, by second intention, 122
  tertiary, by third intention, 122
  wound closure in, 122
  wound contraction in, 120
  wound strength in, 121
Wrist
  compartment syndrome of, 197
  motor examination of, 672, 675
Wrist blocks, anatomy for, 89f, 90f
Wrist bracelet block, 86

X

Xenografts, for burn wound care, 214
Xeroderma pigmentosum, 294

Y

Yersinia, enteric infection with, 440

Z

Zenker's diverticulum, 367
Zinc deficiency, diagnosis and
  treatment of, 26
Zollinger-Ellison syndrome, 352–355,
  353f